VITAMIN E:
BIOCHEMICAL, HEMATOLOGICAL,
AND CLINICAL ASPECTS

ANNALS OF THE NEW YORK ACADEMY OF SCIENCES
Volume 393

VITAMIN E:
BIOCHEMICAL, HEMATOLOGICAL,
AND CLINICAL ASPECTS

Edited by Bertram Lubin and Lawrence J. Machlin

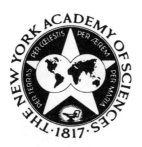

The New York Academy of Sciences
New York, New York
1982

Library of Congress Cataloging in Publication Data

Main entry under title:

Vitamin E, biochemical, hematological, and
   clinical aspects.

   (Annals of the New York Academy of Sciences;
v. 393)
   Proceedings of a conference by the New York
Academy of Sciences held November 11–13, 1981.
   Bibliography: p.
   Includes index.
   1. Vitamin E—Physiological effect—Congresses.
I. Lubin, Bertram, 1939-   . II. Machlin,
Lawrence J., 1927-   . III. New York Academy of
Sciences. IV. Series. [DNLM: 1. Vitamin E—
Congresses.   W1 AN626YL v. 393 / QU 179 V838 1981]
Q11.N5   vol. 393   [QP772.T6]   500s   [612'.399]   82-14414
ISBN 0-89766-176-1
ISBN 0-89766-177-X (pbk.)

SP
Printed in the United States of America
ISBN 0-89766-176-1 (cloth)
ISBN 0-89766-177-X (paper)

ANNALS OF THE NEW YORK ACADEMY OF SCIENCES
VOLUME 393
September 30, 1982

VITAMIN E: BIOCHEMICAL, HEMATOLOGICAL, AND CLINICAL ASPECTS*

Editors and Conference Organizers
BERTRAM LUBIN and LAWRENCE J. MACHLIN

◆

CONTENTS

*This volume is the result of a conference entitled Vitamin E: Biochemical, Hematological, and Clinical Aspects, held on November 11–13, 1981, by The New York Academy of Sciences.

Financial assistance was received from:

- BASF WYANDOTTE CORPORATION
- EASTMAN CHEMICAL PRODUCTS, INC.
- EISAI COMPANY, LTD.
- FOGARTY INTERNATIONAL CENTER, NATIONAL INSTITUTES OF HEALTH
- HENKEL CORPORATION
- HOFFMANN-LA ROCHE, INC.
- NATIONAL HEART, LUNG AND BLOOD INSTITUTE, NIH
- NATIONAL INSTITUTES OF ARTHRITIS, DIABETES, DIGESTIVE AND
    KIDNEY DISEASES, NIH
- OFFICE OF NAVAL RESEARCH
- WYETH LABORATORIES

INTRODUCTION

Bertram Lubin

Children's Hospital Medical Center
Bruce Lyon Memorial Research Laboratory
Oakland, California 94609

Since the last New York Academy of Sciences meeting on vitamin E held 10 years ago, a number of advances in our understanding of this vitamin have been made. We organized this symposium to present current information on the biochemistry, physiology, and role of vitamin E in human disease. We emphasized a review of several potential clinical applications of vitamin E; in particular, those applying to premature infants, to children with intestinal malabsorption, and to patients with hereditary hematologic diseases. An extensive review of the biochemical and physiological effects of vitamin E in cellular elements of blood (i.e., red cells, white cells, and platelets) both normal and abnormal is contained within this publication. In addition, the reader should appreciate the wide spectrum of research directions currently being pursued in regard to the antioxidant and biochemical modulating properties of vitamin E. Advances in free radical technology, coupled with a growing awareness of the physiologic as well as toxic effects of free radicals in biology, have contributed a great deal toward developing systems in which the role of vitamin E can be analyzed. The interplay between free radical biology and prostaglandin metabolism and the effects that vitamin E may have as a modulator for these interactions have enormous implications. Applications of the research advances made in the past 10 years on vitamin E are reflected in the data describing the clinical role of vitamin E in certain human diseases. We are certainly closer to understanding the role of this vitamin in many biological reactions and in human disease. It is clear that this understanding will continue to advance as new technological approaches become available and as we become aware of methods to detect consequences of minimal as well as severe deficiency in humans.

FREE RADICAL BIOLOGY: XENOBIOTICS, CANCER, AND AGING*

William A. Pryor

Department of Chemistry
Louisiana State University
Baton Rouge, Louisiana 70803

INTRODUCTION

It was not very long ago that free radical biology was a rather arcane subject, regarded with disinterest (or even disbelief) by most biologists—a sea of speculation, but few islands of solid fact. Three striking and seminal discoveries have drastically changed this field.

The first was the elucidation by McCord and Fridovich of the nature, function, and role of superoxide dismutase (SOD).[1] In fact, SOD is now the world's most studied enzyme; journal articles, conference proceedings, and books on superoxide chemistry and biology are appearing at a very rapid pace, but we probably are still just seeing the tip of the iceberg.

The second discovery involves the biosynthesis of peroxidic compounds from arachidonic acid—products of what is called the "arachidonate cascade."[2] Not more than 10 years ago, it was thought that lipoxygenase activity was limited to plants and that lipid hydroperoxides were not formed in animal cells. In fact, there was even concern that lipid hydroperoxides in plants might be *in vitro* artifacts and play no role in metabolism. Now it is clear that an array of cyclic and bicyclic peroxides as well as acyclic lipid hydroperoxides not only occur in all animal cells, but play a very critical role in bioregulation and in many vital normal and pathological processes.

The third discovery, although perhaps more distant from traditional biochemical interests, also is having a major impact on current research. It is becoming clear that many important environmental toxins exert their effects through radical-mediated reactions.[3,4] In fact, a majority of the compounds that are positive in the Ames test may involve radical-mediated reactions.

In this article, I will summarize current thinking on the *in vivo* sources of radicals. I will cover both exogenous sources—xenobiotics, pollutants, carcinogens, etc.—and endogenous sources—superoxide systems and the arachidonic cascade. And I will close by making some remarks about the effects of antioxidants on carcinogenesis and on the retardation of aging. Thus, I intend to skate from thick ice to thinner and thinner ice; with good timing, I should fall into the refreshingly cool water just at the end of my talk.

FREE RADICALS DERIVED FROM THE REACTIONS OF XENOBIOTICS

Several mechanisms are available by which xenobiotics—substances foreign to the cell—can react with cellular target molecules to produce damaging

*This work was supported by grants from the National Science Foundation and the National Institutes of Health (HL-16029 and HL-25820). This manuscript is based on the address presented at the symposium banquet.

1

radicals. In this context, it is convenient to divide xenobiotics into four types:

- Toxins that are themselves radicals or contain free radicals (e.g., NO, NO_2, soot, tar, tobacco smoke).
- Toxins that are very reactive and, although they are not radicals themselves, cause radicals to be formed in target molecules (e.g., ozone, singlet oxygen).
- Toxins that interrupt cellular electron flow and by single-electron transfer (SET) reactions form radicals (e.g., CCl_4, nitrofuran drugs, paraquat, bleomycin).
- Toxins that undergo autoxidation to form superoxide and/or hydrogen peroxide (e.g., benzo[a]pyrene, dopa).

THE NITROGEN OXIDES

The nitrogen oxides are the most important example of toxins of the first type, toxins that are themselves free radicals. Both nitrogen dioxide (NO_2) and nitrogen oxide (NO) occur in polluted air; both these species are themselves free radicals and their gas-phase radical chemistry has been the subject of extensive study with the aim of understanding the formation of reactive species in smog.[5]

Cigarette smoke also contains very high concentrations of nitrogen oxides. Fresh undiluted smoke contains up to 1,000 parts per million (ppm) NO_x, largely in the form of NO; on standing, the NO is gradually oxidized by atmospheric oxygen to the more reactive NO_2.[6,7]

Nitrogen dioxide is known to react with polyunsaturated fatty acids (PUFA) in lung lipids *in vivo* and with PUFA *in vitro* to initiate the autoxidation of the unsaturated fatty acid.[3,8-12] The autoxidation of PUFA in lipids damages cellular membranes and causes prelytic damage (such as ion or enzyme leakage from cells) and, ultimately, cell lysis and death. Vitamin E protects PUFA against these effects, both *in vitro* and *in vivo*.

Vitamin E is known to be an effective antioxidant, so its protective effects against NO_2-initiated PUFA autoxidation are not surprising. It may seem surprising, however, that vitamin E can protect a membrane at the levels at which it occurs naturally—about 1 vitamin E molecule per 1,000 lipid molecules. However, vitamin E diffuses relatively rapidly in a membrane. The rate of unimpeded diffusion of species like vitamin E within the lateral plane of a bilayer can be calculated, and it is approximately 10^4 Å/second.[17] Autoxidation of PUFA in a lipid bilayer is kinetically similar to autoxidation in homogeneous solution; the mechanism for PUFA autoxidation is shown below, where LH is a lipid with an allylic hydrogen atom, L· is the allylic radical, LOO· is the lipid peroxyl radical, and LOOH is a lipid or PUFA hydroperoxide. The initiation step is slow; it is the process in which the primordial radicals are produced. (This is, of course, the step that toxins like NO_2 can accelerate.) Once radicals are formed, the two chain

$$LH \xrightarrow[\text{process}]{\text{initiation}} L\cdot \tag{1}$$

$$L\cdot + O_2 \rightarrow LOO\cdot \tag{2}$$

$$LOO\cdot + LH \rightarrow LOOH + L\cdot \tag{3}$$

steps, Equations 2 and 3, occur. Of these two steps, Equation 2 has a rate constant of about 10^8/M per second and is extremely fast if the concentration of dissolved oxygen is about 10^{-4} M. (This is the concentration produced from the diffusion of oxygen into solution from an air atmosphere.) However, Equation 3 has a much smaller rate constant, estimated to be about 60/M per second in bilayers at 30°C.[18] Thus, even under a full atmosphere of air, the chain steps in the autoxidation sequence are sufficiently slow so that lateral diffusion of vitamin E in the bilayer can protect a large number of PUFA molecules from chain autoxidation.

Recently, my group has studied the mechanism of the NO_2 initiation of autoxidation of olefins and PUFA.[8,9] Studies done some years ago by organic chemists, which were performed at very high levels of NO_2, show that NO_2 reacts with olefins by addition to the double bond. (NO_2 exists in equilibrium with its dimer N_2O_4. At high concentrations, the chief species is N_2O_4; at low concentrations, however, it is NO_2.) Our work has shown that at high concentrations, NO_2 does react with simple olefins and PUFA by addition, as shown in Equation 4. However, at the ppm levels of NO_2 actually breathed by humans, NO_2 reacts

$$NO_2/N_2O_4 + \underset{/}{\overset{\backslash}{C}}=\underset{\backslash}{\overset{/}{C}} = NO_2-\overset{|}{\underset{|}{C}}-\overset{|}{\underset{|}{C}}\cdot \tag{4}$$

$$(I)$$

with olefins and PUFA predominantly by abstraction of the allylic hydrogen atom, Equation 5. The same phenomenon is well known for bromine

$$NO_2 + -CH_2-CH=CH- \rightarrow HONO + -\overset{\bullet}{\overline{CH-CH-CH}}- \tag{5}$$

atoms in the bromination of olefins, and the same explanation appears to apply.[19] Addition is thermodynamically favored, but it is reversible, as shown in Equation 4. At low concentrations of NO_2 (or N_2O_4), to trap the initial radical, **I**, the addition step reverses and the slower but irreversible hydrogen abstraction, Equation 5, occurs. These findings appear to have important application in understanding the results of animal inhalation experiments.[20,21]

This hydrogen abstraction process produces nitrous acid as a side product (Equation 5). We have shown that this HONO nitrosates amines, thus leading to a secondary toxin from the inhalation of nitrogen oxides.[8]

REACTIONS OF THE NITROGEN OXIDES WITH HYDROGEN PEROXIDE IN THE LUNG

Both NO and NO_2 are known to react with hydrogen peroxide in the gas phase to produce hydroxyl radicals, Equations 6 and 7.[22] Recently, we have pointed out

$$NO + H_2O_2 \rightarrow HO\cdot + HONO \tag{6}$$

$$NO_2 + H_2O_2 \rightarrow HO\cdot + HONO_2 \tag{7}$$

that these reactions may have important toxicological consequences in the lung when polluted air is breathed.[23,24] For example, cigarette smoke contains high concentrations of NO and NO_2 and also stimulates pulmonary alveolar macrophages (PAM) to produce hydrogen peroxide. Thus, cigarette smoke could produce local conditions in the lung in which NO_x and hydrogen peroxide both occur and the hydroxyl radical is formed.[16] The hydroxyl radical is known to be extremely damaging in biological systems.

It has proven difficult to establish unambiguous evidence for Reaction 6, since NO is rapidly oxidized to the more reactive NO_2 if oxygen is present. However, we find that bubbling purified NO into anaerobic aqueous solutions of phenol containing hydrogen peroxide (and diethylenetriamine pentaacetic acid, DETA-PAC, to eliminate metal-catalyzed decomposition reactions of the hydrogen peroxide) leads to the formation of catechol and hydroquinone, along with many other products. The evidence for Equation 7 is even stronger. Phenol is hydroxylated to catechol and other products by NO_2/H_2O_2 in aerobic aqueous solutions. In addition, linoleic acid (at 10^{-5} M in aqueous buffers) is autoxidized to its conjugated diene hydroperoxide.[24]

Reactions of NO and NO_2 with Thiols

Nitric oxide oxidizes aliphatic thiols or thiophenol in aqueous solutions or emulsions at a very rapid rate, providing the solution is basic enough so that the thiolate anion, RS^-, exists in appreciable concentration.[25] For ordinary thiols, this requires the presence of basic catalysis; however, acidic thiols, such as p-nitrothiophenol, are rapidly oxidized without the need for external base. In aqueous solutions, cysteine and glutathione are very rapidly oxidized to their disulfides, at a pH of 5–10. The NO appears to be converted to hyponitrous acid, which decomposes to N_2O and N_2. Thus, Reaction 8 rapidly oxidizes thiols to disulfides at room temperature and produces only unreactive gases as by-products; therefore, it appears that this reaction may have synthetic utility. From a toxicological viewpoint, it is clear that NO could inactivate thiol-containing enzymes. Cigarette smoke, for example, is known to contain a factor, previously

$$2\,RSH \longrightarrow RSSR \tag{8}$$
$$NO \qquad N_2O + N_2$$

unidentified, that inactivates thiol-containing enzymes, and it is known that externally added cysteine protects. We suggest that this factor could be NO and/or NO_2.[25]

Nitrogen dioxide, being more reactive than NO, reacts with thiols without the necessity of basic catalysis. Again, thiols are converted to the disulfide very rapidly either in organic solvents or in aqueous emulsions or homogeneous solutions. In this case, a green intermediate is rapidly formed as NO_2 is bubbled into a solution of thiophenol, cysteine, etc.; we have identified this green intermediate as the S-nitrosothiol (Equation 9). This species then decomposes (either unimolecularly or upon attack by a thiyl radical) to give the disulfide and NO; the NO can be converted to N_2O_3 if excess NO_2 is present, making the stoichiometry more complex.[25]

$$NO_2 + 2\,RSH \rightarrow RS{-}N{=}O + H_2O \tag{9}$$

$$2\,RS{-}N{=}O \rightarrow RSSR + 2\,NO \tag{10}$$

$$NO + NO_2 \rightarrow N_2O_3 \tag{11}$$

Free Radicals in Cigarette Smoke

We have been studying cigarette smoke as a model for organic combustion products that contain free radicals.[6,7] Soot from urban air, automobile exhaust, unsmoked tobacco, smoked tobacco, and fly ash all contain high concentrations of free radicals. The gas phase of cigarette smoke contains oxygen- and carbon-centered free radicals that are quite reactive and have lifetimes of minutes. The tar phase contains much less reactive free radicals that persist for days. Gas-phase cigarette smoke contains more than 10^{14} free radicals per puff, and both mainstream (the smoke that is inhaled) and sidestream (the smoke that rises into the vicinity) contain similar numbers of radicals. Tar also contains approximately 10^{14} free radicals per puff.

The radicals in gas-phase smoke appear to be primarily reactive oxygen-centered radicals.[6,7] It might have been expected that these reactive oxyradicals would be short lived; however, we find that they have half-lives of about five minutes in the gas phase and travel as much as 180 cm down a pyrex tube with very little decrease in concentration. To explain this paradox, we have suggested that the radicals are continuously formed and destroyed in the gas phase and that a steady state exists. We hypothesize that the slow oxidation of NO to NO_2 produces a continual, low level of the reactive NO_2 free radical. As we have seen above, NO_2 is known to react with olefins to produce carbon-centered free radicals. Olefins and dienes (such as butadiene and isoprene), as well as other reactive species, are present at relatively high concentrations in cigarette smoke. In fact, Dr. M. Tamura in my laboratory has shown in preliminary experiments that nitric oxide (at ppm levels) in air reacts with olefins and dienes in a flowing gas stream to produce oxyradicals that behave similarly to the oxyradicals we identify in gas-phase smoke. Thus, our hypothesis to explain the long lifetimes of gas-phase smoke radicals is that they exist in a steady state as shown below.

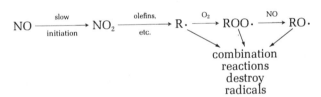

Cigarette tar has been postulated to consist primarily of polynuclear aromatic hydrocarbons (PAH) and other carbonaceous materials. It was originally suggested, therefore, that the persistent free radical in cigarette tar consists of an electron delocalized on a PAH molecule. (A so-called electron in a hole.) For the first time, however, we have been able to extract the tar free radical into homogeneous solution and study its properties there.[6,7] When tar is fractionated, we find that the free radical travels with the fraction of tar containing polyphenolic materials. Polyphenols in tar derive, at least in part, from tobacco leaf pigment, a material that is enzymatically polymerized from phenols in a manner that is similar to the polymerization of dopa to form melanin pigments in animals. In fact, although cigarette tar certainly is not identical to melanin pigments, we find that the electron spin resonance (ESR) characteristics of the cigarette tar radical are very similar to those of the persistent radicals in melanin pigments. Therefore, we have suggested that the cigarette tar radical is a polyphenoxyl radical much like that in melanins. The tobacco leaf pigment fraction of tar is known to have cocarcinogenic properties. Thus, if the tar radical does derive from the tobacco leaf pigment as we propose, then for the first time a possible connection can be suggested between the free radicals in tar and the carcinogenic and/or cocarcinogenic properties of tar.

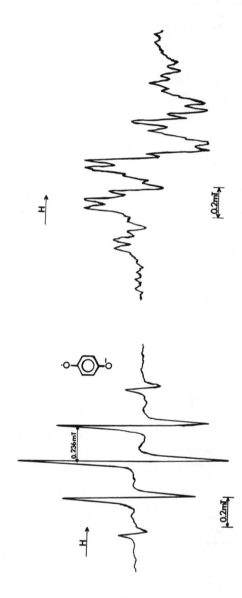

FIGURE 1. Cigarette tar, extracted into alcohol and made slightly alkaline, shows an electron spin resonance signal of the benzene semiquinone radical anion (at left); in about 30 minutes, this signal is replaced by the more complex signal shown at right. The appearance of the semiquinone signal requires the presence of oxygen. We suggest that the ready oxidizability of the hydroquinones in tar explains the cocarcinogenicity of the phenolic fraction of tar. (Unpublished observations of P. I. Premovic, D. F. Church, and W. A. Pryor.)

A Mechanism for Cocarcinogenicity of Phenols

Our work with cigarette tar has led us to suggest a hypothesis for the mode of action of phenolic compounds that are cocarcinogens. As remarked above, cigarette smoke contains a high concentration of phenolic materials and these compounds are very powerful cocarcinogens.[13] We find that if cigarette tar is dissolved in alcohol and then dilute base is added, an extremely strong ESR signal due to the benzene semiquinone radical anion is immediately observed (see FIGURE 1). (This is the first time that a specific free radical has been identified in cigarette tar by ESR or by any other means.)

We suggest that this ready oxidation of hydroquinones is responsible for the strong cocarcinogenic properties of the phenolic fraction of tar. It is known that

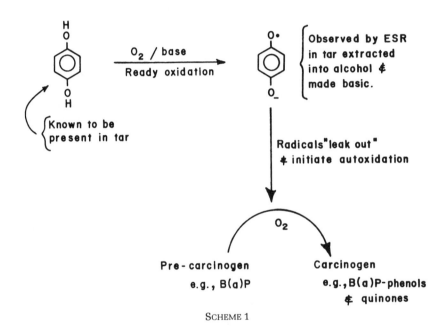

SCHEME 1

systems in which arachidonic acid undergoes enzymatic oxidation to prostaglandins cause the cooxidation of benzo[a]pyrene (BaP) to carcinogenic compounds.[14] Cooxidation is a general phenomenon in the free radical field;[15] when an oxidation-resistant substance is present during the oxidation of an easily oxidized material, the oxidation-resistant compound often is cooxidized along with the more oxidizable material.[15] Thus, our observation of a very strong semiquinone ESR signal from cigarette tar confirms that phenols are present in tar and proves that they are easily air oxidized. As shown in SCHEME 1, the oxidation of phenols produces radicals that can be diverted to attack other materials, such as precarcinogens, and cause them to be cooxidized and thus converted to their carcinogenic state.

Ozone and Free Radicals

Ozone is an example of a toxin that, although not a free radical itself, is able to produce free radicals by reaction with a wide variety of types of organic molecules.[10-12] Ozone is a remarkably reactive molecule; it even reacts with hydrocarbons to form free radicals. Ozone reacts with various other types of molecules (amines, hydroperoxides, etc.) to produce radicals very rapidly even at dry ice temperatures.[26] An extensive body of literature shows that free radical-mediated reactions are responsible for at least part of the pathology caused by breathing ozone at ppm levels that occur in smog.[27,28]

We have recently shown that ozone reacts with PUFA to produce radicals that can be spin trapped using the sensitive ESR spin-trapping technique. The mechanisms for radical production by ozone are complex and are still controversial.[29,30]

Toxin and Drug Metabolism by Electron Transfer

A number of drugs and toxins interrupt cellular electron flow and, by so doing, generate free radicals that may be involved in the drug's action or may produce toxicological consequences. The toxin that has been studied most thoroughly in this regard is carbon tetrachloride.[31,32] Halides of this type, which have high electron affinities, are known to react with solvated electrons in radiation systems by a process that is called "dissociative electron transfer" (Equation 12). The toxic reactions of carbon tetrachloride involve reactions at hepatic cytochrome P_{450}

$$e^- + CCl_4 \rightarrow Cl^- + Cl_3C\cdot \tag{12}$$

sites in a similar manner.[31,32] The trichloromethyl radical that is produced initiates

$$CCl_4 \underset{Fe(II) \quad Fe(III)}{\overset{}{\longrightarrow}} Cl_3C\cdot + Cl^- \tag{13}$$

lipid autoxidation and produces the membrane damage associated with this type of liver toxicity.

Animals given carbon tetrachloride have increased amounts of ethane and pentane in their expired breath; this is considered evidence for the increased production of lipid hydroperoxides. Appropriate PUFA hydroperoxides are known to decompose (via alkoxyl radicals and β-scission) to give ethyl and pentyl radicals; these radicals can be converted to ethane and pentane (along with other products, Equations 14 and 15).[33,34] Vitamin E deficiency also leads to enhanced amounts of expired ethane and pentane.[35]

$$\overset{OOH}{\underset{R-CH-R'}{|}} \rightarrow \overset{O\cdot}{\underset{R-CH-R'}{|}} \rightarrow \begin{array}{c} R-CHO + R'\cdot \\ \text{and} \\ R\cdot + R'-CHO \end{array} \tag{14}$$

$$R\cdot \underset{O_2}{\overset{RH}{\diagup \diagdown}} ROO\cdot \rightarrow \text{Other Products} \tag{15}$$

Radicals from CCl_4 have actually been trapped *in vivo* by the use of phenyl-*tert*-butyl nitroxide (PBN), a well-known spin trap.[36] Interestingly, the toxicity of 2,3,7,8-tetrachlorodibenzo-*p*-dioxin (TCDD), an extremely important and potent compound in the ecosphere, may act via similar free radical reactions; this toxin, with LD_{50} values for rat as low as 50 μg/kg, causes an increase in the age pigment of rat heart at doses as low as 10 μg/kg.[37]

Nifurtimos, a nitrofuran derivative that is used to treat Chagas' disease, appears to function by electron transfer. It increases electron flow from reduced nicotinamide-adenine dinucleotide phosphate (NADPH) to O_2, generates superoxide and hydrogen peroxide, and causes lipid peroxidation.[38] Interestingly, in this case the ESR signal of the nitrofuran radical anion can be observed.[39]

$$ArNO_2 \xrightarrow{\hspace{3cm}} ArNO_2^{\overline{\cdot}} \qquad (16)$$
$$\underset{\text{NADPH} \quad \text{NADP}^+/O_2^{\overline{\cdot}}}{}$$

Bleomycin, BLM, a drug widely used in cancer therapy, is another interesting drug that involves SET, although in a somewhat different manner. It also produces superoxide, which is believed to be crucial to its effectiveness. It complexes both Fe(II) and DNA, and electron transfer from iron to oxygen produces superoxide at the site where damage to DNA can be effectively propagated.[40]

$$BLM + DNA \rightarrow BLM(DNA) \xrightarrow{\text{Fe(II)}} BLM(DNA, Fe(II))$$
$$\qquad\qquad\qquad\qquad\qquad\qquad\qquad\qquad (17)$$
$$\xrightarrow{O_2} BLM(DNA, Fe(III)) \, O_2^{\overline{\cdot}}$$

Another important toxin that is known to undergo electron transfer reactions is the dye methyl viologen, which was discovered to be a herbicide and is used under the name paraquat (PQ^{++}). In the human, paraquat appears not to be metabolized, but to undergo electron transfer cycling in which the free radical form is continually produced and acts as an electron donor. Paraquat is a bipyridylium salt, the reactions of which with oxygen can be symbolized as below.[41]

$$PQ^{++} \xrightarrow{e^-} PQ^{\overline{\cdot}} \qquad (18)$$

$$PQ^{\overline{\cdot}} + O_2 \rightarrow PQ^{++} + O_2^{\overline{\cdot}} \qquad (19)$$

Superoxide generation also can result from the oxidation of hydroquinone-type compounds, QH_2, which can be dehydrogenated in one-electron steps, as shown below. This field, recently reviewed by Borg et al., includes a large number of important drugs such as dopa.[42-45]

$$QH_2 + O_2 \rightarrow QH\cdot + O_2^{\overline{\cdot}} + H^+ \qquad (20)$$

$$QH_2 + O_2^{\overline{\cdot}} + H^+ \rightarrow QH\cdot + H_2O_2 \qquad (21)$$

$$2\,QH\cdot \rightarrow Q + QH_2 \qquad (22)$$

Certain nitroaromatic compounds have found use as radiation sensitizers—

drugs that increase the sensitivity of tumors to radiation therapy.[47,48] These drugs have SET mechanisms for their action, often being reduced instead of oxygen.

$$ArNO_2 \xrightarrow{e^-} ArNO_2\cdot^-$$

SULFUR DIOXIDE AND SULFITE TOXICITY AND ASTHMA

We have found that either sulfur dioxide or bisulfite causes the rapid autoxidation of linoleic acid in aqueous buffers at a pH near neutral.[49] Our studies were done on solutions in which linoleic is 10^{-5} M and where the development of conjugated diene in homogeneous solution can be directly measured. We use diethylene triamine pentaacetic acid (DTPA) to reduce the possibility of iron-catalyzed reactions playing a role. Interestingly, hydrogen peroxide strongly inhibits the autoxidation.

The mechanism for the autoxidation of sulfite involves the SO_3^-, SO_4^-, and SO_5^- radical ions; of these, SO_4^- can abstract hydrogen from ethanol and undoubtedly also from PUFA.[50] Thus, we suggest that PUFA autoxidation is initiated by the autoxidation of sulfite; hydrogen peroxide inhibits because it oxidizes sulfite to sulfate by a nonradical mechanism.[51]

Some asthmatics are extraordinarily sensitive to sulfur dioxide or to bisulfite-type food preservatives.[52-55] It is known that the hydroperoxides of arachidonic acid (AA) are involved in the asthmatic response.[55]

I would like to suggest that sulfite causes the increased rate of conversion of AA to eicosatetraene hydroperoxides (HPETEs), thus explaining the sensitivity of asthmatics to this pollutant.[55] The mechanism of this interaction could involve the initiation of autoxidation of AA by sulfite, as described above. Another possibility might be that sulfite reacts with the epoxide of the HPETEs, forming a product with some properties like the cysteine conjugate SRS-A.[2]

ENDOGENOUS FREE RADICALS: THE GENERATION OF SUPEROXIDE

The above discussion of xenobiotics that lead to the production of superoxide might lead the reader to conclude that this free radical is only produced pathologically; in fact, nothing could be further from the truth. The discovery of enzymatic one-electron reduction of oxygen is surely one of the most striking events in recent enzymology. Interestingly, the trail leading to this enzyme was first discovered in systems involving sulfite.[46] Thus the discovery of SOD involved an early excursion into radical-mediated toxicology.

In a description of their early studies, McCord and Fridovich have reported the events leading to the discovery of the enzyme superoxide dismutase.[1] In November 1969, the isolation and properties of SOD were reported. With this powerful tool, an erroneous dogma could be corrected: one-electron reduction of oxygen, rather than being an unusual event, is now known to occur in almost all aerobic cells.

Members of the Britton Chance group have used a number of techniques to estimate the rate of production of superoxide and hydrogen peroxide in various tissues both *in vitro* and *in vivo*, and to attempt to estimate the rate of "leakage" of these reactive species into the general cellular environment.[56] Although it may be possible to challenge their numbers in particular cases, this must be regarded as most important work. For many years, scientists have wondered whether radicals "leaked" from normal electron transport and could cause pathological changes. Since the question was raised before it was understood that superoxide was a critical species to be looked for, and before SOD was available as a tool to help in the search, a satisfactory answer was not reached in earlier work. However, the Chance group now has produced most interesting data. For example, in living bacteria, hydrogen peroxide is estimated to be 10^{-8} M under usual cell growth conditions. A considerable fraction of the oxygen consumed in the liver is converted to hydrogen peroxide; in the perfused liver, this fraction ranges between 5 and 50%, depending on the supply of peroxisomal substrates.[56,57]

A number of workers, starting with Fridovich and his colleagues,[58] have demonstrated unequivocally that superoxide initiates the autoxidation of PUFA. The mechanism of this reaction has aroused considerable interest, since it is known that superoxide itself is not an oxidizing radical and cannot initiate the chain autoxidation of PUFA. The most widely accepted mechanism currently is the production of the hydroxyl radical in what has been called the "iron-catalyzed" Haber-Weiss mechanism, as shown in Equations 23–25.[59]

$$O_2^{\overline{\cdot}} + Fe(III) \rightarrow O_2 + Fe(II) \tag{23}$$

$$2\,O_2^{\overline{\cdot}} + 2\,H^+ \rightarrow H_2O_2 + O_2 \tag{24}$$

$$Fe(II) + H_2O_2 \rightarrow Fe(III) + HO^- + HO\cdot \tag{25}$$

Thomas and I suggested some years ago that superoxide may react with lipid hydroperoxides to produce initiating radicals by another pathway.[34,60] We showed that superoxide reacts with lipid hydroperoxides to initiate the autoxidation of further lipid. We formulated the mechanism of the interaction between superoxide and a PUFA hydroperoxide, LOOH, as that originally suggested by Peters and Foote in their study of the reaction of superoxide with tert-butyl hydroperoxide, as shown below.[62] Several workers have questioned our conclusions, but they

$$LOOH + O_2^{\overline{\cdot}} \rightarrow LO\cdot + HO^- + O_2 \tag{26}$$

have studied systems very different from the one we used. Our further work in this area has demonstrated that superoxide does indeed initiate the further peroxidation of PUFA that already contains hydroperoxidic impurities,[66] and that this initiation can be demonstrated, as we had shown originally, if the iron-catalyzed Haber-Weiss reaction is blocked through the use of chelating compounds such as DTPA. (Our system also contained 10% ethanol.) However, it now appears doubtful that the mechanism for the superoxide-LOOH reaction is that shown in Equation 26.

Phagocytosis has come under increased study in recent years, following the discovery that the enhanced rate of utilization of oxygen by phagocytes (the "respiratory burst") involves the conversion of oxygen to superoxide and, thence, to hydrogen peroxide. Phagocytes kill bacteria by both an anaerobic and an aerobic mechanism, and neither is understood in any detail as yet.[63,64] However, an attractive hypothesis is that reactive radicals from the superoxide system attack bacterial membranes to destroy them. A criticism of this mechanism that has been raised is that bacterial membranes contain very low concentrations of PUFA.[64] However, the reactive species in the superoxide system probably is the hydroxyl radical, and this species reacts with almost all types of organic molecules with virtually the same rate constant.[61] Thus, the destruction of protein, saturated lipid, or PUFA by hydroxyl radicals is very much a possibility.

PROSTAGLANDINS, INFLAMMATION, AND FREE RADICALS

A rich variety of biologically active compounds are produced from the enzymatic oxidation of arachidonic acid. These compounds include several series of related species; some derive from an endoperoxide-hydroperoxide called PGG, whereas others derive from acyclic lipid hydroperoxides that are called hydroperoxyeicosatetraenoic acid, HPETE.[2] The presence of the HPETE compounds demonstrates that animal cells possess lipoxygenase activity, and that lipid peroxides are probably present in all aerobic animal cells.

McCord originally suggested that inflammation results from the release of superoxide into extracellular fluid during the phagocytosis of leucocytes that are drawn to the site of infection.[75] It now is clear, however, that prostaglandins are involved in the mediation of the inflammatory response.[77-79] Neutrophiles when challenged release arachidonic acid to the cellular environment,[76] and superoxide causes the production of species in the arachidonate cascade. Thus, the inflammatory process initiates the oxidation of arachidonic acid, which produces chemotactic agents that draw more leucocytes to the site.[2,63-65,80]

We had suggested some years ago that malondialdehyde (MDA) detected in the thiobarbituric acid (TBA) test arises from the breakdown of endoperoxides like PGG.[67,68] This suggestion has been confirmed in recent work that shows that TBA-reactive materials in serum are, at least in part, compounds like PGG.[81] The presence of vitamin E may lead to the capture of acyclic peroxyl radicals before they can cyclize, thus reducing the yield of PGG-derived products relative to HPETEs.[82] This suggests a mechanism for the involvement of vitamin E in the production of species that would be active in the inflammatory process.

PRODUCTS OF LIPID PEROXIDATION AND "ACTION AT A DISTANCE"

I have discussed the production of malondialdehyde and its possible origin from oxidative bicyclization of PUFA.[67,68] The role of MDA in free radical pathology may be an important one; Hochstein and Jain and Goldstein et al. have suggested that MDA may be responsible for the increased viscosity of the membrane of red blood cells (RBCs) that leads to their limited lifetime;[69,70] Seligman et al. have suggested a role for MDA in spinal cord trauma following lipid peroxidation; and Mukai and Goldstein have shown that MDA is mutagenic in the Ames test.[72]

In work of this type, a product that results from lipid peroxidation is shown to have toxic properties. The importance of this type of study is in the area that I like to call "action at a distance." The question arises, How can radicals that are produced in one region of the cell diffuse to other parts of the cell, since radicals are extremely reactive? The hydroxyl radical, for example, is only able to diffuse about 10 Å before it reacts. (This is determined from the length of "spurs" in radiation chemistry.) Thus we must ask, Can radicals that are produced in one part of the cell (and presumably in a region where protective enzymes and other species shield the cell from radical damage) diffuse to a distant part (for example, the nucleus) and cause damage? The answer must surely be no in the case of most highly reactive oxyradicals. And yet, we know that radical damage is propagated in the cell.

The answer to this dilemma may be that stable or metastable nonradical products are produced by radical reactions, and these *products* carry the damage to more distant sites. One possible such product is MDA. Another set of products have been identified by Esterbauer and colleagues and by Frankel;[73,74] these are the 2-alkenals and 4-hydroxyl-2-alkenals that result from autoxidation of PUFA. The mechanism for production of 2-alkenals is clear; they result from β-scission of alkoxyl radicals, as shown in Equation 27. However, the mechanism for production of the 4-hydroxyl derivatives is not clear; these 4-hydroxy compounds (such as 4-hydroxy-2-heptenal) are highly cytotoxic.

$$
\begin{aligned}
&\qquad\quad \overset{\text{OOH}}{\underset{|}{}} \qquad\qquad\qquad \overset{\text{O}\cdot}{\underset{|}{}} \\
\text{PUFA} \to\ &\text{R—CH}=\text{CH—CH—R'} \to \text{R—CH}=\text{CH—CH—R'} \qquad\qquad (27)\\
&\qquad\qquad\qquad \to \text{R—CH}=\text{CH—CHO} + \text{R}\cdot
\end{aligned}
$$

CANCER AND FREE RADICALS

A wide variety of antioxidants inhibit tumors induced by a large number of chemical carcinogens in a variety of animals and organs. The data on the protective effects of antioxidants against chemical carcinogenesis are so extensive that the conclusion appears inescapable that the production of tumors by many chemicals somehow involves free radicals.[83] However, the nature of the "somehow" remains very much a mystery. There also are limited data that suggest that the concentrations of free radicals are different in tumor cells than in normal cells, and that electron spin resonance may be useful to detect tumors.[84]

How might free radicals be involved in the production of tumors from chemical carcinogens? There may be a different mechanism for each type of chemical carcinogen.[4,83–89] Some carcinogens are known to involve specific free radical intermediates in their conversion from a precarcinogen to the proximate carcinogen. For example, N-hydroxy-2-acetylaminofluorene is known to be converted to a nitroxyl radical in the course of being converted to a carcinogen.[87,88]

There also may be a somewhat general mechanism for radical-mediated carcinogenesis. For example, leukocytes that produce superoxide are positive in the Ames test,[90] suggesting that the production of superoxide itself may somehow trigger mutations, and some carcinogens are known to be autoxidized and/or metabolized to produce superoxide. Benzoyl peroxide, a compound that is used in many dermatological products, has been shown to be a tumor promoter,[91] again indicating a possible general mechanism relating peroxidic species and chemical carcinogenesis. One possibility for the conversion of polynuclear aromatic hydrocarbons to the carcinogenic state via radicals can be envisioned.[6] Peroxyl radicals are known to epoxidize olefins:

$$
\text{C}=\text{C} + \text{ROO}\cdot \to \text{C}\overset{\text{O}}{\underset{}{\text{—}}}\text{C} + \text{RO}\cdot \qquad\qquad (28)
$$

A similar mechanism can be envisioned for conversion of aromatic compounds to arene oxides; this reaction can be illustrated for benzene, as shown below.

$$
\text{C}_6\text{H}_6 + \text{ROO}\cdot \to \text{C}_6\text{H}_6\text{O} + \text{RO}\cdot \qquad\qquad (29)
$$

There is some evidence that systems that involve peroxyl radicals can epoxidize PAH. For example, Marnett and Reed have shown that the 7,8-diol of benzo[a]pyrene is metabolized to the 7,8,9,10-tetraol by a prostaglandin-oxidizing system,[92] and Ernster and colleagues have found that BaP is oxidized to quinones by peroxidizing systems.[93]

There is some evidence that there may be two mechanisms for the enzymatically catalyzed conversion of PAH such as benzo[a]pyrene to carcinogens: an epoxidation system that yields primarily diols, and a SET system that can give a variety of products including phenols and quinones.[83,94,95] The two types of reactions are illustrated below, using benzene as a simplified PAH for convenience.

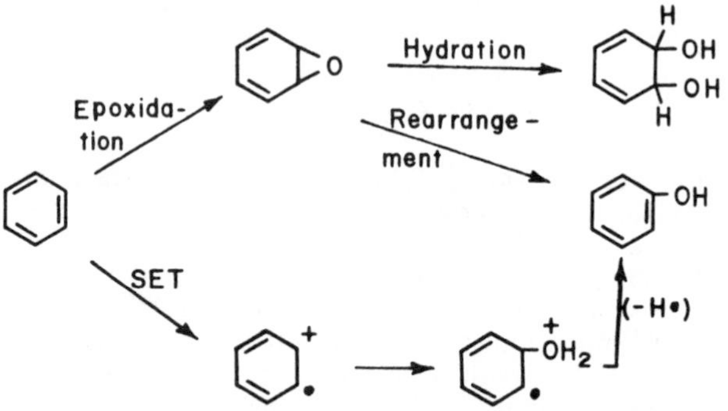

$$(30)$$

Thus, there is evidence to believe that radicals are involved in at least some types of chemical carcinogenesis, and that radical-scavenging agents, usually antioxidants, protect cells against the effects of carcinogens. The detailed mechanisms in most of these processes are not clear as yet.

If antioxidants protect against cancer, then one might speculate on the possible age-extending effects of antioxidants, since cancer is one of the two major life-shortening diseases.

Free Radicals and Aging

Some years ago, Denham Harman conceived the idea that antiradiation drugs might have a life-extending effect on mammals.[96] It was known that radiation damage involves free radical reactions, and radiation-protectant drugs protect against these damaging effects of free radicals. If free radical damage to an organism contributes to aging, then radiation-protectant drugs should extend life span. When Harman first tested this idea using simple radiation drugs such as mercaptoethylamine, his results were greeted with some skepticism. However, in the intervening years a number of workers have duplicated and extended Harman's findings; it now is clear that antioxidants do indeed lengthen the mean life span of mice. Interestingly, vitamin E is without effect, although vitamin E does extend the life span of more primitive organisms.[96-98]

FIGURE 2 shows survivorship curves for populations under various conditions. Curve A is the curve that would result from completely random causes of death.

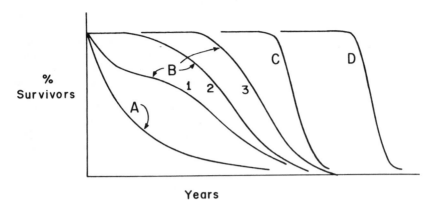

Years

FIGURE 2. Survivorship curves.

This is the first-order kinetic decay curve that is obeyed by radioactive atoms; it also applies to songbirds in the wild. Curves B-1, B-2, and B-3 are the curves that result as better health care begins to exert its effect and more and more of the population lives to a mean age that is characteristic of the species. Curve C results when a large fraction of the species lives healthy lives to an age that corresponds to the maximum that is allowed by the gene pool of the species. Note that there is very little change in the maximum life span during the changes represented by the progression through curves B and C. Curve D is the effect that would be observed if the maximum life span were increased dramatically.

FIGURE 3 shows data for human populations ranging from that in British India to the modern populations of New Zealand and the United States. Note that the

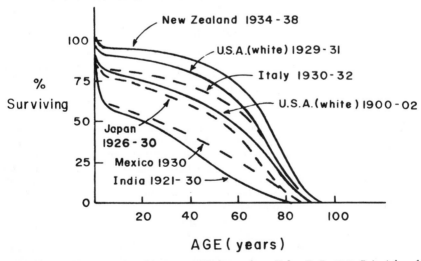

AGE (years)

FIGURE 3. Human survivorship curves. (Redrawn from Kohn, R. R. 1971. *Principles of Mammalian Aging*: 107. Prentice-Hall, Inc. Englewood Cliffs, N.J. Taken from a figure originally in Comfort, A. 1956. *The Biology of Senescence*. Holt, Rinehart, and Winston, Inc. New York, N.Y.)

mean life span has increased very markedly, but very little change in maximum life span has occurred.

FIGURE 4 shows survivorship curves for mice supplied by the Jackson laboratories. These highly inbred animals have some strains that have greatly shortened maximum life spans as well as shorter mean life spans. However, most of the strains, for mice as for men, show the effects of increasing mean life span with little effect on maximum life span.

It is well known that animals that respire faster have shorter life spans. In general, larger animals respire more slowly than do smaller animals and live longer. If respiratory processes produce free radicals, and if some of these "leak out" and produce pathological changes, then one might expect a relation between the rate of respiration and life span.

Recently, Sohal has shown that respiratory rate can be controlled in houseflies by controlling their activity.[98] Flies that are allowed to live in large jars, where

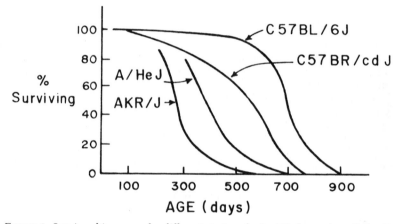

FIGURE 4. Survivorship curves for different strains of mice. (Redrawn from Kohn, R. R. 1971. *Principles of Mammalian Aging*: 108. Prentice-Hall, Inc. Englewood Cliffs, N.J. Taken from a figure in *Biology of the Laboratory Mouse* by the Staff of the Jackson Laboratory, McGraw-Hill Inc., 1966, and copyrighted by McGraw-Hill.)

they can fly, have greatly shortened maximum life spans relative to flies that are kept in small vials that do not allow flight.. The effects are as dramatic as are the well-known effects of caloric restriction or temperature reduction; increases in maximum life span as great as 260% can result. Interestingly, Sohal has also shown that fluorescent age pigment also increases for the flies that are allowed flight during life. Age pigment is thought to be a by-product that results from metabolic activity. This fluorescent pigment was shown by Tappel to contain a chromophore that results from the reaction of MDA (from the cooxidation of PUFA) and nitrogenous materials.[99]

The effects of antioxidant drugs that have been observed by Harman and others are on mean life span, not maximum life span. Antioxidants cannot alter the gene pool and cannot change the life span characteristic for the species. How, then, can they exert their effect?

I believe that they "clean up" the environment of the test animals. They reduce the radical-mediated pathology caused by air-, water-, or food-borne contaminants, thus decreasing the extent of radical damage over the life of the animals, allowing more of them to live closer to the years prescribed for that strain.

They may do one further thing. There is some evidence that strain—physical or psychological—can have effects not unlike those of aging.[100-102] Laboratory animals are kept under conditions of stress, and they also may be subjected to many of the same environmental toxins that pervade the modern world. Perhaps the effects of antioxidants can minimize these effects.

Clearly a "magic bullet" that would reduce the damage to humans from stress due to environmental toxins or to the pressures of modern life would be "a consummation devoutly to be wish'd." To expect such a pill seems rather remote at present, but it is conceivable that such medications could be discovered in the coming years. We must recognize, however, that radical damage probably exerts only a small perturbation on the genetically programmed life span for humans.

Finally, we must return to the function and effects of vitamin E. It is surprising that vitamin E does not extend the mean life span of small animals. Why does the principal antioxidant used in nature not exert an effect on the life span of mammals? This is particularly perplexing, since vitamin E does provide very dramatic protection against such oxidizing threats as hyperbaric pressures of oxygen, ozone, nitrogen dioxide, and other oxidants that normally kill small mammals in exposures of just a few hours or days. Thus, I end with an unanswered question: Why does vitamin E protect animals against above-normal oxidative threats for short periods, but not extend the life span of animals exposed to a normal air atmosphere for all the years of their normal life span? Perhaps when we understand the reasons for this we will feel we have a more complete insight into the function of vitamin E in human metabolism.

REFERENCES

1. McCord, J. M. & I. Fridovich. 1977. Superoxide dismutases: a history. In Superoxide and Superoxide Dismutases. A. Michelson, J. M. McCord & I. Fridovich, Eds.: 1–11. Academic Press, Inc. New York, N.Y.
2. Samuelsson, B., P. W. Ramwell & R. Paolette, Eds. 1980. Advances in Prostaglandin and Thromboxane Research. Volumes 6, 7 & 8. Raven Press. New York, N.Y.
3. Pryor, W. A., J. W. Lightsey & D. G. Prier. 1982. The production of free radicals in vivo from the action of xenobiotics: the initiation of autoxidation of polyunsaturated fatty acids by nitrogen dioxide and ozone. In Lipid Peroxides in Biology and Medicine. K. Yagi, Ed. Academic Press, Inc. New York, N.Y. (In press.)
4. Mason, R. P. 1982. Free radical intermediates in the metabolism of toxic chemicals. In Free Radicals in Biology. W. A. Pryor, Ed. 5(Chapter 6): 161–212. Academic Press, Inc. New York, N.Y.
5. Kerr J. A., J. G. Calvert & K. L. Demerjian. 1976. Free radical reactions in the production of photochemical smog. In Free Radicals in Biology. W. A. Pryor, Ed. 2(Chapter 5): 159–178. Academic Press, Inc. New York, N.Y.
6. Pryor, W. A., K. Terauchi & W. H. Davis, Jr. 1976. Electron spin resonance study of cigarette smoke by use of spin trapping techniques. Environ. Health Perspect. 16: 161–175.
7. Pryor, W. A., D. G. Prier & D. F. Church. 1982. An electron-spin study of mainstream and sidestream cigarette smoke: the nature of the free radicals in gas-phase smoke and in cigarette tar. Environ. Health Perspect. (In press.)
8. Pryor, W. A. & J. W. Lightsey. 1981. Mechanisms of nitrogen dioxide reactions:

initiation of lipid peroxidation and the production of nitrous acid. Science **214:** 435-437.

9. PRYOR, W. A., J. W. LIGHTSEY & D. F. CHURCH. 1982. Reactions of nitrogen dioxide with alkenes and polyunsaturated fatty acids. Addition and hydrogen abstraction mechanisms. J. Am. Chem. Soc. (In press.)

10. PRYOR, W. A. 1980. Methods of detecting free radicals and free radical-mediated pathology in environmental toxicology. *In* Molecular Basis of Environmental Toxicity. R. S. Bhatnagar, Ed.: 3-36. Ann Arbor Science Publishers, Inc. Ann Arbor, Mich.

11. PRYOR, W. A. 1981. Mechanisms and detection of pathology caused by free radicals, tobacco smoke, nitrogen dioxide and ozone. *In* Environmental Health Chemistry. J. D. McKinney, Ed.: 445-466. Ann Arbor Science Publishers, Inc. Ann Arbor, Mich.

12. PRYOR, W. A., D. G. PRIER, J. W. LIGHTSEY & D. F. CHURCH. 1980. Initiation of the autoxidation of polyunsaturated fatty acids by ozone and nitrogen dioxide. *In* Autoxidation in Food and Biological Systems. M. G. Simic & M. Karel, Eds.: 1-16. Plenum Publishing Corp. New York, N.Y.

13. HECHT, S. S., S. CARMELLA, H. MORI & D. HOFFMANN. 1981. A study of tobacco carcinogenesis. Role of catechol as a major cocarcinogen in the weakly acidic fraction smoke condensate. J. Nat. Cancer Inst. **66:** 163-169.

14. MARNETT, L. J. 1981. Polycyclic aromatic hydrocarbon oxidation during prostaglandin biosynthesis. Life Sci. **29:** 531-546.

15. PRYOR, W. A., 1973. Free radical reactions and their importance in biochemical systems. Fed. Proc. **32:** 1862-1869.

16. DOOLEY, M. M. & W. A. PRYOR. 1982. Free radical pathology: inactivation of human -1-proteinase inhibitor by products from the reaction of nitrogen dioxide with hydrogen peroxide. Biochem. Biophys. Res. Commun. **106:** 981-987.

17. THOMPSON, T. E. & C. HUANG. 1977. Dynamics of lipids in biomembranes. *In* Membrane Physiology. T. E. Andreoli, J. F. Hoffman & D. D. Fanestil, Eds.: 34-35. Plenum Medical Book Co. New York, N.Y.

18. BARCLAY, L. R. C. & K. U. INGOLD. 1980. Autoxidation of a model membrane. A comparison of the autoxidation of egg lecithin phosphatidylcholine in water and in chlorobenzene. J. Am. Chem. Soc. **102:** 7792-7794.

19. PRYOR, W. A. 1966. Free Radicals. McGraw-Hill Book Co. New York, N.Y.

20. PARKS, N. J., D. A. KROHN, C. A. MATHIS, J. H. CHASKO, K. R. GEIGER, M. E. GREGOR & N. F. PEEK. 1981. Nitrogen-13 labeled nitrite and nitrate: distribution and metabolism after intratracheal administration. Science **212:** 58-61.

21. GOLDSTEIN, E., N. F. PEEK, N. J. PARKS, H. H. HINES, E. P. STEFFEY & B. TARKINGTON. 1977. Fate and distribution of inhaled nitrogen dioxide in rhesus monkeys. Am. Rev. Respir. Dis. **115:** 403-412.

22. GRAY, D., E. LISSI & J. HEICKLEN. 1972. The reaction of hydrogen peroxide with nitrogen dioxide and nitric oxide. J. Phys. Chem. **76:** 1919-1924.

23. PRYOR, W. A., C. CHOPARD, M. TAMURA & D. F. CHURCH. 1982. Mechanisms of the reactions on nitrogen dioxide and nitrogen radical-mediated damage by cigarette smoke. Fed. Proc. (In press.)

24. CHURCH, D. F., G. CRANK, C. CHOPARD, C. K. GOVINDAN & W. A. PRYOR. 1982. Pulmonary toxicity of nitrogen oxides: the reaction of NO_x with macrophage-derived hydrogen peroxide. Fed Proc. (In press.)

25. PRYOR, W. A., G. CRANK, C. K. GOVINDAN & D. F. CHURCH. 1982. Oxidation of thiols by nitric oxide and nitrogen dioxide: synthetic utility and toxicological implications. J. Org. Chem. **47:** 156-159.

26. PRYOR, W. A. & M. E. KURZ. 1978. Radical production from the interaction of closed-shell molecules. IX. Reaction of ozone with tert-butyl hydroperoxide. J. Am. Chem. Soc. **100:** 7953-7959.

27. MENZEL, D. B. 1976. The role of free radicals in the toxicity of air pollutants (nitrogen oxides and ozone). *In* Free Radicals in Biology. W. A. Pryor, Ed. **2:** 181-202. Academic Press, Inc. New York, N.Y.

28. DUMELIN, E. E., C. J. DILLARD & A. L. TAPPEL. 1978. Breath ethane and pentane as measures of vitamin E protection of *Macaca radiata* against 90 days of exposure to ozone. Environ. Res. **15:** 38-43.

29. PRYOR, W. A., D. G. PRIER & D. F. CHURCH. 1981. Radical production from the interaction of ozone and PUFA as demonstrated by electron spin resonance spin trapping techniques. Environ. Res. **24:** 42–52.

30. PRYOR, W. A., D. G. PRIER & D. F. CHURCH. Detection of free radicals from low temperature ozone-olefin reactions by spin-trapping techniques. (To be submitted.)

31. RECKNAGEL, R. O., E. A. GLENDE, JR. & A. M. HRUSZKEWYCZ. 1977. Chemical mechanisms in carbon tetrachloride toxicity. In Free Radicals in Biology. W. A. Pryor, Ed. **3:** 97–132. Academic Press, Inc. New York, N.Y.

32. REYNOLDS, E. S. & M. T. MOSLEN. 1980. Free-radical damage in liver. In Free Radicals in Biology. W. A. Pryor, Ed. **4:** 49–94. Academic Press, Inc. New York, N.Y.

33. SAGAI, M. & A. L. TAPPEL. 1979. Lipid peroxidation induced by some halomethanes as measured by in vivo pentane production in the rat. Toxicol. Appl. Pharmacol. **49:** 283–291.

34. PRYOR, W. A. 1978. The formation of free radicals and the consequences of their reactions in vivo. Photochem. Photobiol. **28:** 787–801.

35. TAPPEL, A. L. & C. J. DILLARD. 1981. In vivo lipid peroxidation: measurement via exhaled pentane and protection by vitamin E. Fed Proc. **40:** 174–178.

36. MCCAY, P. B., T. NOGUCHI, K. FONG, E. K. LAI & J. L. POYER. 1980. Production of radicals from enzyme systems and the use of spin traps. In Free Radicals in Biology. W. A. Pryor, Ed. **4:** 155–186. Academic Press, Inc. New York, N.Y.

37. ALBRO, P. W., J. T. CORBETT, M. HARRIS & L. D. LAWSON. Effects of 2,3,7,8-tetrachlorobibenzo-p-dioxin on lipid profiles in tissue of the Fischer rat. Chem. Biol. Interactions **23:** 315–330.

38. DOCAMPO, R., S. N. J. MORENO & A. O. M. STOPPANI. 1981. Nitrofuran enhancement of microsomal electron transport, superoxide anion production and lipid peroxidation. Arch. Biochem. Biophys. **207:** 316–324.

39. DOCAMPO, R. 1980. Generation of free radicals from nifurtimos in Trypanosoma cruzi and the mammalian host. In The Host Invader Interplay. H. Van den Bossche, Ed.: 677–681. Elsevier. Amsterdam, the Netherlands.

40. HORWITZ, S. B., E. A. SAUSVILLE & J. PEISACH. 1979. A role for iron in the degradation of DNA by bleomycin. In Bleomycin. S. M. Hecht, Ed.: 170–183. Springer-Verlag. New York, N.Y.

41. AUTOR, A. P. 1977. Biochemical Mechanisms of Paraquat Toxicity. Academic Press, Inc. New York, N.Y.

42. BORG, D. C., K. M. SCHAICH, J. J. ELMORE, JR. & J. A. BELL. 1978. Cytotoxic reactions of free radical species of oxygen. Photochem. Photobiol. **28:** 887–907.

43. BACHUR, N. R. 1979. Anthracycline antibiotic pharmacology and metabolism. Cancer Treatment Rep. **63:** 817–820.

44. BACHUR, N. R., S. L. GORDON, M. V. GEE & H. KON. 1979. NADPH cytochrome P-450 reductase activation of quinone anticancer agents to free radicals. Proc. Nat. Acad. Sci. **76:** 954–957.

45. BACHUR, N. R., S. L. GORDON & M. V. GEE. 1978. A general mechanism for microsomal activation of quinone anticancer agents to free radicals. Cancer Res. **38:** 1745–1750.

46. FRIDOVICH, I. & P. HANDLER. 1958. Xanthine oxidase. III. Sulfite oxide as an ultrasensitive assay. J. Biol. Chem. **233:** 1578–1580.

47. BIAGLOW, J. E. 1981. The effects of ionizing radiation on mammalian cells. J. Chem. Educ. **58:** 144–156.

48. BIAGLOW, J. E. 1980. The effects of hypoxic cell radiosensitizing drugs on cellular oxygen utilization. Pharmacol. Ther. **10:** 283–299.

49. PRYOR, W. A., G. CRANK & C. CHOPARD. 1981. (Unpublished data.)

50. HAYON, E., A. TREININ & J. WILF. 1972. Electronic spectra, photochemistry and autoxidation mechanism of the sulfite-bisulfite-pyrosulfite systems. J. Am. Chem. Soc. **94:** 47–57.

51. MADER, P. M. 1958. Kinetics of the hydrogen peroxide–sulfite reaction in alkaline solution. J. Am. Chem. Soc. **80:** 2634–2639.

52. SHEPPARD, D., A. SAISHO, J. A. NADEL & H. A. BOUSHEY. 1981. Exercise increases sulfur dioxide–induced bronchoconstriction in asthmatic subjects. Am. Rev. Respir. Dis. **123:** 486–491.

53. SHEPPARD, D., W. S. WONG, D. F. UEHARA, J. A. NADEL & H. A. BOUSHEY. 1981. Lower threshold and greater bronchomoter responsiveness of asthmatic subjects to sulfur dioxide. Am. Rev. Respir. Dis. **122:** 873–878.
54. STEVENSON, D. D. & R. A. SIMON. 1981. Sensitivity to ingested metabisulfites in asthmatic subjects. J. Allergy Clin. Immunol. **68:** 26–32.
55. FISH, J. A., M. G. ANKIN, N. F. ADKINSON & V. I. PETERMAN. 1981. Indomethacin modification of immediate-type immunologic airway responses in allergic asthmatic and non-asthmatic subjects. Am. Rev. Respir. Dis. **123:** 609–614.
56. CHANCE, B., H. SIES & A. BOVERIS. 1979. Hydroperoxide metabolism in mammalian organs. Physiol. Rev. **59:** 527–605.
57. FORMAN, H. J. & A. BOVERIS. 1982. Superoxide radical and hydrogen peroxide in mitochondria. *In* Free Radicals in Biology. W. A. Pryor, Ed. **5:** 65–87. Academic Press, Inc. New York, N.Y.
58. KELLOGG, E. W., III & I. FRIDOVICH. 1975. Superoxide, hydrogen peroxide, and singlet oxygen in lipid peroxidation by a xanthine oxidase system. J. Biol. Chem. **250:** 8812–8817.
59. HALLIWELL, B. 1978. Superoxide-dependent formation of hydroxyl radicals in the presence of iron chelates. Is it a mechanism for hydroxyl radical production in biochemical systems? FEBS Lett. **92:** 321–326.
60. THOMAS, M. J., K. S. MEHL & W. A. PRYOR. 1978. The role of the superoxide anion in the xanthine oxidase-induced autoxidation of linoleic acid. Biochem. Biophys. Res. Commun. **83:** 927–932.
61. ANBAR, M. & P. NETA. 1967. A compilation of specific bimolecular rate constants for the reactions of hydrated electrons, hydrogen atoms, and hydroxyl radicals with inorganic and organic compounds in aqueous solution. Int. J. Appl. Radiat. Isot. **18:** 493–523.
62. PETERS, J. W. & C. S. FOOTE. 1976. Chemistry of superoxide ion. II. Reaction with hydroperoxides. J. Am. Chem. Soc. **98:** 873–875.
63. BABIOR, B. M. 1978. Oxygen-dependent microbial killing by phagocytes. N. Engl. J. Med. **298:** 721–725.
64. DECHATELET, L. R. 1979. Phagocytosis by human neutrophils. *In* Phagocytes and Cellular Immunity. H. H. Gadebusch, Ed.: 2–42. CRC Press Inc. Boca Raton, Fla.
65. DEL MAESTRO, R. F., H. H. THAW, J. BJORK, M. PLANKERN & K-E. ARFORS. 1980. Free radicals as mediators of tissue injury. Acta Physiol. Scand. Suppl. **492:** 43–57.
66. THOMAS, M. J., K. S. MEHL & W. A. PRYOR. 1982. The role of superoxide in xanthine oxidase-induced peroxidation of linoleic acid. J. Biol. Chem. (In press.)
67. PRYOR, W. A. & J. P. STANLEY. 1975. A suggested mechanism for the production of malonaldehyde during the autoxidation of PUFA. Nonenzymatic production of prostaglandin endoperoxides during autoxidation. J. Org. Chem. **40:** 3615–3617.
68. PRYOR, W. A., J. P. STANLEY & E. BLAIR. 1976. Autoxidation of polyunsaturated fatty acids. II. A suggested mechanism for the formation of TBA-reactive materials from prostaglandin-like endoperosides. Lipids **11:** 370–379.
69. HOCHSTEIN, P. & S. K. JAIN. 1981. Association of lipid peroxidation and polymerization of membrane proteins with erythrocyte aging. Fed. Proc. **40:** 183–187.
70. GOLDSTEIN, B. D., M. G. ROZEN & M. A. AMORUSO. 1979. Relation of fluorescence in lipid-containing red cell membrane extracts to in vivo lipid peroxidation. J. Lab. Clin. Med. **93:** 687–694.
71. SELIGMAN, M. L., E. S. FLAMM, B. D. GOLDSTEIN, R. G. POSER, H. B. DEMOPOULOS & J. RANSOHOFF. 1977. Spectrofluorescent detection of malonaldehyde as a measure of lipid free radical damage in response to ethanol potentiation of spinal cord trauma. Lipids **12:** 945–950.
72. MUKAI, F. H. & B. D. GOLDSTEIN. 1976. Mutagenicity of malonaldehyde, a composition product of peroxidized polyunsaturated fatty acids. Science **191:** 868–869.
73. SCHAUENSTEIN, E., H. ESTERBAUER & H. ZOLLNER. 1977. Aldehydes in Biological Systems. Pion Limited. London, England. Academic Press, Inc. New York, N.Y.
74. FRANKEL, E. N. 1980. Lipid oxidation. Prog. Lipid Res. **19:** 1.
75. McCORD, J. M. 1974. Free radicals and inflammation: protection of synovial fluid by superoxide dismutase. Science **185:** 529–531.

76. WALSH, C. E., L. R. DeCHATELET, M. J. THOMAS, J. T. O'FLAHERTY & M. WAITE. 1981. Effect of phagocytosis and ionophores on release and metabolism of arachidonic acid from human neutrophils. Lipids **16**: 120–124.
77. HIGGS, G. A., S. MONCADA & J. R. VANE. 1979. The role of arachidonic acid metabolites in inflammation. *In* Advances in Inflammation Research. G. Weissmann, Ed. **1**: 413–418. Raven Press. New York, N.Y.
78. HIGGS, G. A., S. MONCADA & J. R. VANE. 1980. The mode of action of antiinflammatory drugs which prevent the peroxidation of arachidonic acid. Clin. Rheumatic Dis. **6**: 675–693.
79. KUEHL, F. A., JR. & R. W. EGAN. 1980. Prostaglandins, arachidonic acid, and inflammation. Science **210**: 978–984.
80. PEREZ, H. D., B. B. WEKSLER & I. M. GOLDSTEIN. 1980. Generation of a chemotactic lipid from arachidonic acid by exposure to a superoxide-generating system. Inflammation **4**: 313–315.
81. SHIMIZU, T., K. KONDO & O. HAYAISHI. 1981. Role of prostaglandin endoperoxides in the serum thiobarbituric acid reaction. Arch. Biochem. Biophys. **206**: 271–277.
82. PORTER, N. A., L. S. LAHMAN, B. A. WEBER & K. J. SMITH. 1981. Unified mechanism for polyunsaturated fatty acid autoxidation. Completion of peroxy radical hydrogen atom abstraction, beta-scission, and cyclization. J. Am. Chem. Soc. **103**: 6447–6455.
83. TS'O, P. O. P., W. J. CASPARY & R. J. LORENTZEN. 1977. The involvement of free radicals in chemical carcinogenesis. *In* Free Radicals in Biology. W. A. Pryor, Ed. **3**: 251–305. Academic Press, Inc. New York, N.Y.
84. SWARTZ, H. M. 1979. Free radicals in cancer. Ciba Symp. **67**: 107–123.
85. MASON, R. P. 1982. Free radical intermediates in the metabolism of toxic chemicals. *In* Free Radicals in Biology. W. A. Pryor, Ed. **5**(Chapter 6): 161–212. Academic Press, Inc. New York, N.Y.
86. OBERLEY, L. W. & G. R. BUETTNER. 1979. Role of superoxide dismutase in cancer: a review. Cancer Res. **39**: 1141–1149.
87. FLOYD, R. A. & L. M. SOONG. 1977. Obligatory free radical intermediate in the oxidative action of the carcinogen in N-hydroxy-2-acetylaminofluorene. Biochim. Biophys. Acta **498**: 244–249.
88. BARTSCH, H., J. A. MILLER & E. C. MILLER. 1972. N-Acetoxy-2-acetylaminoarenes and nitrosoarenes. 1-Electron nonenzymatic and enzymatic oxidation products of various carcinogenic aromatic acethydroxamic acids. Biochim. Biophys. Acta **273**: 40–51.
89. LORENTZEN, L. & P. O. P. TS'O. 1980. Superoxide induces DNA single strand breaks. Biochimie **19**: 302.
90. WEITZMAN, S. A. & T. P. STOSSEL. 1981. Mutations caused by human phagocytes. Science **212**: 546–547.
91. SLAGA, T. J., A. J. P. KLEIN-SZANTO, L. L. TRIPLETT, L. P. YOTTI & J. E. TROSKO. 1981. Skin tumor-promoting activity of benzoyl peroxide, a widely used free radical-generating compound. Science **213**: 1013–1025.
92. MARNETT, L. J. & G. A. REED. 1979. Peroxidatic oxidation of benzo(a)pyrene and prostaglandin biosynthesis. Biochemistry **18**: 2923–2929.
93. MORGENSTERN, R., J. W. DePIERRE, C. LIND, C. GUTHENBERT, B. MANNERVIK & L. ERNSTER. 1981. Benzo(a)pyrene quinones can be generated by lipid peroxidation and are conjugated with glutathione by glutathione S-transferase B from rat liver. Biochem. Biophys. Res. Commun. **99**: 682.
94. CAVALIERI, E., R. ROTH & E. G. ROGAN. 1976. Metabolic activation of aromatic hydrocarbons by one-electron oxidation in relation to the mechanism of tumor initiation. *In* Carcinogenesis. R. I. Freudenthal & P. W. Jones, Eds. **1**: 181–190. Raven Press. New York, N.Y.
95. RENNEBERT, R., J. CAPDEVILA, N. CHACOS, R. W. ESTABROOK & R. A. PROUGH. 1981. Hydrogen peroxide supported oxidation of benzo(a)pyrene by rat liver microsomal fractions. Biochem. Pharmacol **30**: 843.
96. HARMAN, D. 1982. The free radical theory of aging. *In* Free Radicals in Biology. W. A. Pryor, Ed. **5**(Chapter 8): 255–271. Academic Press, Inc. New York, N.Y.
97. PRYOR, W. A. 1977. Free radicals in biology. The involvement of radical reactions in aging and carcinogenesis. Med. Chem. **5**: 331.

98. SOHAL, R. S. 1981. Metabolic rate, aging, and lipofuscin accumulation. *In* Age Pigments. R. S. Sohal, Ed.: 303–311. Elsevier/North-Holland Biomedical Press. Amsterdam, the Netherlands.

99. TAPPEL, A. L. 1975. Lipid peroxidation and fluorescent molecular damage to membranes. *In* Pathobiology of Cell Membranes. B. F. Trump & A. U. Arstila, Eds. **1:** 145–170. Academic Press, Inc. New York, N.Y.

100. RILEY, V. 1981. Psychoneuroendocrine influences on immunocompetence and neoplasia. Science **212:** 1100–1110.

101. SAGAI, M. & T. ICHINOSE. 1980. Age related changes in lipid peroxidation as measured by ethane, ethylene, butane, and pentane in respired gases of rats. Life Sci. **27:** 731–738.

102. KONTOS, H. A., E. P. WEI, J. T. POVLISHOCK, W. D. DIETRICH, C. T. MAGIERA & E. F. ELLIS. 1980. Cerebral arteriolar damage by arachidonic acid and prostaglandin G_2. Science **209:** 1242–1245.

AN UPDATE ON ANTIOXIDANT THEORY: SPIN TRAPPING OF TRICHLOROMETHYL RADICALS *IN VIVO*

Paul B. McCay, M. Margaret King, J. Lee Poyer,
and Edward K. Lai

Biomembrane Research Laboratory
Oklahoma Medical Research Foundation
Oklahoma City, Oklahoma 73104

and

Department of Biochemistry and Molecular Biology
University of Oklahoma Health Sciences Center
Oklahoma City, Oklahoma 73104

The precise function or functions of α-tocopherol at the molecular level in biological systems have yet to be resolved. Although its free radical–scavenging and singlet oxygen–quenching properties are unquestioned, the extent to which these properties are responsible for its requirement in animals, particularly in young, rapidly growing animals, is not known. A number of structurally unrelated antioxidants appear to substitute for this fat-soluble vitamin, but it is still possible that such antioxidants are simply protecting very minute quantities of α-tocopherol so that effective amounts of the vitamin may reach the essential sites. It appears likely that more than one type of function is involved in the biological manifestations of vitamin E activity.

Tocopherol has been shown to have beneficial effects in a variety of clinical problems including bronchopulmonary dysplasia, retrolental fibroplasia,[1,2] hemolytic anemia associated with iron supplementation,[3] and certain toxic liver injuries.[4] Based on investigations with animal models, the vitamin may play a significant role in prostaglandin metabolism,[5-7] platelet function,[8,9] adrenocortical steroid synthesis,[10,11] erythropoiesis,[12] phagocytosis,[13] T-cell function,[14] autoimmune disease,[15] and inhibition of tumor promotion.[16] In addition, this vitamin may be useful in preventing at least part of the cardiac damage associated with chemotherapy with the anthracycline antibiotic adriamycin.[17,18]

Some of the problems encountered in the investigations of vitamin E function appear to have their basis in conceptual aspects as well as in the experimental conditions employed. An example of the latter is the administration of a single dose of α-tocopheryl acetate intramuscularly or intraperitoneally simultaneously with adriamycin to test the vitamin's effectiveness in ameliorating the cardiopathy and mortality caused by adriamycin cardiotoxicity.[17,19] Very little beneficial effect is observed under those conditions, whereas administration of tocopherol itself, rather than the ester, 24 hours prior to adriamycin treatment provides considerable protection against adriamycin mortality.[18] The esterified form of the vitamin may not have been hydrolyzed in significant amounts in muscle or the peritoneum, and, in addition, when given at the same time as adriamycin, it may not have been incorporated into the critical sites before the damage was inflicted, whereas when the free vitamin was administered well ahead of the adriamycin, significant protection was observed.

23

Another example of a source of conflicting data concerns investigations of the mechanism of toxicity of chlorinated compounds such as CCl_4. Substances with free radical–scavenging properties may be able to provide a measure of protection against that portion of tissue damage caused by CCl_4 if radicals derived from the metabolism of CCl_4 are involved in the mechanism of injury. Whether or not one would see such a protective effect would depend on both the dose size of CCl_4 and the level of antioxidant present in the liver. Hence antioxidants have been reported to have either no effect on liver injury caused by CCl_4 administration[20] or to provide substantial protection.[21] All of these findings may be correct for the experimental conditions employed. In an effort to obtain a better understanding of the effect of α-tocopherol and other antioxidants on the molecular events taking place in the endoplasmic reticulum of the liver (which is the site of the earliest morphological changes in the liver), we have employed a technique recently developed in our laboratory for trapping radicals produced from CCl_4 metabolism in the intact animal. The spin trapping of highly reactive free radicals to form relatively stable radical adducts that can be assayed by electron spin resonance (ESR) has provided direct evidence that the trichloromethyl radical ($\cdot CCl_3$) is formed both *in vitro* by liver microsomes[22] and *in vivo* in the endoplasmic reticulum of the liver.[23] The spin-trapping agent, phenyl-*t*-butyl nitrone (PBN), forms a stable free radical on reacting with the $\cdot CCl_3$ radical

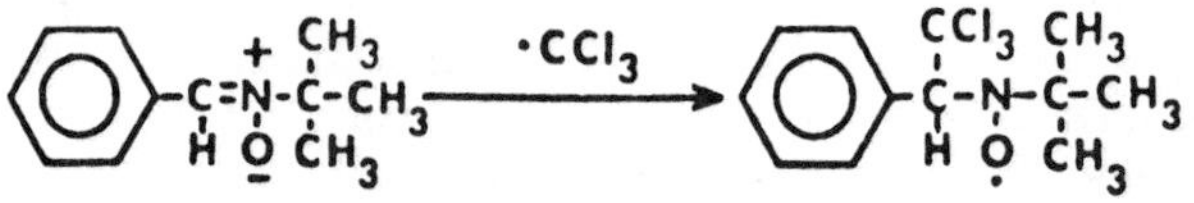

FIGURE 1. Reaction of the spin-trapping agent phenyl-*t*-butyl nitrone with the trichloromethyl radical to form a stable radical adduct. The adduct, which is lipid soluble, can be extracted from biological material with chloroform-methanol 2:1. The radical adduct is stable for several weeks in the lipid extract when stored in the dark at 0°C.

(FIGURE 1), and this radical adduct produces a characteristic signal in an ESR spectrometer (FIGURE 2), which was identified as the adduct of the trichloromethyl radical.[22] Conclusive proof that the initial radical was $\cdot CCl_3$ was obtained by the use of $^{13}CCl_4$. The isotopic carbon is in a position β to the nitrogen atom in the adduct (FIGURE 3), and the resulting effect causes each component of the 6-line spectrum of the ESR signal to split, resulting in a 12-line spectrum. When liver microsomes were incubated with $^{13}CCl_4$, reduced nicotinamide-adenine dinucleotide phosphate (NADPH), and the spin-trapping agent PBN under the conditions shown in FIGURE 2, a 12-line spectrum was obtained indicating that the reaction system was producing $\cdot CCl_3$ radicals (FIGURE 4). We then determined that if rats were given PBN simultaneously with CCl_4 orally or intraperitoneally, the spin-trapped $\cdot CCl_3$ radical could be detected as a strong signal in the lipid extract of liver.[24] The signal was subsequently found to be localized almost entirely in the microsomal subcellular fraction.

Loss of liver microsomal cytochrome P_{450} following exposure to CCl_4 has been shown to occur very quickly. Cytochrome P_{450} is known to be involved in the metabolism of CCl_4 to reactive products.[24] We undertook to determine (1) if a particular form or forms of cytochrome P_{450} were destroyed by CCl_4 treatment, and (2) if any particular form of cytochrome P_{450} was required for the production

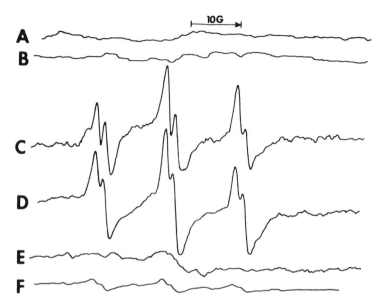

FIGURE 2. Electron spin resonance spectra of liver microsomes oxidizing NADPH in the presence of the spin-trapping agent phenyl-*t*-butyl nitrone and CCl₄ or bromotrichloromethane. The NADPH-generating system, where utilized, was composed of 5 mM glucose-6-phosphate, 0.3 mM NADP, and 0.5 Kornberg units glucose-6-phosphate dehydrogenase per ml of reaction system. All incubation systems contained approximately 1 mg microsomal protein per ml incubation system, 0.14 M phenyl-*t*-butyl nitrone in 0.15 M tris buffer, pH 7.5, all incubated in 1 ml final volume at 24°C plus the following additions and conditions: **A,** 20 μl CCl₄; **B,** the NADPH-generating system and 2 μl CCl₄. In this system, the enzymic activity of the microsomes was inactivated by heating at 65°C for 2 minutes prior to the addition of the NADPH-generating system and PBN; **C,** 20 μl CCl₄ and the NADPH-generating system; **D,** 20 μl bromotrichloromethane and the NADPH-generating system; **E,** the NADPH-generating system; **F,** 5 mM *p*-hydroxymercuribenzoate, 20 μl CCl₄, and the NADPH-generating system. (Reproduced from Reference 22 with the permission of Elsevier Biomedical Press B.V.)

of the trichloromethyl radical. Phenobarbital-treated rats were used in these experiments because the increased content of cytochrome P₄₅₀ in the liver microsomal fraction facilitated observation of certain of these cytochromes following polyacrylamide gel electrophoresis of the solubilized microsomes. Rats were given 75 mg of phenobarbital/kg body weight intraperitoneally in saline

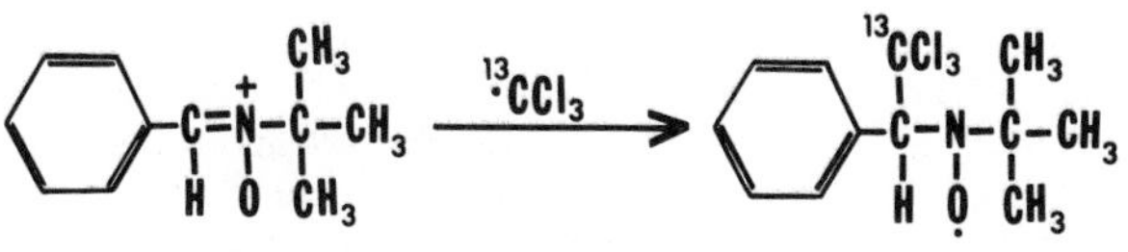

FIGURE 3. Spin trapping of a ¹³C-labeled trichloromethyl radical by phenyl-*t*-butyl nitrone to form the stable ¹³C-labeled radical adduct.

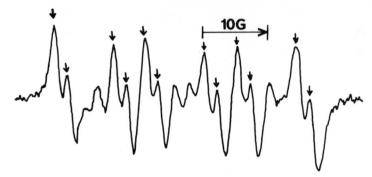

FIGURE 4. Electron spin resonance spectrum of a ^{13}C-labeled radical adduct formed by the reaction of a trichloromethyl radical with phenyl-t-butyl nitrone. Note the 12-line spectrum due to the effect of the ^{13}C-atom β to the nitrogen atom (identified by arrows). The lesser signal of a triplet of doublets is due to the presence of 10% of ^{12}C-carbon tetrachloride present in the ^{13}C-labeled CCl$_4$.

daily for three days. The animals were then given CCl$_4$ orally (0.25 ml/100 g body weight) and then killed at intervals beginning 15 minutes following CCl$_4$ administration. Liver microsomes were prepared, solubilized with sodium dodecyl sulfate (SDS), and subjected to polyacrylamide gel electrophoresis (FIGURE 5). Observation of the polypeptide bands revealed that the first visible change was a decrease in the intensity of band migrating at the 52,000-dalton position (FIGURE 5). By 30 minutes, the loss of this particular band is substantial. One of the polypeptides in rat liver microsomes that is specifically induced by phenobarbital is a P$_{450}$ cytochrome with a molecular weight of 52,000 daltons, and it was reasonable to assume that this was the component that rapidly decreased in microsomes after CCl$_4$ exposure. This led us to consider that this particular form of cytochrome P$_{450}$ was involved in the generation of the ·CCl$_3$ radical, perhaps causing its own destruction. To test that possibility, this form of the P$_{450}$ cytochrome was purified to homogeneity from rat liver microsomes. NADPH-cytochrome P$_{450}$ reductase was also purified, and a reconstituted drug-metabolizing system was assembled as shown in FIGURE 2. When this system was incubated in the presence of the spin-trapping agent PBN, the characteristic 12-line signal was obtained when ^{13}CCl$_4$ was added to the system as in FIGURE 4. Only cytochrome P$_{450}$ fractions containing the 52,000-dalton form produced the ESR signal observed, indicating that only this particular form of cytochrome P$_{450}$ could function in the reaction producing ·CCl$_3$ radicals. If the radicals are integral to the production of liver damage, it would explain the potentiation of liver damage caused by phenobarbital induction since the 52,000-dalton form is primarily induced by phenobarbital.

In considering what may have happened to the 52,000-dalton P$_{450}$ cytochrome that disappeared very early from the slab gels of liver microsomes from CCl$_4$-treated rats, two possibilities arose. One was that production of the radicals by this cytochrome resulted in intense lipid peroxidation in the immediate vicinity of the cytochrome, resulting in a decreased hydrophobic attraction between the protein and the microsomal membrane sufficient to effect the detachment of the cytochrome. However, analyses of microsomal protein content indicated no loss of total protein from the microsomal particles even though the disappearance of the 52,000-dalton cytochrome represented a significant fraction of the total protein. This led us to consider that the cytochrome may have undergone a polymerization

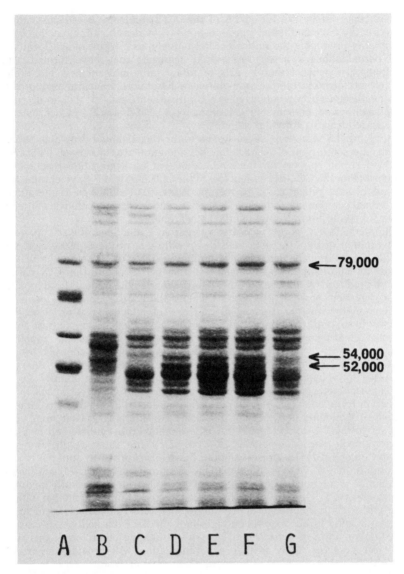

FIGURE 5. SDS-polyacrylamide gel electrophoresis of liver microsomes from phenobarbital-treated rats treated with CCl$_4$ *in vivo*. (**A**) Protein standards (bottom to top): ovalbumin (45,000 daltons), glutamate dehydrogenase (53,000 daltons), catalase (58,000 daltons), bovine serum albumin (68,000 daltons), and NADPH-cytochrome P$_{450}$ reductase (79,000 daltons). Each of the following lanes had wells containing 10 μg of solubilized hepatic microsomal protein from (**B**) β-naphthoflavone-treated rats and (**C**) normal rats. The following lanes had wells containing 10 μg of solubilized hepatic microsomal protein from phenobarbital-treated rats that had been treated with CCl$_4$ and from which the microsomes were prepared at the following times after administering the halocarbon: (**D**) 0 minutes, (**E**)15 minutes, (**F**) 30 minutes, and (**G**) 60 minutes. (Reproduced from Reference 26 with the permission of *Biochemical Pharmacology*.)

process triggered by the formation of the ·CCl$_3$ radicals. A radical-mediated process could have facilitated a protein-protein covalent bonding reaction by the cytochrome producing the radicals. Alternatively, as a result of ·CCl$_3$-initiated lipid peroxidation, a large protein-lipid aggregate may have formed. After modifying the polyacrylamide gels to allow large-molecular-weight protein components to enter a tube gel preparation, electrophoretic separation of proteins from microsomes of rats subjected to CCl$_4$ treatment revealed that an aggregate could be observed, presumably containing the 52,000-dalton P$_{450}$ cytochrome that disappeared from its normal position.

Applying the same type of gel system to the reconstituted drug-metabolizing system, the same type of aggregation phenomenon was observed. This result provided strong support for the conclusion that an aggregation reaction was responsible for the CCl$_4$-dependent loss of the 52,000-dalton P$_{450}$ cytochrome from the endoplasmic reticulum of the rat, and is the first visible sign of alteration of microsomal components following CCl$_4$ treatment, occurring within 30 minutes to 1 hour following administration of the halocarbon.

Supplementation of rats with dietary vitamin E at a level of 0.2% prevented the formation of the aggregate and the specific loss of the 52,000-dalton cytochrome during metabolism of CCl$_4$ in liver of rats in vivo (FIGURE 6). This suggested that the supplemental tocopherol may be scavenging the ·CCl$_3$ radicals that are produced by this cytochrome, thus preventing the radicals from initiating the aggregation process. To probe this possibility, the effect of tocopherol supplementation on the capacity of the liver of intact rats to produce ·CCl$_3$ radicals from orally administered CCl$_4$ was investigated. In contrast to the expected effect, tocopherol supplementation resulted in a greater spin trapping of ·CCl$_3$ radicals (5- to 10-fold) as compared to unsupplemented controls. Because this finding was quite different from the one anticipated, further consideration gave rise to a hypothesis that α-tocopherol must have an affinity for the microenvironment of this cytochrome, protecting it from direct attack by the radicals or from the effects of lipid peroxidation, thus allowing the cytochrome to continue functioning and thereby producing considerably greater numbers of radicals during the time frame of the experiments. Propyl gallate and butylated hydroxyanisole supplementation also produced the same result. Butylated hydroxytoluene (BHT) supplementation, however, resulted in apparently complete inhibition of ·CCl$_3$ production. This seemingly paradoxical result may be explainable when one considers the capacity of BHT for significantly modifying the cytochrome P$_{450}$ content of rat liver microsomes.[25] Supplementation with the other antioxidants mentioned above did not affect liver microsomal cytochrome P$_{450}$ significantly in our experimental animals. If BHT markedly decreases the 52,000-dalton form of cytochrome P$_{450}$ while inducing other forms, this result might be expected. Only further experimentation will provide the insights required to further elucidate this apparently anomalous result.

In summary, α-tocopherol supplementation results in conditions leading to the observation of a very significantly greater number of trapped trichloromethyl radicals from CCl$_4$, yet the elements of the endoplasmic reticulum involved in the production of these radicals are substantially protected from the radicals by the supplementation. In addition, the degree of toxicity of CCl$_4$ treatment is diminished. These observations suggest that production of highly reactive radicals in a tissue may be relatively innocuous if susceptible components vital to the survival of the cell are protected. α-Tocopherol appears to function in this manner very effectively.

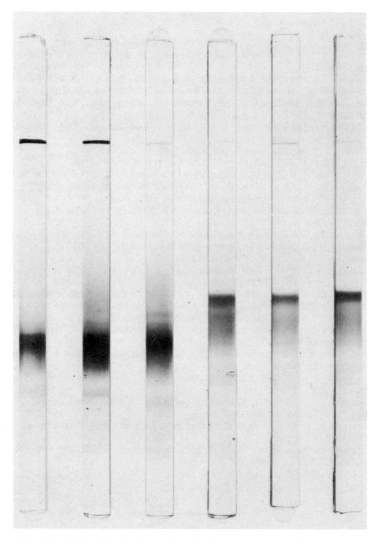

FIGURE 6. Polyacrylamide gel electrophoresis of liver microsomes from rats treated with CCl_4. Rats were administered 125 μl $CCl_4/100$ g body weight in 1.0 ml corn by stomach tube. Two hours later, livers were removed and microsomes prepared and solubilized. (Tube gels are mentioned in order from left to right.) Tube gel electrophoresis followed by staining with Coomassie Blue revealed a large-molecular-weight component that just barely enters the top of the gel (tube gels 1 and 2). The 2% gels, which were used to allow the high-molecular-weight component to enter, resulted in other microsomal proteins prior to administration of CCl_4. Tube gel 3 contained microsomes from a control rat (i.e., not treated with CCl_4). Tube gels 4 and 5 were liver microsomes from two different rats that had been supplemented with vitamin E prior to administration of CCl_4 in the manner described above. Note that the large-molecular-weight component did not form in these rats. Tube gel 6 contained microsomes from a control vitamin E–supplemented rat (i.e., not treated with CCl_4).

REFERENCES

1. PHELPS, D. L. & A. L. ROSENBAUM. 1979. Ophthalmology **86:** 1741–1748.
2. SCHAFFER, D. B., L. JOHNSON, G. E. QUINN & T. R. BOGGS, JR. 1979. Ophthalmology **86:** 1749–1760.
3. JANSSON, L., L. HOLMBERG & R. EKMAN. 1979. Acta Paediatr. Scand. **68:** 705–708.
4. SKAARE, J. U. & I. NAFSTAD. 1978. Acta Pharmacol. Toxicol. **43:** 119–128.
5. RAO, G. H. R., J. M. GERRARD, J. W. EATON & J. G. WHITE. 1978. Photochem. Photobiol. **28:** 845–850.
6. CORNWELL, D. G., J. J. HUTTNER, G. E. MILO, R. V. PANGANAMALA, H. M. SHARMA & J. C. GEER. 1979. Lipids **14**(2): 194–207.
7. FORSTER, W. 1980. Acta Med. Scand. **642:** 47–48.
8. STEINER, M. 1981. Biochim. Biophys. Acta **640:** 100–105.
9. COX, A. C., G. H. R. RAO, J. M. GERRARD & J. G. WHITE. 1980. Blood **55**(6): 907–914.
10. NATHANS, A. H. & A. E. KITABCHI. 1975. Biochim. Biophys. Acta **399:** 244–253.
11. HORNSBY, P. J. 1980. J. Biol. Chem. **255**(9): 4020–4027.
12. FITCH, C. D., G. O. BROWN, JR., A. C. CHOU & N. I. GALLAGHER. 1980. Am. J. Clin. Nutr. **33:** 1251–1258.
13. HARRIS, R. E., L. A. BOXER & R. L. BAEHNER. 1980. Blood **55**(2): 338–343.
14. TANAKA, J., H. FUJIWARA & M. TORISU. 1979. Immunology **38:** 727–734.
15. AYRES, S., JR. & R. MIHAN. 1978. Cutis **21:** 321–325.
16. OHUCHI, K. & L. LEVINE. 1980. Biochim. Biophys. Acta **619:** 11–19.
17. VAN VLEET, J. F. & V. J. FERRANS. 1980. Am. J. Vet. Res. **41**(5): 691–699.
18. MYERS, C. E., W. MCGUIRE & R. YOUNG. 1976. Cancer Treatment Rep. **60**(7): 961–962.
19. VAN VLET, J. R., V. J. FERRANS & W. E. WEIRICH. 1980. Am. J. Pathol. **99**(1): 13–24.
20. MCLEAN, A. E. M. 1967. Br. J. Exp. Pathol. **48:** 632–636.
21. KELLEHER, J., N. P. KEANEY, B. E. WALKER, M. S. LOSOWSKY & M. F. DIXON. 1976. J. Int. Med. Res. **4**(Suppl. 4]: 139–144.
22. POYER, J. L., R. A. FLOYD, P. B. MCCAY, E. G. JANZEN & E. R. DAVIS. 1978. Biochim. Biophys. Acta **539:** 402–409.
23. LAI, E. K., P. B. MCCAY, T. NOGUCHI & K.-L. FONG. 1979. Biochem. Pharmacol. **28:** 2231–2235.
24. POYER, J. L., P. B. MCCAY, E. K. LAI, E. G. JANZEN & E. R. DAVIS. 1980. Biochem. Biophys. Res. Commun. **94**(4): 1154–1160.
25. RIKANS, L. E., D. D. GIBSON, P. B. MCCAY & M. M. KING. 1981. Food Cosmet. Toxicol. **19:** 89–92.
26. NOGUCHI, T., K.-L. FONG, E. D. LAI, L. OLSON & P. B. MCCAY. 1982. Biochem. Pharmacol. **31**(5): 609–614.

DISCUSSION

A. E. KITABCHI (*University of Tennessee, Memphis, Tenn.*): You alluded to the possibility of affinity of tocopherol with protein such as cytochrome P_{450}. Have you in fact done some kinetics to see whether tocopherol is bound?

P. B. MCCAY: No, we haven't. We would like to do that, and we would also like to determine that this particular form of cytochrome is the protein that does most of the binding of the CCl_4, which is also known to be bound during metabolism.

J. G. BIERI (*National Institutes of Health, Bethesda, Md.*): Could you tell us again why the signal is so much larger when you give the tocopherol.

P. B. McCAY: We don't know why, but we postulate that vitamin E may protect the cytochrome that is producing the radical, so that more radicals can be produced before it finally is destroyed by radical attack, therefore allowing for a greater amount of spin trapping during the period of incubation.

In other words, if there is a balance, we would assume there must be a balance between radical production, destruction of the cytochrome, and the amount of antioxidant that might be available to protect the cytochrome.

J. G. BIERI: Did you have animals that were given tocopherol but no CCl_4?

P. B. McCAY: When the spin trapping is done without the CCl_4, one gets no signal.

A. T. QUINTANILHA (*University of California, Berkeley, Calif.*): The signal that you are looking at is in a particular liver homogenate fraction. Have you tried to find out whether the signal may be in other fractions?

P. B. McCAY: The signal is found primarily in the liver microsome fraction; very little is found in any other subcellular fraction.

A. T. QUINTANILHA: It is well known that nitroxide spin labels can be destroyed under certain conditions. It could be that you formed the nitroxide radical and, by some other mechanism, destroyed it before you extracted it.

P. B. McCAY: That's true, but the fact is that you can observe the radical in these microsomes, and the evidence that it is a trichloromethyl radical is reasonably conclusive.

H. H. DRAPER (*University of Guelph, Guelph, Ontario, Canada*): Could you tell us whether this system that you are using is relevant to the mechanisms involved in free radical formation in simple vitamin E deficiency or exposure to agents such as ozone or nitrogen dioxide.

P. B. McCAY: We were not certain that the phenomenon that we're looking at is really involved in the toxicity of tetrachloride, since the destruction of the cytochrome may or may not be involved in this. Since antioxidants, however, do provide some protective action against CCl_4, we would presume this may have some relevance to the toxicity process.

P. MARFEY (*State University of New York, Albany, N.Y.*): Is the effect concentration dependent? Could vitamin E at high concentration decrease the signal by reducing the nitroxide free radical? At first it may enhance the formation and you see a bigger signal, but with higher concentrations you may see reduction of nitroxide free radical by vitamin E.

P. B. McCAY: We have found that BHT removes the signal completely, and we presume that this may be related to the concentration of these various antioxidants in that particular site of the membrane.

MEMBRANE EFFECTS OF VITAMIN E DEFICIENCY: BIOENERGETIC AND SURFACE CHARGE DENSITY STUDIES OF SKELETAL MUSCLE AND LIVER MITOCHONDRIA*

Alexandre T. Quintanilha, Lester Packer,
Joanna M. Szyszlo Davies, Toinette L. Racanelli,
and Kelvin J. A. Davies

*Department of Physiology-Anatomy
and
Membrane Bioenergetics Group
Lawrence Berkeley Laboratory
University of California
Berkeley, California 94720*

Introduction

The biological role of vitamin E has been extensively discussed. Vitamin E has been shown to act as a powerful antioxidant in the lipid matrix where it is located.[1] Vitamin E also seems to be required as a structural component and can provide stability for membranes containing polyunsaturated fatty acids.[2] In addition, vitamin E has been proposed to act as a catalytic or regulatory agent in intermediary metabolism.[3] However, at present no detailed hypothesis exists that provides a comprehensive explanation for the many effects of vitamin E. Since oxidative damage to lipids and proteins will naturally lead to alteration of membrane structure and function, the characterization of such effects may lead to a fuller understanding of the physiological role of vitamin E.

The effect of vitamin E deficiency on tissue oxidation has been the subject of several earlier studies. Excessive rates of respiration from skeletal muscle have been repeatedly demonstrated in nutritional muscular dystrophy produced by deprivation of vitamin E.[4] Although some authors have suggested that the increased oxygen consumption might be due to higher adenosine triphosphatase activity in muscle tissue, they were unable to demonstrate any difference in ATPase activity between muscle and liver homogenates during the early or late stages of vitamin E deficiency.[5] There has been some evidence that vitamin E deficiency uncouples oxidative phosphorylation in muscle homogenates.[6] A recent review of the literature reporting on the enzymatic activities of animals deficient in or supplemented with vitamin E shows different authors claiming contradictory results, thereby adding to the overall state of confusion.[7,8]

We chose to focus our attention on the protective role of vitamin E against membrane damage. Previous work from our laboratory has clearly demonstrated the role of oxidative and photooxidative damage in the mechanisms of inhibition

*This work was supported by a grant from Hoffmann-La Roche, Inc., by the Assistant Secretary for Environment, Office of Health and Environmental Research, Life Sciences Division of the U.S. Department of Energy, under Contract No. W-7405-ENG-48, and by a National Institutes of Health grant GM 24273. K. Davies was recipient of the Chancellor's Patent Fund Award for Research, University of California, Berkeley.

32

of electron transport, and uncoupling of rat liver mitochondria:[9-11] flavin-containing dehydrogenases (e.g., succinate dehydrogenase) were shown to be the most sensitive components of inner mitochondrial membranes to photooxidative damage when incubated at temperatures of 10°C or less. The present study investigates damage to membrane integrity and structure under conditions (temperature of 26°C, with or without illumination, shorter times of incubation) where succinate dehydrogenase is only slightly inactivated. Preparations of liver and muscle mitochondria from control and vitamin E-deficient animals have been used in order to elucidate the differential sensitivity of these membranes to oxidative mechanisms of damage.

METHODS

Animals

Male "Long Evans" rats weighing approximately 100 g each were purchased from Simonsen Laboratories (Gilroy, Calif.).

Diets

Two different diets were purchased from BioServ Inc. (Frenchtown, N.J.). Bio-Mix no. 1331 had less than 1 IU of vitamin E/kg and Bio-Mix no. 1332 had 21 IU of vitamin E (as *all-rac-α*-tocopheryl acetate) per kg. During a period of approximately 100 days, a group of eight rats were fed Bio-Mix no. 1332 and were denoted control animals. Another group of eight rats were fed Bio-Mix no. 1331 and were denoted vitamin E-deficient animals (E−). The severity of vitamin E deficiency in E− rats was assessed by a standard blood hemolysis test.[12] The E− animals exhibited $93\% \pm 3\%$ hemolysis, compared to $10\% \pm 3\%$ hemolysis for controls.

Mitochondrial Preparations

Liver mitochondria were prepared according to established procedures.[13] The isolation medium used was 150 mM mannitol, 75 mM sucrose, 1 mM tris buffer, and 1 mM ethylenediaminetetraacetic acid (EDTA, pH 7.4). For the last centrifugation, the mitochondria were washed in 0.25 M sucrose and finally resuspended in this medium at a concentration of approximately 70 mg protein/ml. Muscle mitochondria were prepared by grinding, trypsin incubation, and homogenization as previously described.[14] They were washed twice in 0.25 M sucrose and resuspended in this medium at a concentration of approximately 35 mg/ml. Protein concentrations were determined by a biuret method.[15]

Illumination Conditions

Incubation of dark and light samples was as previously described.[10] The light source was a battery of 300-W quartz iodide lamps covered by a 400-nm cutoff filter (Corning no. 3389). The net light intensity as measured by an LI-COR LI-185 radiometer was 17 mE/cm^2 per second. For studies of light or dark incubation at

26°C, mitochondrial suspensions (10 ml at 10 mg/ml) were placed in 50-ml Erlenmeyer flasks and slowly shaken in a water bath at 26°C. Dark samples were incubated under the same conditions, but inside flasks covered with aluminum foil.

Absorption spectra of the mitochondrial suspensions at 0.4 mg protein/ml were measured in a dual beam spectrophotometer between 400 nm and 750 nm.

Electron Transport

Rates of oxygen uptake were determined in a Rank oxygen polarograph (Rank Bros., Cambridge, England). Assays were performed at 37°C with 1 mg protein/ml in a medium adapted from that of Dow[16] and consisting of 15 mM KCl, 0.4 mM NAD$^+$ (nicotinamide-adenine dinucleotide) , 45 mM sucrose, 12 mM mannitol, 5 mM MgCl$_2$, 7 mM EDTA, 0.2% bovine serum albumin, 20 mM glucose, 30 mM K$^•$PO$_4$, and 25 mM tris (pH 7.4).[14] Substrates were used at the following concentrations: 20 mM glutamate, 10 mM pyruvate plus 2.5 mM malate, 10 mM succinate plus 4 μM rotenone. State III and IV rates of oxygen consumption and respiratory control ratios (RCR = state III rate of O$_2$ consumption/state IV rate of O$_2$ consumption) were determined according to Chance and Williams,[17] with 0.2 mM adenosine diphosphate (ADP). The uncoupler carbonyl cyanide p-trifluoro-methoxyphenylhydrazone (FCCP) was used at 1 μM. Dicyclohexylcarbodiimide (DCCD, 1 μM) was employed as a blocking agent for the passage of protons across the ATP synthetase complex when measuring the effects of steady-state respiration.

Succinate dehydrogenase activity was measured with phenazine methosulfate as intermediate electron acceptor and dichlorophenolindophenol as final acceptor.[18]

Lipid Peroxidation

Malondialdehyde produced during lipid peroxidation was determined as follows. To 0.2 ml of mitochondrial suspension (equivalent to 2 mg of protein) 0.8 ml of double-distilled water was added, followed by 2 ml of the stock reagent 15% (w/v) trichloroacetic acid; 0.375% (w/v) thiobarbituric acid (TBA), and 0.25 N hydrochloric acid. Lastly, 15 μl of a 2% (w/v) ethanolic solution of butylated hydroxytoluene was added to abolish any metal-catalyzed autooxidation of lipids during heating with the thiobarbituric reagent. The mixture was heated for 15 minutes in a boiling water bath, and after cooling, the flocculent precipitate was removed by centrifugation at 1,000 × g for 10 minutes. The absorbance of the sample was determined at 535 nm against a blank that contained all the reagents minus the mitochondria. The malondialdehyde concentration of each sample was calculated using an extinction coefficient of $1.56 \times 10^5 \cdot M^{-1} \cdot cm^{-1}$.[19]

The detection of lipids containing conjugated dienes was performed as follows. One milliliter of mitochondrial suspension (equivalent to 10 mg protein) was mixed thoroughly with 5.0 ml of chloroform-methanol (2:1), followed by centrifugation at 1,000 × g for five minutes to separate the phases. Of the lower chloroform layer, 3 ml were recovered using a syringe and taken to dryness in a test tube at 45°C under a stream of nitrogen. The lipid residue was dissolved in 1.5 ml of cyclohexane, and the absorbance at 233 nm determined against a cyclohexane blank. The molar extinction coefficient used was $2.52 \times 10^4 \cdot M^{-1} \cdot cm^{-1}$.[19]

Surface Potential

Changes in the electrical surface potential of mitochondria were determined from changes in partitioning between the aqueous and membrane environment of the positively charged paramagnetic amphiphile 4-(decyldimethylammonium)-1-oxyl-2,6,6,6-tetramethyl piperidine bromide (CAT_{10}) and the uncharged spin label 2,2-dimethyl-5,5-methylheptyl-*N*-oxazolidinyloxyl (2N9). Equal volumes of mitochondrial suspensions (10 mg protein/ml) and of a solution of 0.25 M sucrose, 10 mM KPO_4 (pH 7.5), 150 μM CAT_{10} (or 2N9), and 0.5 mM potassium ferricyanide were mixed and allowed to equilibrate for about three minutes. The electron paramagnetic resonance (EPR) spectra of such suspensions were recorded with a Varian E-109E spectrometer.

The partition was defined as the ratio of spin label concentration in the aqueous medium to the concentration on the membrane. These concentrations could be readily determined from the EPR spectra of the spin probes (FIGURE 1).[20,21] Earlier studies have demonstrated that the mitochondrial outer membrane contributes relatively little to the total binding of such spin probes, compared to the inner membrane.[21] Changes in membrane surface potential were estimated as a function of the zero-time partitioning of the probes. The absolute value of the surface potential was not determined, since this would require measurement of the partition of CAT_{10} between the mitochondrial membranes and the aqueous environment at high and zero ionic strength, both of which are technically impossible due to loss of mitochondrial integrity.

Transmembrane Electrical Potentials

Changes in transmembrane potential established by substrate-energized mitochondria were calculated using a tetraphenyl phosphonium electrode.[22] Calculations of transmembrane potentials assumed that tetraphenyl phosphonium distribution between mitochondria and medium followed the Nernst equation and that the mass conservation law applied. Mitochondrial volume was assumed to be 1 μl/mg protein, and final volume was 3 ml. Mitochondrial concentration was 1 mg/ml, tetraphenyl phosphonium concentration of the medium was 5 μM, and tetraphenyl phosphonium concentration in the electrode was 10 μM.

RESULTS

Inactivation of Electron Transport

All mitochondrial samples showed no change in succinate dehydrogenase activity after three hours of incubation in the dark, and even the activity of illuminated samples had decreased by at most 30% (compared to zero-time values), in agreement with earlier results.[10] Significant differences between control and E− samples and between liver and muscle samples could not be ascribed to differences in light absorption, since aerobic suspensions of liver and muscle mitochondria displayed similar absorption spectra. Muscle mitochondrial suspensions absorbed about 10% less light than did liver mitochondria in the whole visible range from 430 to 760 nm. Between 400 and 430 nm, where flavins absorb strongly, both suspensions absorbed comparable amounts of light.

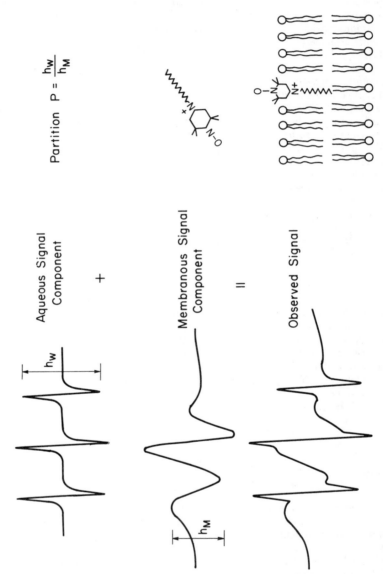

FIGURE 1. Electron paramagnetic resonance spectrum and partition of a CAT probe in the presence of membranes.

Whether differences between liver and muscle mitochondria reflect the *in vivo* state or were caused by isolation procedures was not ascertained.

For the liver mitochondria, in both dark and illuminated samples, state IV rates of respiration remained fairly constant during the first two hours of incubation, decreasing sharply after that. In the case of muscle mitochondria, for both dark and illuminated samples, state IV rates of respiration increased quite substantially during the first hour of incubation, decreasing dramatically thereafter (data not shown). Similar rates of state III respiration were obtained by the

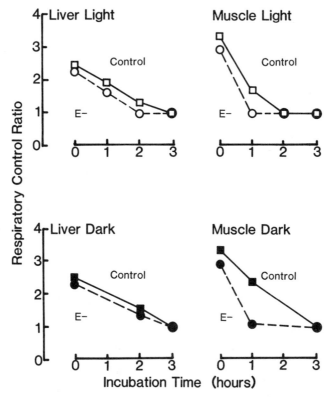

FIGURE 2. Effects of light and dark incubation at 26°C on mitochondrial respiratory control ratios. Standard deviation for respiratory control ratios was ±0.1.

addition of ADP or FCCP. At zero time, state III rates of respiration were similar for control and E− liver mitochondria but were lower in E− muscle mitochondria than in control muscle mitochondria. All samples showed a steady decrease in state III rates of respiration during incubation (data not shown).

Respiratory control ratios during incubation (with or without illumination) were always significantly lower in the E− samples compared to controls, except in the case of liver mitochondria kept in the dark (FIGURE 2).

The levels of malondialdehyde produced during incubation (FIGURE 3) reveal that zero-time levels were always greater in muscle mitochondria than in liver mitochondria (for both control and E− samples). Initial rates of formation and the final concentrations of malondialdehyde present were always larger in illuminated samples. Throughout the incubation, the levels of malondialdehyde were consistently higher in E− samples; furthermore, differences between the concentrations of malondialdehyde found in E− and control samples increased with time of incubation. In general, when malondialdehyde levels increased

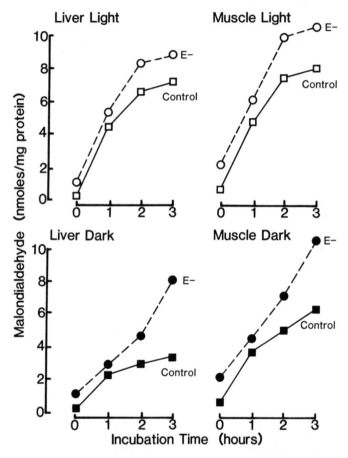

FIGURE 3. Effects of light and dark incubation at 26°C on mitochondrial malondialdehyde concentrations. Standard deviation for malondialdehyde concentrations was ±0.2 nmol/mg.

above about 4–8 nmol/mg protein, mitochondria were uncoupled. The measurement of lipids containing conjugated dienes (TABLE 1) indicated that conjugated diene levels increased with time of incubation and were higher in the E− samples.

When incubated on ice in the dark, only E− muscle mitochondria showed a large decrease in RCR during a three-hour period (FIGURE 4). The decrease in

TABLE 1

MITOCHONDRIAL CONCENTRATIONS OF CONJUGATED DIENES
BEFORE AND AFTER ILLUMINATION AT 26°C

| Mitochondria | | Conjugated Diene Concentration* (nmoles/mg protein) | |
		Zero Time	Two Hours Light
Liver	Control	0.19	0.28
	E Deficient	0.41	0.50
Muscle	Control	0.19	0.56
	E Deficient	0.49	0.99

*Standard deviation for conjugated diene concentration was ±0.05.

RCR could be ascribed almost totally to increases in state IV rates of respiration, indicative of uncoupling. State III rates of respiration did not change significantly during the incubation for either control or E− samples. Attempts were made to alter this pattern of respiratory uncoupling in E− samples by addition of the antioxidant butylated hydroxytoluene (BHT) or the sulfhydryl agent (reduced) glutathione[23] (FIGURE 5). During three hours of incubation, BHT slowed somewhat the rates at which the RCR decreased due to uncoupling of state IV respiration. Both reagents, however, lowered somewhat the levels of malondialdehyde produced.

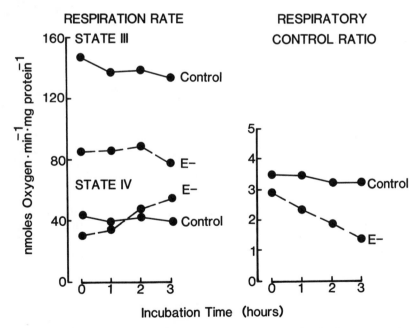

FIGURE 4. Effects of dark incubation at 5°C on muscle mitochondrial state III and IV respiration and respiratory control ratios. Standard deviation for respiration rates was ±5 nmol O_2/mg per minute and for respiratory control ratios was ±0.1.

Uncoupling during Steady-State Respiration

The effect of prolonged steady-state respiration on the coupling of mitochondria was also studied. Mitochondria (1 mg/ml) were incubated in an open Rank oxygen polarograph at 22°C for various lengths of time in the presence of pyruvate plus malate and DCCD. These suspensions were not illuminated. The O_2 concentration in the medium remained approximately 200 μM. At various times during incubation, the oxygen polarograph was capped to enable measurement of basal rates of respiration. Maximal rates of respiration were generated by the addition of FCCP, and the respiratory control index (RCI = uncoupled rate of O_2 consumption/basal rate of O_2 consumption) was calculated. It is clear that the

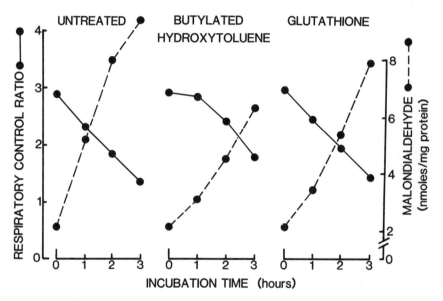

FIGURE 5. Effects of dark incubation at 5°C with antioxidants on muscle mitochondrial respiratory control ratios and malondialdehyde concentrations. Butylated hydroxytoluene was used at 2 μM, and glutathione (reduced) concentration was 1 mM. Standard deviation as in FIGURES 1 and 2.

control samples always exhibited higher RCI than did E− samples (FIGURE 6). Furthermore, after 30 minutes of incubation, the only sample that was almost completely uncoupled (RCI = 1.2) was the E− muscle. All the others still showed an RCI of 2 or higher. Compared to control samples, the E− samples of muscle mitochondria lost their RCI faster than did E− liver mitochondria.

Surface Potentials

Differences in surface potential arising from the outer surface of the inner membrane of muscle and liver mitochondria were observed at zero time and during incubation (with or without illumination) at 26°C (FIGURE 7). Differences in

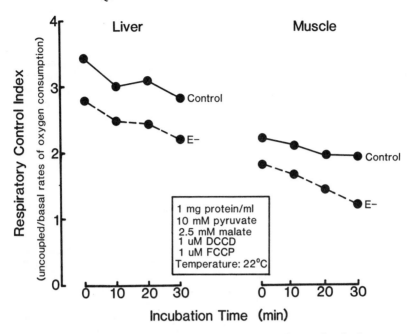

FIGURE 6. Effects of steady-state respiration at 22°C on muscle mitochondrial respiratory control indices. Mitochondria were incubated with pyruvate-malate and DCCD for varying periods. Uncoupled rates were obtained following the addition of FCCP. Standard deviation in respiratory control index was ±0.2.

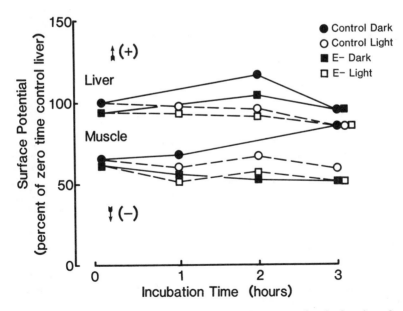

FIGURE 7. Effects of light and dark incubation at 26°C on mitochondrial surface charge density (surface potential). Standard deviation in surface charge density was ±6%.

partitioning of the 2N9 probe between the various samples were negligible, implying that hydrophobic interactions with amphipathic probes were not altered.

Surface potential measurements revealed that the surface potential of muscle mitochondria was always substantially more negative than that of liver mitochondria. We also observed that E− samples exhibited slightly more negative surface potentials than did control samples, both for muscle and liver mitochondria; these differences were, however, not always significant.

Transmembrane Potentials

Changes in transmembrane potential generated during respiration as a function of incubation time (with or without illumination) at 26°C are shown in FIGURE 8. For muscle mitochondria, pyruvate-malate was employed as substrate. In the case of liver mitochondria, transmembrane potentials generated by this substrate were small and succinate was used instead. The results consistently showed that control mitochondria developed a larger transmembrane potential than did E− mitochondria, that muscle mitochondria were more readily inactivated than were liver mitochondria, that when samples were illuminated their capacity to generate transmembrane potentials decreased more rapidly than that of dark samples, and that when E− samples were illuminated loss of transmembrane potential was more rapid than for controls.

DISCUSSION

Vitamin E deficiency has been clinically implicated in muscular and neuromuscular diseases and in the sensitivity of lung, liver, red blood cells, and platelets to damage. Animal models of vitamin E deficiency have proved extremely useful in the study of many of these phenomena.

Muscle versus Liver Mitochondria Susceptibility to Damage

It appears that the effects of vitamin E deficiency in rats include marked increases in mitochondrial sensitivity to damage. This is particularly conspicuous in the case of muscle mitochondria and may well provide a clue as to why vitamin E deficiency causes nutritional muscular dystrophy[24,25] and why, in human clinical studies, it has been implicated in neuromuscular myopathies (see articles by Guggenheim et al. and Muller and Lloyd in this volume). The direct effects of vitamin E on membrane structure have always been hard to assess owing to its low molar ratio in relation to phospholipids (about 1:200 for the inner mitochondrial membrane). The important physiological role of α-tocopherol in protecting inner mitochondrial membranes may arise partially through its antioxidant properties, although its structural stabilizing properties may also be important. Since lipid peroxidation may strongly affect structure and permeability, these two aspects may be closely related.

Surface Potentials

The observation of increased sensitivity of mitochondria with greater negative surface potential to damage—and of small changes in membrane surface charge density accompanying vitamin E deficiency—provides a new and sensitive method with which to investigate further the effect of vitamin E deficiency and surface charge on membrane structure and function.

In accord with previous results from our laboratory,[9-11] the inactivation effects are enhanced by visible light irradiation. These alterations are always more pronounced in the mitochondrial samples with more negative surface potentials (i.e., muscle vs. liver and E– vs. control).

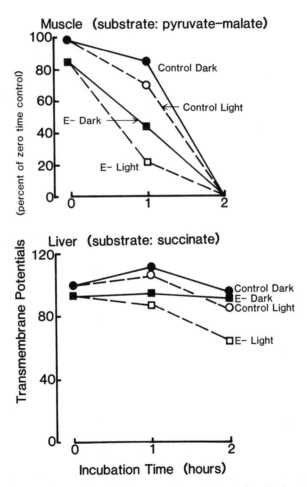

FIGURE 8. Effects of light and dark incubation at 26°C on mitochondrial transmembrane electrical potential. Standard deviation in transmembrane electrical potential was ±5%.

The interrelationship between more negative surface potentials and greater sensitivity to damage may arise from differences in the ionic nature of binding of extrinsic proteins to membranes (see article by Shapiro and Mott in this volume) and from changes in the interaction between intrinsic components in membranes (see article by Sayare et al. in this volume). The effect is particularly clear in the case of muscle vs. liver mitochondria, but is also found for E− mitochondria compared to controls. These differences are maintained during the course of incubation with or without illumination and, although small, are consistent.

Whether lipid peroxidation causes the loss of membrane functional integrity (respiratory control, transmembrane potential) or whether functional losses facilitate lipid peroxidation is not known at present. It is found that, under certain conditions, antioxidants slow down each process.

Temperature Effects

The effect of temperature in the overall inactivation also appears to be important. Earlier experiments performed with liver mitochondria at 10°C showed that the respiratory control ratio was still high after 12 hours of incubation in the dark, and that loss of state III respiration followed succinate dehydrogenase inactivation during illumination.[10] In the present study, we show that when incubated at 26°C, both liver and muscle mitochondria (with or without illumination) lose their respiratory control, and state III rates of respiration decrease by 75% within 3 hours. Since succinate dehydrogenase is only 30% inactivated even in the light, decreased rates of substrate dehydrogenation cannot explain the loss of overall electron transport. It appears possible that decreased state III rates are precipitated by diminished electron transport between respiratory components in the disrupted inner membranes. Clearly, at higher temperatures (26°C), modifications of the electron transport chain and/or the structural integrity of the membrane are more severe than at 10°C. The lack of protective effect of reduced glutathione suggests that sulfhydryl groups are probably not involved in the mechanisms of inactivation. The increased perturbations to membrane integrity at higher temperatures could afford an explanation to some of the damage we observe in muscle following exercise,[26] since it is well known that during physical activity the temperature of muscle tissue increases significantly.[27] Moreover, the decreased levels of latency for cellular enzymes and in respiratory control of mitochondria, and the increased levels of lipid peroxidation and stable tissue radicals, which accompany vitamin E deficiency in rats,[26] may account for the lower exercise-endurance capacity of these animals.

Steady-State Respiration

The effect of steady-state respiration on uncoupling of mitochondria[28] may be related to the well-known superoxide anion generation during state IV respiration.[29] This possibility is especially interesting since E− mitochondria are substantially more sensitive to damage during steady-state respiration than are control mitochondria. Such findings are consistent with an antioxidant role for vitamin E in the mitochondrial membrane. An abstract of some of the studies reported in this work has already appeared.[30]

Summary

Vitamin E deficiency in rats increased the sensitivity of liver and muscle mitochondria to damage during incubation at various temperatures, irradiation with visible light, or steady-state respiration with substrates. In all cases, vitamin E-deficient mitochondria exhibited increased lipid peroxidation, reduced trans-membrane potential, decreased respiratory coupling, and lower rates of electron transport compared to control mitochondria. Muscle mitochondria always showed greater negative inner membrane surface charge density, and were also more sensitive to damage than were liver mitochondria. Vitamin E-deficient mitochondria also showed slightly more negative inner membrane surface charge density compared to controls. The relationship observed between greater negative surface potential and increased sensitivity to damage provides for a new and sensitive method to probe further the role of surface charge in membrane structure and function. Implications of these new findings for the well-known human muscle myopathies and those experimentally induced by vitamin E deficiency in animals are discussed.

Acknowledgment

We thank Dr. E. W. Kellogg III for useful discussions.

References

1. McCay, P. B. & M. M. King. 1980. *In* Vitamin E. L. J. Machlin, Ed.: 289–317. Marcel Dekker, Inc. New York & Basel.
2. Lucy, J. A. 1972. Ann. N.Y. Acad. Sci. **203:** 4–11.
3. Schwartz, K. 1972. Ann. N.Y. Acad. Sci. **203:** 45–52.
4. Hummel, J. P. & D. H. Basinski. 1948. J. Biol. Chem. **172:** 417–422.
5. Jacobs, H. P., S. Rosenblatt, V. M. Wilder & S. Morgulis. 1950. Arch. Biochem. Biophys. **27:** 19–24.
6. Hummel, J. P. 1948. J. Biol. Chem. **172:** 421–426.
7. Corwin, L. M. 1980. *In* Vitamin E. L. J. Machlin, Ed.: 332–347. Marcel Dekker, Inc. New York & Basel.
8. Nelson, J. S. 1980. *In* Vitamin E. L. J. Machlin, Ed.: 397–428. Marcel Dekker, Inc. New York & Basel.
9. Aggarwal, B. B., Y. Avi-Dor, H. A. Tinberg & L. Packer. 1976. Biochem. Biophys. Res. Commun. **69:** 362–368.
10. Aggarwal, B. B., A. T. Quintanilha, R. Cammack & L. Packer. 1978. Biochim. Biophys. Acta **502:** 367–382.
11. Cheng, L. Y. L. & L. Packer. 1979. FEBS Lett. **97:** 124–128.
12. Draper, H. H. & A. S. Csallany. 1970. J. Nutr. **98:** 390–394.
13. Schneider, W. C. & G. H. Hogeboom. 1950. J. Biol. Chem. **183:** 123–128.
14. Davies, K. J. A., L. Packer & G. A. Brooks. Arch. Biochem. Biophys. (In press.)
15. Gornall, A. G., C. J. Bardawill & M. M. David. 1949. J. Biol. Chem. **177:** 751–766.
16. Dow, D. S. 1967. Biochemistry **6:** 2915–2922.
17. Chance, B. & G. R. Williams. 1956. Adv. Enzymol. **17:** 65–134.
18. Singer, T. P. 1974. Methods Biochem. Anal. **22:** 123–175.
19. Buege, J. A. & S. D. Aust. 1978. Methods Enzymol. **52:** 302–310.
20. Castle, J. D. & W. L. Hubbell. 1976. Biochemistry **15:** 4818–4831.
21. Quintanilha, A. T. & L. Packer. 1977. FEBS Lett. **78:** 161–165.

22. KAMO, N., M. MURATSUGA & Y. KOBATAKE. 1979. J. Biol. Chem. **49:** 105–121.
23. CORWIN, L. M. & K. SCHWARTZ. 1963. Arch. Biochem. Biophys. **100:** 385–392.
24. VAN VLEET, J. F., B. V. HALL & J. SIMON. 1968. Am. J. Pathol. **52:** 1967–1971.
25. SWEENEY, P. R., J. C. BUCHANAN-SMITH, F. DE MILLE, J. R. PETTIT & E. T. MORAN. 1972. Am. J. Pathol. **68:** 493–497.
26. DAVIES, K. J. A., A. T. QUINTANILHA, G. A. BROOKS & L. PACKER. (In preparation.)
27. BROOKS, G. A., K. J. HITTELMAN, J. A. FAULKNER & R. E. BYER. 1971. Am. J. Physiol. **221:** 427–431.
28. MCCAY, P. B., P. M. PFEIFER & W. H. STRIPE. 1972. Ann. N.Y. Acad. Sci. **203:** 62–73.
29. CHANCE, B., H. SIES & A. BOVERIS. 1979. Physiol. Rev. **59:** 527–605.
30. QUINTANILHA, A. T., E. W. KELLOGG III & L. PACKER. 1980. Fed. Proc. **39:** 1631.

DISCUSSION

E. R. SIMONS (*Boston University School of Medicine, Boston, Mass.*): I think it's interesting that you find organelle membranes are very sensitive. We've done membrane-potential studies on E-deficient versus normal rats on platelets and on red cells, and find no effect whatsoever.

W. A. PRYOR (*Louisiana State University, Baton Rouge, La.*): Why were the lipid peroxidation products lower in the exercised E-deficient animals?

A. T. QUINTANILHA: We find lower levels of lipid peroxidation in the exercised animals because E-deficient rats cannot run for as long a time as the non-E-deficient animals and are exhausted earlier. So you find the level of TBA-reactive materials to be lower.

W. A. PRYOR: My other question is, What is the free radical whose concentration depends upon exercise and vitamin E level?

L. PACKER: We don't know what the free radicals are.

W. A. PRYOR: What is its G value?

L. PACKER: Well, about two. It may be some sort of ascorbate radical, but we haven't identified it yet.

W. A. PRYOR: But it's not a transition metal, it's an organic radical.

L. PACKER: Yes.

P. B. MCCAY (*Oklahoma Medical Research Foundation, Oklahoma City, Okla.*): Dr. Quintanilha, could you comment on whether you think the cytochrome P_{450} loss may be due to some direct effect of light on the protein or due to lipid peroxidation.

A. T. QUINTANILHA: If you add antioxidants that prevent the formation of TBA reactants, you don't see the destruction of the P_{450}, so we feel that the destruction is probably mediated by lipid peroxidation.

L. PACKER: It's also oxygen dependent, and the inactivation of the P_{450} follows the time course for the increase in lipid peroxidation products.

E. R. SCHWARTZ (*Tufts Medical School, Boston, Mass.*): I'd like to know for how long you exercised the animals and whether you examined the knee joints or the synovial fluid of the animals after conditioning them to a slow pace as compared to sprinting.

L. PACKER: We haven't done any studies on the synovial fluid. With regard to how long we exercised the animal, it depended on whether you mean exercise training or exercise testing.

E. R. SCHWARTZ: The extended duration.

L. PACKER: Endurance-trained animals run for two hours a day for about 10 weeks.

E. R. SCHWARTZ: There might be some pain in your sprinting animals. It would be interesting to look at their joint surfaces and compare them.

L. PACKER: I'd like to make a general statement before we finish. Although we don't know yet precisely how these surface charge changes are related to vitamin E deficiency, it's very clear that surface charge is quite important for the binding of loosely associated proteins with the membrane, and many of these loosely associated proteins with the membrane are extremely important in metabolic activities. I'm not talking now about the intrinsic bioenergetic biological oxidation systems, but all the other metabolic enzymes that are membrane associated. The binding of these enzymes could be altered if you altered surface charge. We think this is an interesting possibility to entertain in terms of understanding the amplification effects of vitamin E on metabolic systems.

KINETICS OF TISSUE α-TOCOPHEROL UPTAKE AND DEPLETION FOLLOWING ADMINISTRATION OF HIGH LEVELS OF VITAMIN E

L. J. Machlin and E. Gabriel

Vitamins and Clinical Nutrition
Hoffmann-La Roche, Inc.
Nutley, New Jersey 07110

A linear relationship has been found between the tocopherol content of tissues and the logarithm of the dose administered when vitamin E is fed to experimental animals.[1-6] This relationship has been demonstrated for plasma,[1,2,4] platelets,[4,5] liver,[1-5] muscle,[1,3,4,6] heart,[1,6] testes,[1,6] spleen,[1] and lung[5] over a wide range of intakes. Some tissues, such as the testes and liver, were much more sensitive to changes in intake than were others, such as the muscle.

Larsson reported that the increase in tocopherol content of muscles of patients with intermittent claudication was proportional to their clinical improvement.[7] Haeger has reported a subjective improvement in such patients after 3–5 months of vitamin E administration and an improvement in arterial blood flow after 12–18 months of treatment.[8] It seems possible that the 12–18 month delay before improvement is observed results from the long time necessary to increase muscle tocopherol after beginning the administration of vitamin E. Bieri studied the effects of the addition of low levels of vitamin E to a diet deficient in vitamin E over a 25-week period in rats,[1] but the effects of higher levels added to an already adequate diet were not investigated. Yang and Desai reported that in rats the α-tocopherol content of the liver and plasma approximately doubled between 8 and 16 months over a wide range of vitamin E intakes,[2] suggesting that α-tocopherol continues to accumulate with time. However, no observations on muscle or other tissues were made. Thus, little information is available on the effects of long-term administration of high levels of vitamin E on tissue concentrations. Whether most tissues continue to accumulate tocopherol with prolonged ingestion of high levels of vitamin E is not known.

MATERIALS AND METHODS

Experiment 1

Mature rhesus monkeys were fed a semipurified diet (casein, sucrose, cellulose, "stripped lard," vitamins and minerals). Groups of four monkeys were fed diets containing either no supplement or 5, 50, or 500 mg/kg of *all-rac-α*-tocopheryl acetate. Plasma vitamin E was determined every 1–2 months for 188 weeks.

Experiment 2

Mature female Sprague Dawley rats were used. Use of mature female animals reduces the influence of tissue growth on tocopherol concentration. At the start of

48

0077–8923/82/0393–0048 $01.75/0 © 1982, NYAS

the experiment and at 1, 2, 4, 8, 14, and 20 weeks of supplementation with 10,000 mg of vitamin E* per kg of laboratory chow,† groups of four animals each were sacrificed and tissues taken for vitamin E analysis. To study the rate of depletion after 8 weeks on the supplemented diets, a group of animals was transferred to the unsupplemented laboratory chow. Then at 1, 2, and 4 weeks after withdrawal of the supplement, four animals were sacrificed for tissue analysis. All animals were sacrificed after an overnight fast, and all tissues were immediately frozen and stored at $-20°C$ until analyzed.

Plasma tocopherol levels were determined by the method of Storer.[9] Heart, muscle, lung, red blood cells, platelets, and brain were analyzed by the procedure of Taylor et al.,[10] while liver and adipose tissue were analyzed by a modification of this procedure as described by Fox and Mueller and Hansen and Warwick, respectively.[11,12]

Experiment 3

The protocol was the same as Experiment 2 except that only 1,000 mg of vitamin E per kg diet were added and groups of six animals each were sacrificed at 0, 1, 4, 9, and 14 weeks after the start of supplementation. After 14 weeks all animals were fed the laboratory chow, and animals were sacrificed for tissue analysis after 1, 2, and 4 weeks on the unsupplemented diet.

Data Summary for Experiments 2 and 3

Generally, there was a linear relationship between time and tissue levels of vitamin E (FIGURES 3, 4, and 5). Accumulation rates were estimated from a line drawn to "best fit" all of the data points. Similarly, depletion rate, calculated as half-life disappearance time, was estimated from a line drawn either through all of the points on the depletion curve or between the starting point and the first point that approximated presupplementation values. Although this calculation method is not completely precise, it still permits certain conclusions based on the large differences observed.

RESULTS

Monkey Studies

When 0 or 5 mg/kg of diet of vitamin E was fed, plasma tocopherol levels decreased to almost negligible values in about 50 weeks (FIGURE 2). With 50 mg/kg, plasma levels remained constant for 3½ years. With 500 mg/kg, there was a relatively rapid increase by 6 weeks, and then a slow but continuous increase for the duration of the experiment. The slope from 6 to 188 weeks was statistically significant.

*Added as all-rac-α-tocopheryl acetate (1 mg is equivalent to 1 IU). All diets were pelleted following addition of supplement.
†Purina Rat Chow, Ralston Purina, St. Louis, Mo. Contained 65 IU/kg vitamin E.

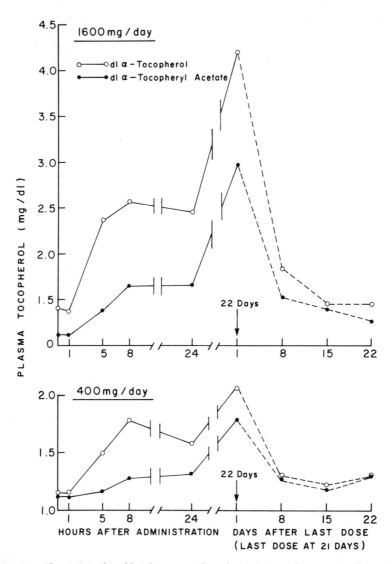

FIGURE 1. Plasma tocopherol levels in man after administration of vitamin E. Three male and three female normal adults were used for each treatment. They were given a single dose of either *all-rac-α*-tocopherol or *all-rac-α*-tocopheryl acetate, and plasma tocopherol was determined at 0, 1, 5, 8, and 24 hours after dosing. The subjects were continued on the same daily intake for 21 more days, and blood tocopherol was again determined at 1, 8, 15, and 22 days after the last intake of supplementary vitamin E. (Based on Baker *et al.*)[9]

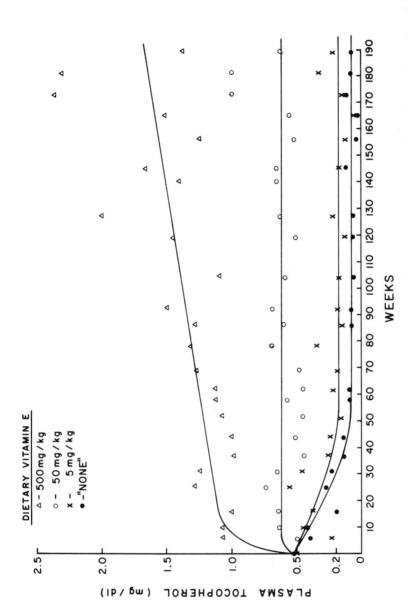

FIGURE 2. Effect of dietary vitamin E on plasma tocopherol levels in the rhesus monkey. Four mature monkeys (three males and one female), which had been fed a commercial diet, were transferred to a semipurified diet at zero time. After administration of ketamine, blood was taken from the cubital vein or femoral artery using EDTA (ethylenediaminetetraacetic acid) as an anticoagulant.

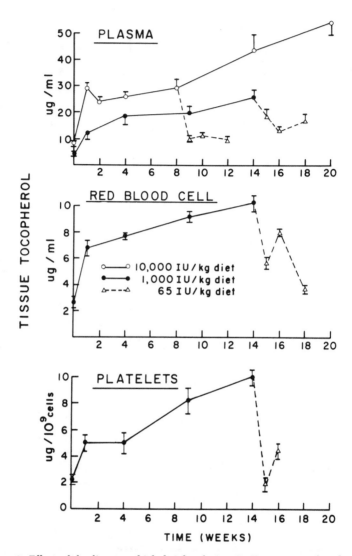

FIGURE 3. Effect of feeding two high levels of vitamin E to mature female rats on tocopherol concentration of plasma, red blood cells, and platelets and its depletion rate following withdrawal of vitamin E supplement from the diet. At the 10,000 mg/kg level (open circles), each point represents the average of four animals; at the 1,000 mg/kg level (filled circles), each point represents the average of six animals. Bar represents standard error.

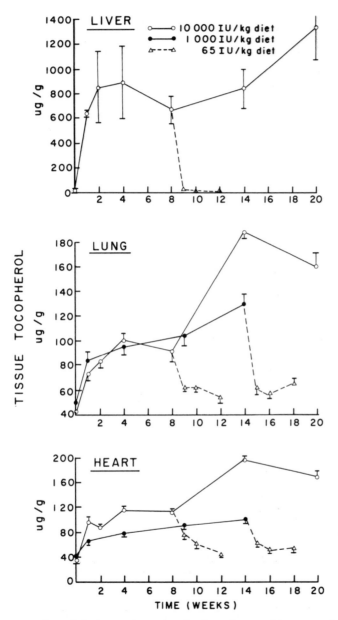

FIGURE 4. Uptake and depletion of tocopherol in liver, lung, and heart. For details, see FIGURE 3.

Rat Studies, Uptake of Tocopherol

One week after the animals were put on the supplemented diet, a rapid increase in the tocopherol level was observed in plasma, red blood cells, platelets, liver, heart, and lung (FIGURES 3 and 4). In contrast, this initial spurt was not as marked in muscle, adipose tissue, or brain (FIGURE 5). Nevertheless, in all tissues there was a progressive increase in tocopherol levels. The tissues of animals on

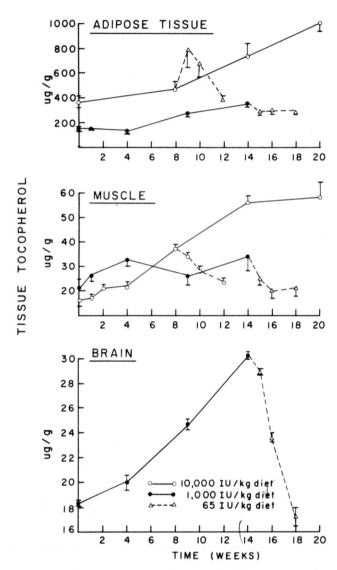

FIGURE 5. Uptake and depletion of tocopherol in adipose tissue, muscle, and brain. For details, see FIGURE 3.

TABLE 1

ACCUMULATION AND DEPLETION RATES OF TOCOPHEROL IN TISSUES

Tissue	Experiment 1 (10,000 mg/kg)		Experiment 2 (1,000 mg/kg)	
	Accumulation Rate (μg/g per day)	Depletion Rate $t_{1/2}$ (days)	Accumulation Rate (μg/g per day)	Depletion Rate $t_{1/2}$ (days)
Plasma	1.8*	1.2	1.0*	3.0
Red Blood Cells	—	—	0.4*	3.0
Platelets	—	—	0.5†	1.4
Liver	41.5	0.8	—	—
Heart	6.8	2.4	3.0	3.1
Lung	7.0	1.3	4.0	1.4
Muscle	2.2	8.2	0.5	6.2
Adipose	32.5	14.8	10.0	14.8
Brain	—	—	0.5	1.4

*μg/ml per day.
†μg/10^9 cells per day.

both levels of vitamin E supplementation showed the same pattern of uptake. Not unexpectedly, the rate of accumulation as well as the maximal levels reached was consistently and considerably higher in the group consuming 10,000 mg/kg of the supplement (FIGURES 3, 4, and 5 and TABLES 1 and 2) than in those fed 1,000 mg/kg. The relative increase in the tocopherol content was higher in liver than in any other tissue (TABLE 2). The accumulation rate of tocopherol was highest in the liver and adipose tissue and lowest in the muscle and brain (TABLE 1).

TABLE 2

RELATIVE SENSITIVITY OF TISSUE TO TOCOPHEROL ADMINISTRATION

Tissue	Tissue Tocopherol Concentration					
	Experiment 1 (10,000 mg/kg)			Experiment 2 (1,000 mg/kg)		
	Minimal*	Maximal*	Ratio of Max/Min	Minimal*	Maximal*	Ratio of Max/Min
Plasma†	8.2	54.0	5.9	4.7	26.4	5.6
Red Blood Cells‡	—	—	—	2.6	10.2	3.9
Platelets§	—	—	—	2.2	10.0	4.5
Liver	22	1,329	60.4	—	—	—
Heart	36	196	5.9	44	101	2.3
Lung	43	189	4.4	50	130	2.6
Muscle	16	58	3.6	21	34	1.6
Adipose	366	1,016	2.8	152	350	2.3
Brain	—	—	—	18	30	1.7

*μg/g.
†μg/ml.
‡μg/ml packed cells.
§μg/10^9 cells.

Rat Studies, Depletion of Tocopherol

With the exception of adipose tissue, the rate of depletion of tocopherol from all tissues was more rapid than the rate of accumulation (FIGURES 3–5). In general, depletion rates were similar in both experiments. The only exception was the plasma level, which decreased more rapidly at the higher level of supplementation (FIGURE 3, TABLE 1).

DISCUSSION

Human Studies

One of the few well-controlled studies with high levels of vitamin E was that of Baker et al. (FIGURE 1).[13] In all four treatments, blood levels peaked at 8 hours after administration and then remained the same or declined slightly by 24 hours. When administration was continued over a 21-day period, plasma levels increased substantially. Blood levels were consistently higher when the free tocopherol was administered rather than tocopheryl acetate. This difference has not been observed when low levels are administered.[14] The higher blood levels attained with tocopherol compared to tocopheryl acetate (FIGURE 1) suggest that hydrolysis of the acetate may be a limiting factor when high levels of the vitamin are administered. This is probably not very important in normal adults, but in subjects with pancreatic insufficiency this difference might be exaggerated. Clinicians may want to consider using free tocopherol for these conditions. The study also demonstrates that there is a considerable increase in plasma levels between 1 and 21 days of administration. Based on these results and those with monkeys (FIGURE 2), it would seem advisable to treat subjects with high levels of the vitamin for at least 1–3 weeks to attain maximal plasma levels.

Rat Studies

Liver and adipose tissue accumulate tocopherol at a much faster rate than do any of the other tissues (TABLES 1 and 2). However, while depletion rate in liver is extremely rapid, that of adipose tissue is extremely slow. This difference in the depletion rate between liver and adipose tissue has been observed previously in rats and guinea pigs.[15,16] In guinea pigs, the rate of release from adipose tissue is so slow that blood levels are not maintained and animals develop a myopathy even though adipose tissue stores are still high.[16] Thus, both studies suggest that liver is the major storage organ for tocopherol and helps maintain plasma levels when the intake of vitamin E becomes inadequate (at least for short time periods).

Because of the extremely slow rate of tocopherol release from adipose tissue, this tissue represents a large, but relatively unavailable, store of the vitamin. Although the vitamin continues to accumulate in adipose tissue with time, its low turnover suggests that analysis of this tissue might provide a useful index of relatively long-term dietary intake of vitamin E. Such an index could be useful in epidemiological studies that attempt to relate vitamin E status to some measure of health. In contrast, liver and plasma levels appear to reflect relatively recent intakes of the vitamin. Fortunately, a reliable procedure for measuring tocopherol by needle biopsy has been developed to study tocopherol kinetics in human adipose tissue.[17]

When 10,000 mg/kg vitamin E was fed (FIGURE 5), the muscle continued to accumulate tocopherol for the duration of the experiment. The trend was the same, but less pronounced, at the lower level of intake. These results suggest that if a significant increase in the tocopherol levels of tissues with slow accumulation rates, such as the muscle and brain, is desired, a prolonged treatment at high levels of intake is necessary. This would be of particular importance in clinical trials with the vitamin. For example, children with severe malabsorption had to be treated with high levels of vitamin E for 3, 6, or 16 months before improvement in neuromuscular symptoms was observed.[18-20] Even if studies are directed at tissues with more rapid accumulation rates, such as the lungs or heart, it would be desirable to continue treatment for at least a few weeks to insure that tissue levels of vitamin E had indeed been elevated.

In the present study tocopherol continued to increase in all tissues examined for the duration of the supplementation. In the study by Yang and Desai, there was a continued increase in both liver and plasma after 8 and 16 months of feeding high levels of vitamin E.[2] These observations suggest that saturation of the tissues with tocopherol is difficult to attain.

Generally, the release of a compound from a tissue is a fixed percentage of its content in the tissue. Therefore, as the tissue content increases, the absolute release rate continues to increase until it is equal to the entry rate, and at that point the tissue concentration remains constant. The observation that tissue concentrations of tocopherol do not plateau suggests that the release rate is limited to an absolute level and is not related to tissue content. The mechanism that controls the release rate must be quite sensitive to small changes in structure, since γ-tocopherol, lacking just one methyl group in the 5 position, is retained much less tenaciously in most tissues than is α-tocopherol.[21,22] Whether release rates are influenced by the presence of specific binding proteins[23-25] in a tissue remains to be determined.

SUMMARY

Following administration of high levels of vitamin E, plasma tocopherol levels in mature humans and monkeys continued to increase with time. In man plasma tocopherol levels were higher when tocopherol rather than tocopheryl acetate was given.

Mature female rats that had been maintained on laboratory chow were put on the diet supplemented with either 1,000 or 10,000 mg/kg of all-rac-α-tocopheryl acetate. All tissues analyzed (plasma, platelets, liver, red blood cells, adipose tissue, heart, lung, skeletal muscle, and brain) continued to increase in tocopherol content for the duration of the supplement (20 weeks). It was concluded that it is difficult to saturate tissue with tocopherol and that not only the level, but the duration, of supplementation with vitamin E influences the concentration of vitamin E in all tissues. Liver and adipose tissue both accumulated tocopherol at a very rapid rate compared to other tissues, but once the chow diet was resumed, liver tocopherol decreased very rapidly and adipose tissue decreased very slowly. The studies suggest that at least for a short time period, the liver is the major available storage organ for tocopherol. When animals were put back on the unsupplemented chow diet, platelet and plasma levels returned to baseline values within 1 week, and red blood cells, heart, muscle, lung, and brain within 4 weeks.

REFERENCES

1. BIERI, J. G. 1972. Kinetics of tissue α-tocopherol depletion and repletion. Ann. N.Y. Acad. Sci. **203**: 181–191.
2. YANG, N. Y. J. & I. D. DESAI. 1977. Effect of high dietary levels of vitamin E on liver and plasma lipids and fat soluble vitamins in rats. J. Nutr. **107**: 1418–1426.
3. MARUSICH, W. L., E. DE RITTER, E. F. OGRINZ, J. KEATING, M. MITROVIC & R. H. BUNNELL. 1975. Effect of supplemental vitamin E in control of rancidity in poultry meat. Poultry Sci. **54**: 831–844.
4. LEHMANN, J. 1979. Relationships among levels of alpha tocopherol in platelets, plasma, and tissues of rats: responses to graded levels of vitamin E. Nutr. Rep. Int. **20**: 685–692.
5. GALLO-TORRES, H. 1980. Transport and metabolism. In Vitamin E, A Comprehensive Treatise. L. J. Machlin, Ed.: 193–267. Marcel Dekker. New York, N.Y.
6. GRIFO, A. P., JR., H. D. EATON, J. E. ROUSSEAU, JR. & L. A. MOORE. 1959. Sensitivity of various tissues of holstein calves to tocopherol intake. J. Anim. Sci. **18**: 232–240.
7. LARSSON, H. & K. HAEGER. 1968. Plasma and muscle tocopherol contents during vitamin E therapy in arterial disease. Pharmacol. Clin. **1**: 72–76.
8. HAEGER, K. 1974. Long-time treatment of intermittent claudication with vitamin E. Am. J. Clin. Nutr. **27**: 1179–1181.
9. STORER, G. B. 1974. Fluorimetric determination of tocopherol in sheep plasma. Biochem. Med. **11**: 71–80.
10. TAYLOR, S. L., M. P. LAMDEN & A. L. TAPPEL. 1976. A sensitive fluorometric method for tissue tocopherol analysis. Lipids **11**: 530–538.
11. FOX, S. H. & A. MUELLER. 1950. The influence of tocopherols on U.S.P. XIV vitamin A assay. J. Am. Pharm. Assoc. Sci. Ed. **39**: 621–623.
12. HANSEN, L. G. & W. J. WARWICK. 1970. A fluorometric micro method for fat tocopherol. Clin. Biochem. **3**: 225–229.
13. BAKER, H., O. FRANK, B. DE ANGELIS & S. FEINGOLD. 1980. Plasma tocopherol in man at various times after ingesting free or acetylated tocopherol. Nutr. Rep. Int. **21**: 531–536.
14. GALLO-TORRES, H. 1980. Absorption. In Vitamin E, A Comprehensive Treatise. L. J. Machlin, Ed.: 170–192. Marcel Dekker. New York, N.Y.
15. GLOOR, U., F. WEBER, J. WURSCH & O. WISS. 1963. Distribution of radioactivity in the rat after administration of ^{14}C dl-α-tocopheryl acetate. Helv. Chim. Acta **46**: 2457–2460.
16. MACHLIN, L. J., J. KEATING, J. NELSON, M. BRIN, R. FILIPSKI & O. N. MILLER. 1979. Availability of adipose tissue tocopherol in the guinea pig. J. Nutr. **109**: 105–109.
17. HATAM, L. & H. J. KAYDEN. Tocopherol levels in needle aspiration biopsies of adipose tissue: normal subjects and abetalipoproteinemic patients. Ann. N.Y. Acad. Sci. (This volume.)
18. UMETSU, D. T., P. COUTURE, H. S. WINTER, B. M. KAGON, M. J. BRESNAN & S. E. LUX. 1980. Degenerative neurological disease in patients with acquired vitamin E deficiency. Pediatr. Res. **14**: 512.
19. GRABERT, B., M. A. GUGGENHEIM, S. RENGEL, P. CHASE & H. E. NEVILLE. 1980. Neuromuscular disease related to chronic vitamin E deficiency. Ann. Neurol. **8**: 217–218.
20. TOMASI, L. G. 1979. Reversibility of human myopathy caused by vitamin E deficiency. Neurology **29**: 1182–1186.
21. GLOOR, J., J. WURSCH, U. SCHWIETER & O. WISS. 1966. Resorption, retention, verteilung und stoffwechsel des dl-α-tocopheramins, d-N-methyl-γ-tocopheramins und des γ-tocopherols in im vergleich zum dl-α-tocopherol bei der Ratte. Helv. Chim. Acta **49**: 2303–2312.
22. PEAKE, I. R. & J. G. BIERI. 1971. Alpha and gamma tocopherol in the rat: in vitro and in vivo tissue uptake and metabolism. J. Nutr. **101**: 1615–1622.
23. CATIGNANI, G. L. 1975. An α-tocopherol binding protein in rat liver cytoplasm. Biochem. Biophys. Res. Commun. **67**: 66–72.

24. KITABCHI, A. E., J. WIMALASENA & J. BARKER. 1980. Specific receptor sites for α-tocopherol in purified isolated adrenocortical cell membrane. Biochem. Biophys. Res. Commun. **96:** 1739–1746.
25. MURPHY, D. J. & R. D. MAVIS. 1981. A comparison of the in vitro binding of α-tocopherol to microsomes of lung, liver, heart and brain of the rat. Biochim. Biophys. Acta **663:** 390–400.

DISCUSSION

M. K. HORWITT (*St. Louis Medical Center, St. Louis, Mo.*): Was the increase in plasma tocopherol levels with time in the monkeys related to the amount of lipid in the plasma?

L. J. MACHLIN: Plasma cholesterol and triglyceride levels were monitored continuously in the monkeys. There was no change with time, so I don't think the lipid levels influenced the results.

J. J. BARBORIAK (*Medical College of Wisconsin, Milwaukee, Wis.*): I was wondering whether at these higher doses of vitamin E, the absorption of vitamin E is somehow affected—or what the excretion part of it is—because not all of it was stored. Also, after giving high levels of vitamin E, does one see the production of deficiency at a faster rate because of an induced higher rate of metabolism?

L. J. MACHLIN: There's very little metabolism of vitamin to excretory metabolites. The Simon's metabolite has been identified as a glucuronate conjugate of tocopheronic acid. This metabolite generally represents less than 1% of the dose administered, even with high levels of intake. So then, since metabolism is minimal, I doubt whether you would see a rebound phenomenon, even after withdrawal of the vitamin. As you increase the intake, the efficiency of absorption goes down and more is excreted in the feces. Once it's absorbed, I don't think there's any significant alteration in metabolism.

L. HOWARD (*Albany Medical College, Albany, N.Y.*): What happens to those adipose tissue stores if you're not only vitamin E depleted but also starved?

L. J. MACHLIN: When we fasted animals for four days, the tocopherol concentration actually went up in the adipose tissue and there was no indication of any increase in the rate of loss upon fasting.

We speculated that tocopherol is primarily in the membrane of the adipocyte and not in the triglyceride part of the cell and that the turnover of membrane tocopherol in this cell is very low.

C. C. REDDY (*Pennsylvania State University, University Park, Pa.*): Regarding vitamin E in liver, do you have any comments on the two proteins that Mavis has recently published? One protein is involved in transfer of vitamin E from cytosol to the microsomes and has a molecular weight of about 34,000. The other one is a cytosolic binding protein with a higher molecular weight. Mavis showed that the binding protein is present in heart, lung, and liver in almost equal amounts, whereas the transfer protein is present only in the liver and absent in the lung and the heart.

L. J. MACHLIN: I would speculate that the importance of the binding proteins would only be apparent with low or nutritional levels of intake, and not when high levels are administered, such as in the present experiments.

P. M. THURLOW (*Duke University Medical Center, Durham, N.C.*): You noted the increased E levels only at the highest dietary intake. What is the relevant actual intake in these animals and which one of the intakes is the most relevant to a real dosage?

L. J. MACHLIN: There were accumulations of vitamin E at both the lower and the higher level of intake. The lower level would be a little more realistic, however. The blood levels with the high level were about 3 mg/dl. These levels are obtained when high levels of vitamin E are given to humans. Therefore, although both were quite high from a dietary standpoint, they may be relevant to humans consuming very high levels.

J. G. BIERI (*National Institutes of Health, Bethesda, Md.*): I think it should be pointed out that 10,000 international units per kilo of diet is 1% of the diet. I'm just wondering if this is really almost a toxic level. Other people have shown in rats and chicks interference with vitamin D or K utilization. With these very high amounts in the liver, did you see fatty liver? Did you look at the liver fat?

L. J. MACHLIN: No we didn't. However, there was no evidence of toxicity in rats fed 1% vitamin E.

UNIDENTIFIED SPEAKER: Are there any known products of vitamin E breakdown that are toxic?

L. J. MACHLIN: The main breakdown product is tocopheryl quinone. Massive amounts of quinone have an anti–vitamin K activity. However, I think these are levels that would never occur even with high level use of the vitamin.

M. P. CARPENTER (*Medical Research Foundation, Oklahoma City, Okla.*): Were there any differences between males and females in the phenomena that you've been seeing? And do you have any data on turnover of tocopherol in adipose tissue?

L. J. MACHLIN: There were no sex differences between blood levels of male and female monkeys. We only used female rats. We have observed a male-female difference in the development of myopathy in an E-deficient rat. We find that the male rats are much more prone to developing muscle degeneration than are the females. If you measure pyruvate kinase as an indicator of dystrophy, the enzyme levels in the male may be five times those of the female.

We have not carried out any turnover studies with the adipose tissue.

M. P. CARPENTER: What is the biological significance of the observation on adipose tissue?

L. J. MACHLIN: Guinea pigs became overtly deficient as manifested by muscle dystrophy even though adipose stores were not depleted. Clearly the rate of release from adipose tissue in this species was insufficient to prevent a vitamin E deficiency. We don't know, of course, whether that's true in humans.

EFFICACY OF VITAMIN E TO PREVENT NITROSAMINE FORMATION

William J. Mergens

Hoffmann-La Roche, Inc.
Roche Chemical Division
Research and Development
Product Development and Applications
Nutley, New Jersey 07110

INTRODUCTION

In the early 1920s, vitamin E was described as a substance important for reproduction in rats,[1] and since then, many studies have detailed the beneficial effects of vitamin E which basically entail its role in the maintenance of the reproductive, central nervous, musculoskeletal, and vascular systems. Numerous reviews dealing with vitamin E deficiencies in man have been written.[2-13] Generally, the function of vitamin E falls into one of two different metabolic roles—first, as a fat-soluble antioxidant; and second, in one or more specific roles related to the metabolism of selenium and sulfur amino acids. The term "vitamin E" has been loosely described as that group of toco and tocotrienol derivatives possessing varying degrees of vitamin activity. The most active of these, α-tocopherol, is the main subject of this presentation, which involves its usefulness in preventing nitrosamine formation. In this role, vitamin E most appropriately falls into the category of fat-soluble antioxidant.

Antioxidants play an important role in the diet as well as *in vivo* toward preventing undesirable and potentially dangerous reactions from being initiated. In fact, in recent years much emphasis on the role of the chemical and biological environment in carcinogenesis has emerged with the suggestion that the majority of all human cancers may be environmentally related. Further weight has been added to this idea with the identification of many carcinogenic substances, such as polynuclear aromatic hydrocarbons, nitrosamines, aflatoxins, etc., in the human environment. Many of these have been found to be present in the diet. One major class of compounds that has been of concern are the nitrosamines. For the most part, they are highly potent animal carcinogens and generally considered potential human carcinogens.

Before discussing the mechanism by which vitamin E is capable of preventing nitrosamine formation, it is important to review some aspects of how nitrosamines themselves are formed.

FORMATION

Basically three things are needed to form a nitroso compound—an amine or amide substrate, a nitrosating agent, and the proper chemical environment. Essentially, it has been demonstrated that all amines—primary, secondary, or tertiary—along with secondary amides are capable of undergoing a nitrosation reaction to yield either a nitrosamine in the case of primary, secondary, or tertiary amines or a nitrosamide in the case of a secondary amide. The reaction of a nitrosating agent with amines is actually a classic, qualitative test. This test was

61

0077-8923/82/0393-0061 $01.75/0 © 1982, NYAS

used to differentiate between primary, secondary, and tertiary amines. The reaction of a nitrosating agent with a primary amine normally leads to deamination products, principally the corresponding alcohol or diene products of the parent amine. However, under certain conditions of catalysis, primary amines can be converted to secondary amines and subsequently nitrosated to form a nitrosamine. Correspondingly, tertiary amines, under the proper conditions, can be dealkylated to form a secondary amine which then can go on to be nitrosated. Generally speaking, secondary amines are the most reactive in their ability to form a nitrosamine. This latter reaction is principally dependent upon the pH of the nitrosating media as well as the pKa of the amine. Firstly, the generation of a nitrosating agent is pH dependent. This equilibrium reaction is in two steps, the first of which is the protonation of nitrite ion to form nitrous acid. Nitrous acid then exists in equilibrium with its anhydrous form, dinitrogen trioxide, which is the actual nitrosating agent (FIGURE 1). This reaction, then, is favored by acidic

$$NO_2^- + H^+ \rightleftharpoons HONO$$

$$2\ HONO \rightleftharpoons N_2O_3 + H_2O$$

$$R_2NH + H^+ \longrightarrow R_2NH_2^+$$

$$\left[R_2NH\right] / \left[R_2NH_2^+\right]$$

FIGURE 1. Some key equilibria for conversion of nitrite to a nitrosating agent. Influence of amine basicity.

conditions. The more reactive form of the amine, on the other hand, is the unprotonated, or free base, form of the amine. Hence, for any given aqueous system the reactivity of an amine, or for that matter an amide, will be dependent upon the pKa of the basic nitrogen. An amine that has a pKa of 4, for example, would be much more susceptible to form a nitrosamine in an aqueous acidic solution than an amine having pKa of 8 or 9. A typical example would be aminopyrine (pKa 5.1), which is much more reactive in this system than dimethylamine (pKa 10.7).

Another condition under which nitrosamines can form is in an alkaline solution. In this environment, chemical reactivity to form a nitrosamine is somewhat different from what we have just discussed. In an alkaline solution, one obviously has the more reactive form of the base present in solution. However, the equilibrium reaction describing the generation of the nitrosating agent from nitrite is by no means favorable. There does exist a situation, however, in which nitrosation reactions rapidly occur, which was described several years ago by Challis et al.[14] This occurs when the nitrosating agent is present as nitrogen dioxide gas or any of its equilibrium counterparts, e.g., N_2O_4, N_2O_3. Conditions that exist in the lung could be very close to that described by Challis, and in vivo nitrosation could be expected to occur at physiological pH's when the lungs are exposed to polluted air. It is not unusual on a high pollution day for the nitrogen oxide (NO_x) content of the atmosphere to rise to near 1–2 parts per million (ppm).

Finally, one last condition under which nitrosamine formation can take place is in the lipophilic phase. The probability of a reaction to occur between an amine and a nitrosating agent is very high since only the more reactive form of the amine (free base) would be soluble in this medium and the pH dependence of the reaction has been eliminated. Most recently, Pryor and Lightsey reported on the enhancing effect that unsaturated fatty acids have on the nitrosation of dicyclo-hexylamine in a lipid medium upon exposure of the system to low level (60 ppm) NO_2.[15]

FIGURE 2 is a summary of much of what we have discussed up to this point. The ordinate is simply the oxidation state of the nitrogen atom in the compound represented, and the abscissa is a schematic of the three different phases in which nitrosation reactions can occur, that is, in aqueous solution, gaseous state, and lipophilic solvents. The shaded area covers those forms of nitrogen oxides that are capable of nitrosating an amine or amide. The main points of this figure are as follows: (a) nitrosation reactions can occur in many different media; and (b) the existence of an equilibrium between these different phases allows the nitrosating agent to migrate as a function of driving force on the given system. The impact of nitrogen oxides in the gas state on aqueous reactions in the lung would be a typical example of the latter. FIGURE 2 also demonstrates the principle by which vitamin E and vitamin C have been employed as nitrosamine blocking agents. The major function of these two vitamins, which in the present sense are really acting as antioxidant compounds, is to reduce a nitrosating agent to a nonnitrosating compound and ultimately inhibit the nitrosation reaction. This inhibition occurs because vitamins E and C can compete effectively with susceptible amines or amides for the nitrosating agent. The major difference between vitamins E and C in the prevention of nitrosamine formation is simply the fact that vitamin E (α-tocopherol) is soluble in the lipid phase and vitamin C (ascorbic acid) serves the same function in the aqueous phase. In principle, then, the mechanism by which vitamin E, and vitamin C for that matter, can prevent nitrosamine formation is one of kinetic competition with the amine for the nitrosating agent.

The reaction product of vitamin C with a nitrosating agent leads to the formation of dehydroascorbic acid, a reaction studied extensively by Dahn et al.[16] Vitamin E, in a very similar fashion, yields α-tocopheryl quinone as the reaction product, which also is the first step in the normal metabolism of α-tocopherol. It should be mentioned that the term "vitamin E" is a description that includes several different chemical moieties, including RRR-α-tocopherol, all-rac-α-tocopherol, and their acetic and succinic esters. Only the unesterified form of vitamin E is effective in inhibiting nitrosation reactions because the oxidation occurs at the free hydroxyl group. All of the studies discussed here have used all-rac-α-tocopherol as the source of vitamin E.

SOURCES OF NITROSATING AGENTS

Many different species are capable of forming a nitrosating agent, for example, nitrite salts, such as sodium nitrite, which are added to meat for color

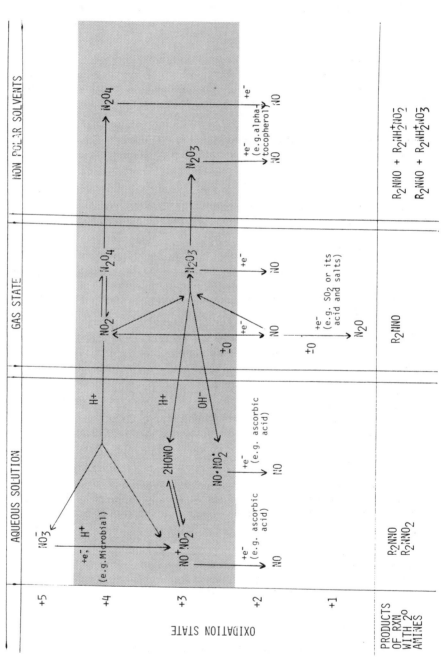

FIGURE 2. Some possible dismutations and transformations of the oxides of nitrogen. Shaded area designates oxidation states of nitrogen capable of nitrosating an amine.

and flavor development as well as control of *Clostridium botulinum*. Nitrate salts present or added in food processing, when coupled with microbiological activity, are readily reduced to nitrite. Fermentation processes, such as pickling or brewing, generally permit microbial conversion of a variety of nitrogen sources, including ammonia and amino acids, to nitrite.

Nitrogen oxides (NO_x), whether derived from "smoking" processes, atmospheric pollution, or direct flame combustion for heating or drying systems, represent a significant source of highly reactive nitrosating agents. The gaseous forms, N_2O_3 and NO_2, are particularly rapid and vigorous in their chemical attack of substrates, even when in alkaline aqueous solution, and extremely rapid when the gases react with substrates in lipid phase.

Transnitrosation also may occur when a nitro or nitroso group in one substance comes into chemical contact under suitable conditions with a substrate that can form a stable nitrosamine. Originally found to be an important source in cosmetics (from Bronopol used as a preservative), transnitrosating agents are getting more attention in mixed and complex chemical systems such as foods.

RELATIONSHIP TO FOOD

One system in which vitamin E has been shown to be effective in preventing nitrosamine formation is the consumer product bacon. Sodium nitrite addition to meat for preservation, particularly against formation of toxin by growth of *Clostridium botulinum*, has been utilized for thousands of years, originating independently in several separate cultures. Of course, originally nitrite was produced from nitrate through microbial reduction in the meat, and nitrate was a contaminant of the sodium chloride. It was not until early in this century that the active meat-preserving component was identified as nitrite and meat producers started adding it directly to cured products. Nitrite also can react with amines in the meat (pyrrolidine, dimethylamine, etc.) to produce carcinogenic nitrosamines. In comminuted meat products, such as frankfurters or similar sausages, it has been shown that sodium ascorbate can prevent nitrosamine formation. A minimum of two moles ascorbate per mole of nitrite is needed. This ascorbate ratio will not interfere with the other desirable functions of nitrite in meat processing, including color formation (nitrosomyoglobin) or antibotulinal control (Perigo effect). In the United States, the trend in such comminuted meat products is to use 120 ppm input of sodium nitrite and 550 ppm of sodium ascorbate.

Bacon, as produced in the United States and prepared for eating by frying, reaches temperatures of about 170°C (for at least a few minutes). This presents a unique problem since the water content is vaporized readily, leaving the residual nitrite in the bacon, which can readily generate the lipid-soluble N_2O_3 nitrosating agent. The amine substrate, presumably proline or pyrrolidine, is present in the collagen fibers buried deep in the thick adipose layer of pork belly used for bacon production. Thus, the nitrosation reaction in bacon takes place primarily in the *fat phase* during the later, high-temperature stages of frying. A lipophilic nitrosamine blocking agent, suitable and safe for foods, was needed to lower the nitrosopyrrolidine (NPYR) content of fried bacon. This, of course, is the basis for much of our work on the use of vitamin E in bacon. FIGURE 3 summarizes several studies that have been performed on bacon in which 500 ppm α-tocopherol has been used to substantially reduce nitrosamine formation in the fried product. NPYR levels were consistently reduced to below 5 ppb (parts per billion).

NITROSATION *IN VIVO*

High dietary intakes of nitrates have been associated with a high rate of gastric cancer in certain sections of the world.[17] This high dietary intake of nitrate can stem from high-nitrate drinking water (Worksop in England and mountainous areas of Colombia, South America)[18,17] and prolonged intakes of high-nitrate vegetables. The pattern appears to involve the microbial reduction of nitrate to nitrite during nonrefrigerated food storage or in the saliva, which ultimately yields a high nitrosation capacity upon ingestion and subsequent acidification in the stomach. Studies are presently under way to attempt reduction of gastric cancer in Colombia by the administration of ascorbic acid and/or α-tocopherol with each meal. The dramatic drop in gastric cancer incidence in the United States over the last few decades has been attributed to the mass use of refrigeration. Before this, food, such as meat, was often stored at ambient or mildly cool

NPYR (PPB) EDIBLE PORTION

COLLABORATOR (PARTICIPANTS)	TYPE	CONTROL(S)	TREATED	DAYS TO FRYING	AVG. TOC. (PPM)
USDA (1)	PILOT	13	5	4	270 (B)
AMI (1)	PILOT	2-8	<1	3	36 (B)
AMI (8)	8-PLANT	4.5 $\pm$ 4.8	1.3 $\pm$ 2.9	14	369 (B)
AMI (5)	PILOT	12.5	4.3	3	268 (S)
		8.0	3.3	14	268 (S)

(B) = BRINE ADDITION

(S) = SPRAY ADDITION

FIGURE 3. Effect of vitamin E on nitrosopyrroline formation in bacon.

temperatures ("ice box") for two to three days. Under these conditions, nitrite rapidly accumulates due to bacterial reduction of nitrate, often accompanied by noticeable flavor changes.

Pickling of vegetables, as a food-preservation method, has been implicated as a cause of the high incidence of esophageal and nasopharyngeal cancer in certain provinces of China.[19] The pickled vegetables appear to have mutagenic substances derived from nitrosation, and at least one N-nitroso compound has been identified.[20]

Kamm *et al.* have studied the *in vivo* inhibition of nitrosamine formation using the rat as a model.[21,22] The simultaneous feeding of aminopyrine and sodium nitrite to the animal leads to the formation of dimethylnitrosamine (DMN) in the acidic environment of the animal stomach. DMN is a liver toxicant, and its formation in the stomach produces an elevation in serum glutamic pyruvic transaminase (SGPT) liver enzyme levels. Using this model, Kamm demonstrated that vitamin E (administered as a water-dispersible form of *all-rac-α*-tocopherol) and, in a separate experiment, vitamin C can completely inhibit the elevation of SGPT when fed at slightly greater than 1 mole/mole of sodium nitrite. He also demonstrated that α-tocopheryl quinone, the oxidation product of *all-rac-α*-tocopherol, was ineffective in the same regimen.

Most recently, the results of a very interesting study on *in vivo* nitrosation have been published by Ohshima and Bartsch.[23] Nitrosoproline had been reported to be noncarcinogenic and nonmutagenic,[24,25] presumably because it is not metabolized *in vivo*. Using the amino acid proline and nitrate (from beet root juice) as the model amine and potential nitrosating agent, respectively, Ohshima and Bartsch have demonstrated several important principles with regard to endogenous nitrosation in man. Firstly, nitrate *is* converted to a nitrosating agent, presumably through the reduction of nitrate to nitrite in the mouth. Secondly, proline is subsequently nitrosated under the acid conditions of the stomach to nitrosoproline. A total of approximately 15 μg nitrosoproline was excreted in the urine over a 24-hour period from an initial dose of 375 mg nitrate and 250 mg proline. The simultaneous ingestion of either 1 g ascorbic acid or 500 mg α-tocopherol inhibited this *in vivo* nitrosation 100% and 50%, respectively. Ascorbic acid totally inhibited while α-tocopherol only partially inhibited the *in vivo* nitrosation of proline. To a first approximation, the molar ratio of blocking agent to potential nitrosating agent was lower for the α-tocopherol experiment than for the ascorbic acid (0.2 to 1). More important, however, and in concert with the main point of this paper, the differences probably lie in the fact that proline is a water-soluble amine and the nitrosation reaction, in this case, is taking place in the aqueous phase. Here, one would expect that ascorbic acid would be the most effective blocking agent to employ. Hence, with respect to the choice of α-tocopherol as a blocking agent to prevent nitrosamine formation, it is not sufficient to know that it is a compound that can effectively react with a nitrosating agent, but one must also consider the environment in which nitrosation occurs.

CONCLUSION

This report has covered a number of points dealing with nitrosamine formation and the principles of inhibition using vitamins E and C. It is an active research sphere, which hopefully will yield an important scientific understanding about the formation of and man's exposure to these and other carcinogens and the possible prevention of environmentally induced cancers.

Much of what has been presented deals with the role of vitamins E and C in preventing nitrosamine formation in foods and *in vivo*. In both systems, vitamin C serves as the water-soluble blocking agent and vitamin E as the lipid or fat-soluble blocking agent. The significance of these roles appears to be twofold. First, it strengthens the importance of the presence of vitamins in the food we eat, not only because of the body's biological need for vitamins, but also because of the influence these two vitamins exhibit in preventing unwanted deterioration of the food we eat prior to ingestion. The second point relates to the *complementary* role these two vitamins exhibit in protecting our food and gastrointestinal environment. Obviously, the question that is being asked is, What is the total role these two vitamins play in the maintenance of good health? From a dietary point of view, then, it is important that the proper level and balance of these two vitamins be defined in preventing not only nitrosamine formation but other undesirable reactions as well. The need for continued study is obvious.

ACKNOWLEDGMENTS

The author wishes to thank Ms. Carol Piascik for her assistance in the preparation of this manuscript.

REFERENCES

1. EVANS, H. M. & K. S. BISHOP. 1922. On the existence of a hitherto unrecognized dietary factor essential for reproduction. Science **56:** 650–651.
2. 1960. "Therapy" with vitamin E. Nutr. Rev. **18:** 227–229.
3. 1974. Supplementation of human diets with vitamin E. Nutr. Rev. Suppl. **32:** 35–38.
4. HORWITT, M. K. 1961. Vitamin E in human nutrition. Borden's Rev. Nutr. Res. **22:** 1–2.
5. HELLSTROM, J. G. 1961. Vitamin E—a review. Med. Serv. J. **17:** 238.
6. HAUBOLD, D. H. & E. HEUER. 1962. On the therapeutic possibilities of vitamin E. Die Kapsel **11:** 37.
7. HERTING, D. C. 1966. Perspective on vitamin E. Am. J. Clin. Nutr. **19:** 210.
8. GERLOCZY, F. 1968. Vitamin E deficiency in men and its mechanism. Orv. Hetil. **109:** 897.
9. DRAPER, H. H. 1969. Vitamin E in human nutrition. In Symposium on the Biochemistry, Assay and Nutritional Value of Vitamin E: 69. Association of Vitamin Chemists. Chicago, Ill.
10. LOSOWSKY, M. S. & J. KELLEHER. 1970. Vitamin E research on man in the United Kingdom. Int. Z. Vitaminforsch. **4:** 107.
11. SHUTE, E. V. 1972. Proposed study of vitamin E therapy. Can. Med. Assoc. J. **106:** 1057.
12. GOODHART, R. S. & M. E. SHILS, Eds. 1973. Modern Nutrition in Health and Disease: Dietotherapy: 1694–1699. Lea & Febiger. Philadelphia, Pa.
13. BIERI, J. G. 1975. Vitamin E. Nutr. Rev. **33:** 161–167.
14. CHALLIS, B. C., A. EDWARDS, R. R. HUNMA, S. A. KRYPTOPOLOUS & J. R. OUTRAM. 1978. Rapid formation of N-nitrosamines from nitrogen oxides under neutral and alkaline conditions. In Environmental Aspects of N-Nitroso Compounds. E. A. Walker, M. Castegnaro, L. Griciute & R. E. Lyle, Eds.: 127–142. International Agency for Research on Cancer. Lyon, France.
15. PRYOR, W. A. & J. W. LIGHTSEY. 1981. Mechanisms of nitrogen dioxide reactions: inhibition of lipid peroxidation and the production of nitrous acid. Science **214:** 435–437.
16. DAHN, H., L. LOEWE & C. A. BUNTON. 1960. Uber die Oxydation von Ascorbinsauer durch salpetrige Saure Tiel VI: Ubersicht und Diskussion der Ergebnisse. Helv. Chim. Acta **43:** 320–323.
17. CUELLO, C., P. CORREA, W. HAENSZEL, G. GORDILLO, C. BROWN, M. ARCHER & S. TANNENBAUM. 1976. Gastric cancer in Colombia. I. Cancer risk and suspect environmental agents. J. Nat. Cancer Inst. **57**(5): 1015–1020.
18. HILL, M. J., G. M. HAWKSWORTH & G. TATTENSALL. 1973. Bacteria, nitrosamines and cancer of the stomach. Br. J. Cancer **28:** 562–567.
19. WEINSTEIN, I. B. 1978. Chemical and viral carcinogenesis. In Cancer in China. H. S. Kaplan & P. J. Tsuchitani, Eds.: 58–73. Alan R. Liss, Inc. New York, N.Y.
20. WEINSTEIN, I. B. 1979. Private communication.
21. KAMM, J. J., T. DASHMAN, A. H. CONNEY & J. J. BURNS. 1973. Protective effect of ascorbic acid on hepatotoxicity caused by nitrite plus aminopyrine. Proc. Nat. Acad. Sci. USA **70:** 747–749.

22. KAMM, J. J., T. DASHMAN, H. NEWMARK & W. J. MERGENS. 1977. Inhibition of amine-nitrite hepatotoxicity by alpha-tocopherol. Toxicol. Appl. Pharmacol. **41:** 575–583.
23. OHSHIMA, H. & H. BARTSCH. 1981. Quantitative estimation of endogenous nitrosation in humans by monitoring N-nitrosoproline excreted in the urine. Cancer Res. **41:** 3658–3662.
24. 1978. IARC Monogr. on the Evaluation of Carcinogenic Risk of Chemicals to Humans **17:** 303–311.
25. MIRVISH, S. S., O. BULAY, R. G. RUNGE & K. PATIL. 1980. Study on the carcinogenicity of large doses of dimethylnitramine, N-nitroso-L-proline, and sodium nitrite administered to drinking water to rats. J. Nat. Cancer Inst. **64:** 1435–1442.

DISCUSSION

V. SRINIVASAN (*National Naval Medical Center, Bethesda, Md.*): You mention an aqueous phase and a lipid phase. Could you elaborate on that a little?

W. J. MERGENS: Tocopherol is usually found in solution in the lipid phase, depending upon the polarity of that lipid and depending upon the presence or absence of emulsifiers in the system. For example, during fat digestion, the tocopherol finds itself within a micelle, either dissolved inside of it or near the polar surface portion of the particle. Depending on whether the hydroxy group of tocopherol is on the surface of the micelle, one could find differences in its ability to interact with a nitrositic agent.

Now when we investigated this particular system, we were using tocopherol and we incorporated tocopherol into the fat phase of that system, which was cetyl alcohol and stearic acid. Cetyl alcohol is relatively polar when one considers the polarity of tocopherol. We found that in that particular system, tocopherol was not sitting at the interface of the micelle but was actually dissolved in this system. If the nitrosating agent was in the aqueous phase and tocopherol solely in the lipid phase, tocopherol would have no effect, because any reactivity would be going on strictly in the aqueous phase and there would be no opportunity for it to even approach a blocking agent.

P. MARFEY (*State University of New York, Albany, N.Y.*): If we were to have a protein terminating with proline, in which case the nitrogen is unprotected, would such prolines be nitrosated and lead to certain pathological consequences?

W. J. MERGENS: You are certainly way ahead of some of the research that's been going on. One of the difficulties in this area is in measuring nitrosation on large molecules. I think that is an excellent thought, because that's where the activity is *in vivo*.

P. MARFEY: Conceivably this would apply to hydroxyproline as well. So proline and hydroxyproline could be considered as potential targets I think.

W. J. MERGENS: Yes.

CLINICAL CONSEQUENCES OF LOW SELENIUM INTAKE AND ITS RELATIONSHIP TO VITAMIN E

O. A. Levander

Beltsville Human Nutrition Research Center
U.S. Department of Agriculture
Science and Education
Beltsville, Maryland 20705

In 1957, Schwarz and Foltz discovered that traces of dietary selenium prevented necrotic liver degeneration in vitamin E-deficient rats.[1] In the late 50s and early 60s, beneficial effects of selenium were observed in several vitamin E-responsive animal diseases of practical agricultural importance, such as white muscle disease in lambs and calves, exudative diathesis in chicks and turkey poults, and hepatosis dietetica in young pigs.[2] In 1969, the essentiality of selenium in its own right was demonstrated because it protected against pancreatic atrophy in vitamin E-supplemented chicks,[3] and improved growth and hair coat in rats fed vitamin E-adequate but selenium-deficient diets over two generations.[4] In 1973, selenium was identified at the active site of glutathione peroxidase,[5] an enzyme that destroys lipid peroxides. That association provided a biochemical rationale for the long-known metabolic relationship between selenium and the fat-soluble antioxidant vitamin E.[6] In 1979, two reports suggested that selenium administration might benefit people with low selenium status.[7,8] In 1980, the Food and Nutrition Board of the National Research Council proposed a safe and adequate range (50 to 200 μg/day) of selenium intake for adults.[9] Others have advocated greater intakes of selenium as a defense against various human diseases such as cancer or cardiovascular disease.[10] We are challenged in the 80s to clarify the true role of selenium in human nutrition and determine the actual relationship of selenium status to human health and disease.

HUMAN SELENIUM INTAKES

The amount of selenium in the food chain depends in large part on the amount of selenium in the soil that is available for uptake by plants.[11] Because plants do not require selenium, plant materials may have a very low selenium content if the level or availability of soil selenium is low. On the other hand, plants will take up large amounts of selenium if the soil selenium content is high and available. For example, levels of selenium ranging from 0.04 to 21.4 μg/g have been found in various wheat samples.[12] Such variation in the selenium content of staple foods leads to great differences in the dietary intake of selenium and in blood selenium levels (TABLE 1). It is difficult to think of another nutrient for which such extremes in dietary intake and blood level have been observed. Those extremes suggest the occurrence of natural deficiencies or excesses of selenium in certain human populations around the world.

0077-8923/82/0393-0070 $01.75/0 © 1982, NYAS

TABLE 1

DIETARY SELENIUM INTAKES AND BLOOD SELENIUM LEVELS AROUND THE WORLD

Country	Dietary Selenium Intake (μg/day)	Blood Selenium Level (ng/ml)
China		
(Keshan disease area)	11	8
New Zealand	28	60–83
Finland	30	56–81
United States	62–216	157–265
Venezuela (Caracas)	218	355
China		
(endemic selenosis area)	4,990	3,180

HUMAN SELENIUM REQUIREMENTS

When the Food and Nutrition Board established its estimated safe and adequate daily dietary intake of selenium,[9] there were few data from human studies to guide such a recommendation. Instead, the board relied upon extrapolation from nutritional experiments with animals. Such an approach in 1976 yielded an estimated human requirement for adults of about 60 μg per day,[13] in good agreement with the board's later adult recommendation of 50 to 200 μg per day with appropriate adjustments for younger age groups (TABLE 2). The range reflects the uncertainty about the human requirement and also allows for any possible benefits from slightly elevated intakes of selenium.[14] Establishment of an upper limit warned consumers about the possible deleterious effects of nutritional abuse ("megadosing") of commercially available selenium supplements.

In order to determine more precisely human selenium requirements, a well-controlled balance trial ("depletion/repletion" study) was carried out in healthy young North American males.[15] After the subjects adjusted to the depletion diet for 12 days, fecal and urinary losses totaled 54 μg/day and selenium balance was quite constant at -21 μg/day. Assuming a selenium absorption of 80% (see below), those men would need a daily selenium intake of about 70 μg to replace excretory losses and maintain body stores. That experimentally derived figure agrees well with that calculated in 1976 and also falls within the safe and adequate range of the Food and Nutrition Board.

TABLE 2

ESTIMATED SAFE AND ADEQUATE DAILY DIETARY INTAKE OF SELENIUM*

	Age (years)	Selenium Intake (μg/day)
Infants	0–0.5	10–40
	0.5–1	20–60
Children	1–3	20–80
	4–6	30–120
	7–11+	50–200
Adults		50–200

*Adapted from Reference 9.

On the other hand, workers in New Zealand estimated that only about 20 μg/day were needed to maintain balance in young women in that country.[16] This lower requirement is probably due to the lower total body pool of selenium in New Zealanders vs. that in North Americans. The New Zealand scientists found no health problems in their population ascribable to habitual consumption of 28–32 μg of selenium/day.[17] No Keshan disease occurred in those areas of China where the dietary selenium intake exceeded 30 μg/day.[18]

When the safe and adequate range was set, little was said about the relative biological availability to humans of selenium in different foods, since such data had not yet appeared. New Zealand women consuming diets furnishing 24 μg of selenium per day absorbed about 80% of their total food selenium intake.[16] But in the case of selenium, absorption does not necessarily mean nutritional availability since several different chemical forms exist in foods and not all of these may be converted with equal efficiency into biologically active forms (e.g., glutathione peroxidase). For example, selenium fed in the form of tuna was less potent than selenium as selenite, beef kidney, or high-selenium wheat in restoring hepatic glutathione peroxidase activity in selenium-depleted rats.[19]

Keshan Disease: A Naturally Occurring Human Selenium Deficiency

Keshan disease, a cardiomyopathy that affects mainly young children and women of child-bearing age, occurs in a broad zone from northeastern to southwestern China.[20] The disease is diagnosed by the following criteria: acute or chronic heart function insufficiency, heart enlargement, gallop rhythm, arrhythmia, electrocardiographic changes, and changes in the heart visible by x-ray examination. The disease has been related to low dietary selenium intake, low blood selenium level, low hair selenium level, decreased blood glutathione peroxidase activity, and decreased urinary excretion of selenium after a loading dose. Moreover, a pronounced prophylactic effect of selenium was observed in an intervention trial involving several thousand children from areas of China in which Keshan disease is common (TABLE 3).[7] In a three-way exchange of samples, we have been able to corroborate the selenium levels reported by Chinese investigators in materials with either low or high contents of selenium (TABLE 4). The results demonstrate the wide range of selenium contents possible in samples from different areas of China (compare, for example, the very low value of rice-flour sample no. 2455, which is from a Keshan disease area, with the

TABLE 3

Prophylactic Effect of Selenium Supplements against Keshan Disease*

Group	Year	Subjects	Total Cases	Deaths
Control	1974	3,985	54	27
	1975	5,445	52	26
Selenium-treated	1974	4,510	10	0
	1975	6,767	7	1
	1976	12,579	4	2
	1977	12,747	0	0

*Adapted from Reference 7.

TABLE 4

COLLABORATIVE SELENIUM ANALYSIS OF SAMPLES FROM THE PEOPLE'S REPUBLIC OF CHINA

Sample Number	Sample Material	Selenium Content ($\mu g/g$)*		
		Beijing Laboratory[†]	Beltsville Laboratory[‡]	South Dakota Laboratory[§]
1454	rice flour	0.082 ± 0.005 (10)	0.083 ± 0.007 (5)	—
2455	rice flour	0.005 ± 0.0004 (8)	0.007 ± 0.004 (7)	—
3052	corn flour	0.028 ± 0.006 (11)	0.027 ± 0.008 (4)	—
122A	coal	84,123 ± 3,525 (17)	—	94,800 ± 1,600 (3)

*Mean ± standard deviation; number of determinations given in parenthesis.
†Keshan Disease Research Group, Institute of Health, Chinese Academy of Medical Sciences, Beijing, China.
‡Vitamin and Mineral Nutrition Laboratory, Human Nutrition Research Center, U.S. Department of Agriculture, Beltsville, Md. 20705.
§Prof. Oscar E. Olson, Biochemistry Section, Department of Chemistry, South Dakota State University, Brookings, S. Dak. 57007.

extremely high value of coal sample no. 122A, which is from a seleniferous zone in China).

While selenium deficiency accounts for many of the features of the disease, certain epidemiologic characteristics are not totally explicable on that basis alone, so secondary factors, such as environmental stressors or viral infection, have been sought. For example, the Chinese scientists found that selenium-deficient mice were much more susceptible than control mice to the cardiotoxic effects of a Coxsackie B_4 virus that had been isolated from a Keshan disease patient.[21] Nutritional cardiomyopathy develops in animals only when their feeds are deficient in both selenium and vitamin E; however, limited surveys indicate that the vitamin E status of the populations in the Keshan disease areas was satisfactory (Xiao Shu Chen, personal communication).

LOW SELENIUM STATUS IN SPECIAL POPULATION GROUPS

Premature Infants

In 1976, Gross described a group of premature infants in the United States whose plasma selenium levels declined from 80 ng/ml during the first week of life to 35 ng/ml after 7 to 8 weeks.[22] Red cell selenium levels and glutathione peroxidase activities declined about 16 and 36%, respectively. Although serum tocopherol levels were considered normal, infants fed a diet rich in polyunsaturated fatty acids and iron showed evidence of increased hemolysis. Gross suggested that insufficient glutathione peroxidase activities might allow free radical reactions in aqueous compartments of cells, which then would lead to hemolytic events.

Children Undergoing Diet Therapy

Lombeck *et al.* in West Germany studied the selenium status of infants and children who had various inborn errors of amino acid metabolism (phenylketonuria and maple syrup urine disease) that require diets that exclude the usual protein foods.[23] These special therapeutic diets, which contain protein hydrolysates or amino acid mixtures, are very low in selenium. Intakes as low as 1 to 5 µg/day have been reported, and such diets are often fed throughout the first decade of life. Serum selenium levels fall from about 40 ng/ml at birth to about 10 ng/ml after 3 to 4 months and stay depressed as long as the therapeutic diet is fed. In patients 1 to 10 years old, median serum selenium values ranged between 12.3 and 14.7 ng/ml, i.e., about 15 to 16% of the normal values for German children. There was no difference in serum vitamin E levels between the treated patients and healthy children of the same age. Selenium content of the hair of dietetically treated children was also depressed: 62 ng/g vs. 429 ng/g for controls. These hair selenium levels are in the range of those observed in the Keshan disease areas in China, and yet the German children thrive. There was no evidence of hematologic, electrocardiographic, or electromyographic abnormalities in the dietetically treated German patients. As already discussed, the Chinese scientists suggested that selenium by itself cannot explain all the epidemiologic aspects of Keshan disease. Although relatively few German children with very low selenium status were studied, their failure to develop any signs of cardiomyopathy also suggests that factors other than selenium are involved in the etiology of Keshan disease.

Total Parenteral Nutrition

In 1979, the Expert Panel on Guidelines for Essential Trace Element Preparations for Parenteral Use of the American Medical Association presented its recommendations for suggested daily intravenous intake of zinc, copper, chromium, and manganese.[24] At the present time, no recommendation exists for the addition of selenium compounds to intravenous feeding fluids even though such preparations contain negligible amounts of the element.[25] Consequently, reports of low selenium status in intravenously fed patients are beginning to appear.

As might be expected, the first such report originated in New Zealand, a country with low selenium soils. Van Rij *et al.* described a 37-year-old female surgical patient from a rural area in the south island where white muscle disease is endemic in sheep.[8] After 30 days of total parenteral nutrition (TPN), she developed bilateral muscular discomfort in her quadriceps and hamstring muscles. At this point, the patient's plasma selenium content had dropped to 9 ng/ml, a level that is associated with selenium-responsive disease in other species. Intravenous supplementation with 100 µg/day of selenium as selenomethionine was begun, and within 7 days muscle pain on active and passive movement disappeared. Selenium balances in six other patients receiving TPN were also measured, and all were markedly negative because of the very low quantities of selenium in the infused diet. Vitamin E status was not determined in any of these patients, but the authors concluded that future studies should consider vitamin E.

A second instance of presumed selenium deficiency in a TPN patient was described as a 43-year-old male residing in the northeastern United States who had been receiving parenteral alimentation for 2 years.[26] Poor selenium status was indicated by low red cell and heart (postmortem) selenium levels and glutathione peroxidase activities. Serum vitamin E levels were also slightly depressed. The patient presented with a dilated cardiomyopathy the histopathologic features of which—focal myocyte loss and scattered fibrous replacement throughout the ventricular subepicardium—were reminiscent of Keshan disease. It was stated that this histopathologic picture was not the same as that of idiopathic congestive cardiomyopathy and was not considered typical of acute or subacute viral myocarditis. The authors concluded that selenium deficiency in this patient resulted from prolonged TPN and was probably accentuated by losses from a chronically draining enterocutaneous fistula and an earlier period of malabsorption.

In a third report, Kay and Knight looked for signs and symptoms of selenium deficiency in 43 adults from the north island of New Zealand (Auckland) during medium to long-term TPN.[27] These workers found that healthy adults in the Auckland area have a mean whole blood selenium level of 79 ng/ml, well below the levels found in North America. In agreement with others, they found that blood selenium may fall to very low levels during TPN and concluded that this decline may be due to prolonged negative selenium balance because of low levels of selenium in the infusate rather than to abnormal renal or extrarenal losses. Although very low levels of both selenium and vitamin E were observed in their patients, none of them complained of any muscular symptoms.

Thus, there are three published reports that discussed signs and symptoms of low selenium status in TPN patients, and each report describes different manifestations of the low selenium state, i.e., muscular pains, dilated cardiomyopathy, and no observable clinical change. This puzzling state of affairs might be explained partially by other complicating factors (e.g., low vitamin E status or adaptation to low selenium intake). Additional work is needed to clarify the role of selenium in total parenteral nutrition.

POSSIBLE ASSOCIATION BETWEEN SELENIUM INTAKE AND CERTAIN HUMAN DISEASES

The rich pathology observed in animals deficient in selenium and vitamin E has given rise to much speculation concerning possible roles for selenium in human health and disease. Its role in Keshan disease is well established, and attempts have been made to link selenium with cancer, heart disease, muscular dystrophy, cystic fibrosis, and other diseases.

The possible connection between selenium intake and cancer was first suggested by the statistical associations made by Shamberger and Frost, which indicated an inverse correlation between blood selenium levels and cancer death rates in certain areas of the United States.[28] This inverse association was noted globally by Schrauzer et al.,[29] but was criticized by Allaway as lacking strength and consistency.[30,31] Although low blood selenium levels have been observed in patients with certain forms of cancer,[32] Robinson et al. concluded that such levels were more likely a result rather than a cause of the cancer.[33] On the other hand, recent experimental cancer studies with rodents have shown that under certain conditions moderate amounts of supplemental selenium can decrease the incidence of virally induced mammary tumors in mice and chemically induced mammary tumors in rats.[34,35] However, significant deleterious interactions of selenium with vitamin C or A have been reported in other carcinogenesis experiments.[36,37] Some investigators have advocated increased intakes of selenium (250–300 μg/day) to fight human cancer,[10] but others doubt that selenium supplements have any practical value against cancer.[38]

Statistical associations have also suggested a possible link between low selenium intake and an elevated incidence of cardiovascular disease.[39] However, a number of studies have shown no difference in tissue selenium levels between patients who died of myocardial infarcts and patients who died of other causes,[40,41] and blood selenium levels of New Zealand hypertensives were similar to those of normotensives.[42] Moreover, some investigators have confused the cardiomyopathy of Keshan disease with the pathology of the degenerative heart disease typical of the West and incorrectly concluded that the Chinese experience with selenium and Keshan disease supports the concept that selenium may play a role in the etiology of arteriosclerosis. On the other hand, the glutathione peroxidase activity of blood platelets is depressed in patients with acute myocardial infarction,[43] and based on the high selenium content of blood platelets, Kasperek et al. suggested that low selenium intakes might increase the risk of thrombotic episodes.[44] Platelet glutathione peroxidase activity is markedly depressed in selenium-deficient rats,[45] and responds rapidly to changes in selenium status.[46] A preliminary human study indicates that sudden increases in dietary selenium intake may influence platelet function.[47]

A biochemical rationale for a possible role of selenium in heart disease is given by considering the physiological balance between thromboxane and prostacyclin, two metabolites of arachidonic acid that control in vivo platelet aggregability. Thromboxane, mainly of platelet origin, is aggregatory and vasoconstrictive, whereas prostacyclin, mainly of vascular origin, is antiaggregatory and vasodilatory. Prostacyclin synthetase is inhibited by low levels of fatty acid hydroperoxides,[48] so it is conceivable that selenium deficiency, by depressing glutathione peroxidase activity, could tip the thromboxane-prostacyclin balance toward the proaggregatory state. Indeed, decreased prostacyclin synthesis was recently reported in aortic rings from selenium-deficient rats.[49] More research is needed to establish whether selenium has any role in the etiology of human heart disease.

When it was shown that vitamin E deficiency caused nutritional muscular dystrophy in animals, several clinicians tried vitamin E or some of its metabolites as a cure for human muscular dystrophy, but without success.[50] Likewise, when selenium deficiency was discovered to play a role in the development of white muscle disease in sheep or cattle, it was natural to suggest a possible role for the element in human muscular dystrophy. However, attempts to link selenium with human dystrophy have generally been disappointing. For example, two recent reports found no difference in blood glutathione peroxidase activity between dystrophic patients and controls.[51,52] Robinson et al. could not demonstrate any effect of daily selenium supplements on the fibromuscular rheumatism that affects certain residents of the low-selenium areas of the south island of New Zealand.[53]

Cystic fibrosis is a particularly frustrating disease for medical researchers because a suitable animal model is not available. On the basis of limited data, Wallach and Garmaise suggested that cystic fibrosis was due to a perinatal selenium deficiency.[54] However, more extensive surveys carried out since then showed that whole blood or serum selenium levels of cystic fibrosis patients were not in the deficiency range and whole blood glutathione peroxidase activity was considered normal.[55-57] Also, a workshop held at the National Institutes of Health concluded that there was no direct evidence to support the concept that selenium is a causative factor in cystic fibrosis.[58]

BIOCHEMICAL RELATIONSHIP BETWEEN SELENIUM AND VITAMIN E

When selenium was discovered to be a component of glutathione peroxidase, it was possible to propose a biochemical mechanism that linked its metabolic role with that of vitamin E.[6] These two nutrients were considered part of the body's antioxidant defense system, vitamin E as a lipid-soluble antioxidant and selenium as a part of glutathione peroxidase. In addition to its role in destroying hydrogen peroxide, glutathione peroxidase was thought to reduce fatty acid peroxides in the lipid bilayer of the cell membrane to the corresponding alcohols, thereby preventing further oxidative deterioration. However, there are now a number of observations that seem inconsistent with the latter idea. First of all, glutathione peroxidase appears unable to utilize fatty acid peroxides esterified in phospholipid as a substrate even though it acts effectively on fatty acid peroxide salts or free fatty acid peroxides.[59] Second, a glutathione-dependent, heat-labile factor that protects against lipid peroxidation in membranes but that is not glutathione peroxidase has been found in rat liver cytosol.[59,60] Third, Burk and associates have reported effects of selenium on the hepatic metabolism of heme or on the toxicity of diquat that are not readily explained on the basis of changes in glutathione peroxidase activity.[61,62] Finally, Burk and Gregory have recently described a selenoprotein in rat liver and plasma that is distinct from glutathione peroxidase.[63] All of these observations suggest biochemical roles for selenium in addition to that of glutathione peroxidase. Certainly, the occurrence of numerous selenoenzymes in various microorganisms gives ample biological precedent for multiple metabolic roles of selenium in mammals.[64] Additional research is needed to clarify the metabolic interactions of selenium and vitamin E.

SUMMARY

Great differences in dietary selenium intake have resulted in naturally occurring human selenium deficiencies and toxicities in certain parts of the world. Most North American diets, however, provide levels of selenium that fall within the estimated safe and adequate range of intake (50 to 200 μg/day for adults) as established by the U.S. National Research Council. Low selenium status may develop in individuals fed certain therapeutic diets or given total parenteral nutrition. Attempts have been made to link low selenium intake with cancer and heart disease, but additional research is needed in this area. Selenium, as a constituent of glutathione peroxidase, plays a role in the antioxidant defense systems of the body, but other metabolic roles for selenium may yet be discovered.

REFERENCES

1. SCHWARZ, K. & C. M. FOLTZ. 1957. Selenium as an integral part of factor 3 against dietary necrotic liver degeneration. J. Am. Chem. Soc. **79:** 3292–3293.
2. National Research Council, Committee on Animal Nutrition, Subcommittee on Sele-

nium. 1971. Selenium in Nutrition. National Academy of Sciences. Washington, D.C.

3. THOMPSON, J. N. & M. L. SCOTT. 1969. Role of selenium in the nutrition of the chick. J. Nutr. **97:** 335–342.
4. McCoy, K. E. M. & P. H. WESWIG. 1969. Some selenium responses in the rat not related to vitamin E. J. Nutr. **98:** 383–389.
5. ROTRUCK, J. T., A. L. POPE, H. E. GANTHER, A. B. SWANSON, D. G. HAFEMAN & W. G. HOEKSTRA. 1973. Selenium: biochemical role as a component of glutathione peroxidase. Science **179:** 588–590.
6. HOEKSTRA, W. G. 1975. Biochemical function of selenium and its relation to vitamin E. Fed. Proc. **34:** 2083–2089.
7. Keshan Disease Research Group. 1979. Observations on effect of sodium selenite in prevention of Keshan disease. Chinese Med. J. **92:** 471–476.
8. VAN RIJ, A. M., C. D. THOMPSON, J. M. McKENZIE & M. F. ROBINSON. 1979. Selenium deficiency in total parenteral nutrition. Am. J. Clin. Nutr. **32:** 2076–2085.
9. National Research Council. 1980. Recommended Dietary Allowances, Ninth Revised Edition. National Academy of Sciences. Washington, D.C.
10. SCHRAUZER, G. N. & D. A. WHITE. 1978. Selenium in human nutrition: dietary intakes and effects of supplementation. Bioinorg. Chem. **8:** 303–318.
11. ALLAWAY, W. H. 1973. Selenium in the food chain. Cornell Vet. **63:** 151–170.
12. SCHROEDER, H. A., D. V. FROST & J. J. BALASSA. 1970. Essential trace metals in man: selenium. J. Chronic Dis. **23:** 227–243.
13. LEVANDER, O. A. 1976. Selenium in foods. *In* Selenium-Tellurium in the Environment: 26–53. Industrial Health Foundation. Pittsburgh, Pa.
14. MERTZ, W. 1981. Vitamins and minerals. *In* Human Nutrition Research—BARC Symposium Number 4. G. R. Beecher, Ed.: 49–66. Allanheld, Osmun, & Co. Totowa, N.J.
15. LEVANDER, O. A., B. SUTHERLAND, V. C. MORRIS & J. C. KING. 1981. Selenium balance in young men during selenium depletion and repletion. Am. J. Clin. Nutr. **34:** 2662–2669.
16. STEWART, R. D. H., N. M. GRIFFITHS, C. D. THOMSON & M. F. ROBINSON. 1978. Quantitative selenium metabolism in normal New Zealand women. Br. J. Nutr. **40:** 45–54.
17. THOMSON, C. D. & M. F. ROBINSON. 1980. Selenium in human health and disease with emphasis on those aspects peculiar to New Zealand. Am. J. Clin. Nutr. **33:** 303–323.
18. CHEN, X., G. YANG, J. CHEN, X. CHEN, Z. WEN & K. GE. 1980. Studies on the relations of selenium and Keshan disease. Biol. Trace Element Res. **2:** 91–107.
19. DOUGLASS, J. S., V. C. MORRIS, J. H. SOARES, JR. & O. A. LEVANDER. 1981. Nutritional availability to rats of selenium in tuna, beef kidney, and wheat. J. Nutr. **111:** 2180–2187.
20. Keshan Disease Research Group. 1979. Epidemiologic studies on the etiologic relationship of selenium and Keshan disease. Chinese Med. J. **92:** 477–482.
21. BAI, J., S. Q. WU, K. Y. GE, X. J. DENG & C. Q. SU. 1980. The combined effect of selenium deficiency and viral infection on the myocardium of mice (preliminary study). Acta Acad. Med. Sinicae **2:** 29–31.
22. GROSS, S. 1976. Hemolytic anemia in premature infants: relationship to vitamin E, selenium, glutathione peroxidase, and erythrocyte lipids. Semin. Hematol. **13:** 187–199.
23. LOMBECK, I., K. KASPEREK, L. E. FEINENDEGEN & H. J. BREMER. 1981. Low selenium state in children. *In* Selenium in Biology and Medicine. J. E. Spallholz, J. L. Martin & H. E. Ganther, Eds.: 269–282. AVI Publishing Co. Westport, Conn.
24. AMA Department of Foods and Nutrition. 1979. Guidelines for essential trace element preparations for parenteral use. J. Am. Med. Assoc. **241:** 2051–2054.
25. ZABEL, N. L., J. HARLAND, A. T. GORMICAN & H. E. GANTHER. 1978. Selenium content of commercial formula diets. Am. J. Clin. Nutr. **31:** 850–858.
26. JOHNSON, R. A., S. S. BAKER, J. T. FALLON, E. P. MAYNARD, J. N. RUSKIN, Z. WEN, K. GE & H. J. COHEN. 1981. An occidental case of cardiomyopathy and selenium deficiency. N. Engl. J. Med. **304:** 1210–1212.

27. KAY, R. G. & G. S. KNIGHT. 1981. Selenium in human nutrition. Abstract, New Zealand Workshop on Trace Elements in New Zealand: 16. University of Otago. Dunedin, New Zealand.
28. SHAMBERGER, R. J. & D. V. FROST. 1969. Possible protective effect of selenium against human cancer. Can. Med. Assoc. J. **100:** 682.
29. SCHRAUZER, G. N., D. A. WHITE & C. J. SCHNEIDER. 1977. Cancer mortality correlation studies. III. Statistical associations with dietary selenium intakes. Bioinorg. Chem. **7:** 23–34.
30. ALLAWAY, W. H. 1972. An overview of distribution patterns of trace elements in soils and plants. Ann. N.Y. Acad. Sci. **199:** 17–25.
31. ALLAWAY, W. H. 1978. Perspectives on trace elements in soil and human health. In Trace Substances in Environmental Health. D. D. Hemphill, Ed. **12:** 3–10. University of Missouri Press. Columbia, Mo.
32. SHAMBERGER, R. J., E. RUKOVENA, A. K. LONGFIELD, S. A. TYTKO, S. DEODHAR & C. E. WILLIS. 1973. Antioxidants and cancer. I. Selenium in the blood of normals and cancer patients. J. Nat. Cancer Inst. **50:** 863–870.
33. ROBINSON, M. F., P. J. GODFREY, C. D. THOMSON, H. M. REA & A. M. VAN RIJ. 1979. Blood selenium and glutathione peroxidase activity in normal subjects and in surgical patients with and without cancer in New Zealand. Am. J. Clin. Nutr. **32:** 1477–1485.
34. SCHRAUZER, G. N., D. A. WHITE & C. J. SCHNEIDER. 1978. Selenium and cancer: effects of selenium and of the diet on the genesis of spontaneous mammary tumors in virgin inbred female C_3H/St mice. Bioinorg. Chem. **8:** 387–396.
35. IP, C. & D. K. SINHA. 1981. Enhancement of mammary tumorogenesis by dietary selenium deficiency in rats with a high polyunsaturated fat intake. Cancer Res. **41:** 31–34.
36. JACOBS, M. M. & A. C. GRIFFIN. 1979. Effects of selenium on chemical carcinogenesis. Comparative effects of antioxidants. Biol. Trace Element Res. **1:** 1–13.
37. THOMPSON, H. J., L. D. MEEKER & P. J. BECCI. 1981. Effect of combined selenium and retinyl acetate treatment on mammary carcinogenesis. Cancer Res. **41:** 1413–1416.
38. GRIFFIN, A. C. 1979. Role of selenium in the chemoprevention of cancer. Adv. Cancer Res. **29:** 419–442.
39. SHAMBERGER, R. J., C. E. WILLIS & L. J. MCCORMAK. 1978. Selenium and heart disease. III. Blood selenium and heart mortality in 19 states. In Trace Substances in Environmental Health. D. D. Hemphill, Ed. **12:** 59–63. University of Missouri Press. Columbia, Mo.
40. MASIRONI, R. & R. PARR. 1976. Selenium and cardiovascular diseases: preliminary results of the WHO/IAEA joint research programme. In Selenium-Tellurium in the Environment: 316–325. Industrial Health Foundation. Pittsburgh, Pa.
41. WESTERMARCK, T. 1977. Selenium content of tissues in Finnish infants and adults with various diseases and studies on the effects of selenium supplementation in neuronal ceroid lipofuscinosis patients. Acta Pharmacol. Toxicol. **41:** 121–128.
42. THOMSON, C. D., H. M. REA, M. F. ROBINSON & F. O. SIMPSON. 1978. Selenium concentrations and glutathione peroxidase activities in blood of hypertensive patients. Proc. Univ. Otago Med. School **56:** 1–3.
43. WANG, Y. X., K. BOCKER, H. REUTER, J. KIEM, K. KASPEREK, G. V. IYENGAR, F. LOOGEN, R. GROSS & L. E. FEINENDEGEN. 1981. Selenium and myocardial infarction: glutathione peroxidase in platelets. Klin. Wochenschr. **59:** 817–818.
44. KASPEREK, K., G. V. IYENGAR, J. KIEM, H. BORBERG & L. E. FEINENDEGEN. 1979. Elemental composition of platelets. III. Determination of Ag, Au, Cd, Co, Cr, Cs, Mo, Rb, Sb, and Se in normal human platelets by neutron activation analysis. Clin. Chem. **25:** 711–715.
45. BRYANT, R. W. & J. M. BAILEY. 1980. Altered lipoxygenase metabolism and decreased glutathione peroxidase activity in platelets from selenium-deficient rats. Biochem. Biophys. Res. Commun. **92:** 268–276.
46. MORRIS, V. C. & O. A. LEVANDER. 1981. Response of platelet glutathione peroxidase (GSH-Px) activity in rats fed selenite or high-selenium yeast (Se-Y). Fed. Proc. **40:** 902.
47. BRYANT, R. W., J. M. BAILEY, J. C. KING & O. A. LEVANDER. 1981. Altered platelet

glutathione peroxidase activity and arachidonic acid metabolism during selenium repletion in a controlled human study. *In* Selenium in Biology and Medicine. J. E. Spallholz, J. L. Martin & H. E. Ganther, Eds.: 395–399. AVI Publishing Co. Westport, Conn.

48. MONCADA, S. & J. R. VANE. 1979. Arachidonic acid metabolites and the interactions between platelets and blood vessel walls. N. Engl. J. Med. **300:** 1142–1147.

49. BULT, H., P. VAN DEN BOSCH, R. VAN DEN BOSCH, A. VAN HOYDONCK & A. G. HERMAN. 1981. Selenium deficiency impairs the biosynthesis of prostacyclin in rat aorta. Thromb. Haemostasis **46:** 272.

50. HARRIS, P. L. & K. E. MASON. 1956. Alpha-Tocohydroquinone and muscle dystrophy. Am. J. Clin. Nutr. **4:** 402–407.

51. HUNTER, M. I. S., M. S. BRZESKI & P. J. DE VARE. 1981. Superoxide dismutase, glutathione peroxidase, and thiobarbituric acid–reactive compounds in erythrocytes in Duchenne muscular dystrophy. Clin. Chim. Acta **115:** 93–98.

52. BURRI, B. J., S. G. CHAN, A. J. BERRY & S. K. YARNELL. 1980. Blood levels of superoxide dismutase and glutathione peroxidase in Duchenne muscular dystrophy. Clin. Chim. Acta **105:** 249–255.

53. ROBINSON, M. F., D. R. CAMPBELL, R. D. H. STEWART, H. M. REA, C. D. THOMSON, P. G. SNOW & I. H. W. SQUIRES. 1981. Effect of daily supplements of selenium on patients with muscular complaints in Otago and Canterbury. N. Z. Med. J. **93:** 289–292.

54. WALLACH, J. D. & B. GARMAISE. 1979. Cystic fibrosis: a perinatal manifestation of selenium deficiency. *In* Trace Substances in Environmental Health. D. D. Hemphill, Ed. **12:** 469–476. University of Missouri Press. Columbia, Mo.

55. LLOYD-STILL, J. D. & H. E. GANTHER. 1980. Selenium and glutathione peroxidase levels in cystic fibrosis. Pediatrics **65:** 1010–1012.

56. CASTILLO, R., C. LANDON, K. ECKHARDT, V. MORRIS, O. LEVANDER & N. LEWISTON. 1981. Selenium and vitamin E status in cystic fibrosis. J. Pediatr. **99:** 583–585.

57. UNDERWOOD, B. A. 1980. Personal communication.

58. HUBBARD, V. S., G. BARBERO & H. P. CHASE. 1980. Selenium and cystic fibrosis. J. Pediatr. **96:** 421–422.

59. McCAY, P. B., D. D. GIBSON & K. R. HORNBROOK. 1981. Glutathione-dependent inhibition of lipid peroxidation by a soluble, heat-labile factor not glutathione peroxidase. Fed. Proc. **40:** 199–205.

60. BURK, R. F., M. J. TRUMBLE & R. A. LAWRENCE. 1980. Rat hepatic cytosolic glutathione-dependent enzyme protection against lipid peroxidation in the NADPH-microsomal lipid peroxidation system. Biochim. Biophys. Acta **618:** 35–41.

61. CORREIA, M. A. & R. F. BURK. 1978. Rapid stimulation of hepatic microsomal heme oxygenase in selenium-deficient rats: an effect of phenobarbital. J. Biol. Chem. **253:** 6203–6210.

62. BURK, R. F., R. A. LAWRENCE & J. M. LANE. 1980. Liver necrosis and lipid peroxidation in the rat as the result of paraquat and diquat administration—the effect of selenium deficiency. J. Clin. Invest. **65:** 1024–1031.

63. BURK, R. F. & P. E. GREGORY. 1982. Some characteristics of ^{75}Se-P, a selenoprotein found in rat liver and plasma, and comparison of it with seleno-glutathione peroxidase. Arch. Biochem. Biophys. **213:** 73–80.

64. STADTMAN, T. C. 1980. Selenium-dependent enzymes. Ann. Rev. Biochem. **49:** 93–110.

DISCUSSION

P. B. McCAY (*Oklahoma Medical Research Foundation, Oklahoma City, Okla.*): I would like to comment on the explanation you gave us for glutathione peroxidase protection against lipid peroxidation. I think some other explanation may be necessary. We've been able to show that glutathione peroxidase will not reduce lipid peroxides in membrane to lipid alcohols. Furthermore, purified glutathione peroxidase apparently has no influence on lipid peroxidation. I think maybe the protection comes about through keeping the levels of hydrogen peroxide low. Glutathione peroxidase will reduce fatty acid hydroperoxides in aqueous solution to alcohols, but this to the best of our knowledge does not happen in membranes.

O. A. LEVANDER: I think that the fact that we have enzymes in our cells that purposely create lipid peroxides—such as lipoxygenase, which is then reduced by the glutathione peroxidase in cytosol—indicates a more subtle and perhaps more exciting role for this enzyme than just protecting against the oxidative damage.

W. A. PRYOR (*Louisiana State University, Baton Rouge, La.*): In these patients who are selenium deficient, is there some abnormality in their sulfur amino acid chemistry?

O. A. LEVANDER: Many people with Keshan disease have multiple nutritional problems, and it wouldn't be surprising if they were low in sulfur amino acid intake. Much of their protein is coming from soy, for example, which is somewhat low in sulfur amino acids.

G. J. HANDELMAN (*University of California, Santa Cruz, Calif.*): It has been shown that if rats are given two sources of selenium either from selenomethionine or from selenite and if the diet is also low in sulfur amino acids, the animals cannot use the selenium from selenomethionine to make glutathione peroxidase. They can only use selenium from selenomethionine to make glutathione peroxidase if there is a high availability of methionine. If, however, the animals are given selenite, then they make normal levels of glutathione peroxidase regardless of the levels of dietary protein.

O. A. LEVANDER: I agree. Apparently animals and presumably people who are low in sulfur amino acids have this problem as well as a lack of precursor for glutathione in the glutathione peroxidase reaction.

G. J. HANDELMAN: The high levels of methionine in the diet of New Zealanders might explain why selenium deficiency is not observed even with the low intakes reported in New Zealand.

O. A. LEVANDER: Quite so.

H. W. SEEGER (*Justus-Liebig University, Giessen, Federal Republic of Germany*): I don't know whether it is related, but it is known that adriamycin, which is associated with lipid peroxidation, also causes cardiomyopathy. Do you think there might be a parallel with the cardiomyopathy of selenium deficiency?

O. A. LEVANDER: Yes, possibly.

K. C. BHUYAN (*Mount Sinai School of Medicine, New York, N.Y.*): I would like to give a word of caution. We and other investigators have reported that selenium at a dose 5 to 10 times higher than the requirement produces cataracts in rats and mice. We can produce cataract by a single injection of 20 micromoles of selenium per kilo body weight.

I also wanted to ask you, Why are New Zealanders immune to selenium deficiency?

O. A. LEVANDER: Unless there's some sort of long-term adaptation that takes place in people, we don't know. Or as Dr. Handelman suggested, perhaps the high intake of animal protein and sulfur amino acids helps in their situation. I don't think that this is very clear, and we're trying to look at the different areas—New Zealand, Finland, and China—and find out why you get such different patterns in the three countries.

UNIDENTIFIED SPEAKER: What is the synergism between selenium and vitamin E? Is selenium involved in protecting vitamin E, or is vitamin E involved in protecting selenium? In addition to the glutathione peroxidase, selenium is also known to be present in several other proteins. What is known about them?

O. A. LEVANDER: The two nutrients can spare one another. For example, the selenium requirement for chickens is decreased by increasing the amount of vitamin E in the diet. As far as other biological roles for selenium, there are three well-characterized bacterial enzymes that are now known to contain selenium, and I think it's just a matter of time until we find more mammalian proteins.

R. J. SOKOL (*Children's Hospital Medical Center, Cincinnati, Ohio*): In the patients with phenylketonuria, was the amount of vitamin E in their diet examined? And were glutathione peroxidase levels done?

O. A. LEVANDER: The vitamin E levels were considered sufficient. They did do glutathione peroxidase determinations, and these did decrease after birth.

INTRODUCTION

Lewis A. Barness

Department of Pediatrics
University of South Florida
College of Medicine
Tampa, Florida 33620

Nervous system dysfunctions were a group of striking abnormalities noted in early studies of vitamin E–deficient states. Examples included encephalomalacia in young chicks[1] and muscle dystrophy in rabbits.[2] Extensive research in animals attempted to relate vitamin E deficiency to dystrophy in humans; but all measurements in humans were normal and, clinically or biochemically, no detectable response was noted in dystropic children to vitamin E supplementation.

In the early 1950s, Andersen and Mike, followed by others, reported improvement in muscle strength in children with cystic fibrosis—a condition known to have poor vitamin E absorption—when supplemented with oral water-soluble vitamin E preparations.[3] Andersen and others related this to a lipofuscin-stained material in muscles, a substance also found in E-deficient animals, ceroid. Similarly staining material was found in adults with malabsorption, and this was termed "brown-bowel" syndrome.

Children with abetalipoproteinemia were shown to have very low levels of vitamin E due to lack of carrier proteins.[4] They were known to develop severe nervous system abnormalities, reversible in some with large doses of vitamin E. In the 1950s, also, retrolental fibroplasia was noted in baby rats.[5] This was followed by treatment with vitamin E, but this was before the relationship of oxygen to retrolental fibroplasia was recognized.

For a time, the nervous and muscle system effects and their treatment with pharmacological doses of vitamin E escaped the tendency to confuse deficiency states with excess use of vitamin E in nondeficient states to prevent symptoms. Nonetheless, reports of prevention of aches and pains with vitamin E, usually by testimonial, have stimulated the use of large doses of vitamin E in nondeficient individuals.

It is refreshing that this conference includes not only nervous system abnormalities in humans, a system with possibilities of benefiting from fat-soluble antioxidants, but also other disease states that may respond to vitamin E supplementation.

REFERENCES

1. PAPPENHEIMER, A. M. & M. GOETTSCH. 1931. A cerebellar disorder in chicks, apparently of nutritional origin. J. Exp. Med. **53:** 11–16.
2. MILHORAT, A. T. 1954. Therapy in muscular dystrophy. Med. Ann. D.C. **23:** 15–22.
3. ANDERSEN, D. H. & E. M. MIKE. 1955. Diet therapy in celiac syndrome. J. Am. Diet. Assoc. **31:** 340–346.
4. KAYDEN, H. J. & R. SILBER. 1965. The role of vitamin E deficiency in the abnormal autohemolysis of acanthocytosis. Trans. Assoc. Am. Physicians **78:** 334.
5. CALLISON, E. C. & E. CRENT-KELLES. 1981. Abnormalities of eye (retrolental fibroplasia) occurring in young vitamin E deficient rats. Proc. Soc. Exp. Biol. Med. **76:** 295–297.

PROGRESSIVE NEUROMUSCULAR DISEASE IN CHILDREN WITH CHRONIC CHOLESTASIS AND VITAMIN E DEFICIENCY: CLINICAL AND MUSCLE BIOPSY FINDINGS AND TREATMENT WITH α-TOCOPHEROL*

Mary Anne Guggenheim,†‡ Steven P. Ringel,‡
Arnold Silverman,†§ Brian E. Grabert,†¶
and H. E. Neville‡

*School of Medicine
University of Colorado Health Sciences Center
Denver, Colorado 80262*

INTRODUCTION

Although it is more than 50 years since vitamin E was discovered, only since 1965 has the importance of this small, fat-soluble molecule in human nutrition been documented.[1,2] Neuropathologic and myopathic abnormalities have been recognized in children at risk for E deficiency for more than 20 years.[3-6] Recently, neuromuscular disease in children has been related to chronic E deficiency.[7-11]

This report describes the clinical findings and muscle pathology in four children with a progressive neuromuscular disease and chronic vitamin E deficiency. Parenteral (intramuscular) administration of all-rac-α-tocopherol (α-T) was necessary to normalize serum E concentrations in three patients, and one patient responded to high doses of oral vitamin E.

PATIENTS AND METHODS

Four patients were identified with congenital liver disease of varying types resulting in cholestasis who had progressive deterioration of coordination and gait. Extensive evaluations of these four patients were carried out in the Pediatric Clinical Research Center (CRC) of University Hospital of the University of Colorado between October 1978 and October 1981. All laboratory studies were performed by the pediatric microchemistry–CRC laboratory or other specialized University Hospital laboratories. Serum α-T was determined by a spectrophotometric method requiring less than 0.5 cm serum.[12] All vitamin E levels are expressed as mg/g cholesterol as suggested by Farrell.[13]

Muscle specimens were obtained by open biopsy of the quadriceps in three

*This work was supported in part by grants from the General Clinical Research Centers Program of the Division of Research Resources, National Institutes of Health (Grant RR-69), by the Muscular Dystrophy Foundation of America, and by Roche Laboratories.
†Department of Pediatrics.
‡Department of Neurology.
§Address correspondence to Denver General Hospital, West 8th Avenue & Cherokee, Denver, Colo. 80204.
¶Address correspondence to 2131 North Tejon, Colorado Springs, Colo. 80907.

children and by excision of a lateral abdominal muscle at the time of open liver biopsy in the fourth. One specimen was mounted in gum tragacanth and quick frozen in isopentane immersed in liquid nitrogen. Ten-micron serial sections were stained with a battery of 14 histochemical reactions,[14] including modified trichomes, hematoxylin and eosin, Verhoff-van Giessen, nicotinamide-adenine dinucleotide-tetrazolium (NADH-TR), alkaline phosphatase, acid phosphatase, periodic acid-Schiff (PAS), oil red o, sudan black, myofibrillar adenosine triphosphatase (ATPase) at pH 9.4, 4.6, and 4.2, nonspecific esterase, and phosphorylase. A second specimen was fixed in 3% glutaraldehyde, embedded in Epon, thin sectioned with a Porter Blum III microtome, and examined using a Hitachi AE6 electron microscope. Therapeutic trials utilized commercially available water-dispersible α-T acetate (Aquasol®), an emulsified oral preparation of α-T, and α-T as a 50 mg/cc alcohol solution for intramuscular use. The latter two preparations were supplied by Roche Laboratories. All aspects of the study were reviewed and

TABLE 1

DETAILS OF NEUROMUSCULAR DISEASE*

Patient	1	2	3	4
Age when neurologic symptoms began (by history)/age when examined	6/7 years	11–12/14 years	7–8/16 years	5/6½ years
Ataxia: truncal	+ + +	+ +	+	+ + +
appendicular	+ +	+ +	+ + +	+ +
Ophthalmoplegia (supranuclear)	+	+ +	+ +	+ + +
Deep tendon reflexes	absent	absent	absent	absent
Muscle strength	N	+ (occasional fasciculations)	N (bilateral pes cavus)	N
Sensation: vibration	+ + +	+ + +	+ + +	+ + +
position sense	+	+	N	N
other	N	slight ↓ to light touch distally	moderate ↓ light touch distally	N
Serum vitamin E prior to treatment (N = 3–15 mg/g cholesterol)	0.85–2.33	0.17–0.74	0.73–2.06	0.17–0.32

*+ = mildly abnormal; + + = moderately abnormal; + + + = severely abnormal; and N = normal.

approved by the Human Subjects Committee of the University of Colorado School of Medicine, and written parental consent obtained.

RESULTS

TABLE 1 summarizes the neurologic findings and pretreatment vitamin E levels in the four patients. The neuromuscular disease consisted of a progressive ataxia, which varied in severity from difficulty with tandem gait to inability to walk. All had an ophthalmoplegia (supranuclear type) with loss of volitional upward gaze; Patients 2, 3, and 4 had additional oculomotor abnormalities. All had complete areflexia, severe loss of vibratory sensation in both arms and legs, and other minor abnormalities. All are mentally normal and attending school, where they do average to excellent academic work. Despite mildly increased retinal pigmentation, all have normal visual acuity and electroretinograms done in two patients were normal.

Laboratory tests showed evidence of chronic cholestasis and a general tendency for malabsorption of fat-soluble vitamins. Low prothrombin times correctable by vitamin K (in 2/4 patients), borderline low concentrations of vitamin A (in 2/4), and consistently low serum carotene levels (4/4) were found. Pretreatment serum concentrations of vitamin E were repeatedly low in all four patients (TABLE 1), and the red blood cell (RBC) hemolysis test—a functional screen of vitamin E deficiency—was consistently elevated (19–65%, normal = <10%). Normal laboratory studies included serum immunoglobulins, lipoproteins, phytanic acid, thyroid studies, cortisol and adrenocorticotrophic hormone (ACTH), folate, B_{12}, lactate, pyruvate, cerebrospinal fluid protein, urinary amino and organic acids, and leukocyte lysosomal enzymes.

Electromyography and motor and sensory nerve conduction studies were done on all four patients. Patient 1 had slightly decreased conduction velocity in one median nerve (35 m/second) and unobtainable sural nerve conduction. Three other nerves studied in her and multiple studies in both upper and lower extremities in the other three patients showed normal motor and sensory conduction rates.

MUSCLE PATHOLOGY

Conventional histological reactions (modified trichrome, hematoxylin and eosin, Verhoff-van Giessen) revealed abundant basophilic flecks within most muscle fibers including muscle spindles on all four patients. The flecks were positive with the nonspecific esterase and acid phosphatase reactions and were strongly autofluorescent (yellow). They were also PAS-positive and frequently stained dark with the NADH-TR reaction. FIGURE 1 demonstrates these histochemical findings. In one patient, the muscle also showed considerable variation in fiber size, necrosis, and regeneration. In this specimen the flecks were frequently fused into larger deposits and occasionally there was central necrosis. No increase in fat, connective tissue, or inflammatory cells was noted. Oxidative reactions revealed minor disruption of the intermyofibrillar network in all patients and occasional dark-staining angular fibers. Myofibrillar ATPase series revealed type 1 predominance and early-fiber-type grouping. Normally myelinated nerve was noted in all biopsies, but no studies of peripheral nerve were done.

By electron microscopy, the abnormal flecks were densely osmiophilic, circular or oblong-shaped inclusions surrounded by a limiting membrane and located between myofibrils. Numerous membranous whorls, autophagic vacuoles, and areas of Z-band streaming were also seen. FIGURE 2 shows these findings.

TREATMENT WITH α-TOCOPHEROL

In an attempt to normalize the consistently low concentrations of serum E, we initially gave large oral doses (up to 4 g per day) of α-T acetate. Although in all patients serum vitamin E values tended to increase slightly, only Patient 3 attained a normal serum concentration. The other three patients were given brief trials of a special emulsified form of α-T (doses up to 1,000 mg per day) without

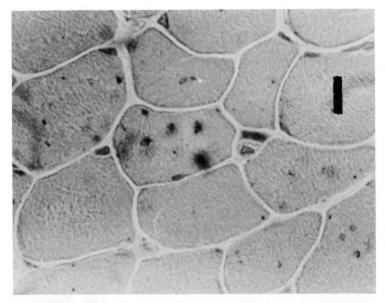

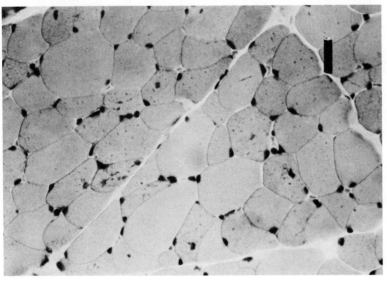

FIGURE 1. Ten-micron serial cryostat sections of muscle. **Left:** Abundant basophilic flecks are seen within most muscle fibers and are readily distinguishable from larger subsarcolemmal nuclei. Hematoxylin and eosin, ×389.5; bar = 25 μ. **Right:** These flecks are strongly positive with the acid phosphatase reaction. ×900; bar = 10 μ.

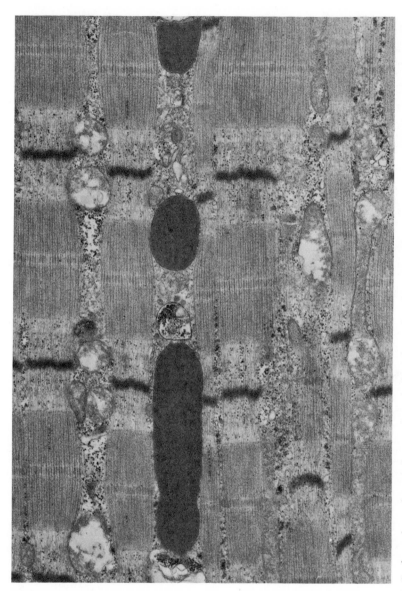

FIGURE 2. Oval membrane-bound electron-dense bodies of 1-3 μ length seen on electron microscopy of longitudinally sectioned muscle. These bodies correspond to the cytoplasmic inclusions of FIGURE 1.

improvement. Because animal data show that co-ingestion of medium-chain triglycerides (MCT) may improve E absorption,[15] this was tried in two patients. They immediately developed severe steatorrhea, and the MCT was stopped.

There are no available guidelines for the use of intramuscular α-T in children other than premature infants. Therefore, we obtained pharmacokinetic data on three patients following a standard intramuscular dose. Using these results we calculated the dose and frequency of intramuscular injections required to maintain a serum E steady state in the therapeutic range. In these three patients

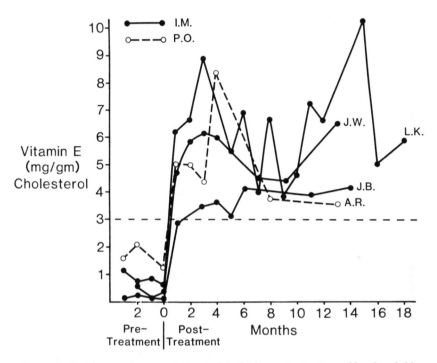

FIGURE 3. Serial concentrations of vitamin E in the four patients. Normal level in children is <3 mg/g cholesterol. Open circles indicate one patient treated with 1,000–1,200 units per day of tocopheryl acetate perorally. Closed circles indicate three patients given intramuscular α-tocopherol. Doses (mg/kg per 24 hours) based on individualized pharmacokinetic data were LK = 1.12; JW = 1.42; and JB = 0.55.

there was wide variation in serum half-life of E (26–114 hours), but all had similar volume of distribution (0.37–0.42 L/kg). Pretreatment values and results of both oral and intramuscular vitamin E supplementation are summarized in FIGURE 3.

RESPONSE TO TREATMENT

All patients have shown definite neurologic improvement since treatment with intramuscular E. Patient 1 was unable to walk, even with support, and moved around by crawling. She now walks distances of several blocks with minimal support, and has recently walked short distances alone. Patient 4 was "bouncing off the walls" prior to treatment and falling frequently. After six months of effective E replacement, she now walks steadily and will attempt to run. Her severe ophthalmoplegia is slightly better. The ophthalmoplegia in Patient 2 is no longer present. Upper extremity deep tendon reflexes (DTRs) are hypoactive but obtainable in all four patients, but DTRs have not yet been elicited in the legs. Without question the two younger patients have had the greatest functional improvement. No deterioration of any aspects of the disease has occurred in any of the four patients, nor have any new abnormalities occurred. During the time of therapeutic trials of E, no other changes in medications or vitamin supplements given these children were made. No adverse reactions to the intramuscular administration of α-T were seen. In addition to neurologic improvement, RBC hemolysis promptly returned to normal.

DISCUSSION

The evidence is strong that the neuromuscular disease described in this paper may be due to chronic vitamin E deficiency. All other known causes of progressive ataxia and ophthalmoplegia in these patients were excluded. All four children had chronic and severe E deficiency secondary to persistent cholestasis. The clinical findings in these patients are identical to those reported in other children with cholestasis and chronic E deficiency.[8-10] Similar neurologic manifestations occur in patients with Bassen-Kornzweig disease, who have chronic E deficiency resulting from genetically determined absence of β-lipoproteins.[7,15,16]

The morphologic abnormalities in the muscle of our patients are similar to changes that can be induced in animals with dietary E deficiency.[17-20] The muscle findings are like those reported by Gomez et al. in a young woman with progressive ataxia, areflexia, retinal degeneration, and loss of posterior column sensation who had underlying cholestatic disease.[21] Although serum E was not measured, the nature of the patient's biliary disease would suggest chronic E deficiency.

Four other children whom we have examined (all 6 years of age or older) who have cholestasis but normal levels of E have a normal neurologic examination. In other younger children (under 5 years of age) in whom we have found low levels of vitamin E due to chronic cholestasis, the neurologic examination is normal except for occasional hyporeflexia.[22]

Finally, normalization of serum E levels, without any other therapeutic modification, has not only arrested the previously progressive neurologic deterioration, but resulted in definite improvement.

We suspect that neuraxonal dystrophic changes in the brain, spinal cord, and dorsal root underlie the neurologic deficits in our patients. Neuraxonal changes and demyelination of the posterior columns have been noted in animals with experimental E deficiency, in children with malabsorption states that predispose to low E values, and in the children described by Rosenblum and coworkers who have the same clinical syndrome as do our patients.[6,10,19,23-25] The morphologic abnormalities noted in the muscle of our patients do not appear to relate directly to the clinical symptoms, although one patient had elevated serum creatinine phosphokinase (CPK) levels.

The autofluorescent inclusions noted in the muscle fibers (including spindles) of all four patients are distinctive, and should suggest the diagnosis of E deficiency. Similar inclusions were described in two previous patients with presumptive E deficiency,[21,26] but not noted in a third case.[8] Since the flecks stain basophilic with conventional histologic reactions, they are easily confused with internal nuclei. Histochemistry readily confirms the lysosomal nature of the lipochrome pigment.[27] The presence of identical membranous whorls, mitochondrial remnants, and inclusion bodies ultrastructurally in both our patients and in E-deficient animals suggests that the pathogenesis of the muscle lesions is related to lipid peroxidation of membranes.[17,18,27] Significant muscle necrosis was present in only one of our patients and resembled the proteolysis noted in E-deficient animals.[19]

It appears likely that the developing neuromuscular system is more susceptible to damage by E deficiency than is the adult system. Ataxia and paresis developed slowly in adult rats made E deficient,[23] whereas similar pathology occurred much more rapidly in young weanling rats.[19] These observations would explain why no definite human disease in E-deficient adults has been identified.[1,28,29] Most of the disease states that predispose to severe chronic E deficiency (cystic fibrosis, other malabsorption states, congenital cholestasis, and abetalipoproteinemia) are present in early infancy.

The potential reversibility of this neuromuscular disease is unknown. Our patients did not develop neurologic abnormalities until 5 to 15 years despite the almost certain fact that they were E deficient since infancy. Similar observations have been made by others.[7,9,10,30] The neuropathologic abnormalities described in E-deficient patients are more pronounced in the older children, suggesting a slowly progressive process.[6] Nelson *et al.* found only partial reversibility of axonal changes in three monkeys made E deficient for 30–33 months and then supplemented for 2 months prior to sacrifice.[25] So far, our clinical observations suggest that the disease may be more easily reversed in younger children.

A review of the literature and our experience indicate that oral supplementation seldom reverses E deficiency secondary to cholestatic disease.[3,8–10,31–33] The supplemental use of water-dispersible vitamin preparations of A, D, K, and E is part of the routine medical management of children with chronic cholestasis. Indeed, the four children reported here were on such supplemental therapy from infancy. It is apparent that one cannot assume that normalization of serum levels of these vitamins has been achieved (even when given in a water-dispersible form) unless confirmed by specific laboratory testing. Why some cholestatic patients poorly absorb vitamin E is unclear at this time. It is theoretically possible that cholestyramine, which is often given to these patients, may further impair E absorption. Only two of our four patients were taking cholestyramine on a regular basis prior to the onset of neurologic symptoms.

Intramuscular α-tocopherol therapy for children who cannot achieve normal serum levels with oral supplementation may be indicated. Individualized pharmacokinetic data helped us determine the correct dosage schedule in order to maintain a steady-state serum level of E. At the present time the intramuscular use of E is restricted to experimental use, although this vitamin has previously been used parenterally in both preterm infants and children without adverse effects.[15,34,35]

Summary

We have studied four children (ages 6 to 17 years) with chronic cholestasis who developed a slowly progressive neuromuscular disease characterized by ataxia, dysmetria, areflexia, loss of vibratory sensation, and a variable ophthalmo-plegia. Serum vitamin E concentrations were low in all patients prior to treatment (0.17–2.0 mg/g cholesterol, normal >3 mg/g). Muscle histochemical studies showed prominent yellow autofluorescence, basophilic cytoplasmic inclusions which stain with esterase and acid phosphatase, and occasional necrotic fibers. Ultrastructural findings consisted of increased number and size of membrane-bound dense bodies (lysosomes), membranous whorls, and autophagic vacuoles. Intramuscular injections of all-rac-α-tocopherol (0.55–1.42 mg/kg per 24 hours based on individualized pharmacokinetic data) were required in three patients to achieve normal serum vitamin E values. High-dose (32 mg/kg per 24 hours) oral supplementation was effective in one patient. After normalization of serum vitamin E concentrations for 12 to 20 months, the neurologic disease has improved in all four patients.

ACKNOWLEDGMENTS

Patient 4 was referred by Dr. John Lilly. Special thanks to Ginny Jackson, R.N., who assisted in the ambulatory clinical research on these patients, to Kathy Bell for secretarial support, and to Peter Chase, M.D., whose laboratory performed the initial determinations of vitamin E.

REFERENCES

1. BINDER, H. J., D. C. HERTING, V. HURST, S. C. FINCH & H. M. SPIRO. 1965. Tocopherol deficiency in man. N. Engl. J. Med. **273:** 1289–1297.
2. HORWITT, M. K. 1980. Therapeutic uses of vitamin E in medicine. Nutr. Rev. **38:** 105–113.
3. WEINBERG, T., H. H. GORDON, E. H. OPPENHEIMER & H. M. NITOWSKY. 1958. Myopathy in association with tocopherol deficiency in a case of congenital biliary atresia and cystic fibrosis of the pancreas. Am. J. Pathol. **34:** 565.
4. SUNG, H. J. 1964. Neuraxonal dystrophy in mucoviscidosis. J. Neuropathol. Exp. Neurol. **23:** 567–583.
5. NELSON, J., C. FITCH, V. FISCHER, et al. 1978. Progressive neuropathologic lesions with vitamin E deficiency in mammals including man. J. Neuropathol. Exp. Neurol. **37:** 666.
6. SUNG, J. H., S. H. PARK, A. R. MASTRI & W. J. WARWICK. 1980. Axonal dystrophy in the gracile nucleus in congenital biliary atresia and cystic fibrosis (mucoviscidosis): beneficial effects of vitamin E therapy. J. Neuropathol. Exp. Neurol. **39:** 584–597.
7. MULLER, D. P. R., J. K. LLOYD & A. C. BIRD. 1977. Long-term management of abetalipoproteinemia: possible role for vitamin E. Arch. Dis. Child. **52:** 209–214.
8. TOMASI, L. G. 1979. Reversibility of human myopathy caused by vitamin E deficiency. Neurology **29:** 1182–1186.
9. UMETSU, D. T., P. CONTURE, H. S. WINTER, B. M. KAGAN, M. J. BRESNAN & S. E. LUX. 1980. Degenerative neurologic disease in patients with acquired vitamin E deficiency. Pediatr. Res. **14:** 512.
10. ROSENBLUM, J. L., J. P. KEATING, A. P. PRENSKY & J. S. NELSON. 1981. A progressive, disabling, neurologic syndrome in children with chronic liver disease: a possible result of vitamin E deficiency. N. Engl. J. Med. **304:** 503–508.
11. GRABERT, B. E., M. A. GUGGENHEIM, S. P. RINGLE, H. P. CHASE & H. E. NEVILLE. 1980. Neuromuscular disease related to chronic vitamin E deficiency. Ann. Neurol. **8:** 217.

12. HANSEN, L. G. & K. W. J. WARWICK. 1969. A fluorometric micromethod for serum vitamins A and E. Am. J. Clin. Pathol. **51:** 538–541.
13. FARRELL, P. M., S. L. LEVINE, M. D. MURPHY & A. J. ADAMS. 1979. Plasma tocopherol levels and tocopherol-lipid relationships in a normal population of children as compared to healthy adults. Am. J. Clin. Nutr. **31:** 1720–1726.
14. DUBOWITZ, V. & M. H. BROOKE. 1973. Muscle Biopsy: A Modern Approach. W. B. Saunders Co. Ltd. London, England.
15. AZIZI, E., J. L. ZAIDMAN, J. ESCHAR & A. STEINBERG. 1978. Abetalipoproteinemia treated with parenteral and oral vitamins A and E, and with medium chain triglycerides. Acta Pediatr. Scand. **67:** 797–801.
16. HERBERT, P. N., A. M. GOTTO & D. S. FREDRICKSON. 1978. Familial lipoprotein deficiency. *In* The Metabolic Basis of Inherited Disease. J. H. Stanbury, D. S. Wyngaarden & D. S. Fredrickson, Eds.: 544–588. McGraw-Hill. New York, N.Y.
17. WEST, W. T. 1963. Muscular Dystrophy of Vitamin E Deficiency in Man and Animals. G. H. Boune & M. N. Golaz, Eds.: 368–405. Hafner. New York, N.Y.
18. HAWES, E. L., H. M. PRICE & J. M. BLUMBERG. 1964. The effects of a diet producing lipochrome pigment (ceroid) on the ultrastructure of skeletal muscle in rats. Am. J. Pathol. **45:** 599–631.
19. MACHLIN, L. J., R. FILIPSKI, J. NELSON, L. R. HORN & M. BRIN. 1977. Effects of a prolonged vitamin E deficiency in the rat. J. Nutr. **107:** 1200–1208.
20. NELSON, J. S. 1980. Pathology of vitamin E deficiency. *In* Vitamin E, A Comprehensive Treatise. L. J. Machlin, Ed.: 397–428. Marcel Dekker. New York, N.Y.
21. GOMEZ, M. R., A. G. ENGEL & P. J. DYCK. 1972. Progressive ataxia, retinal degeneration, neuromyopathy, and mental subnormality in a patient with true hypoparathyroidism, dwarfism, malabsorption and cholelithiasis. Neurology **22:** 849–855.
22. GUGGENHEIM, M. A., V. JACKSON & J. LILLY. 1981. Unpublished observations.
23. PENTSCHEW, A. & K. SCHWARZ. 1962. Systemic axonal dystrophy in vitamin E deficient adult rats. Acta Neuropathol. **1:** 313–334.
24. GELLER, A., F. GILLES & H. SHWACHMAN. 1977. Degeneration of fasiculus gracilis in cystic fibrosis. Neurology **27:** 185–187.
25. NELSON, J. S., C. D. FITCH, V. W. FISHER, G. O. BROUN & A. C. CHOU. 1981. Progressive neuropathologic lesions in vitamin E–deficient rhesus monkeys. J. Neuropathol. Exp. Neurol. **40:** 166–186.
26. ROTT, E., G. DELPRE & V. KADRIH. 1977. Abetalipoproteinemia (Bassen-Kornzweig syndrome). Acta Neuropathol. (Berlin) **37:** 255–258.
27. HADLOW, W. J. 1973. Myopathies of animals. *In* The Striated Muscle. C. M. Pearson & F. K. Mostofi, Eds.: 364–409. Williams & Wilkins. Baltimore, Md.
28. 1976. Vitamins in search of a disease. J. Am. Med. Assoc. **201:** 195. (Editorial.)
29. BIERI, J. G. & P. M. FARRELL. 1976. Vitamin E. Vitam. Horm. **34:** 31–75.
30. FRYDMAN, M., *et al.* 1981. Neurologic syndrome in liver disease. N. Engl. J. Med. **305:** 108. (Letter to the editor.)
31. NITOWSKY, H. M., M. CORNBLUTH & H. H. GORDON. 1956. Studies of tocopherol deficiency in infants and children. II. Plasma tocopherol and erythrocyte hemolysis in hydrogen peroxide. Am. J. Dis. Child. **92:** 164–174.
32. MULLER, D. P. R., J. T. HARRIES & J. K. LLOYD. 1974. The relative importance of the factors involved in the absorption of vitamin E in children. Gut **15:** 966–971.
33. NITOWSKY, H. M., H. H. GORDON & J. T. TILDON. 1956. Studies of tocopherol deficiency in infants and children. IV. The effect of α-tocopherol on creatinuria in patients with cystic fibrosis of the pancreas and biliary atresia. Bull. Johns Hopkins Hosp. **98:** 361–371.
34. GRAEBER, J. E., L. A. BUTLER, M. L. WILLIAMS & F. A. OSKI. 1976. The use of intramuscular vitamin E in the premature infant. Optimum dose and iron interaction. Pediatr. Res. **10:** 377.
35. GROSS, S. J. 1979. Vitamin E and neonatal bilirubinemia. Pediatrics **64:** 321–323.

H. J. KAYDEN (*New York University School of Medicine, New York, N.Y.*): I'm obviously very intrigued by the relationship of the disease you described to abetalipoproteinemia. I'm interested in the comparison between the two groups of children you talked about—those that seemed to mimic the same disorder but did not have neurologic disease and had higher vitamin E levels and those that developed neurologic disease. I wondered if you could tell us a little bit about absorption of vitamin E in your groups. Are chylomicrons actually formed in these children? What degree of fat malabsorption do they have? And lastly, in the lipoprotein distribution, I wondered whether there is any distinction between the two groups in the quantity of what we call lipoprotein X.

M. A. GUGGENHEIM: There was no apparent change between the lipoproteins in normal children or these children with cholestasis. They all had what seemed to be the normal amounts of β-lipoproteins. It is our assumption—though we have no data and have not studied these children from the point of view of biliary secretion either qualitatively or quantitatively—that small amounts of vitamin E are absorbed in some children even though they have biliary obstruction. We assume that cholestasis is not an all or none phenomenon, that there are both qualitative and quantitative aspects, and it is only some types of cholestasis that totally prevent absorption even of a small amount of vitamin E. It may just be that very small amounts will do the job. These children did not have overt steatorrhea.

C. C. TANGNEY (*Rush University, Chicago, Ill.*): I have a few questions to ask you, one in reference to the observations of gait and incoordination. Did you also look at blood or plasma selenium levels?

M. A. GUGGENHEIM: No, we've not done that.

C. C. TANGNEY: During the period before supplementation, did you also notice increased platelet levels in these children?

M. A. GUGGENHEIM: Yes, many of them had thrombocytosis, and several of them normalized following treatment with vitamin E.

C. C. TANGNEY: With regard to the intramuscular treatment, what form of vitamin E was used? Was it the free α-tocopherol form or the esterified form?

M. A. GUGGENHEIM: We used the free alcohol, *all-rac-α*-tocopherol specially prepared for parenteral use by Roche Laboratories.

C. C. TANGNEY: And roughly what was the range of dose per day?

M. A. GUGGENHEIM: It averaged 1 mg per kilo per day, but the range was something like 0.5 to 1.8.

C. C. TANGNEY: Are there any other particular vitamins or nutrients that you add to the supplementation phase?

M. A. GUGGENHEIM: These children are often supplemented with vitamin K when they have bleeding difficulties. They seem able to absorb large amounts of vitamins A and D, if those are given in large enough amounts orally. It seems as though vitamin E is poorly absorbed by the oral route in a certain subgroup of children with cholestasis no matter how much you supplement them. These children must be treated with parenteral vitamin E.

M. K. HORWITT (*St. Louis Medical Center, St. Louis, Mo.*): May I inquire whether you followed the creatinine in the urine and whether creatinuria, if present, was reversed by the therapy you used?

M. A. GUGGENHEIM: We did not measure creatinine levels in the urine. We noticed increased CPK in the serum. This is hard to follow in the children who get daily intramuscular injections. One child who responded to oral treatment and whose CPK was originally high had a fall in CPK to normal.

M. K. HORWITT: It may be difficult, but you might consider in future studies following the erythrocyte lifetime.

M. A. GUGGENHEIM: Yes. I would add that I have the definite impression that there are probably 50 to 100 such patients around the country, most of whom are not yet being treated.

I. D. DESAI (*University of British Columbia, Vancouver, B.C., Canada*): First I want to compliment you for demonstrating all the classical biochemical symptoms of vitamin E deficiency in real case studies, including lipofuscin and fluorescence. I have some questions regarding the assessment of vitamin E status. You have expressed some of your values as milligrams of vitamin E per gram of cholesterol, and I wonder what the justification was for this expression. There are other ways of expressing vitamin E that are much more dependable and accurate, such as milligram per gram of plasma lipids or perhaps on the basis of plasma or blood volume.

M. A. GUGGENHEIM: The measurement is actually performed on a volume of plasma. The expression of E per gram of serum cholesterol is calculated. Dr. Farrell has pointed out that this expression is probably important, especially as these children have variable serum lipid and serum cholesterol levels. The cholesterol in these children is proportionate to the total lipids and was a more convenient measurement for us to perform.

I. D. DESAI: Did you also calculate the E values based upon milligram of vitamin E per gram plasma lipid? And did you find any relationship to E per cholesterol levels?

M. A. GUGGENHEIM: There is a definite difference in one child if you calculate the vitamin E as milligram per deciliter of serum. It looks like her vitamin E levels are higher than the normal range. However, she has significant hyperlipidemia and hypercholesterolemia. Her vitamin E actually just barely falls within the normal range when you look at it based upon her cholesterol level.

J. NIXON (*Linus Pauling Institute, Palo Alto, Calif.*): I was curious about the intramuscular injections and the fact that you were able to achieve a normal range but it plateaued in that range. Is there any indication that in that particular patient, or possibly other patients, you get altered metabolism or accelerated metabolism of vitamin E?

M. A. GUGGENHEIM: Our initial doses were calculated to achieve a steady state. For almost two years in one patient, the E level has remained remarkably constant except, as occasionally happens, when we run out of the injectable form of E, in which case the serum level drops. It would appear that wherever the vitamin E is going, that process is remaining constant.

R. J. SOKOL (*Children's Hospital Medical Center, Cincinnati, Ohio*): I was wondering if I might be able to answer a couple of the questions that you were asked in terms of the vitamin E absorption data. We're studying several children similar to this, and in five out of the six in whom we have done interluminal bile acid determinations of samples from a duodenal aspirant, there were very, very small, almost nondetectable, bile acids even after stimulation of gallbladder contraction. Fecal fat excretion in these children is usually about 15 to 20%, whereas normally it is somewhere in the range of 5 to 10%. Children with cystic fibrosis who aren't treated have two or three times that in terms of fat malabsorption. The degree of vitamin E malabsorption doesn't seem to necessarily correlate with the degree of fat malabsorption or the degree of bile acids in the intestine.

EVALUATION OF VITAMIN E DEFICIENCY IN CHILDREN WITH LUNG DISEASE*

Philip M. Farrell, Elaine H. Mischler, and Gary R. Gutcher

Department of Pediatrics
University of Wisconsin
Madison, Wisconsin 53792

INTRODUCTION

After approximately four decades of research on human tocopherol levels, one might expect that a reliable definition of vitamin E deficiency should have been established and widely accepted by now. The importance of accurate assessment of vitamin E status stems from a need to determine human requirements for this nutrient; this is accomplished in part by population surveys of tocopherol levels. In addition, patients with disorders leading to malnutrition, such as malabsorption syndromes and cancer, need to be assessed accurately. Although biopsy of adipose tissue can be helpful,[1] the most convenient approach is to analyze blood samples. As reviewed by Farrell, there have been numerous nutritional surveys of healthy individuals in which blood samples have been used for analysis of either plasma or serum tocopherol.[2] Usually total tocopherols have been measured colorimetrically, although the most abundant and active isomer, α-tocopherol, has occasionally been measured after thin-layer or high-pressure liquid chromatography. In clinical evaluations of vitamin E status, the reported blood tocopherol levels have often been accompanied by peroxide hemolysis test results.[3,4] Despite many investigations of human E status, however, confusion persists as to the best means of diagnosing vitamin E deficiency in patients.

On the basis of data obtained from evaluating normal and malnourished children and adults, Horwitt et al. have concluded that blood tocopherol concentrations alone may be misleading and cause erroneous interpretations.[5] Their data indicate the dependency of plasma or serum tocopherol concentrations on the level of circulating lipids. Other reports have appeared that confirm the advantages of a blood lipid reference base,[6,7] rather than the expression of results per unit volume of serum or plasma. Nevertheless, this problem in establishing an adequate definition of vitamin E deficiency does not seem to be widely appreciated, as judged from a review of recent reports on the vitamin E status of pediatric patients.[8-10] As a consequence, many patients have been described as vitamin E deficient when in reality they may be normal.

The necessity of using a blood lipid reference base for tocopherol concentrations is especially evident in data obtained from the study of young children.[6] Therefore, this report emphasizes observations on tocopherol-lipid relationships in pediatric populations. Coincidentally, the two major groups of children that are susceptible to low vitamin E levels, namely, premature infants and patients with cystic fibrosis (CF), are also likely to have pulmonary disease and to require supplemental oxygen. This may have implications relating to pulmonary oxygen toxicity in view of reports on the importance of lung antioxidants.[11] In addition to

*This research was supported by grants from the Cystic Fibrosis Foundation and the National Heart, Lung and Blood Institute, National Institutes of Health (Pulmonary SCOR Award 1-P50-HL-27358-01).

96

data on vitamin E status, a summary will be presented of results obtained from a comprehensive evaluation of the possible effects of tocopherol deficiency in children, particularly hematologic assessment of CF patients.

The conclusion emerging from our work concerns the inadequacy of attempting to evaluate vitamin E status of abnormal subjects by blood tocopherol concentrations alone. Regardless of whether serum, plasma, or erythrocytes are used, it seems essential to determine at least tocopherol concentrations (preferably tocopherol isomers) and some measure of circulating lipids (preferably total lipids). Furthermore, it is highly desirable to measure erythrocyte hemolysis *in vitro*.

METHODS

Subjects

Our studies have included four distinct populations: prematurely delivered infants during the first week of life, children between the ages of 3 months and 12 years who were generally in good health with no manifestations of chronic disease as described previously,[6] patients with cystic fibrosis,[3] and normal adolescents and adults. The diagnosis of cystic fibrosis was established firmly by the presence of at least three of the four standard criteria for the disease: positive family history, pancreatic insufficiency, chronic obstructive pulmonary disease, and elevated sweat electrolytes.[12] For purposes of this investigation, the patients with cystic fibrosis were divided into three subgroups. The first consisted of patients who had clinical or laboratory evidence of pancreatic insufficiency with variable degrees of malabsorption and who were not receiving supplementary tocopherol. The second subgroup was comprised of patients with pancreatic insufficiency who had been placed on supplements of water-miscible *all-rac-α*-tocopheryl acetate. The third subgroup consisted of patients who were not taking supplementary vitamin E and who demonstrated intact digestive function, as seen in approximately 15% of cystic fibrosis patients.[3]

Samples Obtained for Analysis

Informed consent was obtained from all patients and control subjects participating in the study. Blood samples, obtained in the fasting state either by venipuncture or from an arterial catheter, were mixed with anticoagulant [heparin or ethylenediaminetetraacetic acid (EDTA)] and were centrifuged within two hours. The red blood cells (RBCs) were then analyzed immediately, while the plasma was often frozen before extraction of lipids.

Analytical Methods

Measurement of tocopherol was performed on plasma according to a modification of a colorimetric method that utilizes $FeCl_3$ and bathophenanthroline as the chromogenic reagent.[3,6] Correction was made for plasma carotenoids, which were measured in the sample by first reading the absorbance at 450 nm. In some instances, tocopherol isomers were first separated, generally by thin-layer chromatography using the method of Bieri and Prival with a solvent system of benzene-ethanol (99:1).[13] Total plasma lipids were determined by the technique of de La Huerga et al.,[14] which we had previously modified in order to use smaller volumes than described in the original procedure.[6] Cholesterol concentrations were measured using the enzymatic method of Roeschlan et al.[15] The hemolysis test was performed with fresh saline-washed erythrocytes incubated without agitation as 5% suspensions in hydrogen peroxide (2% initial concentration). After three-hour incubations at 37°C, samples were centrifuged and the absorbance of the supernatant at 575 nm measured to determine the extent of hemoglobin release. Additional suspensions were incubated in distilled water to produce total hemolysis and obtain a reference hemoglobin value for expression of results. Accordingly, peroxide hemolysis data are expressed as the percent of total hemoglobin detected in the erythrocyte suspensions incubated with distilled water. This technique was adapted from that of Horwitt et al.[16] and is described in detail elsewhere;[3] the test yields less than 5% hemolysis with suspension of red cells taken from healthy adults with normal blood tocopherol concentrations.

Erythrocyte Survival

This was evaluated by measuring the half-life of ^{51}Cr-labeled, autologous erythrocytes. The specific procedure employed was method C recommended by the International Committee for Standardization in Hematology.[17] Labeling with radiochromium was carried out with 10-ml samples of venous blood mixed with acid-citrate dextrose; approximately 1 μCi of ^{51}Cr was added per kg of body weight. Blood samples of 5 ml volume were drawn one hour after injection and every two or three days until a total of 12 specimens were available for determination of radioactivity. Data obtained were corrected for chromium elution, which was found to be the same for vitamin E–deficient erythrocytes and control subjects.

RESULTS

Total tocopherol concentrations as mg/dl plasma are shown in FIGURE 1 for children ranging from 3 months to 12 years of age. From these data, it is readily apparent that no association can be established between the concentration of tocopherol and the age of the subjects studied. Our results indicated that more than one-third of the children had concentrations below 0.5 mg/dl, the traditionally accepted lower limit of normal.[2] None of these children, however, showed abnormal peroxide hemolysis test results, i.e., all values were 1 or 2%. The mean ± standard error (SE) tocopherol concentration was 0.59 ± 0.3 mg/dl for 39 children, which is significantly (p < 0.001) less than the value of 0.79 ± 0.04 mg/dl obtained for 22 adults evaluated concurrently.

As shown in FIGURE 2, tocopherol concentrations correlated with total plasma lipids in both the children and adults; however, as reported elsewhere,[6] the values for children did not show a significant correlation with plasma cholesterol concentrations. The total lipid values were lower (p < 0.005) in the pediatric population, namely, 484 ± 12 versus 549 ± 14 mg/dl. Although the ratio of milligrams tocopherol per gram of total lipid was also slightly lower in children (1.22 ± 0.06) compared to adults (1.38 ± 0.08), it is clear that plasma tocopherol values parallel lipid concentrations and that lower blood lipids in the pediatric population can influence the level of circulating vitamin E.

Data obtained from the study of patients with cystic fibrosis are shown in TABLES 1–3. It was found that subjects with pancreatic insufficiency who received no vitamin E supplements showed not only low levels of total tocopherol (TABLE 1) and α-tocopherol,[3] but also reduced tocopherol-lipid ratios. Thus, CF patients show an average ratio that is less than half the mean of the control group (0.65 versus 1.64 mg/g; $p < 0.001$). This occurred despite a reduction in total plasma lipids in the CF patients. Peroxide hemolysis test results were generally quite abnormal in the CF patients, but not always. From a review of individual values presented in TABLE 2, it is apparent that some patients with "low" tocopherol concentrations show normal or nearly normal peroxide hemolysis test results. Examination of total plasma lipids and tocopherol-lipid ratios in individual patients indicates that a more reliable assessment of vitamin E status can be

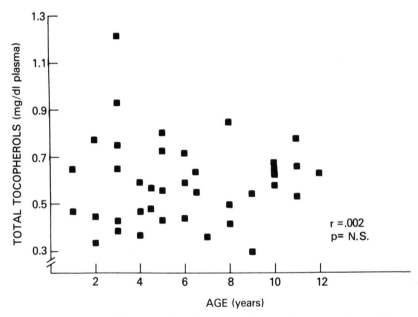

FIGURE 1. Total plasma tocopherol concentrations as related to age ($r = 0.002$).

obtained by taking lipid concentrations into account. For instance, Patient 5 showed a total tocopherol concentration of 0.219 mg/dl plasma, total lipids of 279 mg/dl, producing a tocopherol-lipid ratio of 0.785, and a peroxide hemolysis result of 8% (just above the upper limit of normal). Similarly, Patient 10 showed a tocopherol concentration of 0.210 mg/dl, a total lipid level of 193 mg/dl, thus a tocopherol-lipid ratio of 1.09, while the hemolysis in peroxide was only 6%. Both of these patients would have traditionally been considered severely deficient based on tocopherol concentrations of 0.219 and 0.210 mg/dl, but these would have been misleading.

Patients with cystic fibrosis who manifested pancreatic insufficiency and were taking supplements of vitamin E were found to have normal plasma concentrations of tocopherol (TABLE 1), as noted in a previous study.[3] Examination

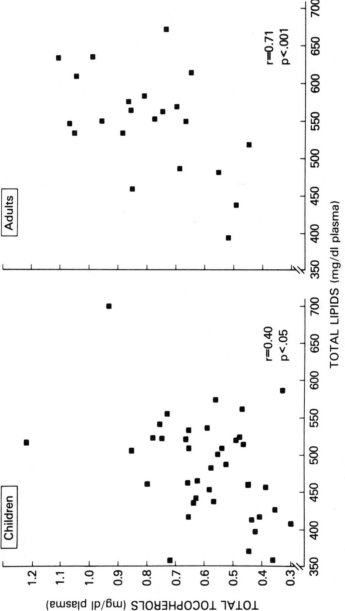

FIGURE 2. The relationship between plasma tocopherol concentrations and total lipid values in children and adults.

TABLE 1

ASSESSMENT OF VITAMIN E IN CYSTIC FIBROSIS (CF) PATIENTS*

	Controls	CF (PI − E)†	CF (PI + E)‡
Population	17	14	12
Total Tocopherol (mg/dl plasma)	0.840 ± 0.034	0.237 ± 0.026§	0.975 ± 0.132
Total Lipid (mg/dl plasma)	527 ± 22	374 ± 23§	409 ± 44¶
Tocopherol:Lipid	1.64 ± 0.09	0.65 ± 0.07§	2.59 ± 0.31‖
% RBC Hemolysis	1.5 ± 0.6	37.0 ± 7.0§	0.94 ± 0.2

*Table includes mean ± SE.
†CF patients with pancreatic insufficiency who were not taking vitamin E supplements.
‡CF patients with pancreatic insufficiency who were taking oral supplements of water-miscible *all-rac-α*-tocopheryl acetate (50–200 IU/day).
§Compared to control group, p < 0.001.
¶Compared to control group, p < 0.02.
‖Compared to control group, p < 0.005.

of total lipid concentrations and tocopherol-lipid ratios, however, reveals that these patients actually had unusually high levels of circulating vitamin E, with a mean ± SE ratio of 2.59 ± 0.31 (p < 0.005 compared to the value of 1.64 ± 0.09 in the controls).

It has previously been reported that the deficiency of vitamin E in CF patients is attributable to malabsorption associated with pancreatic insufficiency, rather than dietary deficiency.[3] The data presented in TABLE 3 on five subjects with intact pancreatic function support this hypothesis. In particular, these five patients showed normal values of total tocopherol concentration and total lipids, thus a normal tocopherol-lipid ratio. Furthermore, there were no abnormalities in peroxide hemolysis and all were on normal diets.

TABLE 2

VITAMIN E STATUS OF CYSTIC FIBROSIS PATIENTS WITH PANCREATIC INSUFFICIENCY*

Patient Number	Age (years)	Total Tocopherol (mg/dl plasma)	Total Lipids (mg/dl plasma)	E:Lipid Ratio†	% Hemolysis (in H_2O_2)
1	1	0.126	391	0.322	78
2	2	0.251	437	0.574	25
3	12	0.156	477	0.327	59
4	14	0.222	559	0.563	43
5	14	0.219	279	0.785	8
6	15	0.401	495	0.810	29
7	15	0.255	337	0.757	14
8	15	0.324	441	0.734	36
9	18	0.139	359	0.387	39
10	20	0.210	193	1.09	6
11	20	0.125	296	0.422	68
12	21	0.206	420	0.490	81
13	25	0.230	293	0.784	28
14	29	0.455	429	1.06	4

*None of these patients were taking supplements of vitamin E.
†Ratio of milligrams tocopherol per gram of total plasma lipids.

TABLE 3

VITAMIN E STATUS OF CYSTIC FIBROSIS PATIENTS WITHOUT MALABSORPTION

Age (years)	Total Tocopherol (mg/dl plasma)	Total Lipids (mg/dl plasma)	E:Lipid Ratio*	% Hemolysis (in H_2O_2)
13	0.741	659	1.12	2.2
14	0.842	527	1.60	1.2
15	0.673	479	1.40	1.4
22	1.35	762	1.77	0.3
25	1.20	728	1.64	0.7
Mean	0.960	631	1.51	1.2
SE	0.130	55.3	0.11	0.32

*Ratio of milligrams tocopherol per gram of total plasma lipids.

A limited number of premature infants susceptible to respiratory disease were studied during the first week of life. As shown in TABLE 4, very low levels of total plasma lipids were found—in fact, approximately half the concentration found in the controls. These infants also exhibited "low" tocopherol concentrations in most instances (mean = 0.335 mg/dl), but variable tocopherol-lipid ratios. It is evident, however, from TABLE 4 that some of the infants had abnormally high levels of peroxide-induced hemolysis, whereas others were less than 5%. Tocopherol-lipid ratios averaged 0.92 mg/g in these infants.

Our studies on the *effects of vitamin E deficiency* have focused on the neuromuscular system and possible hematologic abnormalities in CF patients with low tocopherol-lipid ratios. These results have previously been reported in detail and revealed no consistent evidence of either neurologic disease or muscle

TABLE 4

VITAMIN E STATUS OF THREE-DAY-OLD PREMATURE INFANTS*

Patient Number	Gestational Age (weeks)	Total Tocopherol† (mg/dl plasma)	Total Lipids (mg/dl plasma)	E:Lipid Ratio‡	% Hemolysis (in H_2O_2)
1	27	0.291	271	1.07	1.8
2	28	0.481	475	1.01	10.1
3	28	0.379	639	1.69	1.8
4	29	0.279	477	0.58	4.5
5	29	0.545	543	1.00	1.0
6	29	0.275	207	1.33	2.2
7	31	0.177	284	0.62	47.0
8	31	0.223	339	0.66	69.2
9	32	0.240	307	0.78	62.6
10	33	0.203	281	0.72	39.5
11	34	0.577	680	0.85	60.0
12	34	0.473	366	1.29	1.3
13	35	0.262	441	0.59	3.8
14	35	0.285	432	0.66	22.4

*These infants did not receive oral or parenteral tocopherol before assessment.

†Determined after high-pressure liquid chromatography[23] as the sum of α-, β-, and γ-isomers.

‡Ratio of milligrams tocopherol per gram of total lipid.

necrosis.[2,3] In particular, plasma creatine phosphokinase (CPK) activities, which are markedly elevated in tocopherol-deprived animals with nutritional myopathy and in humans with genetic muscular dystrophy, were found to be normal in 48 of 50 CF patients evaluated while vitamin E deficient. Furthermore, muscle biopsies from the quadriceps femoris of 4 CF patients (including the 2 with high CPK levels) revealed no necrosis or fragmentation of muscle fibers, despite the absence of detectable tocopherol in these tissues.[2] Hematologic studies, however, were more revealing. In addition to abnormal hemolysis *in vitro* during peroxide exposure (TABLES 1 and 2, Reference 3), vitamin E–deficient erythrocytes showed abnormal survival *in vivo* as measured with ^{51}Cr-labeled cells. The $t_{1/2}$ values for 19 CF patients (with decreased tocopherol levels) ranged from 16 to 29 days with a mean $\pm$ SE of 22.4 $\pm$ 0.9 days compared to 25–35 days and 28.0 $\pm$ 0.5 days in 28 control subjects (p < 0.001). Six patients were available for repeat ^{51}Cr-RBC survival measurements after supplementation with oral tocopherol. This subgroup exhibited a significant increase (p < 0.001) in $t_{1/2}$ from 19.0 $\pm$ 1 (pretreatment value) to 27.6 $\pm$ 0.9 days. Despite this evidence of shortened erythrocyte survival, it should be noted that the degree of abnormality in $t_{1/2}$ values is not sufficient to produce frank hemolytic anemia (^{51}Cr-RBC $t_{1/2}$ values in hemolytic diseases are approximately 5–15 days). Thus, Farrell *et al.* found no evidence of clinically significant hemolysis in vitamin E–deficient patients and no change in hematologic indices such as the hematocrit after supplementation with tocopherol.[3]

DISCUSSION

From this work and studies published previously,[5-7] there are several implications concerning methods for clinical evaluation of vitamin E status. Because blood specimens are universally available from patients, in contrast to tissue biopsies including those from adipose sites, investigation of human vitamin E status is generally limited to analysis of plasma (or serum) and erythrocytes. On the basis of data presented herein, it is clear that circulating tocopherol concentrations alone may be misleading and result in erroneous interpretations. In particular, many patients with less than 0.5 mg/dl, the traditional lower limit of normal, cannot be regarded as "deficient" in vitamin E since there is no evidence of insufficient antioxidant based on evaluation of erythrocyte stability in hydrogen peroxide. Although this measure of peroxide-induced hemolysis is an imperfect test, a normal result implies an adequate level of intracellular antioxidants.

Study of premature infants over more than three decades has obviously led to erroneous interpretations regarding vitamin E status.[2] These infants initially have very low levels of circulating lipid because of the relatively ineffective transport of fat across the placenta. It should also be mentioned that premature infants and cystic fibrosis patients evaluated in our studies tend to be low in linoleic acid[18,19] and may have less polyunsaturated fatty acid susceptible to oxidation. Both plasma and red cell fractions demonstrate significantly reduced linoleate, along with other biochemical evidence of essential fatty acid deficiency.[19] Thus, it is important to carry out further studies with these patients and establish their tocopherol status and requirements in relationship to lipid metabolism. Because of recent reports suggesting beneficial effects of vitamin E treatment for infants with retrolental fibroplasia and bronchopulmonary dysplasia,[20,11] such studies are urgently needed. Furthermore, there is a current tendency to treat these infants with intravenous polyunsaturated fatty acid (PUFA), which could influence not only lipid levels but also tocopherol requirements.

In view of tocopherol concentration data that have yielded erroneous information about vitamin E status (without concurrent lipid measurements), Horwitt et al. suggested "that no one ever again report a serum tocopherol level without presenting simultaneous data on the serum lipids."[5] Their recommendation was that total lipids be determined, rather than one of the subfractions which can fluctuate more than total lipid levels. Our results from assessment of pediatric populations (FIGURE 2 and Reference 6) indicate that total lipid values are superior to cholesterol concentrations. It might be argued that measurement of total plasma lipids introduces greater complexity than is needed for clinical evaluation of vitamin E status and that the procedure is not sufficiently precise. However, we have found that the method of de La Huerga et al. is not difficult, nor does it require more than 0.1 ml of plasma or serum.[14] Therefore, we support the conclusion of Horwitt et al.[5] and reiterate the current recommendation that blood tocopherol concentrations be reported using a lipid reference base. Although this is especially important in studies dealing with pediatric subjects and patients with malabsorption, there is also a risk of erroneous interpretations in carrying out population surveys in adults without measuring lipid values. This was made clear in a report by Farrell and Bieri describing 28 megavitamin consumers, when highly variable triglyceride concentrations were found.[7]

The proposal that tocopherol-lipid ratios be utilized to assess nutritional status corresponds to the mechanism of tocopherol transport in blood, since circulating vitamin E is carried with lipoproteins according to the fat concentration of the various fractions.[21] This provides part of the rationale for using a lipid reference base in expressing results on circulating tocopherol levels. In addition, there is a large body of evidence from animal studies indicating that vitamin E requirements should be related to polyunsaturated fat, especially linoleic acid intake.[22] More fundamentally, information described elsewhere in this volume on the biological role of vitamin E provides further justification for expressing tocopherol concentrations in relationship to a lipid reference base. Tocopherols are unusual among the essential nutrients because of their protective role, especially with regard to oxidation of membrane lipid constituents. In essence, vitamin E serves a defensive function by blunting the impact of the environment on the organism's vital cells. However, because the adequacy of any defense must be measured against the applied offense, it is probably more meaningful to utilize a definition of vitamin E *sufficiency* rather than "deficiency." Thus, what may be most relevant is not the absolute amount of vitamin E present in a given compartment or cell, but whether that amount is sufficient to protect membrane lipids against the stress of peroxidation. By relating the *protector* (vitamin E) to the *protected* (lipid), and taking into account the magnitude of anticipated oxidation processes, it should be possible to achieve a quantitative definition of human vitamin E *sufficiency* that is more reliable than plasma tocopherol concentrations.

On the basis of results obtained in a study of hospitalized patients, Horwitt et al. concluded that a ratio above 0.8 mg tocopherol per gram of total lipid in serum should be considered a sign of sufficient vitamin E nutrition.[5] Subsequently, Farrell et al. identified several children with ratios of 0.6–0.8 who did not show abnormal peroxide hemolysis test results.[6] Data presented in TABLE 2, however, indicate that a ratio of 0.8 can be associated with abnormal hemolysis test results.

Therefore, it must be concluded that additional data are needed to determine what value of tocopherol-total lipid should be established as the lower limit of normal. Ideally, future studies should utilize measurement of tocopherol isomers by high-pressure liquid chromatography.[23] Because unsaturated fatty acids are particularly vulnerable to oxidation, the ratio of α-tocopherol to PUFA may eventually provide a more accurate index of vitamin E sufficiency than using total lipid as the denominator. Furthermore, erythrocyte vitamin E levels related to PUFA might be a helpful index, even though there is normally a rapid equilibrium between plasma and the red blood cell fraction.[24] Finally, it is recommended that along with tocopherol and lipid determinations, one should routinely assess erythrocyte antioxidant in clinical evaluations of vitamin E status by utilizing a test such as the peroxide hemolysis procedure.

SUMMARY

The clinical assessment of vitamin E status has traditionally depended upon measurement of tocopherol concentrations in plasma or serum, with 0.5 mg/dl being used as the lower limit of normal. This approach can be supplemented by measurement of tocopherol in erythrocytes or by evaluating their susceptibility to hemolysis in the presence of hydrogen peroxide. Data obtained during the last decade indicate that tocopherol concentrations in blood samples may be misleading, and that tocopherol-lipid ratios are more reliable indicators of vitamin E status. In our studies, small populations of healthy children have been evaluated, along with infants and children with a variety of chronic diseases. Of interest is the observation that premature infants susceptible to lung disease, who often require high levels of inspired oxygen, and children with cystic fibrosis who have chronic obstructive pulmonary disease are almost invariably below 0.5 mg tocopherol per deciliter plasma. A substantial number, however, show no abnormality in peroxide-induced erythrocyte hemolysis. Expression of the tocopherol data per gram of total lipid indicates that many children with "low" tocopherol concentrations per unit volume of plasma are *not* deficient in vitamin E, but rather are above 0.8 mg/g, the ratio of tocopherol to lipid previously reported as the lower limit of normal.

ACKNOWLEDGMENTS

We thank Drs. John Bieri, Joseph Fratantoni, Robert Wood, and Paul di Sant'Agnese for collaborating on aspects of this research involving patients with cystic fibrosis. The expert technical assistance of D. Jeannette Brown and Sze-Mei Lau is also greatly appreciated.

REFERENCES

1. HATAM, L. & H. J. KAYDEN. Tocopherol levels in needle aspiration biopsies of adipose tissue: normal subjects and abetalipoproteinemic patients. Ann. N.Y. Acad. Sci. (This volume.)
2. FARRELL, P. M. & L. J. MACHLIN. 1980. *In* Vitamin E, A Comprehensive Treatise. L. J. Machlin, Ed.: 519–620. Marcel Dekker. New York, N.Y.

3. FARRELL, P. M., J. G. BIERI, J. F. FRATANTONI, R. E. WOOD & P. A. DI SANT'AGNESE. 1977. The occurrence and effects of vitamin E deficiency: a study in patients with cystic fibrosis. J. Clin. Invest. **6**: 233-241.
4. GROSS, S. & D. K. MELHORN. 1972. Vitamin E, red cell lipids and red cell stability in prematurity. Ann. N.Y. Acad. Sci. **203**: 141-162.
5. HORWITT, M. K., C. C. HARVEY, C. H. DAHM, JR. & M. T. SEARCY. 1972. Relationship between tocopherol and serum lipid levels for determination of nutritional adequacy. Am. J. Acad. Sci. **203**: 223-236.
6. FARRELL, P. M., S. L. LEVINE, M. D. MURPHEY & A. J. ADAMS. 1978. Plasma tocopherol levels and tocopherol-lipid relationships in a normal population of children as compared to healthy adults. Am. J. Clin. Nutr. **31**: 1720-1726.
7. FARRELL, P. M. & J. G. BIERI. 1975. Megavitamin E supplementation in man. Am. J. Clin. Nutr. **28**: 1381-1386.
8. CASTILLO, R., C. LANDON, K. ECKHARDT, V. MORRIS, O. LEVANDER & N. LEWISTON. 1981. Selenium and vitamin E status in cystic fibrosis. J. Pediatr. **99**: 583-585.
9. BELL, E. F. & L. J. FILER, JR. 1981. The role of vitamin E in the nutrition of premature infants. Am. J. Clin. Nutr. **34**: 414-422.
10. GRAEBER, J. E., M. L. WILLIAMS & F. A. OSKI. 1977. The use of intramuscular vitamin E in the premature infant. J. Pediatr. **90**: 282-284.
11. EHRENKRANZ, R. A., B. W. BONTA, R. C. ABLOW & J. B. WARSHAW. 1978. Amelioration of bronchopulmonary dysplasia after vitamin E administration. N. Engl. J. Med. **229**: 565-569.
12. WOOD, R. E., T. F. BOAT & C. F. DOERSHUK. 1976. State of the art—cystic fibrosis. Am. Rev. Respir. Dis. **113**: 833-878.
13. BIERI, J. G. & E. L. PRIVAL. 1965. Serum vitamin E determined by thin-layer chromatography. Proc. Soc. Exp. Biol. Med. **120**: 554-557.
14. DE LA HUERGA, J., C. YESINICK & H. POPPER. 1953. Estimation of total serum lipids by a turbidimetric method. Am. J. Clin. Pathol. **23**: 1163-1167.
15. ROESCHLAN, P. L., E. BERNT & W. GRUBER. 1974. Enzymatic determination of total cholesterol in serum. Z. Klin. Chem. Klin. Biochem. **12**: 226.
16. HORWITT, M. K., C. C. HARVEY, G. D. DUNCAN & W. C. WILSON. 1956. Effects of limited tocopherol intake in man with relationship to erythrocyte hemolysis and lipid oxidation. Am. J. Clin. Nutr. **4**: 408-419.
17. The International Committee for Standardization in Hematology. 1971. Recommended methods for radio-isotope red cell survival studies. Blood **38**: 378-386.
18. HUBBARD, V. S., G. D. DUNN & P. A. DI SANT'AGNESE. 1977. Abnormal fatty acid compositions of plasma lipids in cystic fibrosis—a primary or secondary defect? Lancet **2**: 1302-1304.
19. FRIEDMAN, Z., A. DANON, M. T. STAHLMAN & J. A. OATES. 1976. Rapid onset of essential fatty acid deficiency in the newborn. Pediatrics **58**: 640-649.
20. HITTNER, H. M., L. B. GODIA, A. J. RUDOLPH, J. M. ADAMS, J. A. GARCIA-PRATS, Z. FRIEDMAN, J. A. KAUTZ & W. A. MONACO. 1981. Retrolental fibroplasia: efficacy of vitamin E in a double-blind clinical study of preterm infants. N. Engl. J. Med. **305**: 1365-1371.
21. BIERI, J. G. & P. M. FARRELL. 1976. Vitamin E. Vitam. Horm. **34**: 31-75.
22. WITTING, L. A. 1972. The role of polyunsaturated fatty acids in determining vitamin E requirement. Ann. N.Y. Acad. Sci. **203**: 192-198.
23. BIERI, J. G., T. L. J. TOLLIVER & G. L. CATIGNANI. 1979. Simultaneous determination of α-tocopherol and retinol in plasma or red cells by high pressure liquid chromatography. Am. J. Clin. Nutr. **32**: 2143-2149.
24. POUKKA, R. K. & J. G. BIERI. 1970. Blood α-tocopherol: erythrocyte and plasma relationships in vitro and in vivo. Lipids **5**: 757-761.

DISCUSSION

L. A. BARNESS (*University of South Florida, Tampa, Fla.*): It's my recollection that ceroid has been reported in the muscle of cystic fibrosis patients before α-tocopherol treatment.

P. M. FARRELL: Although ceroid pigment has been observed in smooth muscle, we did not find ceroid pigment deposition in the muscle of our patients.

G. J. HANDELMAN (*University of California, Santa Cruz, Calif.*): I think you've given a demonstration of the need for tocopherol to total lipid ratios, at least in children, that is unequivocally convincing. However, I've done some work with adults, and I've found the tocopherol to cholesterol ratio works extremely well with plasma values of 0.8 or greater. The total lipid assays have been very difficult for me to do. Can you tell us just a little bit about how you do your total lipid assay.

P. M. FARRELL: The procedure we've used is a turbidometric method carried out on total lipid extract. It correlates very well with the summation of the lipid subfractions in plasma, and it has been satisfactory from our point of view. You won't find clinical hospital laboratories doing this, however, because they tend to measure cholesterols or triglycerides.

I also think that in adults, unless there are abnormalities in lipid concentrations of plasma, you won't generally have difficulty in assessing tocopherol status. It's more the abnormal patients and children that present problems.

H. J. KAYDEN (*New York University School of Medicine, New York, N.Y.*): I'd agree to the last comment that you made that in adults, the direct measurement of tocopherol is probably as valuable as tocopherol-lipid ratios. It's in the children where changes in lipid level affect this ratio. I did want to comment, however, about all the effort that's being put forth in studying CF children. I suggest that an adipose tissue biopsy, which you did not comment on, might be something to add to your armamentarium in assessing the total tocopherol value. We've published a method, as has Jack Bieri, on high-pressure liquid chromatography that is quite sensitive. The posters will show this afternoon that this can be done on an adequate adipose tissue sample obtained by a simple needle aspiration technique. This makes it possible to measure not only the tocopherol levels but also the fatty acid distribution in the adipose tissue.

P. M. FARRELL: I want to point out, though, the major difficulty in obtaining the adipose tissue from premature infants. The deposition of adipose tissue is a late-gestational phenomenon—the last six to eight weeks—and I don't think it's going to help with premature infants. It may help with patients who have malabsorption.

I. D. DESAI (*University of British Columbia, Vancouver, B.C., Canada*): I'm happy to see that you are reemphasizing the usefulness of E to total lipids as an assessment method. However, we are still not clear on the cutoff line for normal. Should it be 0.6 or 0.8 mg/g total lipid with respect to infants? Are you still stressing 0.8?

P. M. FARRELL: I think that's a good question. I don't know where to draw the line. It must be somewhere between 0.6 and 1, but it is not clear where the line ought to be drawn. The value will likely depend on other indices of lipid status, such as polyunsaturated fatty acids. Even though 0.6–1.0 is broad, you'd rather have a margin of safety and for now should probably use a ratio of 1.0.

L. PACKER (*University of California, Berkeley, Calif.*): Thinking as a cell physiologist, it seems to me that in addition to having blood lipid E values and having good data on red cell hemolysis, it would be nice if we could go a step further and have in addition the actual amount of E in the lipids of the membrane of the particular cell involved—red cell or other cell membrane.

P. M. FARRELL: This is an important point. We've based quite a lot on the percentage of the hemolysis and hydrogen peroxide, but that's really not an ideal approach.

VITAMIN E AND INTRAVENTRICULAR HEMORRHAGE IN THE NEWBORN

Malcolm L. Chiswick, John Wynn,* and Nancy Toner

Department of Neonatal Medicine
North Western Regional Perinatal Center
St. Mary's Hospital
Manchester, M13 0JH, England

INTRODUCTION

One function of vitamin E (α-tocopherol) is to protect cell membranes against lipid peroxidation. Plasma vitamin E levels are lower in the newborn compared with adults,[1,2] and at birth the red blood cells (RBCs) of normal preterm and term babies have an increased susceptibility to hemolysis by hydrogen peroxide (H_2O_2).[3,4] A hemolytic anemia responsive to vitamin E has been described in vitamin E-deficient prematurely born babies, aged 6 to 10 weeks, fed proprietary formulas.[5] It is not surprising, because of its position in cellular function, that diverse roles have been suggested for vitamin E in the newborn, including protection against hyperbilirubinemia,[6] retrolental fibroplasia,[7] and bronchopulmonary dysplasia.[8] In a preliminary study designed to assess the efficacy of intramuscular vitamin E in increasing plasma vitamin E levels and reducing H_2O_2 hemolysis in preterm newborn babies, we made the unexpected observation that treated babies had a reduced incidence of intraventricular hemorrhage (IVH) compared with nontreated controls, and this is the subject of the present report.

PATIENTS AND METHOD

We studied 35 premature babies who were without major congenital malformation and who were cared for in the neonatal medical unit of this hospital during a 10-month period. Their gestational ages ranged from 25 to 36 weeks, and their birth weights from 550–1,750 g. Thirty (85.7%) had respiratory distress defined as a respiratory rate greater than 60 per minute and thoracic cage retraction on inspiration persisting for longer than 4 hours after birth. Those babies did not receive milk during the first 4 days of life, and their fluid needs were met by intravenous 10% dextrose (60–150 ml/kg per day). The remaining 5 babies received SMA-Gold Cap Milk (Wyeth Laboratories, Slough, England) by the nasogastric route, 60–150 ml/kg per day. Fourteen of the 35 babies were randomly selected to receive 20 mg per kg vitamin E (Ephynal, F. Hoffmann-La Roche and Co. Ltd., Basel, Switzerland) within 24 hours of birth and thereafter at daily intervals for a total of four doses. The concentration of the vitamin E solution was 100 mg per 2 ml, and individual doses greater than 0.5 ml were divided and given into two different injection sites to avoid a local inflammatory reaction. The 21 nontreated babies served as a control group.

A specimen of venous or arterial blood (1.5 ml, heparinized) was taken from each control baby within 24 hours of birth (day 0) and from treated babies

---

*Department of Obstetrics.

109

0077-8923/82/0393-0109 $01.75/0 © 1982, NYAS

TABLE 1

CAUSES OF RESPIRATORY DISTRESS

	n	Percent
IRDS	19	54.3
IRDS—congenital pneumonia	6	17.1
Congenital pneumonia	2	5.7
IRDS—pulmonary hemorrhage	2	5.7
Transient tachypnea	1	2.9
	30	85.7

immediately before they received their first dose of vitamin E (day 0). Further specimens were taken from each baby at daily intervals for three days (days 1, 2, and 3). Plasma vitamin E (total tocopherol) concentration was measured in each specimen using a calorimetric method in which ferrous ion produced by the reduction of ferric ion by vitamin E is used as an index of plasma vitamin E concentration.[9] The susceptibility of the red blood cells to peroxidation was measured in each specimen by the hydrogen peroxide (H_2O_2) hemolysis test using the method originally described by Rose and György and modified by Gordon, Nitowsky, and Cornblath.[10,11] Unless otherwise indicated, the paired or unpaired Student t-test was used for the statistical analysis of results.

RESULTS

Respiratory distress was present in 30 babies (85.7%), and the most common cause was idiopathic respiratory distress syndrome (IRDS) (TABLE 1). The mean birth weight and gestational age of babies in the treated and control groups were similar, and there was no significant difference in the incidence of birth asphyxia, respiratory distress, and the need for positive pressure ventilation for longer than 12 hours in the two groups (TABLE 2). The mean ± standard deviation (SD) plasma vitamin E level on day 0 was similar in treated (0.64 ± 0.2 mg per 100 ml) and

TABLE 2

CLINICAL DESCRIPTION, BIRTH WEIGHTS, AND GESTATIONAL AGES
OF VITAMIN E-TREATED BABIES AND CONTROLS

	Vitamin E (n = 14)		Control (n = 21)	
	n	Percent	n	Percent
Onset of respiration >1 minute*	10	71.4	14	66.7
Five-minute Apgar score <6	6	42.9	6	28.6
Respiratory distress	13	92.9	17	81.0
PPV >12 hours†	9	64.3	15	71.4
Birth weight (kg) (mean ± SD)	1.21 ± 0.29		1.25 ± 0.33	
Gestational age (weeks) (mean ± SD)	29.1 ± 3.3		29.3 ± 3.3	

*Spontaneous respiration not established within one minute of birth.
†Positive-pressure ventilation required for longer than 12 hours.

untreated babies (0.56 ± 0.2 mg per 100 ml). Thereafter treated babies had a pronounced rise in mean vitamin E levels in contrast to the stable low levels in untreated babies. The mean vitamin E level was significantly higher in treated babies on days 1, 2, and 3 ($p < 0.001$) (FIGURE 1). There was no correlation between plasma vitamin E levels and gestational age on day 0. However, the mean ± SD vitamin E level on day 0 in babies less than 30 weeks gestation (0.5 ± 0.19 mg per 100 ml) was lower compared with the more mature babies (0.72 ± 0.17 mg per 100 ml) ($p < 0.02$). The mean ± SD H_2O_2 hemolysis fell sharply in treated babies from 28.7% ± 17.4% on day 0 to 3.1% ± 1.9% on day 3, whereas the control babies had no significant change in mean ± SD H_2O_2 hemolysis from day 0 (31.5% ± 16.5%)

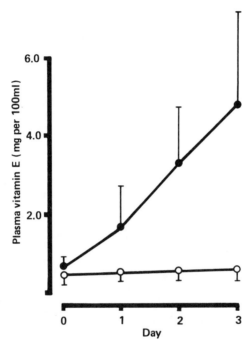

FIGURE 1. Mean ± SD plasma vitamin E levels in vitamin E–treated babies (filled circles) and controls (open circles). (All figures in this article © University Department of Medical Illustration, Royal Infirmary, Manchester, M13 9WL, England. Reproduced with permission.)

to day 3 (33.0% ± 15.4%). Treated babies had a significantly lower mean H_2O_2 hemolysis on day 1 ($p < 0.01$) and on days 2 and 3 ($p < 0.001$) compared with the control group (FIGURE 2).

Mortality and the incidence of IVH in treated and control groups are shown in TABLE 3. One of the 2 babies in the treated group who died had bilateral IVH at necropsy, but permission for necropsy was declined in the other baby, who died with intractable respiratory failure at 12 days. All the other deaths in the study occurred within 5 days of birth. All 6 control babies who died had IVH at necropsy, and 3 survivors had IVH diagnosed by the presence of an increasing

TABLE 3

MORTALITY AND INCIDENCE OF INTRAVENTRICULAR HEMORRHAGE
IN VITAMIN E-TREATED AND CONTROL BABIES

	Mortality		IVH	
	n	Percent	n	Percent
Vitamin E treated (n = 14)	2	14.3	2*	14.3
Control (n = 21)	6	28.6	9	42.9

*Includes one baby who died and did not have a necropsy.

head circumference and computerized tomography (CT) findings of dilated ventricles containing blood clots (1 baby); convulsions and uniformly blood-stained cerebrospinal fluid and CT confirmation of IVH (1 baby); and convulsions, a tense anterior fontanel, and uniformly bloodstained cerebrospinal fluid (1 baby). The 10 babies with IVH were all less than 30 weeks gestation. When only those babies less than 30 weeks gestation were considered, the incidence of IVH in the treated group (22.2%) was lower than in the control group (69.2%), even when it was assumed that the treated baby who did not have a necropsy suffered an IVH ($p < 0.05$, Fisher exact test) (TABLE 4). That patient was excluded in the further analysis of results.

Babies with and without IVH had a similar mean plasma vitamin E level on day 0. Thereafter those without IVH had a sharp rise in mean vitamin E levels whereas the mean level remained relatively low in those who suffered IVH (FIGURE 3.) The mean ± standard error of the mean (SEM) plasma vitamin E level on day 2 was significantly higher in babies who escaped IVH (2.07 ± 0.46 mg per 100 ml) compared with those who suffered IVH (0.6 ± 0.23 mg per 100 ml) ($p < 0.05$) (FIGURE 3). The contrast in vitamin E levels in babies with and without IVH was even more pronounced when only those babies less than 30 weeks gestation were considered. In those very premature babies without IVH, the rise in mean plasma vitamin E levels was significant from day 0 to day 1 ($p < 0.05$) and from day 1 to day 2 ($p < 0.01$) and the mean ± SEM vitamin E level on day 2 (2.58 ± 0.6 mg per 100 ml) was higher compared with those who suffered IVH (0.6 ± 0.11 mg) ($p < 0.025$) (FIGURE 4). At no time was there a significant difference in the mean H_2O_2 hemolysis result between babies with and without IVH.

TABLE 4

MORTALITY AND INCIDENCE OF INTRAVENTRICULAR HEMORRHAGE IN VITAMIN E-TREATED AND CONTROL BABIES LESS THAN 30 WEEKS GESTATION

	Mortality		IVH	
	n	Percent	n	Percent
Vitamin E treated (n = 9)	2	22.2	2*	22.2
Control (n = 13)	6	46.2	9	69.2†

*Includes one baby who died and did not have a necropsy.
†p < 0.05 (versus treated babies, Fisher exact probability test).

However, only those without IVH had a significant reduction in the mean H_2O_2 hemolysis from day 0 to day 1 (p < 0.02) and from day 1 to day 2 (p < 0.05) (FIGURE 5).

DISCUSSION

Plasma vitamin E levels in umbilical cord blood and in the newborn are lower compared with maternal levels, but most investigators have not shown significant

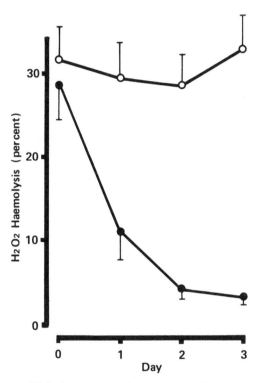

FIGURE 2. Mean ± SD hydrogen peroxide (H_2O_2) hemolysis (percent) in vitamin E–treated babies (filled circles) and controls (open circles).

differences in mean vitamin E levels at birth between preterm and mature babies.[1,2] Changes in plasma vitamin E after birth depend in part on the dietary intake of vitamin E and polyunsaturated fatty acid (PUFA).[12,13] Whether or not clinically normal preterm and term babies can be said to be truly vitamin E deficient is partly a question of semantics. Dju, Mason, and Filer showed that in fetuses and the newborn there was a positive linear relationship between total body tocopherol and lipid stores.[14] Others have shown a positive correlation between cord blood vitamin E levels and β-lipoprotein,[14] cholesterol,[16] and PUFA[17] concentrations, suggesting that the relatively low vitamin E levels in the

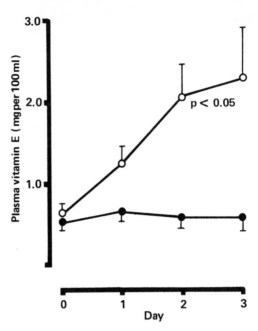

FIGURE 3. Mean ± SEM plasma vitamin E levels in babies with (filled circles) and without (open circles) intraventricular hemorrhage.

newborn may primarily reflect a low placental transport capacity of these lipids. One function of vitamin E is to protect the lipid membrane of cells from peroxidation, and irrespective of a definition of vitamin E deficiency, it is certain that the red blood cells of apparently normal preterm and term babies have increased H_2O_2 hemolysis, which is corrected by treatment with vitamin E.[3,4] Furthermore, a hemolytic anemia has been described in preterm babies that is associated with low circulatory levels of vitamin E and is reversed by treatment with vitamin E.[5] The present study confirms that the low plasma vitamin E levels at birth can be increased by vitamin E administration while rendering the RBCs less susceptible to H_2O_2 hemolysis. Although we observed no correlation between plasma vitamin E levels and gestational age, we did note that very premature babies less than 30 weeks gestation had a significantly lower mean plasma vitamin E concentration compared with more mature babies.

Neonatal intensive care, particularly ventilatory support, has contributed to the widely reported improved survival rates of very premature babies. However, one factor that limits both their survival and the long-term prognosis of survivors is IVH, which is prone to occur during the first week of life, particularly in babies born very prematurely. Many factors apart from prematurity are thought to contribute to the etiology of IVH,[18] including hypoxemia, hypercapnia, increase in cerebral blood flow, and the rapid correction of blood pH by hyperosmolar alkali solutions. It is therefore not surprising that babies with respiratory distress are prone to IVH. The population of babies in the present study had an increased risk of IVH by virtue of the high incidence of respiratory distress and the large proportion of babies less than 30 weeks gestation. An unexpected finding was a lower incidence of IVH in babies less than 30 weeks gestation who had been given vitamin E supplements. The incidence of clinical factors that might influence the occurrence of IVH—such as birth asphyxia, respiratory distress, and its severity as judged by the need for positive pressure ventilation—was similar in the vitamin E-treated and control groups, as was the mean gestational age of babies in the two groups. The lower incidence of IVH in the treated group cannot be explained on the basis of a reduced susceptibility. Babies under 30 weeks gestation with or without IVH had a similar mean plasma vitamin E level in the first 24 hours after birth; thereafter those who escaped IVH had a sharp rise in the mean level, whereas in those who suffered IVH the vitamin E level remained stable and low. This is in keeping with vitamin E exerting a protective effect against IVH in preterm babies. The changes in H_2O_2 hemolysis are more difficult to interpret. It is true that a significant reduction in mean H_2O_2 hemolysis occurred only in the groups of babies without IVH, but those groups had rather high mean H_2O_2 hemolysis values in the first 24 hours. Babies with IVH subsequently did have a higher mean H_2O_2 hemolysis result compared with unaffected babies, but this difference was not significant.

The origin of IVH is periventricular bleeding emanating from small vessels, predominantly immature capillaries in the subependymal germinal matrix.[18] The

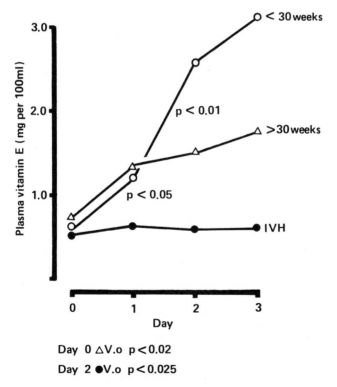

Day 0 △V.o $p < 0.02$
Day 2 ●V.o $p < 0.025$

FIGURE 4. Mean plasma vitamin E levels in babies without intraventricular hemorrhage less than 30 weeks gestation (open circles), more than 30 weeks gestation (open triangles), and in those with intraventricular hemorrhage (filled circles).

hemorrhage ruptures through the ependyma into the ventricles. There are many reports suggesting that vitamin E has an antipurpuric action in animals and humans, including newborn babies.[19-22] The precise mechanism of this action is not very well understood. It is speculative that in some examples of purpura, vitamin E reduces capillary fragility by protecting the endothelial membrane from lipid peroxidation. The relationship between vitamin E and platelets is complex and paradoxical. Thrombocytosis and platelet hyperaggregability are features of vitamin E deficiency in infancy and are reversed by vitamin E

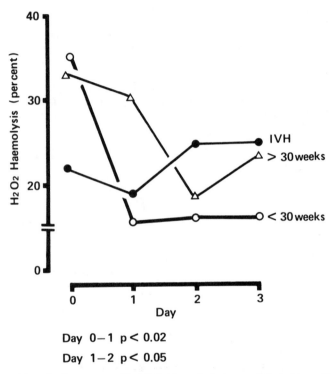

Day 0−1 p< 0.02
Day 1−2 p< 0.05

FIGURE 5. Mean hydrogen peroxide (H_2O_2) hemolysis (percent) in babies without intraventricular hemorrhage less than 30 weeks gestation (open circles), more than 30 weeks gestation (open triangles), and in those with intraventricular hemorrhage (filled circles).

treatment.[23] Vitamin E excess may also inhibit platelet aggregation.[24] The results of our study support a hypothesis that vitamin E deficiency contributes to the etiology of IVH in babies born very prematurely. The immature capillary walls of the germinal layer might be unstable as a result of lipid peroxidation. Germinal layer hemorrhage and IVH are uncommon in stillborn babies.[25] The normal arterial P_{O_2} of a fetus is only 25 mm Hg or less, and one may speculate that capillary membranes may be relatively protected against lipid peroxidation in utero. Further support for vitamin E protecting against IVH comes from the veterinary sciences. In 1931, Pappenheimer and Goettsch described a cerebellar disorder in chicks probably caused by vitamin E deficiency.[26] Edema, necrosis, and hemorrhage were the pathological hallmarks. Subsequently it was established that nutritional encephalopathy was a feature in growing chicks with incompletely mature brains fed diets deficient in vitamin E and enriched with linoleic acid. The microcirculation of the central nervous system (CNS) is primarily involved, and progressive endothelial cell changes occur including lysosomal activity.[27] The latter is of interest in the light of vitamin E's role, in combination with selenium, in stabilizing lysosomes and preventing lipid peroxidation of membranes of subcellular organelles.[28] Another related vitamin E deficiency disease occurring in fetal hamsters is spontaneous hemorrhagic necrosis of the CNS.[29] The initial lesion does indeed involve the subependymal vasculature in 12- or 13-day-old fetuses, and progression to IVH and CNS necrosis is moderated by treatment of the dams with vitamin E.

Further studies in premature babies will elucidate whether our findings can be repeated or whether they were chance observations. We are currently conducting a randomized trial of vitamin E in preterm babies less than 1,750 g birth weight, using daily ultrasound examination of the head so that the earliest stages of germinal layer hemorrhage and its progression may be identified. Vitamin E is a relatively safe drug,[30,31] and should it prove to be beneficial in the prevention of IVH, prior treatment of mothers in premature labor or before elective cesarean section is possible so that babies might benefit from higher vitamin E levels from birth.

ACKNOWLEDGMENTS

We are very grateful to F. Hoffmann-La Roche and Co. Ltd., Basel, Switzerland, for the gift of Ephynal. We thank Mrs. M. O'Donnell for her secretarial help.

REFERENCES

1. MOYER, W. T. 1950. Vitamin E levels in term and premature newborn infants. Pediatrics **6:** 893–896.
2. WRIGHT, S. W., L. J. FILER, JR. & K. E. MASON. 1951. Vitamin E blood levels in premature and full term infants. Pediatrics **7:** 386–393.
3. GYÖRGY, P., G. COGAN & C. S. ROSE. 1952. Availability of vitamin E in the newborn infant. Proc. Soc. Exp. Biol. Med. **81:** 536–538.
4. MACKENZIE, J. B. 1954. Relation between serum tocopherol and hemolysis in hydrogen peroxide of erythrocytes in premature infants. Pediatrics **13:** 346–351.
5. OSKI, F. A. & L. A. BARNESS. 1967. Vitamin E deficiency: a previously unrecognized cause of hemolytic anemia in the premature infant. J. Pediatr. **70:** 211–220.
6. GROSS, S. J. 1979. Vitamin E and neonatal bilirubinaemia. Pediatrics **64:** 321–323.
7. JOHNSON, L., D. SCHAFFER & T. R. BOGGS, JR. 1974. The premature infant, vitamin E deficiency and retrolental fibroplasia. Am. J. Clin. Nutr. **27:** 1158–1173.
8. EHRENKRANZ, R. A., B. W. BONTA, R. C. ABLOW & J. B. WARSHAW. 1978. Amelioration of bronchopulmonary dysplasia after vitamin E administration. N. Engl. J. Med. **299:** 564–569.
9. MARTINEK, R. G. 1964. Method for determination of vitamin E (total tocopherols) in serum. Clin. Chem. **10:** 1078–1086.
10. ROSE, C. S. & P. GYÖRGY. 1952. Specificity of hemolytic reaction in vitamin E deficient erythrocytes. Am. J. Physiol. **168:** 414–420.
11. GORDON, H. H., H. M. NITOWSKY & M. CORNBLATH. 1955. Studies of tocopherol

deficiency in infants and children. I. Hemolysis of erythrocytes in hydrogen peroxides. Am. J. Dis. Child. **90:** 669–681.

12. WILLIAMS, M. L., R. J. SHOTT, P. L. O'NEAL & F. A. OSKI. 1975. Role of dietary iron and fat on vitamin E deficiency anemia of infancy. N. Engl. J. Med. **292:** 887–890.

13. VILLALAZ, R. A., N. TONER & M. L. CHISWICK. 1981. Dietary vitamin E and polyunsaturated fatty acid (PUFA) in newborn babies with physiological jaundice. Early Hum. Dev. **5:** 145–150.

14. DJU, M. Y., K. E. MASON & L. J. FILER, JR. 1952. Vitamin E (tocopherol) in human fetuses and placentae. Etudes Néo-Natales **1:** 49–60.

15. HÅGÅ, P. & G. LUNDE. 1978. Selenium and vitamin E in cord blood from preterm and full term infants. Acta Paediatr. Scand. **67:** 735–739.

16. JAGADEESAN, V. & K. PREMA. 1980. Plasma tocopherol and lipid levels in mother and umbilical cord; influence on birthweight. Br. J. Obstet. Gynaecol. **87:** 908–910.

17. MARTINEZ, F. E., A. L. GONCALVES, S. M. JORGE & I. D. DESAI. 1981. Vitamin E in placental blood and its inter-relationship to maternal and newborn levels of vitamin E. J. Pediatr. **99:** 298–300.

18. PAPE, K. E. & J. S. WIGGLESWORTH. 1979. Haemorrhage, Ischaemia and the Perinatal Brain. Spastics International Medical Publications. William Heinemann Medical Books, London, and J.B. Lippincott Co., Philadelphia.

19. SKELTON, F., E. SHUTE, H. G. SKINNER & R. A. WAUD. 1946. Anti-purpuric action of α-tocopherol (vitamin E). Science **103:** 762.

20. MINKOWSKI, A. 1950. La resistance vasculaire du nouveau-né et la prévention des hémorragies cerebro-méningées du prématuré. Ann. Paediatr. **174:** 80–86.

21. BECKMANN, R., H. JATZKO & J. SCHNEIDER. 1963. Klinische und experimentelle Befunde über den Einfluss von α-Tocopherol (Vitamin E) auf die Capillarresistenz bei Neugeborenen. Klin. Wochenschr. **41:** 1043–1048.

22. FUJII, T. 1972. The clinical effects of vitamin E on purpuras due to vascular defects. J. Vitaminol. **18:** 125–130.

23. LAKE, A. M., M. J. STUART & F. A. OSKI. 1977. Vitamin E deficiency and enhanced platelet function: reversal following E supplementation. J. Pediatr. **90:** 722–725.

24. STUART, M. J. & F. A. OSKI. 1979. Vitamin E and platelet function. Am. J. Pediatr. Hematol. Oncol. **1:** 77–82.

25. HARCKE, H. T., R. L. NAEYE, A. STORCH & W. A. BLANC. 1972. Perinatal cerebral intraventricular hemorrhage. J. Pediatr. **80:** 37–42.

26. PAPPENHEIMER, A. M. & M. GOETTSCH. 1931. A cerebellar disorder in chicks, apparently of nutritional origin. J. Exp. Med. **53:** 11–26.

27. NELSON, J. S. 1980. Pathology of vitamin E deficiency. In Vitamin E, A Comprehensive Treatise. L. J. Machlin, Ed.: 407–413. Marcel Dekker. New York, N.Y.

28. COMBS, G. F., JR., T. NOGUCHI & M. L. SCOTT. 1975. Mechanisms of action of selenium and vitamin E in protection of biological membranes. Fed. Proc. **34:** 2090–2095.

29. KEELER, R. F. & S. YOUNG. 1979. Role of vitamin E in the aetiology of spontaneous hemorrhagic necrosis of the central nervous system of fetal hamsters. Teratology **20:** 127–132.

30. ZIPURSKY, A., R. A. MILNER, V. S. BLANCHETTE & M. A. JOHNSTON. 1980. Effect of vitamin E therapy on blood coagulation tests in newborn infants. Pediatrics **66:** 547–550.

31. 1981. Safety of vitamin E therapy in low birthweight infants. Nutr. Rev. **39**(3): 121–123.

DISCUSSION

M. A. GUGGENHEIM (*University of Colorado Medical Center, Denver, Colo.*): We've done quite a bit of work with germinal matrix hemorrhage and IVH in

Denver—not relating to vitamin E, I might say. I have two questions relating to your obviously tentative conclusions. One has to do with time and the other has to do with other risk factors, both of which have received a lot of attention. You alluded to timing these hemorrhages. We and a number of others around the country have done sequential studies with ultrasound; and indeed it appears that the vast majority of the initial germinal matrix hemorrhage occurs within that first 24 hours, certainly by 36 hours. Since you mentioned in your protocol that often the first injection was given within 24 hours, I wonder if indeed the hemorrhage might already have occurred and, therefore, if the vitamin E response is an epi phenomenon.

The second question relates to looking more carefully at other possible risk factors. For instance, a number of studies now suggest the extreme importance of volume expansion as a pathogenic factor.

M. L. CHISWICK: To answer the second question first, a retrospective review of the case notes included an estimation of the total volumes received by these infants expressed per kilogram body weight per day in the two groups of babies. It was similar in both the treated and control groups. However, that will not exclude sudden bolus injections and sudden volume expansion. I agree with your point.

Regarding your first question, the relationship of the timing of the bleeding, yes, you are so right. It could well be that the first dose of vitamin E in some of these babies was in fact given after the subependymal hemorrhage started, and we have some preliminary results from our ultrasound studies. We studied a total of about 32 babies, approximately 16 in each group. If you lump together subependymal bleeding—the very earliest stage with no hemorrhage—and compare that with babies that had what we call grade II hemorrhage or more—that means bleeding into the ventricles themselves—our preliminary ultrasound studies show that there is a reduced incidence, not of subependymal bleeding, but of intraventricular bleeding in babies that have been supplemented with vitamin E. It's preliminary, and it's not significant statistically yet.

R. E. OLSON (*St. Louis University School of Medicine, St. Louis, Mo.*): Dr. Chiswick, on the point of other risk factors, did you evaluate the vitamin K status of these infants?

M. L. CHISWICK: No, all our babies are given one milligram of vitamin K at birth.

A. ANGEL (*University of Toronto, Toronto, Ont., Canada*): Two clinical questions. Would you recommend that mothers of infants at risk, for example, cesarean section, diabetic mothers, be supplemented with vitamin E to increase available E to the baby *in utero*? And second, for premature infants on a nutrient prescription given Intralipid that contains α-tocopherol, do you think that that is a therapeutic advantage?

M. L. CHISWICK: As far as supplementing mothers is concerned, I wouldn't dream of suggesting that they ought to be. I'm speculating that if our second study confirms an association between vitamin E treatment in the baby and a reduction of intraventricular hemorrhage, then we could go on to supplement mothers. But I don't think the evidence is strong enough at present.

Regarding your other question, yes, the tocopherol in Intralipid is interesting, but certainly on our unit we do not give babies Intralipid in the first weeks of life. It's only when they are developing chronic respiratory illness and feeding difficulties that we go on to total parenteral nutrition. And by that time, the problem of IVH isn't a major problem inasmuch as it has already occurred.

L. A. BARNESS (*University of South Florida, Tampa, Fla.*): I would like to caution about vitamin E in Intralipid. Some is tocopherol, but most of it is not

α-tocopherol. It's a bunch of other stuff and does not prevent hemolysis in the premature infant.

P. M. FARRELL (*University of Wisconsin, Madison, Wis.*): Just two related points as far as Intralipid is concerned. There are a number of neonatal units that are infusing Intralipid without giving vitamin E supplements, and this may turn out to be quite risky because of the marginal tocopherol status in these patients. The fact is, I think, that 80 to 90% of the tocopherol is γ rather than α in the Intralipid.

Another point. Just because a mother takes supplements of tocopherol, this will not necessarily mean that the fetus or the newborn will have a higher concentration of tocopherol, because of the relatively inefficient transport of lipid and fat-soluble substances across the placenta.

M. L. CHISWICK: Right. What I had in mind, in fact, was the intravenous injection of large doses of vitamin E during premature labor, where the situation might be different and transfer might occur more readily.

N. J. M. CARRASCO (*Albany Medical College, Albany, N.Y.*): My first question concerns the relationship of IVH to other risk factors, such as osmotic shifts, correction of acid-base balance, and also the degree of hypoxemia that might have persisted during your assisted ventilation. Can you give us this information on your two groups.

M. L. CHISWICK: Yes, but only in a crude retrospective way. We looked at the blood gas charts of the babies, and in unventilated babies we calculated the mean arterial P_{O_2}, the mean arterial CO_2, and the mean pH. There was no significant difference in the two groups, but retrospective studies such as this are fraught with problems.

N. J. M. CARRASCO: My second question is, How did you pick your dose of vitamin E?

M. L. CHISWICK: In the literature, this dose has been used in at least three previous papers. The investigators have found that it has reduced the initial hydrogen peroxide hemolysis test results.

I. D. DESAI (*University of British Columbia, Vancouver, B.C., Canada*): I want to support Dr. Farrell's concern that injecting mothers with vitamin E is by no means going to increase the concentration of E in the newborn unless it's injected into the placenta itself.

R. L. BAEHNER (*Indiana University, Indianapolis, Ind.*): Dr. Chiswick, did you have an opportunity to look at the total granulocyte counts? Ohe at Rhode Island has done some work to show that respiratory distress in some newborns is perhaps related to leucocyte aggregation in the lung. This might occur in other areas, which in turn might lead to endothelial damage through release of free radicals from granulocytes.

M. L. CHISWICK: We didn't look at granulocyte counts.

VITAMIN E AND TOTAL PARENTERAL NUTRITION*

Peter M. Thurlow and John P. Grant†

Department of Surgery
Duke University Medical Center
Durham, North Carolina 27710

Study of vitamin E requirements during total parenteral nutrition (TPN) has been complicated by the rarity of and difficulty in defining vitamin E deficiency in humans. Though normal adults possess extensive body stores of vitamin E, patients requiring TPN may have depleted vitamin E stores due to chronic malnutrition. With the initiation of TPN, dietary intake is interrupted and intravenous vitamin E supplementation is limited, placing these patients at risk of developing vitamin E deficiency. Though few tests for human vitamin E deficiency exist, platelet hyperaggregation and *in vitro* peroxide-induced hemolysis have been correlated with low plasma vitamin E concentrations in children.[1] Such correlations are complicated, however, by the influence of dietary unsaturated fatty acid intake on plasma vitamin E and by other factors known to influence platelet aggregation, such as essential fatty acid deficiency (EFAD), a state commonly seen during TPN.[2-5]

In this study we evaluated two groups of patients for development of vitamin E deficiency during TPN support. One group received fat-free TPN supplemented with *all-rac-α*-tocopherol, and the other group received TPN supplemented with 1 to 2 liters of a 10% fat emulsion per week. Our objectives were to determine the incidence of vitamin E deficiency during TPN based on plasma vitamin E concentration, abnormal platelet aggregation, and increased *in vitro* peroxide-induced hemolysis. In addition, using a water-miscible form of *all-rac-α*-tocopherol, the requirements for vitamin E were determined as well as possible effects of EFAD and intravenous fat administration upon those requirements.

MATERIALS AND METHODS

Forty-three patients referred to the Duke Nutritional Support Service with projected TPN requirements of at least two weeks without surgery were studied after informed consent was obtained. Initial nutritional assessment—including weight, triceps skin-fold thickness, arm muscle area, creatinine excretion, serum albumin and transferrin, and reactivity to common skin test antigens[6]—allowed calculation of Mullen's prognostic nutritional index (PNI), which has been useful in the evaluation of the presence and severity of malnutrition [PNI = % risk of postoperative complication = 158 − 16.6 (albumin) − 0.78 (triceps skin-fold thickness) − 0.2 (transferrin) − 5.8 (delayed hypersensitivity score)].[7]

Patients were divided into two groups, an early group (A) of 19 and a later group (B) of 24 patients. Group A did not receive routine intravenous fat emulsion. Serum fatty acids were monitored weekly for evidence of essential fatty acid deficiency by the ratio of 5,8,11-eicosatrienoic acid to arachidonic acid (triene-tetraene ratio). Intralipid 10% (Cutter Laboratories), 1.0 liter per week, was given

*Supported by National Institutes of Health Fellowship No. 1F32AM06160-01A1.
†Author to whom reprint requests should be addressed.

in this group when the triene-tetraene ratio became greater than 0.4 or upon failure to gain weight after prolonged fat-free TPN even with a normal triene-tetraene ratio. Group B patients routinely received 1.0 liter per week of an intravenous fat emulsion (Intralipid, 10%), increasing to 1.5–2.0 liters per week if EFAD developed despite fat supplementation. All patients received the same standard TPN solution containing 4.2% crystalline amino acids (Freamine II, McGaw Laboratories) and 25% dextrose to provide 1.8 to 2.1 times basal energy requirements (estimated from the Harris-Benedict formula), along with appropriate electrolytes and minerals. Daily vitamin supplementation in both groups included 2.5 IU vitamin E with vitamins A, D, and B-complex vitamins as ½ ampule Multi-Vitamin Infusion (MVI) (USV Laboratories, Inc.) mixed in the TPN solution. Group A patients received an additional 50 mg vitamin E intravenously daily using an experimental water-miscible form of all-rac-α-tocopherol (Hoffmann-La Roche Inc., Nutley, N.J., IND no. 14927) if abnormal platelet aggregation was observed or plasma vitamin E concentrations remained below 0.5 mg% for one week during TPN. Two of the Group B patients also received additional all-rac-α-tocopherol in the TPN solution when platelet hyperaggregation persisted even after Intralipid supplementation.

TABLE 1

UNDERLYING DISEASE PROCESS IN PATIENTS REQUIRING TPN*

	Group A	Group B
Inflammatory bowel disease	2	2
Enterocutaneous fistula	3	8
Short bowel syndrome	3	0
Cancer	6	7
Radiation enteritis	2	0
Small bowel obstruction	2	0
Peptic ulcer disease or pancreatitis	3	7

*Some patients were included more than once, due to multiple underlying diseases.

Weekly measurements of plasma vitamin E concentration, platelet aggregation, in vitro peroxide-induced hemolysis, and triene-tetraene ratios were made. Plasma vitamin E was measured colorimetrically according to the method of Quaife et al.[8] Plasma E concentrations less than 0.5 mg% were considered to represent a deficiency state. In vitro peroxide-induced hemolysis was performed according to the method of Binder et al.,[9] except for the use of 1% rather than 2% hydrogen peroxide for the red blood cell incubations. Hemolysis greater than 10% was considered abnormal. Triene-tetraene ratios were measured by gas liquid chromatography of hexane-extracted saponified serum by the method of Gerhardt and Gehrke.[10] Ratios greater than 0.4 have generally been accepted as a biochemical indicator of EFAD.[3,11] Platelet aggregation studies were performed on a BIO/DATA Corp. PAP-3 platelet aggregation profiler following standard methods.[12] Threshold concentrations of adenosine diphosphate (ADP) and epinephrine required to produce irreversible aggregation were determined using freshly mixed dilutions of ADP and epinephrine (Sigma Chemical Co., St. Louis, Mo.) ranging from 50 to 0.05 μM. Irreversible aggregation was observed with between 2 and 5 μM of either ADP or epinephrine in platelet-rich plasma (PRP) from a group of normal volunteers. Abnormal platelet aggregation (hyperaggrega-

TABLE 2

MEAN PLASMA VITAMIN E CONCENTRATIONS IN PATIENTS WITH NORMAL VERSUS
ABNORMAL PLATELET AGGREGATION AND PEROXIDE-INDUCED HEMOLYSIS

	Test Results		
Test	Normal	Abnormal	p
Platelet aggregation	0.71 ± 0.03*	0.40 ± 0.4	<0.001
Peroxide-induced hemolysis	0.64 ± 0.04	0.56 ± 0.05	NS

*Mean vitamin E concentration in mg per 100 ml $\pm$ SEM.

tion) was therefore defined as irreversible aggregation in response to less than 1 μM ADP or epinephrine.

RESULTS

The mean PNI following initial nutritional assessment was $58.7 \pm 10.2\%$ for Group A and $71.7 \pm 4.05\%$ for Group B [mean $\pm$ standard error of the mean (SEM), p < 0.05 by t-test], indicating the presence of moderate to severe malnutrition in both groups. The underlying disease processes leading to TPN are shown in TABLE 1. Results of initial platelet function, peroxide-induced hemolysis, and plasma vitamin E concentrations are presented in TABLES 2 and 3. Mean plasma vitamin E concentration for all patients was 0.59 mg%, with half of the patients having concentrations less than 0.5 mg%. TABLE 2 gives mean plasma vitamin E concentrations in patients with normal versus abnormal platelet aggregation and in vitro peroxide-induced hemolysis. Plasma vitamin E concentrations were significantly lower in patients with abnormal platelet aggregation but not in those with abnormal peroxide-induced hemolysis. TABLE 3 relates the incidence of abnormal platelet aggregation or peroxide-induced hemolysis to plasma vitamin E concentrations. Half the patients tested exhibited platelet hyperaggregation and abnormal peroxide-induced hemolysis as well as vitamin E deficiency. Contingency table analysis, however, demonstrated only platelet hyperaggregation to be correlated with vitamin E deficiency ($\chi^2 = 30$, p < 0.001). Intravenous all-rac-α-tocopherol supplementation in Group A and in two patients in Group B significantly increased plasma vitamin E concentrations and corrected abnormal

TABLE 3

ABNORMAL PLATELET AGGREGATION AND PEROXIDE-INDUCED RED CELL HEMOLYSIS IN
PATIENTS WITH NORMAL VERSUS LOW PLASMA VITAMIN E CONCENTRATIONS

Plasma Vitamin E Concentration (mg%)	Abnormal Platelet Aggregation	Abnormal Peroxide-Induced Hemolysis
<0.5 (low)	21/22 (95%)*	12/23 (52%)*
>0.5 (normal)	3/23 (13%)	11/16 (69%)
	p < 0.001†	NS†

*Number abnormal of total patients tested, (x) = percent abnormal.
†By χ^2 analysis.

TABLE 4

CHANGES IN SERUM VITAMIN E CONCENTRATION, PLATELET AGGREGATION, AND
PEROXIDE-INDUCED RED CELL HEMOLYSIS WITH 50 MG/DAY α-TOCOPHEROL
SUPPLEMENTATION TO ROUTINE, FAT-FREE TPN

	Before TPN	After TPN with Vitamin E Supplementation	p
Plasma vitamin E concentration (mg% ± SEM)	0.523 ± 0.06	1.25 ± 0.13	<0.001
Platelet aggregation (abnormal/total, % abnormal)	10/11 (91%)	4/11 (36%)*	<0.001
Peroxide-induced red cell hemolysis (normal/abnormal, % abnormal)	8/10 (80%)	0/10 (0%)	<0.001

*All 4 not correcting had EFAD.

peroxide-induced hemolysis and platelet hyperaggregation, with the exception of four patients, all of whom also had EFAD (TABLE 4).

TABLE 5 summarizes results in 11 of the 24 patients in Group B who remained on fat-supplemented TPN long enough for repeat platelet aggregation and peroxide-induced hemolysis testing. In these patients, neither plasma vitamin E, platelet aggregation, nor peroxide-induced hemolysis changed significantly with one to two liters of intravenous fat emulsion per week. Of the 24 Group B patients, EFAD was observed at least once during TPN in 7 patients despite routine fat supplementation. TABLE 6 gives all platelet aggregation results, triene-tetraene levels, and vitamin E concentrations in Group B, including more than one set of results per patient. The relationship between vitamin E deficiency and abnormal platelet aggregation observed in Group A patients existed only in the absence of EFAD in Group B patients. In the presence of EFAD, the incidence of platelet hyperaggregation was independent of plasma vitamin E concentration.

Five of the seven patients in Group B with EFAD remained on TPN and intravenous fat emulsions long enough for multiple plasma vitamin E, platelet aggregation, peroxide-induced hemolysis, and triene-tetraene ratio determinations. One had normal plasma vitamin E concentrations and platelet aggregation

TABLE 5

CHANGES IN PLASMA VITAMIN E CONCENTRATION, PLATELET AGGREGATION, AND
PEROXIDE-INDUCED RED CELL HEMOLYSIS WITH ADDITION OF 1 TO 2 LITERS FAT
EMULSION PER WEEK TO ROUTINE TPN

	Before TPN	After TPN with Lipid Emulsion	p
Plasma vitamin E concentration (mg% ± SEM)	0.55 ± 0.07	0.61 ± 0.07	NS
Platelet aggregation (abnormal/total, % abnormal)	7/10 (70%)	5/10 (50%)	NS
Peroxide-induced red cell hemolysis (abnormal/total, % abnormal)	9/11 (82%)	10/11 (91%)	NS

throughout his clinical course (enterocutaneous fistulae following an abdominal gunshot wound), and EFAD was corrected by 1.0 liter of fat emulsion weekly. Another had severe vitamin E deficiency (0.25 mg%) and platelet hyperaggregation throughout his TPN course (for Crohn's disease), yet EFAD was corrected with 1.0 liter of fat emulsion weekly. The other three patients, all with enterocutaneous fistulae (two following abdominal surgery for benign disease, and one following resection of a colon carcinoma), exhibited initial vitamin E deficiency, EFAD, and platelet hyperaggregation. Supplementation with up to 2.0 liters fat emulsion weekly for one month corrected the plasma vitamin E deficiency in all three but did not correct EFAD or platelet hyperaggregation. Addition of 50 mg intravenous *all-rac-α*-tocopherol daily in two of the three patients raised vitamin E concentrations further, but EFAD and platelet hyperaggregation again persisted. One of these two then received 100 mg intravenous *all-rac-α*-tocopherol per day, which raised plasma vitamin E concentration to 1.63 mg% and corrected platelet hyperaggregation, though EFAD persisted despite 1.5 liters of fat emulsion per week. The other patient underwent operative closure of her enterocutaneous fistula and normalized platelet function and EFAD on an oral diet, though

TABLE 6

EFFECT OF ESSENTIAL FATTY ACID DEFICIENCY ON PLATELET AGGREGATION*

	Normal Triene-Tetraene Ratio		High Triene-Tetraene Ratio	
	Normal E†	Low E	Normal E	Low E
Normal platelet aggregation	20	1	2	0
Platelet hyperaggregation	3	12	13	6
p (χ^2)	<0.00001		NS	

*Combined results of all determinations of triene-tetraene ratios, platelet aggregation, and vitamin E concentrations in Group B patients (more than one set of results per patient).
†Low E <0.5 mg%.

plasma vitamin E concentration dropped to the presupplementation level. The third patient also corrected platelet function upon resumption of an oral diet. The clinical courses of the two patients with EFAD who received both fat emulsion and *all-rac-α*-tocopherol are shown in FIGURE 1.

DISCUSSION

The population of malnourished patients receiving TPN provides an opportunity for the study of vitamin E deficiency and its interaction with EFAD. Half of our moderately to severely malnourished patients receiving TPN were found to have deficient plasma vitamin E concentrations, platelet hyperaggregation, and abnormal peroxide-induced hemolysis. Vitamin E deficiency in humans has traditionally been defined by increased *in vitro* peroxide-induced hemolysis.[9] The patients tested here exhibited an incidence of abnormal peroxide-induced hemolysis similar to the incidence of vitamin E deficiency (~50%), but the two did not correlate with each other (TABLES 2 and 3). The lack of correlation implies a

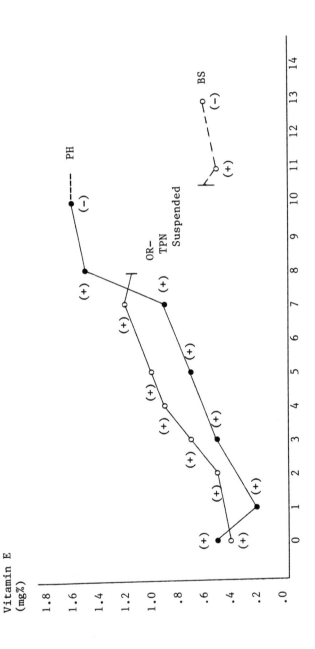

FIGURE 1. Clinical course of two patients (PH, BS) with enterocutaneous fistulae. Intralipid 1.5 l/week and 1.0 l/week (BS only); all-*rac*-α-tocopherol 50 mg/day and 100 mg/day (PH only). Open circles, BS; closed circles, PH; (+), abnormal aggregation; (−), normal aggregation; solid line, triene-tetraene ratio > 0.4 (EFAD); dashed line, triene-tetraene ratio < 0.4.

more general defect in the red cell membrane than that caused by vitamin E deficiency alone. Platelet hyperaggregation, on the other hand, did correlate with vitamin E deficiency in the absence of EFAD, confirming similar results in children with cystic fibrosis.[13] Correction of both platelet and red blood cell abnormalities by intravenous all-rac-α-tocopherol confirms a role for vitamin E in the stabilization of both cell membranes.

In the absence of oral intake, vitamin E intake during TPN is easily quantitated. Fat-free TPN with standard vitamin supplementation provides 2.5 mg vitamin E per day. This level of vitamin E support during TPN has been associated with slowly decreasing plasma vitamin E concentrations.[11] The addition of 25 mg all-rac-α-tocopherol in previous studies has raised plasma vitamin E concentrations to the low normal range (0.8 mg%).[14,15] In this study, addition of 50 mg all-rac-α-tocopherol per day raised plasma vitamin E concentrations to high normal (1.2 mg%) and corrected abnormal platelet aggregation and peroxide-induced hemolysis in the absence of EFAD. It therefore appears that 25 to 50 mg of vitamin E are required during fat-free TPN in the absence of EFAD instead of the current recommended daily allowance (RDA) of 5–15 mg.

Routine addition of 1.0 to 2.0 liters of intravenous fat emulsion per week (Intralipid, 10%) during TPN adds another 12–24 mg of γ-tocopherol,[16] increasing the daily infusion of vitamin E from 2.5 mg in MVI to 4 to 6 mg total, similar to the RDA for vitamin E. This amount of vitamin E supplementation, however, did not significantly change plasma vitamin E concentrations in our experience, nor did it correct abnormal platelet aggregation or peroxide-induced hemolysis in Group B patients. This result could be due to metabolic ineffectiveness of γ-tocopherol or to increased vitamin E requirements with infusion of fat emulsions during TPN. The latter would be consistent with animal studies in which vitamin E requirements were proportional to dietary intake of unsaturated fatty acids.[2] The former has been well documented, with γ-tocopherol exhibiting only a fraction of the metabolic activity of α-tocopherol.[16] The colorimetric assay used in this study measures total tocopherols and does not distinguish between γ- and α-tocopherol. A functional vitamin E deficiency might therefore develop during Intralipid-10% emulsion administration in spite of normal plasma vitamin E concentrations, which is consistent with the observed abnormal platelet aggregation and increased peroxide-induced hemolysis that persisted despite up to two liters of Intralipid-10% weekly. Use of a different fat emulsion (Liposyn, Abbott Laboratories) with a vitamin E content that is both greater (20 mg/liter) and entirely α- rather than γ-tocopherol[16] might give different results than those observed here with Intralipid.

The failure of 50 mg all-rac-α-tocopherol daily to correct platelet hyperaggregation in two patients after prolonged fat emulsion administration implies either an even greater vitamin E requirement during fat emulsion administration or a separate platelet defect due to EFAD that is unresponsive to vitamin E. Such platelet abnormalities have been reported with EFAD. Neonates receiving fat-free TPN who have developed EFAD have been found to develop platelet hypoaggregation.[4] However, adults with EFAD due to malabsorption exhibit increased platelet "stickiness" analogous to the platelet hyperaggregation seen in most patients with EFAD during TPN.[5] The combination of high carbohydrate intake and elevated serum insulin during fat-free TPN effectively blocks lipolysis, isolating tissue essential fatty acid stores. As a consequence, EFAD typically occurs in from one week in neonates to four weeks in adults.[3] Whether platelet essential fatty acid stores—the basic source of platelet prostaglandins that initiate aggregation—are subject to similar modification by TPN is not known, making effects on platelet aggregation unpredictable. However, EFAD due to the malabsorption of cystic fibrosis has been associated with increased serum prostaglandin levels.[17] Extrapolation of such findings to platelets would explain platelet hyperaggregation during EFAD due to increased platelet prostaglandin production. The persistence of EFAD and platelet hyperaggregation despite up to 2.0 liters fat supplementation per week in several patients with enterocutaneous fistulae in Group B implies either an increased fat requirement or inefficient fat utilization during TPN. Inefficient fat utilization might occur with a coexisting carnitine deficiency, as fatty acid transport is carnitine dependent. Alternatively, by analogy with animal experiments showing prostaglandin production directly proportional to linoleic acid levels when linoleic acid intake is high,[18] the persistence of platelet hyperaggregation despite fat supplementation could be due to elevated platelet prostaglandin production with the high linoleic acid content of the fat emulsion. This may become increasingly important with the growing use of intravenous fat emulsion for a caloric as well as an essential fatty acid source during TPN, supplying as much as 30% of calories as fat.[19] Clearly, platelet hyperaggregation during TPN is correlated with vitamin E deficiency only in the absence of EFAD. The use of platelet aggregation patterns for the study of vitamin E deficiency must take potentially coexisting EFAD into consideration.

The clinical significance of vitamin E deficiency lies in its potential role in venous thrombosis, a postoperative complication occurring in as many as 30% of general surgical patients.[20] Of the classic Virchow's triad of venous thrombosis, perioperative venous stasis is most important, but vessel injury and hypercoagulation states may contribute significantly.[21] Platelet hyperaggregation similar to that seen here with vitamin E deficiency and EFAD has been reported in both the normal postoperative state and in acute thrombosis,[22] and may reflect a hypercoagulable state. Despite the platelet abnormalities present in half the patients studied here, no clinically overt venous thrombosis was observed, a likely result of the often clinically silent nature of venous thrombosis as well as its low incidence at our institution.[21] Studies of central venous thrombosis during TPN show an incidence of 30% by venography, though less than 5% of cases are clinically evident.[23,24] Just as early regimens for the prophylaxis of postoperative venous thrombosis included vitamin E,[25] so may pharmacologic inhibition of platelet aggregation by vitamin E aid in the prevention of venous thrombosis during TPN, especially in the presence of vitamin E deficiency and possibly EFAD.

CONCLUSIONS

1. Vitamin E deficiency manifested by low serum concentrations and platelet hyperaggregation may be present in up to 50% of malnourished patients receiving TPN.

2. The traditional peroxide-induced hemolysis test for vitamin E deficiency lacks specificity in this population.

3. Daily supplementation during fat-free TPN with 25 to 50 mg all-rac-α-tocopherol intravenously provides an effective means of correcting, and likely preventing, vitamin E deficiency, an amount significantly greater than the current RDA.

4. A standard intravenous fat emulsion used to supplement TPN—Intralipid 10%—contains insufficient metabolically active vitamin E to meet requirements.

5. EFAD is associated with platelet hyperaggregation independently of vitamin E deficiency.

SUMMARY

Vitamin E and essential fatty acid status were examined in two groups of patients, one receiving fat-free total parenteral nutrition (TPN) with intravenous all-rac-α-tocopherol for vitamin E deficiency and the other receiving routine intravenous fat (Intralipid, 10%) emulsions with TPN to supply both fatty acid and vitamin E requirements. Initial evaluation of both groups revealed a 50% incidence of vitamin E deficiency, platelet hyperaggregation, or in vitro H_2O_2-induced hemolysis. Only platelet hyperaggregation correlated significantly with vitamin E deficiency. Supplementation with all-rac-α-tocopherol corrected platelet hyperaggregation and H_2O_2-induced hemolysis; daily dosage requirements of 25–50 mg (fat-free TPN) or more (with intravenous fat) suggest increased vitamin E requirements during TPN. Intravenous fat emulsion did not correct the platelet and red blood cell abnormalities, a result of either increased vitamin E requirements or low α-tocopherol-equivalent content of the emulsion. Essential fatty acid deficiency (EFAD) was observed in seven patients with an associated platelet hyperaggregation independent of vitamin E deficiency. Prolonged TPN for enterocutaneous fistulae in three patients was associated with persistent EFAD and platelet hyperaggregation despite up to 2.0 liters of intravenous fat emulsion weekly.

ACKNOWLEDGMENTS

The authors are grateful for the use of the laboratory facilities of Dr. J. Anderson, Department of Hematology, for platelet studies; to the laboratory of Dr. J. Moylan for fatty acid studies; to K. Trexler, R.Ph. and S. Emerson, R.Ph. for TPN formulations; and to P. Jarrett and S. Curtas, R.N. for aid in laboratory and clinical studies.

REFERENCES

1. LAKE, M. A., M. J. STUART & F. A. OSKI. 1977. Vitamin E deficiency and enhanced platelet function: reversal following E supplementation. J. Pediatr. **90:** 722–725.
2. WITTING, L. A. 1972. The role of polyunsaturated fatty acids in defining vitamin E requirements. Ann. N.Y. Acad. Sci. **203:** 192–198.
3. GOODGAME, J. T., S. F. LOWRY & M. F. BRENNAN. 1978. Essential fatty acid deficiency in total parenteral nutrition: time course of development and suggestions for therapy. Surgery **84:** 271–277.
4. FRIEDMAN, Z., et al. 1977. Platelet dysfunction in the neonate with essential fatty acid deficiency. J. Pediatr. **90:** 439–443.
5. PRESS, M. J., et al. 1974. The correction of essential fatty acid deficiency and "sticky" platelets in man by the cutaneous administration of sunflower oil. Clin. Sci. **46:** 13P.
6. GRANT, J. P., P. CUSTER & J. P. THURLOW. 1981. Current techniques of nutritional assessment. Surg. Clin. North Am. **61:** 437–464.
7. MULLEN, J. L. 1981. Consequences of malnutrition in the surgical patient. Surg. Clin. North Am. **61:** 465–488.
8. QUAIFE, M. S., W. S. SCRIMSHAW & O. H. LOWRY. 1949. A micromethod for assay of total tocopherol in blood serum. J. Biol. Chem. **180:** 1229–1235.

9. BINDER, H. J., *et al.* 1965. Tocopherol deficiency in man. N. Engl. J. Med. **273:** 1289–1297.
10. GERHARDT, V. O. & G. W. GEHRKE. 1972. Rapid microdetermination of fatty acids in biological materials by gas-liquid chromatography. J. Chromatogr. **143:** 335–344.
11. FLEMING, C. R., L. M. SMITH & R. E. HODGES. 1976. Essential fatty acid deficiency in adults receiving total parenteral nutrition. Am. J. Clin. Nutr. **29:** 976–983.
12. COLLER, B. S. 1979. Platelet aggregation by ADP, collagen and vistocetin: a critical review of methodology and analysis. *In* CRC Handbook Series in Clinical Laboratory Sciences: Hematology. R. M. Schmidt, Ed. **1:** 381–396. CRC Press, Inc. Boca Raton, Fla.
13. STUART, M. J. & F. A. OSKI. 1979. Vitamin E and platelet function. Am. J. Pediatr. Hematol. Oncol. **1:** 77–82.
14. THURLOW, P. M. & J. P. GRANT. 1980. Vitamin E deficiency and platelet hyperaggregation during total parenteral nutrition. Surg. Forum **31:** 105–107.
15. THURLOW, P. M. & J. P. GRANT. 1980. Vitamin E, essential fatty acids and platelet function during TPN. J. Parenteral Enteral Nutr. **4:** 584.
16. BELL, E. F. & L. J. FILER. 1981. The role of vitamin E in the nutrition of premature infants. Am. J. Clin. Nutr. **34:** 414–422.
17. CHARC, H. P. & J. DUPONT. 1978. Abnormal levels of prostaglandins and fatty acids in blood of children with cystic fibrosis. Lancet **2:** 236–238.
18. DUPONT, J., M. M. MATHIAS & P. T. CONNALLY. 1978. Prostaglandin synthesis as a function of dietary linoleate concentration. Fed. Proc. **37:** 445.
19. JEEJEBHOY, K. W., *et al.* 1976. Total parenteral nutrition at home: studies in patients surviving 4 months to 5 years. Gastroenterology **71:** 943–953.
20. KAKKAR, V. V. 1975. Deep vein thrombosis: detection and prevention. Circulation **51:** 8.
21. SCHOLZ, P. M., R. H. JONES & D. C. SABISTON. 1979. Prophylaxis of thromboembolism. Adv. Surg. **13:** 115–143.
22. YAMAZAKI, H., *et al.* 1980. Consumption of larger platelets with decrease in adenine nucleotide content in thrombosis, disseminated intravascular coagulation and postoperative state. Thromb. Res. **18:** 77–88.
23. AXELSSON, K. & F. EFSEN. 1978. Phlebography in long-term catheterization of the subclavian vein. Scand. J. Gastroenterol. **13:** 933–938.
24. VALERIO, D., J. K. HUSSEY & F. W. SMITH. 1981. Central venous thrombosis associated with intravenous feeding—a prospective study. J. Parenteral Enteral Nutr. **5:** 240–242.
25. OCHSNER, A., *et al.* 1950. Newer concepts of blood coagulation, with particular reference to postoperative thrombosis. Ann. Surg. **131:** 652–665.

DISCUSSION

H. W. SEEGER (*Justus-Liebig University, Giessen, Federal Republic of Germany*): What form of intravenous α-tocopherol did you use?

P. M. THURLOW: An emulsified form as supplied by Hoffmann-La Roche. A small amount of alcohol was used to make it soluble in the TPN solution. It was given directly with the rest of the nutrients. The vitamin is stable in this formulation.

D. H. HWANG (*Louisiana State University, Baton Rouge, La.*): Did you equalize platelet counts in the vitamin E–deficient group and the control group? Vitamin E deficiency can increase platelet counts and that can affect platelet aggregation.

P. M. THURLOW: Standard procedures for platelet aggregation studies include the adjustment of platelet counts to 300,000/mm³.

D. H. HWANG: My second question is, Could you correct abnormality of platelet aggregation by adding vitamin E *in vitro*?

P. M. THURLOW: Yes.

D. H. HWANG: Could you elaborate on how much vitamin E you added and in what form?

P. M. THURLOW: In a small group of patients using concentrations of tocopherol similar to those present *in vivo*, these aggregation changes were reversible to normal levels.

D. H. HWANG: I'd like to note that supplemental addition of vitamin E to rat PRP or vitamin E-deficient groups does not affect platelet aggregation.

M. K. HORWITT (*St. Louis Medical Center, St. Louis, Mo.*): It's obvious that giving vitamins intravenously has an advantage in terms of nutritional requirements, assuming of course you have normal subjects. Obviously these subjects were not normal, and so it raises a point. I'd like to know which of the solutions you used to get the estimate of 25 mg to give you 0.8 mg/dl plasma. Was it Intralipid or was it Liposyn?

P. M. THURLOW: This was accomplished during fat-free TPN.

M. K. HORWITT: Were these subjects on intravenous feeding before this period?

P. M. THURLOW: For several days. Long enough to determine that they had abnormal platelet and red cell E levels.

M. K. HORWITT: The dose of vitamin E you gave is so much higher than our current RDA.

P. M. THURLOW: I think that's largely going to be a function of the preexisting E-deficiency state in these patients. It may also be a consequence of increased requirements during TPN. My data can't be used to differentiate between those two possibilities.

L. HOWARD (*Albany Medical College, Albany, N.Y.*): The E-total lipid is probably the worst index in these patients. Since they do have constant feedings, their triglycerides can be anywhere. I suspect that E-cholesterol ratios would be much more useful.

P. M. THURLOW: In point of fact, any number of denominators change in rather divergent directions during TPN, and therefore, we used absolute levels.

L. HOWARD: One of the problems that we all have is coming up with something that is specific for E status. Certainly peroxide hemolysis is not very specific, and you confirmed that in your patients, it didn't seem to be a good expression. Did you look at the other factors that could influence membrane stability, such as selenium or essential fatty acids?

P. M. THURLOW: We did not study selenium.

L. HOWARD: The use of Dr. Holman's triene-tetraene ratio is not terribly useful in these patients. Perhaps this is because intravenous high polyunsaturated fatty acid solutions can very readily suppress eicosatrienoic acid. One could fairly readily restore the arachidonic acid levels, and yet even giving as much as 15% of the calories as polyunsaturated fat doesn't necessarily restore linoleic levels. Did you look at the total fatty acid pattern either in the red cells or in the plasma of your patients?

P. M. THURLOW: No we did not. I think my data indicate that this ratio is a relatively good predictor of platelet aggregation abnormalities.

L. HOWARD: It doesn't necessarily tell us whether or not these patients have normal levels of essential fatty acids.

P. M. THURLOW: It is, however, the best test available at present.

P. M. FARRELL (*University of Wisconsin, Madison, Wis.*): What was the amount of linoleic acid administered to your patients as Intralipid and what was the average total calories per day?

P. M. THURLOW: Roughly 2,500 calories per day. Therefore approximately 5% of the calories are given as linoleic acid.

M. STEINER (*The Memorial Hospital, Pawtucket, R.I.*): I'm somewhat surprised at the platelet effects that you have found in these patients. You should be cautious in your interpretation since the individuals you were treating had many different diseases that can influence platelet aggregation. I think to relate your findings to vitamin E status alone may be somewhat overstating the case.

P. M. THURLOW: I would agree in general. However, if that were the case, then the correlation between vitamin E deficiency and platelet hyperaggregation would probably not be so strong. There were a number of patients in the study who had normal vitamin E levels, and these patients had normal platelet aggregation.

L. JOHNSON (*University of Pennsylvania, Philadelphia, Pa.*): I would like to suggest with reference to the use of the hydrogen peroxide fragility test that perhaps it would be better to measure the red blood cell malondialdehyde content. It may be a better indication of vitamin E status.

P. M. THURLOW: We have measured platelet malondialdehyde levels, using methods reported by Dr. Stewart, in most of the Group A patients. However, while these levels were slightly elevated with respect to values reported in the literature, they did not change, nor were they correlated, with the presence or absence of vitamin E deficiency. Furthermore, they did not change with tocopherol supplementation.

EFFECT OF LARGE ORAL DOSES OF VITAMIN E ON THE NEUROLOGICAL SEQUELAE OF PATIENTS WITH ABETALIPOPROTEINEMIA

David P. R. Muller

Institute of Child Health
London, WC1N 1EH, United Kingdom

June K. Lloyd

St. George's Hospital Medical School
London SW17, United Kingdom

INTRODUCTION

Abetalipoproteinemia is a rare condition with less than 50 reported cases.[1] The clinical features were first described by Bassen and Kornzweig in 1950;[2] and in 1960, three groups of investigators independently demonstrated the total absence of beta (low-density) lipoprotein from the plasma of affected individuals.[3-5] Subsequently it was shown that apoprotein B, the major apoprotein of low-density lipoprotein, was undetectable.[6]

Three distinct genetic conditions have now been described in which there is a complete absence of betalipoprotein from plasma. Firstly, a recessively inherited condition (classical abetalipoproteinemia) in which the primary abnormality is thought to be defective synthesis of apoprotein B, although the possibility of a defect in the intracellular assembly of lipoproteins containing apoprotein B, or their secretion, cannot be ruled out. Secondly, the homozygous form of familial hypobetalipoproteinemia, which has an autosomal dominant mode of inheritance and in which defective synthesis of apoprotein B has been demonstrated in heterozygotes;[7] and finally, a normotriglyceridemic form of abetalipoproteinemia in which only the production of the hepatic species of apoprotein B is affected.[8]

The clinical and biochemical features of recessively inherited abetalipoproteinemia and homozygous hypobetalipoproteinemia appear to be identical, and in this paper the term abetalipoproteinemia will be used to cover both disorders. Only one case of normotriglyceridemic abetalipoproteinemia has been reported to date;[8] the clinical and biochemical features are different from the other conditions, and this disorder will not be considered further.

As a result of the absence of apoprotein B, not only low-density lipoproteins but also very low-density lipoproteins and chylomicrons cannot be formed, and the lack of these three major lipoproteins results in greatly reduced concentrations of plasma lipids. The defective chylomicron formation causes triglyceride to accumulate within enterocytes and impairs the major transport route for fat absorption.

Fat malabsorption together with the striking abnormality of red cell shape, acanthocytosis, is present from birth, and the condition commonly presents in early infancy with steatorrhea and failure to thrive. An ataxic neuropathy and pigmentary retinopathy tend to develop toward the end of the first decade or in later childhood and adolescence, and have been the presenting features in some cases.

The pathogenesis of the neurological and retinal abnormalities remains

133

0077-8923/82/0393-0133 $01.75/0 © 1982, NYAS

uncertain. One hypothesis is that these features result from prolonged deficiency of a fat-soluble compound normally transported by an apoprotein B–containing lipoprotein. Vitamin E, which normally relies on chylomicrons for its absorption and low-density lipoprotein for its transport, could be such a substance. In the human, low concentrations of plasma vitamin E are found in many disorders of fat malabsorption but the most severe deficiency occurs in abetalipoproteinemia in which the vitamin is undetectable in plasma.[9,10] Abetalipoproteinemia thus provides a good model for studying the effects of vitamin E deficiency in man.

The possible efficacy of large oral doses of vitamin E in the management of abetalipoproteinemia was first suggested in 1977 in a report of eight patients followed for periods of 3 to 15 years.[11] We now report our findings on the same patients after a further 6 years.

Patients and Methods

The earlier details of the eight patients and their treatment have been reported.[12,11] The current ages and details of the vitamin therapy and its duration are summarized in Table 1. Family studies on all patients suggest that Case 7 has the homozygous form of familial hypobetalipoproteinemia, and confirm that the other cases have recessively inherited abetalipoproteinemia.

We are indebted to Dr. P. H. Neligan (Ninewells Hospital and Medical School, Dundee, United Kingdom) for recent information on Case 8. The most recent clinical examinations on all the other patients were carried out by one of us (JKL). The current nerve conduction studies and ophthalmological investigations on Cases 1, 4, 5, and 6 and Case 7 were performed by Drs. J. M. B. Payan and D. Taylor respectively (The Hospital for Sick Children, Great Ormond Street, London, United Kingdom) and on Case 8 by Drs. J. A. R. Lenman and A. K. Tulloch (Ninewells Hospital and Medical School, Dundee, United Kingdom); recent tests on Cases 2 and 3 have not been done.

Vitamin E status was assessed by measuring plasma vitamin E concentration and by in vitro tests of red cell hemolysis (either autohemolysis or peroxide hemolysis) as described previously.[10] All other biochemical analyses were carried out by established methods.

Results

The progress of the patients in terms of growth, neurological, visual, and intellectual function is summarized in Table 2, which gives the condition at diagnosis, at follow-up in 1975, and the current status.

Growth

Growth rate has been satisfactory in all patients since dietary treatment was instituted, and Cases 1, 5, 6, and 7 showed good "catch up" growth.[12] Of the patients whose height remains on or below the third centile, Case 2 had obstructive uropathy with renal calculi necessitating several operations in early infancy, Case 3 is of Chinese origin and his short stature is genetically determined, and Case 8 was not diagnosed until the age of 7 years. Cases 6–8 have

TABLE 1

CURRENT AGES AND TREATMENT OF PATIENTS

Case Numbers*	Initials	Sex	Age				Treatment					
			At Diagnosis		Current		Vitamin E†			Vitamin A		Vitamin K
			Year	Month	Year	Month	Duration		Current Dose (mg/kg per day)	Duration		Current Dose (IU/day)	Current Dose (IU/day)
							Year	Month		Year	Month		
1	SJ	F	0	1	11	3	11	1	55	11	1	20,000	30
2	MJ	M	0	3	14	4	14	1	48	14	1	20,000	45
3	KM	M	0	5	12	0	11	7	82	11	7	10,500	1.5
4	LG	F	0	11	10	5	9	6	64	9	6	25,000	5
5	MS	F	1	1	12	10	11	6	30	11	6	25,000	5
6	SW	M	1	7	17	7	14	2	88	16	0	29,000	10
7	CS	F	1	5	23	6	14	9	55	22	1	20,000	5
8	AL	M	7	3	25	3	15	0	70	18	0	25,000	10

*Case numbers are the same as in the previous report.[11] Cases 1 and 2 are siblings.

†As all-rac-α-tocopheryl acetate.

TABLE 2

LONG-TERM PROGRESS IN ABETALIPOPROTEINEMIA*

Case No.	Growth						Neurological Status					
	Height (D)	Centile		Weight (D)	Centile		Clinical			Nerve Conduction		
		1	2		1	2	D	1	2	D	1	2
1	3	15	10	3	25	10	N	N	N	—	N	N
2	<3	3	3	<3	10	10	N	N	N	N	—	—
3	<3	3-10	3	<3	<5	<3	N	N	N	—	N	—
4	10	10	10	<3	3	3-10	N	N	N	N	N	N
5	3	75	75	<3	50	50	Hypotonic Absent KJ, AJ	N	N	—	—	N
6	10	50	50	<3	10	25	Absent KJ, AJ	Absent KJ, AJ Reduced vibration	Absent KJ, AJ Reduced vibration	N	Normal motor reduced sensory	Reduced sural and radial action potentials otherwise N
7	10	90	90	10	75	90	Absent KJ, AJ	Absent KJ, AJ	Absent KJ, AJ	—	N	Reduced sural action potential otherwise N
8	<3	<3	<3	<3	<3	<3	Ataxia areflexia pes cavus	Less ataxic areflexia pes cavus	Slightly ataxic areflexia pes cavus	Reduced motor	N	N

all passed through normal puberty, and pubertal development is proceeding normally in Case 5. The other children have not yet entered puberty.

Neurological and Visual Function

Cases 1–5 (the younger children, aged 10–14 years) have no detectable neurological or visual abnormalities as assessed clinically and by electrodiagnostic techniques. These children had all received supplementary vitamins, including large oral doses of vitamin E (as all-rac-α-tocopheryl acetate), from about the time of diagnosis (before one year in Cases 1–4, from 16 months in Case 5).

Cases 6–8, although receiving large doses of vitamin A and other vitamin supplements from the time of diagnosis, did not receive large doses of vitamin E until aged 3½, 8¾, and 10¼ years respectively.

In Case 6, deep tendon reflexes at knee and ankle could not be elicited at the time of diagnosis and remain absent. He was first noted to have some impairment of vibration sense in both upper and lower extremities at the age of 11 years, and this abnormality has persisted. At the most recent examination (age 17½ years), he had in addition minimal defects of proprioception in his left arm and leg. At the age of 11, sensory action potentials were reduced in amplitude; and at age 17½, the amplitudes of the sural and radial nerve action potentials remain reduced. Retinal appearances and visual function have remained normal.

Case 7 had absent deep tendon reflexes at knee and ankle at diagnosis, and

TABLE 2 (cont.)

Ophthalmoscopy			Visual Function			Intellectual Development		
D	1	2	D	1	2	D	1	2
N	N	N	—	—	N	N	N. school	N. school
N	N	N	—	—	—	N	N. school	N. school
N	N	N	—	—	—	—	N	N. school
N	N	N	—	N	N	—	IQ 80	IQ 85 N. school
N	N	N	—	—	N	Delayed development	N	N. school
N	N	N	N	N	N	? N	IQ 90–100	Car repairer further education
N	Slight pigmentary retinopathy	Pigment unchanged angioid streaks	—	N	N	N	N	Univ. degree Teacher
Pigmentary retinopathy	Unchanged	Unchanged	Abnormal EOG, ERG	N	N	IQ 65	Employed sheltered workshop	Same

*Symbols are as follows: D, at diagnosis; 1, at follow-up in 1975;[11] 2, at follow-up in 1981; N, normal; IQ, intelligence quotient; KJ, knee jerks; AJ, ankle jerks; EOG, electrooculogram; ERG, electroretinogram.

these have not returned. Otherwise clinical examination has not revealed any abnormalities. Electrodiagnostic tests of nerve conduction at the age of 23½ years showed a minimal reduction in amplitude of the sural nerve action potential. At the age of 5 years (before vitamin E administration was started), slight peripheral pigmentary retinopathy was observed in both eyes and there was minimal diminution of dark adaptation. Since then the pigmentation has not increased and all electrodiagnostic tests of retinal function have been normal. At the most recent examination, angioid streaking in both fundi was noted; the significance of this is uncertain.

In Case 8 the diagnosis was not made until the age of 7¼ years, at which time he had absent deep tendon reflexes, marked pes cavus, moderate ataxia, and a marked pigmentary retinopathy affecting both the periphery and macula in both eyes. By the age of 10 years, just before vitamin E treatment was started, the ataxia had become more marked, motor nerve conduction was delayed, and electrodiagnostic tests of retinal function were abnormal. At the age of 19 years, his ataxia was less marked, motor nerve conduction was normal, and, although the pigmentary retinopathy was unchanged, the electrodiagnostic tests had become normal.[11] At the most recent examination (age 25¼), he was found to have a wide-based and high-stepping gait but no unsteadiness on turning, Romberg's sign was positive, deep tendon reflexes remained absent, and vibration sense was diminished at the right elbow and both wrists and ankles. Motor and sensory nerve conduction velocities were normal. Ophthalmoscopic examination showed no change in the pigmentary retinopathy; electrodiagnostic tests remained normal.

Intellectual Development

Cases 1–5 are all attending normal schools; Case 4 had an intelligence quotient (IQ) of 80 at the age of 4½ years, and this has remained unaltered. Case 6 attended normal school but had reading delay and was found to have an IQ of 90–100. He is currently employed as an apprentice motor repairer and attends further education classes. Case 7 attended university and obtained a degree in education; she teaches in a secondary school. Case 8 had an IQ of 65 at the time of diagnosis, attended a special school, and is now in full-time employment making chairs in a sheltered workshop.

Other Features

Case 7 has had occasional episodes of supraventricular paroxysmal tachycardia since the age of about 14 years; treatment with digoxin has occasionally been needed, but attacks are currently infrequent and of short duration.

Compliance with Vitamin Therapy

In Cases 4–7, all the evidence indicates good compliance over the years. Red cell hemolysis was generally normal, and when on occasions the values were high, these could be corrected by an increase in the oral dose of vitamin E to keep pace with growth. Plasma concentrations of vitamin E have frequently been detectable up to 5.5 μmol/l. The variations in plasma vitamin E and red cell hemolysis in Case 7 over 15 years are shown by way of example in FIGURE 1. Measurements of the other fat-soluble vitamins (A, D, and K) have likewise been satisfactory.

In Case 3, language problems (his family speaks only Cantonese) have made assessment difficult and it has not been possible to carry out regular tests of red cell hemolysis. Plasma vitamin E concentrations have, however, varied between trace levels and 5.4 μmol/l, and the levels of other vitamins have been normal. Case 8 had the prescribed therapy up to the age of about 18 years, but compliance is now less good and increasing alcohol consumption has become a problem. Cases 1 and 2 are known to have had erratic vitamin intakes throughout the years. They have, however, been seen at least every three months, and general assessment together with regular estimations of the fat-soluble vitamins indicates fair overall compliance.

DISCUSSION

Herbert et al., in their comprehensive review of 43 cases of abetalipoproteinemia, state that the neuromuscular manifestations of the condition are "devastating," that at least a third of affected children develop a symptomatic neurological disorder during the first decade of life, and that virtually all have demonstrable ataxia by the age of 20.[1] There are no reports of spontaneous improvement of neurological function in untreated patients.

Our findings in eight patients for periods ranging from 9½ to 22 years suggest that therapy has influenced the outcome and that vitamin E has played a major role. In all the patients, estimations of plasma vitamin E concentrations and red cell hemolysis have indicated that the vitamin can be absorbed if large enough

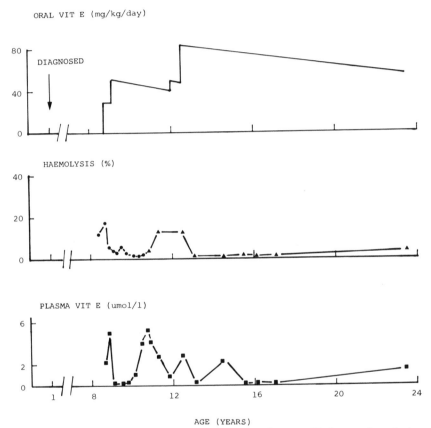

FIGURE 1.   Response of Case 7 to oral vitamin E supplements. Circles, autohemolysis—normal < 5%. Triangles, peroxide hemolysis—normal < 10%. Reference range for plasma vitamin E is 11.5–35.0 μmol/l.

doses (of the order of 100 mg/kg per day) are given. None of the five youngest patients, now aged 10½ to 14 years, who all had large oral supplements of vitamin E from early infancy, have developed any retinal or neurological signs. Case 5 had, in fact, absent deep tendon reflexes at the time of diagnosis; these reflexes have subsequently returned and have remained normal.

In the three older patients, vitamin E therapy was not given until later. In

Cases 7 and 8, retinal and neurological signs were already present when vitamin E was started and at a time when both children had received vitamin A and dietary treatment for some years.

Case 7, who is the patient originally described by Salt et al.,[5] is the only patient in our series who may have homozygous familial hypobetalipoproteinemia.[1] It could be argued that her excellent condition at the age of 23 years represents a different natural history in this condition from that exhibited by classical abetalipoproteinemia. As only four patients with homozygous hypobetalipoproteinemia have been described to date,[1] the progression of the neurological and ophthalmological lesions in this disorder is not well documented. The fact that our patient had absent deep tendon reflexes at the time of diagnosis and developed retinal pigmentation at the age of 5 years indicates that the retinopathy and neuropathy can occur at an early age, and there is no reason to believe that these features would not have been progressive if untreated. Case 8 showed undoubted improvement in neurological and visual functioning after vitamin E was started, and this has been maintained. Only Case 6 appears to have developed minimal neuropathy while receiving vitamin E, and he has not deteriorated clinically over the past 6 years.

Reports of the efficacy of large doses of vitamin E in ameliorating the neuroophthalmological features of abetalipoproteinemia have also been made by other investigators. Azizi et al. recorded marked improvement in the ataxic gait and scotopic vision of an 11-year-old girl after treatment with parenteral and oral vitamin E,[13] and follow-up over 5½ years showed stabilization of her condition with no further changes. Miller et al. described a patient who, at the age of 22 years, had progressive neurological and retinal lesions but since the administration of large doses of vitamin E showed little or no progression of the neurological disorder.[14] Herbert et al. in their review also refer to three other patients who are now in their early 30s, who have been receiving long-term oral vitamin E, and who have not developed retinal or serious neurological lesions.[1]

If the progressive neurological and retinal lesions in abetalipoproteinemia result from a chronic lack of vitamin E, similar features might be expected in other diseases in which prolonged and severe vitamin E deficiency occurs. Apart from abetalipoproteinemia, the most severe deficiency has been found in patients with chronic liver disease.[10] Tomasi has reported a 7-year-old boy with chronic liver disease who developed both a myopathy and neurological lesions, and whose neuropathy improved during 16 months of treatment with large oral doses of a water-soluble preparation of vitamin E at the same time as the plasma vitamin E concentrations increased.[15] More recently, a progressive neurological syndrome in six children with chronic liver disease who had reduced plasma concentrations of vitamin E has been described.[16] Neuropathological studies in two of these cases showed similar lesions to those described in the vitamin E–deficient adult rat and growing monkey.[17-19]

Chronic vitamin E deficiency also occurs in cystic fibrosis, and severe axonal dystrophy in the gracile nucleus has been found at autopsy in patients with this disorder.[20] Recently Sung et al. reported a decrease in the incidence of axonal dystrophy in patients who had been supplemented with vitamin E.[21] A spinocerebellar disorder with features similar to those in untreated abetalipoproteinemia has been described in four adult patients (two with cystic fibrosis and two with chronic liver cirrhosis) who had undetectable or trace concentrations of plasma vitamin E.[22] In one of these patients, regular intramuscular injections of vitamin E (100 mg/week) over a two-year period have resulted in normal plasma vitamin E concentrations and clinical improvement.

There is, therefore, evidence that vitamin E is important for normal neurological functioning and that large oral doses of vitamin E may prevent the development of neurological lesions in abetalipoproteinemia. Established lesions in abetalipoproteinemia and other conditions associated with chronic severe vitamin E deficiency may also be improved by vitamin E therapy.

ACKNOWLEDGMENTS

We thank Drs. M. Baber, C. C. Forsyth, G. Hesling, G. Katz, and D. Trounce for referring the patients to us. We also thank Prof. O. H. Wolff for his advice and encouragement and Hoffmann-La Roche and Co. for their continued interest in our studies.

REFERENCES

1. HERBERT, P. N., A. M. GOTTO & D. S. FREDRICKSON. 1978. Familial lipoprotein deficiency. In The Metabolic Basis of Inherited Disease. J. B. Stanbury, J. B. Wyngaarden & D. S. Fredrickson, Eds.: 544–588. McGraw Hill. New York, N.Y.
2. BASSEN, F. A. & A. L. KORNZWEIG. 1950. Malformation of the erythrocytes in a case of atypical retinitis pigmentosa. Blood 5: 381–387.
3. LAMY, M. J., J. FRÉZAL, J. POLONOVSKI & J. REY. 1960. L'absence congénitale de betalipoproteins. C. R. Soc. Biol. (Paris) 154: 1974–1978.
4. MABRY, C. C., A. M. DIGEORGE & V. H. AUERBACH. 1960. Studies concerning the defect in a patient with acanthocystosis. Clin. Res. 8: 371.
5. SALT, H. B., O. H. WOLFF, J. K. LLOYD, A. S. FOSBROOKE, A. H. CAMERON & D. V. HUBBLE. 1960. On having no betalipoprotein; a syndrome comprising abetalipoproteinaemia, acanthocytosis and steatorrhoea. Lancet 2: 325–329.
6. GOTTO, A. M., R. I. LEVY, K. JOHN & D. S. FREDRICKSON. 1971. On the nature of the protein defect in abetalipoproteinemia. N. Engl. J. Med. 284: 813–818.
7. SIGURDSSON, G., A. NICOLL & B. LEWIS. 1977. Turnover of apolipoprotein-B in two subjects with familial hypobetalipoproteinemia. Metabolism 26: 25–31.
8. MALLOY, M. J., J. P. KANE, D. A. HARDMAN, R. L. HAMILTON & K. B. DALAL. 1981. Normotriglyceridemic abetalipoproteinemia. Absence of the B-100 apolipoprotein. J. Clin. Invest. 67: 1441–1450.
9. KAYDEN, H. J., R. SILBER & C. E. KOSSMANN. 1965. The role of vitamin E deficiency in the abnormal autohemolysis of acanthocytosis. Trans. Assoc. Am. Physicians 78: 334–342.
10. MULLER, D. P. R., J. T. HARRIES & J. K. LLOYD. 1974. The relative importance of the factors involved in the absorption of vitamin E in children. Gut 15: 966–971.
11. MULLER, D. P. R., J. K. LLOYD & A. C. BIRD. 1977. Long-term management of abetalipoproteinaemia. Possible role for vitamin E. Arch. Dis. Child. 52: 209–214.
12. LLOYD, J. K. & D. P. R. MULLER. 1972. Management of abetalipoproteinaemia in childhood. In Protides of the Biological Fluids. H. Peeters, Ed.: 331–335. Pergamon Press. Oxford & New York.
13. AZIZI, E., J. L. ZAIDMAN, J. ESHCHAR & A. SZEINBERG. 1978. Abetalipoproteinemia treated with parenteral and oral vitamin A and E and with medium chain triglycerides. Acta Paediatr. Scand. 67: 797–801.
14. MILLER, R. G., C. J. F. DAVIS, D. R. ILLINGWORTH & W. BRADLEY. 1980. The neuropathy of abetalipoproteinemia. Neurology 30: 1286–1291.
15. TOMASI, L. G. 1979. Reversibility of human myopathy caused by vitamin E deficiency. Neurology 29: 1182–1186.
16. ROSENBLUM, J. L., J. P. KEATING, A. L. PRENSKY & J. S. NELSON. 1981. A progressive neurologic syndrome in children with chronic liver disease. N. Engl. J. Med. 304: 503–508.

17. PENTSCHEW, A. & K. SCHWARZ. 1962. Systemic axonal dystrophy in vitamin E deficient adult rats: with implication in human neuropathology. Acta Neuropathol. **1:** 313–334.
18. MACHLIN, L. J., R. FILIPSKI, J. NELSON, L. R. HORN & M. BRIN. 1977. Effects of prolonged vitamin E deficiency in the rat. J. Nutr. **107:** 1200–1208.
19. NELSON, J. S., C. D. FITCH, V. W. FISCHER, G. O. BROWN & A. C. CHOW. 1981. Progressive neuropathological lesions in vitamin E deficient rhesus monkeys. J. Neuropathol. Exp. Neurol. **40:** 166–186.
20. SUNG, J. H. 1964. Neuroaxonal dystrophy in mucoviscidosis. J. Neuropathol. Exp. Neurol. **23:** 567–583.
21. SUNG, J. H., S. H. PARK, A. R. MASTRI & W. J. WARWICK. 1980. Axonal dystrophy in the gracile nucleus in congenital biliary atresia and cystic fibrosis (mucoviscidosis): beneficial effect of vitamin E therapy. J. Neuropathol. Exp. Neurol. **39:** 584–597.
22. ELIAS, E., D. P. R. MULLER & J. SCOTT. 1981. Spinocerebellar disorders in association with cystic fibrosis or chronic childhood cholestasis and virtually undetectable serum concentrations of vitamin E. Lancet **2:** 1319–1322.

DISCUSSION

H. J. KAYDEN (*New York University School of Medicine, New York, N.Y.*): As the original proponent of the use of vitamin E in treatment of patients with abetalipoproteinemia, this report is most gratifying; and we can add a number of patients who received tocopherol supplementation for some 17 and 18 years. I think it is important to identify that it is only those patients caught early in life, long before there is established disease, that the vitamin can truly cause reversal of the abnormal neurologic disease. Unfortunately, we found two patients who were undiagnosed, unrecognized—two sisters in their early 30s with abetalipoproteinemia with devastating neurologic disease, and administration of tocopherol has not made any significant change in their neurologic state.

In addition, I think it would be appropriate to indicate that the studies that Dr. Illingworth, Dr. Connor, and Dr. Miller have carried out recommending very large doses of tocopherol for amelioration of symptoms need to be correlated with long-term follow-up of neurologic disease. If one takes the measurement of tocopherol levels of the red cell, one finds that in patients with abetalipoproteinemia, it is not possible to raise the levels of the red cell by oral administration much beyond perhaps 50% of what one calls a normal value. Nonetheless, correction of hemolysis occurs at levels far below that. We've been interested in looking at the adipose tissue concentration of patients with abetalipoproteinemia—individuals who have been on long-term supplementation of tocopherol. In comparing these to normal, in patients supplemented with levels of approximately 800 mg to 1 g of tocopherol per day, their levels run about 10 to 20% of what is present in the normal population.

On the other hand, in the one patient that Dr. Illingworth sent us—an adipose tissue biopsy who has been receiving approximately 100 mg/kg per day—the tocopherol level in the adipose tissue was similar to that of a normal. The third condition that you did not discuss in any detail was the normal triglyceridemic abetalipoproteinemic patient of Drs. Malloy and Kane, who absorbs vitamin E perfectly normally and whose report in the *Journal of Clinical Investigation* indicates that her ataxia was corrected during the time she had tocopherol. On a relatively low dose for these subjects of 400 mg per day, her adipose tissue content is really quite high. So it does seem to me that it's essential to give these patients very large oral doses for a very prolonged period of time and perhaps the only guide that one has to the response from therapy actually is changes in their neurologic status.

D. P. R. MULLER: Thank you very much, Dr. Kayden. We would wholeheartedly agree.

R. J. SOKOL (*Children's Hospital Medical Center, Cincinnati, Ohio*): Do you have any idea on which fractions in serum the tocopherol is transported in these patients, since their low-density lipoprotein concentration is so low if detectable at all? Do you think it's bound to albumin?

D. P. R. MULLER: We have no data. But there are some data in the literature to suggest that quite a high proportion of what is present is carried on high-density lipoprotein.

E. R. LOEW (*Cornell University, Ithaca, N.Y.*): In the last subject that you outlined for us, you indicated that prior to vitamin E supplementation, the electroretinogram and the electroocculogram were abnormal and that there was a pigmentary retinopathy. Following therapy with vitamim E, the ERG and EOG assumed a normal appearance; however, the pigmentary retinopathy remained. Were visual fields done on the child before and after supplementation and were thresholds measured?

D. P. R. MULLER: They have been done, but I'd have to look back at the data. Visual fields were normal before and after supplementation with vitamin E.

M. A. GUGGENHEIM (*University of Colorado Medical Center, Denver, Colo.*): It was in large part your published work that led us to try to treat the patients I reported. As a neurologist, I'm interested in the eye movements. This has been a consistent finding in the acquired vitamin E deficiency neuromuscular disease reported by both Rosenblum and Keating. Would you comment on your patients please.

D. P. R. MULLER: As far as I'm aware, the one patient in our study that was affected didn't have ophthalmoplegia. But ophthalmoplegia has been reported in the literature. The retinal pigmentation invariably found in untreated abetalipoproteinemia is, however, a rare finding in patients with chronic liver disease.

I think one may have to be careful in extrapolating from all the groups in terms of the eye symptoms as there may be differences between the groups. But it seems that the neurological features appear to be very similar.

M. A. GUGGENHEIM: Would you have any comments on the underlying neuropathology?

D. P. R. MULLER: Since I'm not a neuropathologist, there are people in the audience much more capable of commenting on this. However, it does seem that there is a selective loss of the larger-caliber myelinated fibers. This seems to be a consistent finding in one patient with abetalipoproteinemia, in the deficient animal states, and in patients with chronic liver disease.

G. J. HANDELMAN (*University of California, Santa Cruz, Calif.*): It's clear that identifying these patients before they are one year old is going to make them completely normal. How can a physician recognize a child with abetalipoproteinemia prior to one year of age?

D. P. R. MULLER: What is interesting is that although abetalipoproteinemia is very rare, it's one of those conditions that pediatricians are certainly aware of. Therefore, if a child presents with fat malabsorption, the pediatrician tends to think of abetalipoproteinemia as one of the possible causes. It is, of course, very easy to rule out by taking some blood onto a slide and looking for spiky red cells or by doing a serum cholesterol or electrophoretic strip.

UNIDENTIFIED SPEAKER: Two questions. One is, Do you think the myopathy is simply a denervation phenomenon or a separate entity dependent on vitamin E availability? And what is the relationship between abetalipoproteinemia and the neuropathology of Friedreich's ataxia and vitamin E?

D. P. R. MULLER: I may stand to be corrected by others in the audience, but to my knowledge a myopathy has not been described in abetalipoproteinemia. In terms of Friedreich's ataxia, the clinical features are very similar indeed, and also this loss of the large-caliber myelinated fibers seems to be common to the two conditions. So there are very great similarities.

UNIDENTIFIED SPEAKER: In abetalipoproteinemia, increase in muscle enzymes has been observed. In one patient that we've had the opportunity to follow for five years on E supplementation, the increased creatine phosphokinase, lactate dehydrogenase, aspartate transaminase, etc., improved.

D. P. R. MULLER: Thank you very much.

R. L. BAEHNER (Indiana University, Indianapolis, Ind.): When you corrected the vitamin E levels and returned them to normal, was this associated with any improvement in the shape change of the red cell? Did the acanthocytes no longer persist in the circulation?

D. P. R. MULLER: They still persisted. There was no change in the shape of the acanthocytes.

VITAMIN E AND RETROLENTAL FIBROPLASIA: ULTRASTRUCTURAL SUPPORT OF CLINICAL EFFICACY*

Frank L. Kretzer, Helen M. Hittner,† A. Tim Johnson,
Rekha S. Mehta, and Louis B. Godio‡

Cullen Eye Institute
Baylor College of Medicine
Houston, Texas 77030

INTRODUCTION

As differentiation proceeds peripherally from the optic disc, the avascular human retina thickens and stratifies and the inner retina becomes spatially removed from its choroidal oxygen source. Mesenchymal spindle cells, which arise from division of cells in the hyaloid artery, then invade the nerve fiber layer and slowly migrate toward the ora serrata, forming the vanguard of the vasoformative elements. The spindle cells differentiate into endothelial cells forming the rear guard, which advances behind the vanguard toward the ora serrata. The interface between the vanguard and the rear guard is the site of the future shunt.[1] Vascularization reaches the ora serrata only at term. There is a 360° circumferential area of vanguard in the retina at <36 weeks gestational age,[2] containing an apron of spindle cells.[3] It is the nascent vessels adjacent and posterior to the shunt that proliferate in retrolental fibroplasia (RLF).[4]

In 1956, Kinsey identified oxygen as the primary etiological factor in RLF.[5] The pathophysiology of RLF is oxygen-induced constriction of the existing arterioles in the rearguard retina and obliteration of the nascent capillaries posterior to the shunt. There is then an intraretinal proliferation of new vessels from existing endothelial cells, which can be seen clinically between three and four weeks. At some unknown time, there is a proliferation of the vanguard spindle cells in the nerve fiber layer. From existing capillaries, there can be intravitreal neovascularization.[4] When this occurs, it becomes clinically significant at six to eight weeks.[6,7]

Three controlled clinical studies have been reported claiming efficacy of vitamin E in reducing the severity of RLF.[7-9] These studies by Owens and Owens, Johnson et al., and Hittner et al. imply that vitamin E does not prevent RLF, but reduces the severity of the retinopathy that occurs.

This paper reports the data generated from 21 whole-eye donations from infants enrolled in the 1980 and 1981 clinical studies.[7,10] It is the first documentation of the ultrastructure of human retinal spindle cells in the preterm, high-risk infant. It elucidates the preclinical changes in the vanguard, modulated by vitamin E, that prime the nascent retinal vasculature in the rear guard to proliferate in RLF.

*Supported by grants from the Retina Research Foundation, the Retinitis Pigmentosa Foundation, the National Institutes of Health (EY 02607), and the University of Houston (HOPTFC 1319).
†Also affiliated with the Department of Pediatrics.
‡College of Optometry, University of Houston, Houston, Texas 77004.

145

MATERIALS AND METHODS

Clinical Studies

The 1980 and 1981 studies were performed in the Texas Children's Hospital Neonatal Intensive Care Unit, Houston, Texas.[7,10] These studies enrolled 250 infants who arrived on the first day of life, were ≤1,500 grams at birth weight, and were in respiratory distress. In 1980, 150 infants were enrolled double-blind via a random number table into either a control or treatment group. The former received 5 mg vitamin E/kg body weight orally and daily, while the latter received 100 mg vitamin E/kg body weight.[7] The vitamin E (all-rac-α-tocopherol as water-miscible emulsion) was supplied by Hoffmann-La Roche, Inc. In 1981, all 100 infants received 100 mg/kg body weight,[10] and the vitamin was purchased from U.S.V. Laboratories (all-rac-α-tocopheryl acetate as water-miscible emulsion). Plasma vitamin E levels[11] were determined on days 2, 4, and 7 and weekly thereafter until age 5 weeks.

The McCormick classification of RLF was employed throughout in which grade I is neovascularization of the retina; grade II, neovascularization extending into the vitreous; and grade III, vitreal neovascularization plus increased dilatation and tortuosity of the vessels of the posterior pole.[12] No infant was allowed to advance to grade IV, which is retinal detachment. Any infant found to have RLF grade III was removed from the study and treated surgically. Indirect ophthalmoscopic examinations were initiated at the third week and continued weekly until the RLF regressed or required surgical treatment (RLF grade ≥III). Since RLF generally does not develop fully until prior to 8 weeks of life, those infants dying before this time were excluded from the statistical analysis.

The RLF score as defined by Hittner et al. assigns 0–2 points for each of the five RLF risk factors [gestational age, oxygen duration and level, intraventricular hemorrhage (IVH), sepsis, and birth weight].[7] Totals of 0–2 predict minimal; 3–6, moderate; and 7–10, severe risk for development of RLF. This RLF score was calculated at three weeks to allow the factors of oxygen duration and level, sepsis, and IVH to have their clinical influence. Thus, those RLF scores assigned before three weeks because of death at earlier points are merely speculative.

Morphological Studies

From the 250 infants enrolled in the clinical study, 10 resulted in whole-eye donations, which were studied ultrastructurally. One additional infant received control levels of vitamin E at the Jefferson Davis Hospital, Houston, Texas, and was referred to the Texas Children's Hospital for treatment of bilateral RLF III, but died of pulmonary complications two weeks following a scleral buckling procedure on one eye. The untreated eye is included in this ultrastructural study. Whole-eye donations were granted within one to five hours postmortem.

The intact globes were immediately submerged in buffered 2% glutaraldehyde–2% formalin for 1 hour. The globes were then opened with a cut anterior to the ora serrata, and the anterior and posterior hemispheres were fixed in cold, buffered 2% glutaraldehyde for 12 hours. Segments of the nasal and temporal vanguard retina were isolated and processed for transmission electron microscopy,[13] such that each segment began at the ora serrata and extended centrally into the most peripheral vascularized retina. Thick sections (0.5 μ) were stained with toluidine blue, and photographed at 25× on a Zeiss PMIII. Light micrographs (730×) of expanses of peripheral retina were assembled into montages. As per the stereological methods of Weibel,[14] a grid meshwork on clear acetate paper was placed randomly over areas of the nerve fiber layer. The nature of every intersect was determined as either extracellular vacuoles, non-spindle cell cytoplasm, or spindle cell cytoplasm. These data were used to calculate the volume of the nerve fiber layer that was occupied by spindle cells.

Thin sections (400 Å) were cut, and low-magnification (4,000×) montages of continuous expanses of the vanguard were assembled. In such retinal expanses, the morphology of the spindle cells could be elucidated. To establish the three-dimensional topography of spindle cells in the nerve fiber layer, nasal and temporal vanguard segments were processed for scanning electron microscopy.

Where clusters of spindle cells with adjacent plasma membranes occurred, electron micrographs were taken and printed at a final magnification of 40,000×. From these micrographs, the contribution of gap junctions to the total surface area of the spindle cell plasma membrane was calculated using a Zeiss Videoplan. On each micrograph, either <10% (minimal), 10–30% (intermediate), or >30% (maximal) of the plasma membrane surface was differentiated into gap junctions. This information was expressed for each infant as the percentage of micrographs included in each of the three categories.

RESULTS

Clinical Studies

TABLE 1 summarizes the clinical data for all infants enrolled in the 1980 and 1981 studies.[7,10] The percentage incidence of RLF was 60 to 65. Oral, uninterrupted, daily treatment dosages of vitamin E were found to significantly suppress RLF ≥III (p < 0.03 in 1980 but not in 1981, p < 0.12). In addition, a multivariate analysis considering vitamin E and all five RLF risk factors simultaneously indicated that the treatment dose significantly suppressed the severity of RLF overall (p = 0.012 and 0.003 in 1980 and 1981, respectively). In the control group, the average serum vitamin E level was 0.6 mg/100 ml. The 1980 and 1981 treatment groups were not clustered because the average plasma vitamin E level was 1.2 mg/100 ml in 1980 as compared to 1.8 mg/100 ml in 1981. This difference was related to the utilization of two different vitamin E preparations.

The postpartum ages of the 11 infants (A–K) included in the morphological analysis are shown in FIGURE 1. Three infants (A, B, and C) were from the 1980 control population, and 1 other control infant (D) was referred from another hospital. Three infants (F, I, and K) were from the 1980 treatment population, and 4 infants (E, G, H, and J) were from the 1981 protocol. TABLE 2 lists the clinical parameters of these 11 infants. All infants were between 25 and 29 weeks gestational age and thus had absence of vascularization in the vanguard region, except for infants J and K, where the retinopathy had regressed and vessels had developed anterior to the shunt. All infants were in severe respiratory distress and received continuous oxygen throughout life, dying at 1 day to 19 weeks postpartum age. Those RLF scores that are in parentheses are for infants who died at <25 days, and thus their scores are an extrapolation of the clinical events to the time of death. Infants who died at <25 days had no clinical RLF grade, although this in no way represents the maximum that could have evolved.

TABLE 1
SUMMARY OF CLINICAL STUDIES

Parameters	1980		1981
	Control	Treatment	Treatment
Enrolled	76	74	100
Died <8 weeks	25	24	31
Survived >8 weeks	51	50	69
Vitamin E (mg/kg per day) (oral dose given)	5*	100*	100†
Vitamin E (mg/100 ml) (average plasma level measured)	0.6	1.2	1.8
RLF grade (McCormick)			
0	18	18	28
I	22 (43)‡	28 (56)	33 (48)
II	6 (12)	4 (8)	6 (9)
≥III	5 (10)	0 (0)	2 (3)
RLF incidence (percent)	65	64	60
Significance of vitamin E efficacy			
Univariate analysis		<0.03	<0.12
Multivariate analysis		= 0.012	= 0.003
Infants studied ultrastructurally	A, B, C, D§	F, I, K	E, G, H, J

*Vitamin E (all-rac-α-tocopherol) supplied by Hoffmann-La Roche, Inc.
†Vitamin E (all-rac-α-tocopheryl acetate, Aquasol E) purchased from U.S.V. Laboratories.
‡Numbers in parentheses indicate percent.
§Infant referred from outside hospital.

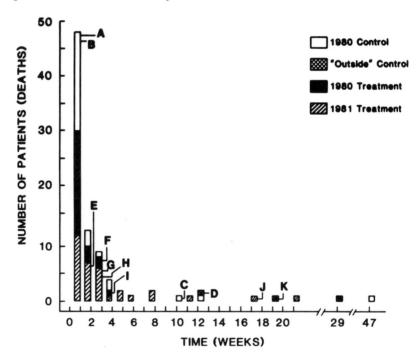

FIGURE 1. Number of infant deaths in the 1980 and 1981 clinical studies as a function of postpartum age (weeks). The letters indicate infants from whom whole-eye donations were obtained postmortem.

Morphological Studies

Light micrograph montages of continuous expanses of both nasal and temporal peripheral retina were used to determine the spindle cell volume in the nerve fiber layer in all 21 eyes. The vanguard retina was homogeneous in structure and nonvascularized in infants A through I. In infants J and K, the vasculature extended anterior to the shunt. All quadrants in any given infant were indistinguishable with regard to spindle cell density or morphology. The spindle cells formed an apron that anastomosed around the Muller and ganglion cells (FIGURES 2A and 3). In the retinas of control infants C and D, the spindle cells had proliferated and formed stacked profiles demarcated by columns of Muller cell processes (FIGURE 2B and C). The light microscopic parameters of the vanguard spindle cells in the nerve fiber layer are summarized in TABLE 3.

TABLE 2

CLINICAL PARAMETERS OF PRETERM, HIGH-RISK INFANTS

Infant	GA (weeks)	RLF Risk Factors*			BW (grams)	RLF Score†	RLF Grade‡ (McCormick)	Postpartum Age at Death
		O₂	IVH	Sepsis				
Control								
A	28	cont	1	—	950	(6)	—	1 day
B	28	cont	4	—	1,060	(6)	—	5 days
C	26	cont	4	+	625	10	III	10 weeks
D	27	cont	0	—	900	6	III	12 weeks
Treatment								
E	28	cont	0	—	790	(5)	—	10 days
F	26	cont	4	—	830	(8)	—	15 days
G	29	cont	4	—	940	(7)	—	19 days
H	27	cont	4	—	940	(8)	—	20 days
I	25	cont	0	+	760	(8)	—	25 days
J	28	cont	0	—	1,040	4	I	17 weeks
K	27	cont	0	—	1,030	5	I	19 weeks

*GA is gestational age; BW is birth weight.
†Numbers in parentheses are projected scores.
‡Minus signs indicate no clinical manifestation of RLF.

In all control and treatment infants, the nerve fiber layer was laced with extracellular vacuoles between adjacent Muller and ganglion cell processes. Such vacuoles were postmortem artifacts, although there was no direct relationship between postmortem delay in obtaining the eyes and the extent of vacuoles. Extensive vacuolization thickened the nerve fiber layer and compressed adjacent cytoplasm. Therefore, calculations of total nerve fiber volume including and excluding this parameter are given, although only the former are used in this paper. The nerve fiber layer in control infants C and D (FIGURE 2B and C) was occupied by a significantly ($p < 0.001$) greater volume of spindle cells than that of control infants A and B (FIGURE 2A). The percentage of the nerve fiber volume occupied by spindle cells was similar in all treatment infants (E–I) (FIGURE 3) and was not statistically different from control infants A and B ($p = 0.51$).

The scanning electron micrographs shown in FIGURE 4 demonstrate the three-dimensional stacking of spindle cells in the vanguard nerve fiber layer of

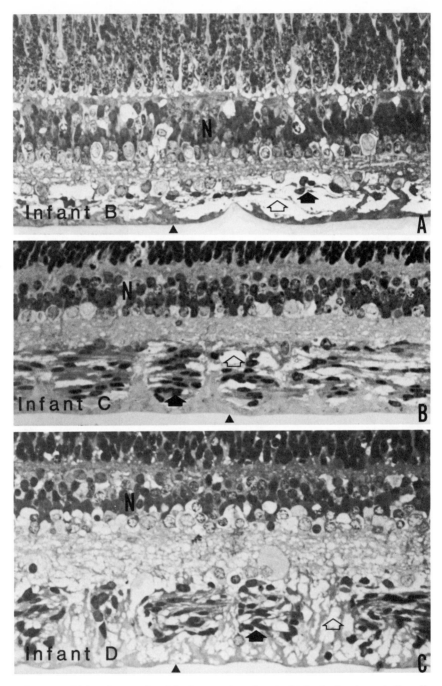

FIGURE 2. Light micrographs of the inner retina of control infants showing spindle cells (black arrows) in the nerve fiber layer with vacuoles (white arrows). Inner nuclear layer (N), retina-vitreous interface (black triangles). 450×.

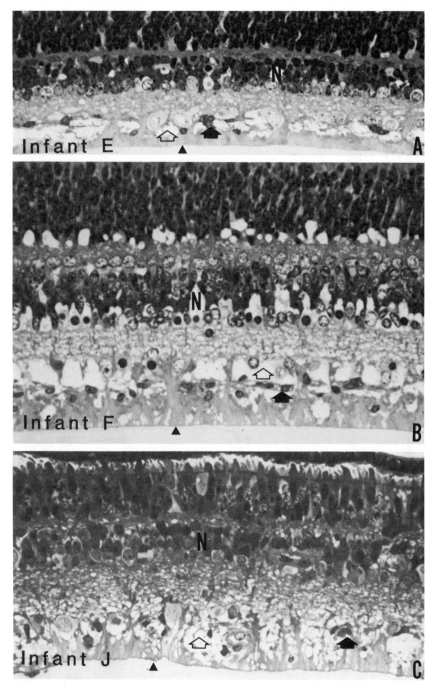

FIGURE 3. Light micrographs of the inner retina of treatment infants showing spindle cells (black arrows) in the nerve fiber layer with vacuoles (white arrows). Inner nuclear layer (N), retina-vitreous interface (black triangles). 450×.

control infant C with development of grade III RLF (FIGURE 4A). This contrasts with the scarcity of spindle cells in the nerve fiber layer of treatment infant K, who developed grade I RLF (FIGURE 4B).

In all quadrants in both control and treatment populations, the spindle cells uniformly contained oblate nuclei with dispersed chromatin, aggregations of glycogen granules (FIGURE 5A), bloated rough endoplasmic reticulum filled with osmiophilic material (FIGURE 5B), few mitochondria, inconspicuous Golgi apparatus, and no basal lamina. In control infants A and B, who survived for 1 and 5 days, respectively, the spindle cells showed few surface microvilli (FIGURE 6A), although in infants C and D, who survived for 10 and 12 weeks, respectively, the spindle cells contained numerous microvilli (FIGURE 6B). The same trend occurred throughout the age spectrum of the seven treatment infants. The spindle cells in those infants who survived for <25 days (infants E-I) possessed few

TABLE 3

LIGHT MICROSCOPY PARAMETERS OF THE VANGUARD SPINDLE CELLS
IN THE NERVE FIBER LAYER

| | | | | % Spindle Cell Volume of Nerve Fiber Layer | | |
| | | Stereological Strikes | | | | |
Infant	Vacuoles	Non-Spindle Cells	Spindle Cells	Excluding Vacuoles	Including Vacuoles	Eyes Obtained (hours postmortem)
Control						
A	887	955	107	10.1	5.5	3
B	716	927	89	8.8	5.1 (2A)*	1
C	463	727	1,390	65.7	53.9 (2B)	4
D	1,090	1,225	1,070	46.6	31.6 (2C)	4
Treatment						
E	169	718	63	8.1	6.6 (3A)	3
F	1,073	1,934	169	8.0	5.3 (3B)	4
G	542	744	41	5.2	3.1	2
H	224	908	57	5.9	4.8	3
I	329	875	118	11.9	8.9	1
J	582	1,068	68	6.0	4.0 (3C)	5
K	871	1,095	25	2.2	1.3	3

*Numbers in parentheses refer to FIGURES 2 and 3.

microvilli (FIGURE 6C), while in those infants who survived for 17 and 19 weeks (infants J and K), the spindle cells had extensive surface microvilli (FIGURE 6D), which was comparable to the density of microvilli seen in the oldest control infants.

TABLE 4 contains data regarding the percent of the total surface area of the spindle cell plasma membrane that has differentiated into gap junctions ("gap junction area"). In the control group, the micrographs of infant A all contained minimal gap junction area (FIGURE 7A); in infant B, all showed maximal gap junction area (FIGURE 7B); in infant C, there was a mixture of minimal and intermediate gap junction areas (FIGURE 8A); and in infant D, all had minimal gap junction area (FIGURE 8B). In the treatment groups, infants E-I contained mixtures of minimal, intermediate, and maximal gap junction areas (FIGURE 9A). However, in no instance did a treatment infant show the maximal gap junction proliferation

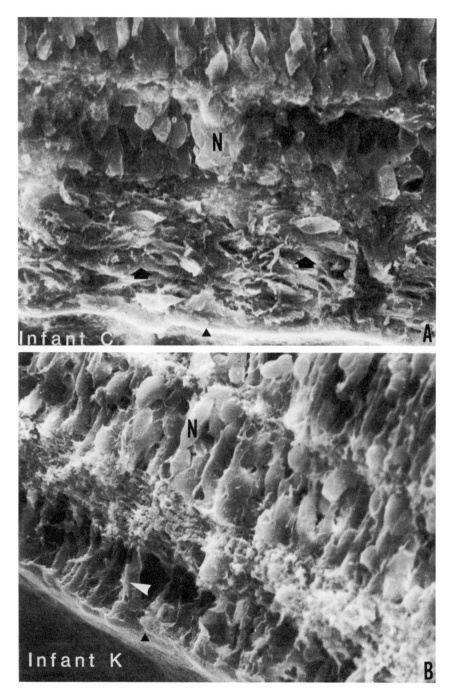

FIGURE 4. Scanning electron micrographs comparing spindle cell density (black arrows) in the nerve fiber layer of control (A) and treatment (B) infants who survived for ≥ 10 weeks. Inner nuclear layer (N), Muller cell processes (white arrowhead), retina-vitreous interface (black triangles). 1,200×.

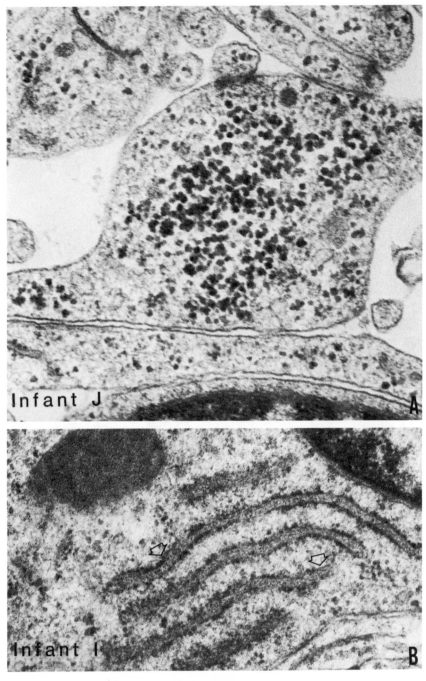

FIGURE 5. Electron micrographs demonstrating the cytoplasmic characteristics of spindle cells in the nerve fiber layer. (A) Glycogen granules (white arrowhead). (B) Bloated rough endoplasmic reticulum with osmiophilic content (arrows). 60,000×.

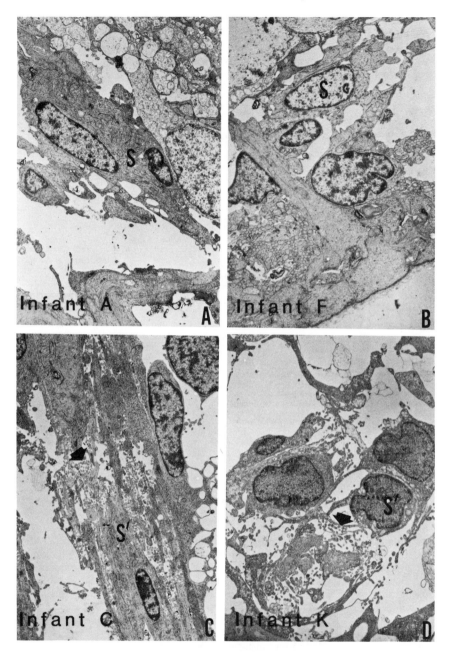

FIGURE 6. Electron micrographs comparing activated (trend II) spindle cells (S) with few surface microvilli and mature (trend III) spindle cells (S') with numerous microvilli (arrows). Micrographs A and C are control infants. Micrographs B and D are treatment infants. 4,000×.

that was seen in control infant B. Infants J and K showed homogeneously minimal gap junction area (FIGURE 9B).

The relationships among the gap junction area, percentage of the nerve fiber volume occupied by spindle cells, postpartum age, gestational age, and RLF scores are shown in FIGURE 10.

DISCUSSION

When multivariate analysis is used, the 1980 and 1981 clinical studies indicate that vitamin E significantly reduces RLF severity.[7,10] However, when single variate analysis, which does not consider the factors of immaturity, illness, and

TABLE 4

ULTRASTRUCTURAL PARAMETERS OF THE VANGUARD SPINDLE CELLS
IN THE NERVE FIBER LAYER

| | | | Gap Junction Density* | | | Gap Junction Area | | |
| | Scanning | Surface | | | | | Range | |
Infant	Electron	Microvilli	<10%	10–30%	>30%	Average	Low	High
Control								
A	apron	− (6A)†	100	0	0 (7A)	1.8	0.5	2.6
B	apron	−	0	0	100 (7B)	43.8	39.8	57.4
C	stacked (4A)	+ (6B)	40	60	0 (8A)	11.9	6.7	22.4
D	stacked	+	100	0	0 (8B)	2.5	0.0	7.2
Treatment								
E	apron	−	50	50	0	12.4	6.8	23.6
F	apron	− (6C)	10	30	60 (9A)	31.8	8.9	61.8
G	apron	−	90	10	0	5.9	0.0	14.1
H	apron	−	0	30	70	22.9	10.7	32.4
I	apron	−	20	40	40	28.9	3.8	79.8
J	apron	+	100	0	0 (9B)	1.9	1.1	3.4
K	apron (4B)	+ (6D)	100	0	0	0.5	0.0	1.1

*Percentage of micrographs containing <10% (minimal), 10–30% (intermediate), >30% (maximal) gap junction area.
†Numbers in parentheses refer to FIGURES 4 and 6–9.

oxygen administration, is used, the effect of vitamin E appears to be significant in the 1980 study ($p \leq 0.03$) but not in the 1981 study ($p \leq 0.12$), where two clinical failures occurred. The ultrastructural data presented in this paper explain the gestational age–dependent response of spindle cells to a vitamin E–modulated suppression of the preclinical proliferation of gap junctions. Thus, there is an explanation for clinical failures of infants of gestational age ≤ 27 weeks. The working hypothesis is that the linkage of spindle cells by gap junctions inhibits migration of new vessels, primes spindle cell proliferation anterior to the shunt, and triggers neovascularization posterior to the shunt.

Gap junctions are specialized areas of adjacent plasma membranes involved in communication between cells. By transmission electron microscopy, gap junctions appear as areas of close plasma membrane apposition.[15] The concept of rapid modulation (within 48 hours) of the size and distribution of gap junctions in

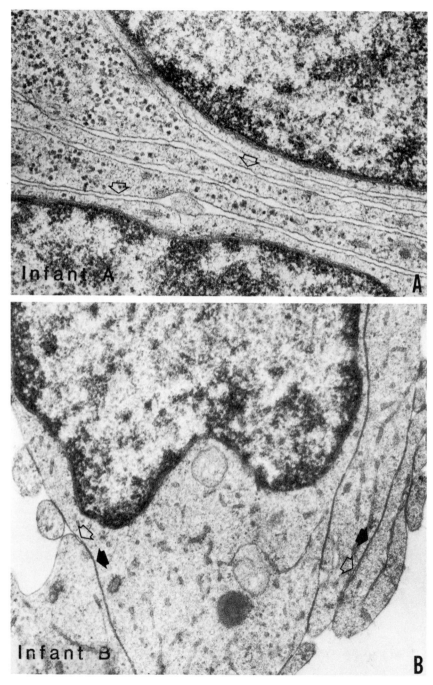

FIGURE 7. Electron micrographs comparing the extent of gap junction area between spindle cells in control retinas in the embryologic state (trend I) (A) and maximal activation state (trend II) (B). Nonfused plasma membranes (white arrows), gap junction areas (black arrows). 40,000×.

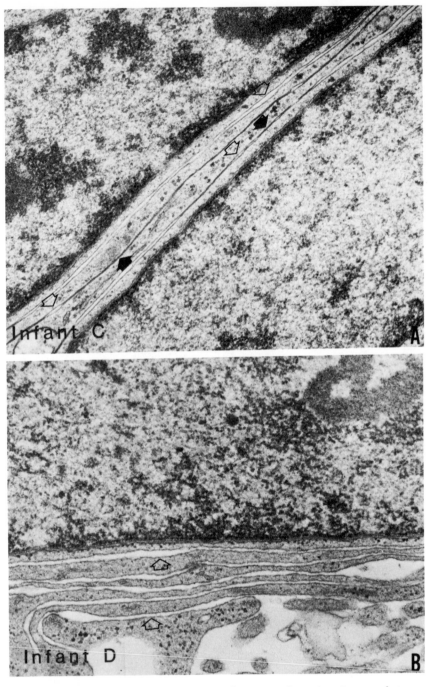

FIGURE 8. Electron micrographs comparing the extent of gap junction area between mature (trend III) spindle cells in control infants. Nonfused plasma membranes (white arrows), gap junction areas (black arrows). 40,000×.

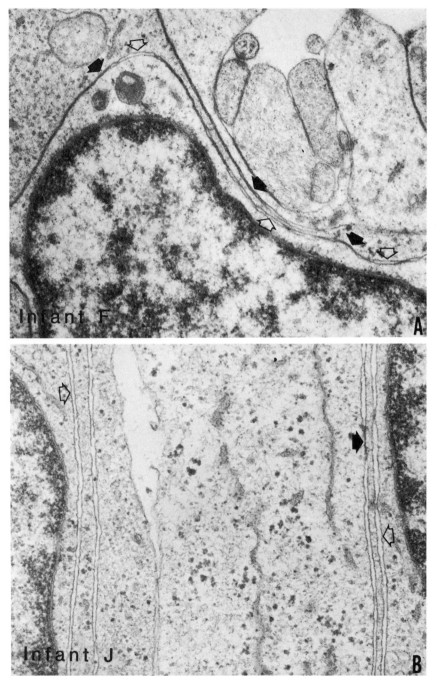

FIGURE 9. Electron micrographs comparing the extent of gap junction area between spindle cells in treatment retinas at activation (trend II) (A) and maturation (trend III) (B). Nonfused plasma membranes (white arrows), gap junction area (black arrows). 40,000×.

developing systems is exemplified by experimental use of hormones, hepatecto-my, and vitamins. In hypophysectomized *Rana pipiens* larvae, thyroid hormone administration led to a 20-fold increase in gap junction area between differentiat-ing ependymoglial cells within 20–40 hours.[16] Following partial hepatectomy in rats, gap junctions between remaining liver cells completely disappeared by 28 hours, but by 48 hours had reappeared and were indistinguishable in size and distribution from those in control animals.[17] In organ culture of 14-day chick embryo shank skin, vitamin A–induced mucous metaplasia was accompanied by gap junction increase that was maximal at one day.[18]

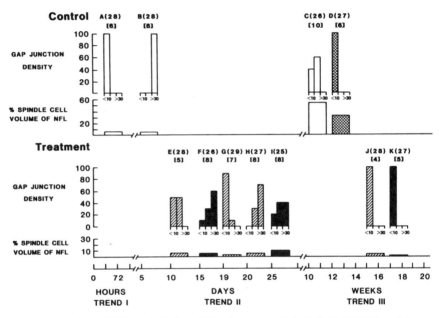

FIGURE 10. Control infants A, B, C, and D and treatment infants E, F, G, H, I, J, and K are plotted as a function of postpartum age. For each infant, both the gap junction density and the percentage volume of the nerve fiber layer that is occupied by spindle cells are given. In the lowest line, the data are partitioned into embryonic trend I (in hours), activation trend II (in days), and maturation trend III (in weeks). For each infant, the gestational age in weeks appears in parenthesis and the total RLF score appears in brackets.

In the preterm infant, an increase in gap junction area could be an immediate cellular response when the retinal environment changes from hypoxia *in utero* to hyperoxia at birth.[9] Since the preterm is known to have low levels of vitamin E,[19] free oxygen radicals could induce lipid peroxidations,[20] which alter membrane surface properties and trigger gap junction formation. If treatment levels of vitamin E are given orally at day one, these plasma vitamin E levels[7,21] effectively suppress such potential increases in gap junction area in infants who are ≥ 27 weeks gestational age (infants B and E).

The data regarding gap junction area (TABLE 4) are grouped into three trends: embryologic, activation, and maturation. Trend I represents the embryologic state of the spindle cells where juxtaposed plasma membranes contain minimal gap junction area (infant A). This is confirmed by the absence of gap junctions between embryonic spindle cells in the parallel rat model at >15 days.[22] Trend II is the activation phase of the spindle cells in which there is an increase in gap junction area prior to spindle cell proliferation (infants B and E-I). The magnitude of this activation appears to be modulated by treatment levels of vitamin E and immaturity. Trend III is a down modulation of the gap junction area in maturing spindle cells, which can occur after extensive spindle cell proliferation (infants C and D) or as the spindle cells become a minimal retinal component (infants J and K).

The spindle cells in retinas of preterm infants given continuous oxygen because of respiratory distress show an immediate increase in gap junction area. The kinetics of this increase cannot be resolved by these data, but by five days of continuous oxygen and control levels of vitamin E, there is a uniform hyperoxic response of the cells toward maximal gap junction area (infant B). This increase in gap junction area is suppressed by treatment levels of vitamin E, as documented by treatment infant E who had significantly lower gap junction area ($p < 0.005$) than age-matched infant B. This suppression is not an all-or-none phenomenon (infants E-I) (FIGURE 10). Immaturity may explain the variability of RLF severity in preterms exposed to equal oxygen administration. As younger gestational age infants are kept alive, treatment levels of vitamin E alone cannot suppress the initial increase in gap junction area. Since the plasma level of oral vitamin E takes seven days to reach a maximum,[7,22] vitamin E therapy must start at day one. The retina is known to sequester natural antioxidants,[23] but the exact retinal level of vitamin E during the first days of life is unknown. Any increase above the depressed base plasma level of the preterm infant[19] is ultrastructurally demonstrated to be beneficial in suppressing gap junction proliferation.

If vitamin E is used therapeutically only after the first clinical manifestations of RLF,[24] trend II activation has already occurred, and shunt activation and spindle cell proliferation have been cellularly triggered. There are clinical instances in which the prophylactic administration of continuous, daily treatment levels of vitamin E was not given. One infant in the 1980 study developed necrotizing enterocolitis, and vitamin E was stopped from 2 to 4 weeks of age. The vitamin E treatment in another nonstudy infant was reduced to control levels at 8 weeks of age by a neonatologist because only RLF I had developed. In several nonstudy infants, vitamin E treatment was not initiated until age 1 to 2 weeks because routine oral feedings had not begun. All cases subsequently developed RLF III. This emphasizes the potentially long duration of trend II and favors the continuous, daily administration of high levels of vitamin E until clinical regression is evidenced by growth of retinal vessels past the shunt.[25] However, in very high-risk, preterm infants (infant F, 26 weeks and 830 grams; infant I, 25 weeks and 760 grams), continuous, high-dose vitamin E cannot suppress gap junction proliferation, and thus there are clinical failures.

Spindle cell proliferation occurs during trend III and is related to the RLF score. Although this RLF score was empirically created,[7] it appears to predict the different extent of spindle cell proliferation in control infants C and D (FIGURE 2B and C). Infant C was assigned an RLF score of 10 and died at 10 weeks postpartum age with the spindle cells occupying 54% of the nerve fiber volume. This contrasts with infant D, whose RLF score was 6 and who died at 12 weeks postpartum age with significantly fewer ($p < 0.001$) spindle cells in the nerve fiber layer (32% volume). Thus, there is ultrastructural support for differences between the moderate risk and severe risk categories established by this RLF score.

The presence of microvilli extending from spindle cells appears to be related to postpartum age. All control or treatment infants <25 days postpartum (infants A, B, and E–I) had smooth contoured spindle cells (FIGURE 6A and C). Only those control and treatment infants >10 weeks postpartum (infants C, D, J, and K) had spindle cells with numerous surface microvilli (FIGURE 6B and D), whether the spindle cells were a minimal or an extensive retinal component. There was also no relationship between the number of microvilli and the increase in gap junction area (TABLE 4) (infants B and F–I).

This is the first time that the ultrastructural parameters of human spindle cells have been documented. In the embryologic state, they are not linked by gap junctions, display minimal surface microvilli, and secrete no basal lamina. Their cytoplasm contains bloated rough endoplasmic reticulum with a dense osmiophilic content and numerous glycogen granules, which explain their periodic acid-Schiff (PAS)–positive staining in light microscopy preparations.[4] In these infants, the spindle cells form a continuous, uniform apron in advance of the nascent retinal vasculature. This apron extends to the ora serrata by 25 weeks gestational age. In infant H, the inner retina had not differentiated peripherally and there were no spindle cells in these regions. Therefore, spindle cells extend anteriorly only after a morphological nerve fiber layer exists.

There is a need for an animal model in which the human condition can be more closely analyzed. In the fetal rat,[22] the process of spindle cell migration into the nerve fiber layer prior to angiogenesis is identical to that observed in humans. However, premature (>15 day) rats have not survived for vitamin E and oxygen modulation experiments. The rabbit and kitten have inner retinal vascularizations that proliferate from endothelial cells,[26,28] and thus, there are no mesenchymal spindle cell precursors despite intravitreal neovascularization in response to oxygen administration. Furthermore, in the kitten there is never any retinal separation or cicatricial RLF but only a slow remodeling of the retinal vasculature.[24,27]

The data base of this paper is pathologic material that was derived from human sources, and thus, exactly matched control and treatment infants could not be obtained at the ideal times. Material from a few critical times still has to be obtained. Specifically, the eyes from a few very young infants (<4 days) should be obtained to confirm that the spindle cells initially have minimal gap junction area, that is, that trend I is a consistent phenomenon. Some young infants (4–15 days) should be obtained to determine trend II kinetics. Finally, numerous eyes from infants who survive longer than 4 weeks with RLF scores from 7 to 10 must be studied to determine the effectiveness of vitamin E in modulating maturation events of trend III. In this study, no eyes from any treatment infant with an RLF score from 7 to 10 have been obtained. Little "control" pathologic material is anticipated, since the efficacy of vitamin E has been established and high-dose, daily, oral vitamin E is part of routine care of the high-risk, preterm infant at the Texas Children's Hospital.

ACKNOWLEDGMENTS

The authors acknowledge the photographic expertise of Alexander Kogan, the laboratory assistance of Evelyn Brown and Dorothy Carr, the discussions with Ramon L. Font, M.D., the critical evaluation of the text by Michael Osato, Ph.D., and David Hunter, and the efforts of the nurses, pediatric house officers, and neonatology fellows and academic staff of the Texas Children's Hospital and the Jefferson Davis Hospital, Houston.

REFERENCES

1. ASHTON, N. 1970. Retinal angiogenesis in the human embryo. Br. Med. Bull. **26:** 103–106.
2. PATZ, A. 1969. Retrolental fibroplasia. Surv. Ophthalmol. **14:** 1–29.
3. FOOS, R. Y. & S. M. KOPELOW. 1973. Development of retinal vasculature in paranatal infants. Surv. Ophthalmol. **18:** 117–127.
4. FOOS, R. Y. 1975. Acute retrolental fibroplasia. Albrecht von Graefes Arch. Klin. Exp. Ophthalmol. **195:** 87–100.
5. KINSEY, V. E. 1956. Retrolental fibroplasia: cooperative study of retrolental fibroplasia and the use of oxygen. Arch. Ophthalmol. **56:** 481–543.
6. PALMER, E. A. 1981. Optimal timing of examination for acute retrolental fibroplasia. Ophthalmology **88:** 662–668.
7. HITTNER, H. M., L. B. GODIO, A. J. RUDOLPH, J. M. ADAMS, J. A. GARCIA-PRATS, Z. FRIEDMAN, J. A. KAUTZ & W. A. MONACO. 1981. Retrolental fibroplasia: efficacy of vitamin E in a double-blind clinical study of preterm infants. N. Engl. J. Med. **305:** 1365–1371.
8. OWENS, W. C. & E. U. OWENS. 1949. Retrolental fibroplasia in premature infants. II. Studies on the prophylaxis of the disease: the use of alpha tocopheryl acetate. Am. J. Ophthalmol. **32:** 1631–1637.
9. JOHNSON, L., D. SCHAFFER & T. R. BOGGS, JR. 1974. The premature infant, vitamin E deficiency and retrolental fibroplasia. Am. J. Clin. Nutr. **27:** 1158–1173.
10. HITTNER, H. M., L. B. GODIO, M. E. SPEER, A. J. RUDOLPH, M. M. TAYLOR, C. BLIFELD & F. L. KRETZER. Retrolental fibroplasia: further clinical evidence and ultrastructural support for efficacy of vitamin E in the preterm infant. Pediatrics. (Submitted for publication.)
11. HANSEN, L. G. & W. J. WARWICK. 1966. A fluorometric micro method for serum tocopherol. Am. J. Clin Pathol. **46:** 133–138.
12. MCCORMICK, A. Q. 1977. Retinopathy of prematurity. Curr. Probl. Pediatr. **7:** 1–28.
13. KRETZER, F. L., H. M. HITTNER & R. MEHTA. 1981. Ocular manifestations of Conradi and Zellweger syndromes. Metab. Pediatr. Ophthalmol. **5:** 1–11.
14. WEIBEL, E., G. KISTLER & W. SCHERLE. 1966. Practical stereological methods for morphometric cytology. J. Cell Biol. **30:** 23–38.
15. HERTZBERG, E. L., T. S. LAWRENCE & N. B. GILULA. 1981. Gap junctional communication. Annu. Rev. Physiol. **43:** 479–491.
16. DECKER, R. S. 1976. Hormonal regulation of gap junction differentiation. J. Cell Biol. **69:** 669–685.
17. YEE, A. G. & J. P. REVEL. 1978. Loss and reappearance of gap junctions in regenerating liver. J. Cell Biol. **78:** 554–564.
18. ELIAS, P. M. & D. S. FRIEND. 1976. Vitamin-A-induced mucous metaplasia. An *in vitro* system for modulating tight and gap junction differentiation. J. Cell Biol. **68:** 173–188.
19. FARRELL, P. M. 1979. Vitamin E deficiency in premature infants. J. Pediatr. **95:** 869–872.
20. KORNBRUST, D. J. & R. D. MAVIS. 1980. Relative susceptibility of microsomes of lung, heart, liver, kidney, brain and testes to lipid peroxidation: correlation with vitamin E content. Lipids **15:** 315–322.
21. BELL, E. F., E. J. BROWN, R. MINNER, J. C. SINCLAIR & A. ZIPURSKY. 1979. Vitamin E absorption in small premature infants. Pediatrics **63:** 830–832.
22. SHAKIB, M., L. F. DE OLIVEIRA & P. HENKIND. 1968. Development of retinal vessels. II. Earliest stages of vessel formation. Invest. Ophthalmol. **7:** 689–700.
23. ROBISON, W. G., T. KUWABARA & J. G. BIERI. 1979. Vitamin E deficiency and the retina: photoreceptor and pigment epithelial changes. Invest. Ophthalmol. Vision Sci. **18:** 683–690.
24. PHELPS, D. L. & A. ROSENBAUM. 1979. Vitamin E in kitten oxygen-induced retinopathy. II. Blockage of vitreal neovascularization. Arch. Ophthalmol. **97:** 1522–1526.
25. FLYNN, J. T., G. E. O'GRADY, J. HERRERA, B. J. KUSHNER, S. CANTOLINO & W. MILAM. 1977. Retrolental fibroplasia. I. Clinical observations. Arch. Ophthalmol. **95:** 217–223.

26. ASHTON, N., B. TRIPATHI & G. KNIGHT. 1972. Effects of oxygen on the developing retinal vessels of the rabbit. I. Anatomy and development of the retinal vessels of the rabbit. Exp. Eye Res. **14:** 214–220.
27. PHELPS, D. L. & A. ROSENBAUM. 1977. The role of tocopherol in oxygen-induced retinopathy: kitten model. Pediatrics **59:** 998–1005.
28. MICHAELSON, I. C. 1948. Vascular morphogenesis in the retina of the cat. J. Anat. **82:** 167–174.

DISCUSSION

S. J. GROSS (*Duke University Medical Center, Durham, N.C.*): What do you do with the very high-risk babies you describe when you can't put anything through the gastrointestinal tract? This certainly isn't an uncommon problem.

F. L. KRETZER: That's correct. These patients have all been given vitamin E by the oral route. There has been no problem with the development of necrotizing enterocolitis. There were two control and two treatment cases with necrotizing enterocolitis in the 1980 and 1981 studies. For instance, one child was removed from vitamin E because of enterocolitis from days 10 to 20 and went on to develop a very severe retinopathy. Apparently the spindle cells are more sensitized at 27 to 30 weeks. But these data have to be given a multivariate analysis. It's too simplistic to say it's only gestational age.

K. C. BHUYAN (*Mount Sinai School of Medicine, New York, N.Y.*): The way I understood it, when you expose the premature infant to high oxygen tension, the vessels respond with constriction even to the extent of obliteration?

F. L. KRETZER: That's correct.

K. C. BHUYAN: In your classification, I didn't hear you stating that. What you said was vasodilation and proliferation.

F. L. KRETZER: Dr. Hittner, do you want to comment on the classification?

H. M. HITTNER: The immediate vasoconstriction that you see with regard to administration of oxygen is not in the McCormick classification. The McCormick classification describes the neovascularization in the retina (I) and in the vitreous (II) and the late visual dilatation that occurs in the posterior pole (III). The vasoconstriction that Dr. Bhuyan is talking about is not in the McCormick system.

K. C. BHUYAN: Have you seen cataracts in these cases?

H. M. HITTNER: No. Not at all.

K. C. BHUYAN: Is there any change of photoreceptor atrophy?

F. L. KRETZER: Some of the children we've looked at are so immature that in the peripheral retina, the outer segments still have not been developed. But I think you can see from the light microscopy that there is no atrophy or reduction in the number of photoreceptor nuclei, there's no change in the synaptology if it has developed that far peripherally, and there's certainly no toxicity of the ganglion cells. So with regard to retinal ultrastructure, that's not affected.

A. E. KITABCHI (*University of Tennessee, Memphis, Tenn.*): Is there background retinopathy in these children or is it all proliferative retinopathy?

F. L. KRETZER: Proliferative in the two cases of RLF III.

A. E. KITABCHI: How do you contrast these with diabetic proliferative retinopathy? Do you have fluorescein leakage in the anterior chamber?

H. M. HITTNER: Diabetic and RLF leakage of vessels is similar. Dr. Flynn has documented leakage of fluorescein from the shunt and has specified that growth of the vessels past the shunt indicates early regression. We and others have documented that in the anterior segment, the iris vessels also leak.

L. JOHNSON (*University of Pennsylvania, Philadelphia, Pa.*): Dr. Kretzer, I think it's important to remember the levels of vitamin E that were present in your two groups. In your control group, your mean level was 0.6 mg%, and in your treatment group, in the range of 1.8 mg%?

F. L. KRETZER: 1.2–1.8 mg%.

L. JOHNSON: Could you comment later on the kind of formulas that you are giving the infants and also what the [umbilical] cord levels of vitamin E were. The infants that we are now treating in a control fashion—the placebo infants—most of them had mean serum E levels in the range of 1.8 mg%.

F. L. KRETZER: How old are those infants?

L. JOHNSON: The babies are born with cord blood levels of 0.6 mg%, but there has been quite a change, at least in this part of the country, in the E nutrition in the population in general. And I think that is important in interpreting results of control studies.

The other thing I would like to say is that we were sorry, along with you, that you found that some babies did develop severe RLF in the treatment group. We found two infants—who were maintained quite well on higher levels of serum vitamin E than you had with an oral preparation—who had bad RLF. We hoped that with the parenteral preparation given early, we could prevent this.

F. L. KRETZER: It's not an all-or-none phenomenon. I don't think you can ever ask for vitamin E to be one hundred percent effective in suppressing retinopathy. The efficacy comes maximally in those children age 27, 28, and 29 weeks. Those at 25 and 26 weeks are at maximal risk for developing RLF even under treatment conditions.

H. M. HITTNER: I might just comment that the two failures we had were both at 27 weeks gestational age, weighed less than 790 grams, had always been on oxygen, and had intraventricular hemorrhage. These were very, very sick babies.

L. JOHNSON: I think you are seeing an example of RLF that is greatly complicated by things other than hyperoxia, because even levels of 5 mg% vitamin E persistently will not prevent this.

F. L. KRETZER: That's why I think the multivariate analysis is so crucial.

M. K. HORWITT (*St. Louis Medical Center, St. Louis, Mo.*): Dr. Johnson has already commented on a point I want to raise, and that's the difference in the plasma levels between the two groups. You had a 50% difference. What were the compounds used in the second series?

F. L. KRETZER: The first was *all-rac-α*-tocopherol in propylene glycol polyascorbate-80.

M. K. HORWITT: Well that's the *all-rac* compound then. Was the other one something else?

F. L. KRETZER: The other compound was *all-rac-α*-tocopheryl acetate (Aquasol E).

K. C. HAYES (*Harvard School of Public Health, Boston, Mass.*): I'm trying to contemplate the cell biology of your observations. Would you care to comment on whether or not you think that tocopherol has a primary effect on the gap junctions or if it is a secondary phenomenon.

F. L. KRETZER: The surface area of the gap junctions can be modulated within a short period of time. This is a very common biological phenomenon. It can be hormone modulated, with thyroid hormone. It can be increased by *in vitro* tissue culture when you add vitamin A. Now whether vitamin E is a modulator or whether it prevents the lipid peroxidation that changes the membrane fluidity and this allows the connexin to aggregate, is not known.

K. C. HAYES: Let me just press you, Dr. Kretzer, on this same point. What hypothesis of vitamin E action best explains this embryological effect on gap junction development in children?

F. L. KRETZER: At the gap junction, as the spindle cells normally exist in the hypoxic condition *in utero*, spindle cells continue to form endothelial cells and the vasculature continues to develop normally. However, if you put that infant into the hyperoxic situation of continuous oxygen therapy, you could then speculate that there might be lipid peroxidation of those membranes, changes in lipid fluidity, aggregation of those isolated connexin areas into maximal gap junction areas, and this becomes a new population of spindle cells that are not primed for endothelial differentiation.

K. C. HAYES: But is there evidence of this peroxidation in this particular step?

F. L. KRETZER: As far as I know, no one has isolated these spindle cells and seen a change in the polyunsaturated lipid content.

K. C. HAYES: I only raise this question because there still is a genetic regulatory hypothesis for vitamin E action that is illustrated in rotifer differentiation and the induction of certain enzymes in animals as a function of vitamin E status. The mechanism underlying these effects of vitamin E is not settled yet.

H. R. D. WOLF (*Justus-Liebig University, Giessen, Federal Republic of Germany*): I want to come back to your point concerning vascular leakage. I wanted to ask you if there is any evidence for occurrence of vascular leakage in adult tissues.

H. M. HITTNER: The vascular leakage in the shunt that you're talking about occurs at eight weeks of life. That's a late phenomenon. This gap junction phenomenon that we are talking about occurs in the first five days of life. There's no leakage at that time.

TISSUE α-TOCOPHEROL LEVELS IN NORMAL, OBESE, AND HYPERLIPEMIC RATS

G. L. Catignani and P. A. Fuller

Department of Food Science
North Carolina State University
Raleigh, North Carolina 27650

A direct relationship of plasma tocopherol levels to tissue tocopherol levels in normolipemic animals has been reported.[1] In addition it is known that altered plasma total lipid alters plasma tocopherol.[2] It would be expected then that altered plasma lipids would alter plasma tocopherol and, hence, tissue tocopherol. Although decreased plasma lipids decrease tissue tocopherol,[3,4] elevated plasma lipids in Zucker obese rats did not elevate tissue tocopherol.[4] The failure of tissue to accumulate α-tocopherol was attributed primarily to the degree of adiposity that the animals exhibited. Zucker obese rats also exhibited a hyperlipemia; thus, distinguishing the effect of hyperlipemia from those of obesity was not possible with this animal model. Therefore study was undertaken to determine the effects of hyperlipemia in the absence of obesity on the level of α-tocopherol in rat tissue.

Male Zucker obese and normal littermates were used throughout the study. Animals were maintained on AIN-76A complete diet containing 50 mg/kg RRR-α-tocopheryl acetate. Obese and normal rats were pair fed using complete diet. Obese rats were given an additional portion of a vitamin E-free diet daily.

Plasma and red blood cell tocopherol levels were determined by the method of Bieri et al.,[5] and tissue tocopherol levels were determined by a method developed in this laboratory. Briefly, frozen tissues were ground in anhydrous Na_2SO_4 (6 g to 1 g of tissue) in a cold mortar and pestle, divided into equal portions, extracted with hexane, and treated as above for plasma. Tocopherol was added to one portion, and recoveries calculated. Tissues were analyzed for total lipid content by the procedure of Folch et al.,[6] and plasma lipid levels were analyzed by a modified procedure of Knight et al.[7]

Zucker obese rats, which exhibit both hyperlipemia and obesity, and normal littermates injected with Triton WR-1339 to induce hyperlipemia alone were used as models. Normal littermates served as controls. Plasma total lipid and plasma tocopherol values increased significantly in both models. Neither model exhibited the increase in tissue tocopherol levels known to accompany the increase in plasma tocopherol levels in normolipemic animals. Previous literature had suggested that adiposity was the primary cause of the failure of tissues to accumulate α-tocopherol.[4] By use of the chemical-induced hyperlipemic model, it was demonstrated that the tissue α-tocopherol levels were not elevated even in the absence of excess adiposity. Thus hyperlipemia alone produced the observed effects on tissue tocopherol level. A direct relationship of tissue tocopherol to degree of hyperlipemia or to levels of plasma tocopherol was not observed. Instead it was found that the parameter that defines the role of plasma levels both for tocopherol and for total lipid to tissue levels of α-tocopherol was the α-tocopherol to total lipid ratio in plasma. Over a ratio range of 0.77 to 9.07 (normal, obese, and hyperlipemic animals), the tissue levels of α-tocopherol of both testes and lungs gave a correlation coefficient of 0.88.

The total lipid in these tissues was not different when compared to controls. The data suggest that tissue and plasma α-tocopherol exchange in a passive manner with partitioning being determined by the level of total lipid in each compartment. The use of plasma α-tocopherol–total lipid ratio to assess tocopherol status has been suggested[2] but has not found widespread use in either clinical or survey settings. The α-tocopherol to total lipid ratio gives the best estimate of tissue tocopherol levels and thus should be employed routinely where a questionable tocopherol status is suspected. The use of this ratio may be particularly judicious for the assessment of tocopherol status in hyperlipemic individuals.

REFERENCES

1. BIERI, J. G. 1972. Ann. N.Y. Acad. Sci. **203:** 181.
2. HORWITT, M. K., C. C. HARVEY, C. H. J. DAHM & M. T. SEARCY. 1972. Ann. N.Y. Acad. Sci. **203:** 223.
3. DAVIES, T., J. KELLEHER, C. L. SMITH, B. E. WALKER & M. S. LOSOWSKY. 1972. J. Lab. Clin. Med. **79:** 824.
4. BIERI, J. G. & R. P. EVARTS. 1975. Proc. Soc. Exp. Biol. Med. **149:** 500.
5. BIERI, J. G., T. J. TOLLIVER & G. L. CATIGNANI. 1979. Am. J. Clin. Nutr. **32:** 2143.
6. FOLCH, J., M. LEES & G. H. S. STANLEY. 1957. J. Biol. Chem. **226:** 497.
7. KNIGHT, J. A., S. ANDERSON & J. M. RAWLE. 1972. Clin. Chem. **18:** 199.

THE ROLE OF VITAMIN E IN THERAPY OF CATARACT IN ANIMALS*

Kailash C. Bhuyan, Durga K. Bhuyan, and Steven M. Podos

Department of Ophthalmology
Mount Sinai School of Medicine
City University of New York
New York, New York 10029

Oxidative damage to the crystalline lens is a common occurrence in the majority of cataracts. It is our hypothesis that toxic metabolites of oxygen, such as O_2^-, H_2O_2, OH·, and $^1O_2$, are the triggering agents in cataractogenesis.[1,2] From studies on animal models of cataract, we have found that H_2O_2 is increased in aqueous humor as a result of decreased primary enzymatic defenses against O_2^- and H_2O_2.[1-5] The secondary defenses, such as ascorbic acid of lens, aqueous humor, and vitreous humor and glutathione (GSH) of lens, are also lowered in cataracts. Evidence of peroxidative damage to the lenticular plasma membrane lipids, as indicated by increased malondialdehyde (MDA) formation in cataracts, has been observed.[4-6] Similar biochemical alterations were seen in the senile cataracts of the human.[6] Since the biological antioxidant α-tocopherol (vitamin E) is capable of minimizing lipid damage from peroxidation in cellular membranes,[7] we investigated its efficacy in the therapy of cataracts in animals.

Two different experimental models of cataract were used. Cataract was induced in healthy, just-weaned Dutch rabbits by feeding them 0.2–0.4% 3-amino-1H-1,2,4-triazole (3-aminotriazole) in the diet or in drinking water, following our previously reported technique.[2,3] Morphologically, cataracts were classified as stages 1 through 5 depending on the severity of changes and the density of opacification as seen by slit-lamp biomicroscopy. When multiple vacuoles appeared in the equatorial zone with a trace posterior cortical opacity (stage 2), 3-aminotriazole was withdrawn from the diet or drinking water; and in a group of such rabbits, therapy of cataract was started by administering *all-rac-α*-tocopherol (Hoffmann-La Roche, Inc.), 50 mg/kg body weight intramuscularly daily, for 5–16 weeks. In another group of rabbits having stage 2 cataract, vitamin E, 100 mg daily for 2–3 weeks, was given orally as a capsule. Another identical group of rabbits was maintained as controls without therapy. FIGURE 1 shows that in the control group, cataract advanced to stage 4 or 5, in which the lenticular opacity increased to a complete zonular form, in 10 to 16 weeks after 3-aminotriazole feeding. In the experimental rabbits on therapy for 2 to 16 weeks, the cataract was arrested in about 50% of animals.

At the end of therapy, H_2O_2 and ascorbic acid concentrations in ocular humors were determined by their respective oxidation and reduction reactions with 2,6-dichlorophenolindophenol as described in earlier reports.[1,2,4,5] MDA of lens was estimated by its condensation reaction with 2-thiobarbituric acid,[4-6,8] and the vitamin E content of aqueous humor, vitreous humor, and lens was estimated by Dr. Lawrence J. Machlin using a high-pressure liquid chromatography technique. We confirmed that in rabbits, α-tocopherol reaches the aqueous humor, vitreous

*This investigation was supported by U.S. Public Health Service Grants RO1.EY03012, EY01867, and EY03651 from the National Eye Institute, National Institutes of Health.

humor, and lens after its parenteral administration as a single dose of 50 mg/kg body weight intramuscularly daily for 4–5 days (unpublished data). The data given in TABLE 1 show that in untreated experimental rabbits having cataract, there was a two- to threefold increase of H_2O_2, a 60% decrease of ascorbic acid of aqueous humor and vitreous humor, and a twofold increase of MDA of lens, as compared to the controls. However, in vitamin E–treated rabbits, these altered biochemical parameters were restored close to the levels observed in eye tissues of control rabbits.

The second model for cataract was induced in three- to four-day-old Sprague-Dawley rats by injecting Na_2SeO_3 subcutaneously as a single dose of 20 μmoles/kg body weight. The morphology of cataract was classified as stages 1 through 7. When a trace opacity was observed in the nuclear zone (stage 1a or 1b), therapy was begun in groups of such rats by administering *all-rac-α*-tocopherol, 50 mg/kg body weight as a single intraperitoneal injection daily, or a supplement of *all-rac-α*-tocopheryl acetate, 2.5 g/kg in the diet for three to six weeks. In each group, control littermate rats were maintained with placebo. Though the effects of vitamin E treatment on the morphology of cataract in rat were inconclusive, the treatment caused a significant decrease in H_2O_2 of aqueous humor to 0.05 ± 0.01 mM [mean ± standard deviation (SD), 10 groups of five to six rats each] as compared to 0.15 ± 0.05 mM (12 groups) in placebo-injected littermates. Similarly, after therapy there was reduction in MDA of lens by about 40% (p < 0.001).

A prior report shows retardation of sugar-induced cataract *in vitro* by vitamin E.[9] Our experimental evidence demonstrates that parenterally administered

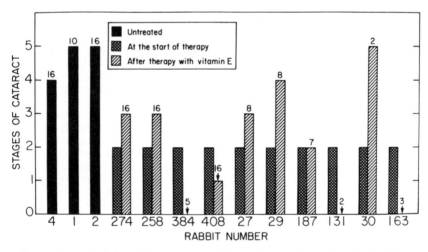

FIGURE 1. Effect of vitamin E treatment on the morphology of 3-aminotriazole-induced cataract in rabbit. Therapy with vitamin E was started with a dose of 50 mg/kg body weight intramuscularly daily, except for rabbits 131, 30, and 163, which received an oral dose of 100 mg vitamin E daily. Figure on top of each column indicates weeks. Cataract was graded as stage 1, separation of posterior lens suture with vacuoles at either end, lamellar separation, and trace posterior opacity (1+); stage 2, findings of stage 1, multiple vacuoles in ring form at the equator, and increased posterior cortical opacity (2+); stage 3, partial disappearance of vacuoles and extension of cortical opacity (3+) to the equator; stage 4, few scattered vacuoles at the equator and light complete zonular opacity (4+); or stage 5, complete disappearance of vacuoles and dense zonular opacity (5+), nucleus still clear.

TABLE 1

EFFECT OF VITAMIN E *In Vivo* ON SOME BIOCHEMICAL PARAMETERS
IN CATARACT INDUCED IN RABBIT BY 3-AMINOTRIAZOLE

Biochemical Constituents of Eye	Control Rabbit with Normal Lens	Experimental Rabbit with Early Cataract (Stage 2)	
		No Treatment	α-Tocopherol*
Aqueous humor			
H_2O_2 (mM)	0.05 ± 0.01 (4)†	0.14 ± 0.02 (4)‡	0.04 ± 0.01 (4)‡
Ascorbic acid (mM)	1.17 ± 0.14 (4)	0.38 ± 0.03 (4)	1.01 ± 0.35 (4)
Vitreous humor			
H_2O_2 (mM)	0.03 ± 0.003 (4)	0.06 ± 0.004 (4)	0.02 ± 0.01 (4)
Ascorbic acid (mM)	0.41 ± 0.07 (4)	0.17 ± 0.05 (4)	0.42 ± 0.12 (4)
Lens			
MDA (nmol/g wet weight)	1.21 ± 0.17 (8)	2.63 ± 0.24 (8)	1.76 ± 0.25 (8)

*In a dose of 50 mg/kg body weight administered intramuscularly daily for 2–16 weeks.
†Mean ± SD, number of rabbits or lenses studied given in parentheses.
‡$p < 0.001$ for all the results given in columns three and four.

vitamin E is capable of arresting the progression of 3-aminotriazole-induced cataract *in vivo* in about 50% of rabbits and reversing the cataract in some animals. In addition, vitamin E in rabbit or rat is capable of reducing some biochemical changes occurring in the eyes of animals with cataract. Thus we conclude that vitamin E is effective in the therapy of certain forms of cataract in the rabbit.

REFERENCES

1. BHUYAN, K. C. & D. K. BHUYAN. 1977. Regulation of hydrogen peroxide in eye humors: effect of 3-amino-1*H*-1,2,4-triazole on catalase and glutathione peroxidase of rabbit eye. Biochim. Biophys. Acta **497**: 641–651.
2. BHUYAN, K. C. & D. K. BHUYAN. 1978. Superoxide dismutase of the eye: relative functions of superoxide dismutase and catalase in protecting the ocular lens from oxidative damage. Biochim. Biophys. Acta **542**: 28–38.
3. BHUYAN, K. C., D. K. BHUYAN & H. M. KATZIN. 1973. Amizol induced cataract and inhibition of lens catalase in rabbit. Ophthalmic Res. **5**: 236–247.
4. BHUYAN, K. C., D. K. BHUYAN & S. M. PODOS. 1981. Selenium induced cataract: biochemical mechanism. *In* Selenium in Biology and Medicine. J. E. Spallholz, J. L. Martin & H. E. Ganther, Eds. (Chapter 40): 403–412. Avi Publishing Company, Inc. Westport, Conn.
5. BHUYAN, K. C., D. K. BHUYAN & S. M. PODOS. 1981. Cataract induced by selenium in rat. II. Increased lipid peroxidation and impairment of enzymatic defense against oxidative damage. IRCS Med. Sci. **9**: 195–196.
6. BHUYAN, K. C., D. K. BHUYAN & S. M. PODOS. 1981. Evidence of increased lipid peroxidation in cataracts. IRCS Med. Sci. **9**: 126–127.
7. LUCY, J. A. 1972. Functional and structural aspects of biological membranes; a suggested structural role for vitamin E in the control of membrane permeability and stability. Ann. N.Y. Acad. Sci. **203**: 4–11.
8. DAHLE, L. K., E. H. HILL & R. T. HOLMAN. 1962. The thiobarbituric acid reaction and the autoxidations of polyunsaturated fatty acid methyl esters. Arch. Biochem. Biophys. **98**: 253–261.
9. CREIGHTON, M. O. & J. R. TREVITHICK. 1979. Cortical cataract formation prevented by vitamin E and glutathione. Exp. Eye Res. **29**: 689–693.

THE NEUROPATHOLOGY OF CHRONIC VITAMIN E DEFICIENCY IN MAN AND OTHER MAMMALS*

James S. Nelson

Department of Pathology
Washington University School of Medicine
St. Louis, Missouri 63110

Nervous system lesions in mammals with chronic vitamin E deficiency have been delineated most extensively in rats. Other mammals including primates have been studied to a limited extent. Dystrophic axons occur postmortem in medullary sensory relay nuclei of children with lipid malabsorption and putative vitamin E deficiency associated with cystic fibrosis or congenital biliary atresia. Degeneration of the gracile fasciculus has been described in cystic fibrosis. These retrospective studies have not been correlated with a clinical neurological disorder.

We have studied nervous system lesions in vitamin E–deficient rats and rhesus monkeys and in two children with congenital biliary atresia, documented low serum vitamin E levels, and a progressive neurological disorder.[1-3] In this report the neuropathologic lesions in the experimental animals and humans are compared. The relationship between the neuropathologic lesions in the children and the accompanying neurologic syndrome is demonstrated.

Experimental animals were fed purified vitamin E–deficient diets for 1-3 years. Control animals were fed identical diets supplemented with vitamin E. The children were two males dying at ages 5 and 8 years with congenital biliary atresia. Serum vitamin E levels, despite treatment, remained very low throughout the life of the patients. At 4 years of age, the older child had developed a progressive neurologic disorder including loss of deep tendon reflexes, posterior column signs, gait disturbance, and abnormal extraocular movements. An identical neurologic syndrome has been observed in five other patients in our institution with congenital biliary atresia and low serum vitamin E levels.

Paraffin and plastic sections of the central and peripheral nervous system were examined using the following stains: hematoxylin and eosin, Luxol Fast Blue–periodic acid Schiff (myelin), Sevier-Munger (axons), Holzer (astrocytes), and alkaline toluidine blue (sural nerve). Individual osmicated fibers were teased from the sural nerves of two deficient monkeys and the two children, and examined by light microscopy. The frequency distribution of myelinated fiber diameters per mm^2 of endoneurium and the number of myelinated fibers per mm^2 of endoneurium (fiber density) in the sural nerves of monkeys and humans were determined using photographic enlargements of the sural nerves, a planimeter, a Zeiss TGZ 3 particle-size analyzer, and a programmable calculator.

These studies demonstrated a progressive systematized sensory axonopathy affecting large-caliber myelinated axons in the vitamin E–deficient rats, monkeys, and humans. The lesions were most severe in the distal segments of the axon. The most extensive lesions were found in the posterior or dorsal columns. Dystrophic axons were numerous in humans and rats and infrequent in monkeys.

*Supported by U.S. Public Health Service Grant NS 11277 and by a grant from Hoffmann-La Roche, Inc.

Nerve cell bodies were only slightly affected. Neurogenic patterns of skeletal muscle atrophy are absent. The neurologic syndrome in the older child correlates closely with the neuropathologic lesions observed at autopsy. The vitamin E-deficient rat is a convenient experimental model for neuropathologic studies of vitamin E deficiency applicable to humans.

REFERENCES

1. MACHLIN, L. J., R. FILIPSKI, J. NELSON, L. HORN & M. BRIN. 1977. Effects of a prolonged vitamin E deficiency in the rat. J. Nutr. **107:** 1200–1208.
2. NELSON, J. S., C. D. FITCH, V. W. FISCHER, G. D. BROUN, JR. & A. C. CHOU. 1981. Progressive neuropathologic lesions in vitamin E-deficient rhesus monkeys. J. Neuropathol. Exp. Neurol. **40:** 166–186.
3. ROSENBLUM, J. L., J. P. KEATING, A. L. PRENSKY & J. S. NELSON. 1981. A progressive neurologic syndrome in children with chronic liver disease. N. Engl. J. Med. **304:** 503–508.

PLASMA HIGH-DENSITY LIPOPROTEIN CHOLESTEROL AND VITAMIN E SUPPLEMENTS

Joseph J. Barboriak, Kaup R. Shetty, Ahmed Z. El-Ghatit, and John H. Kalbfleisch

Medical College of Wisconsin and
Wood Veterans Administration Medical Center
Milwaukee, Wisconsin 53193

An inverse association between the blood levels of high-density lipoprotein cholesterol (HDLC) and the extent of coronary artery occlusion has been reported by several groups of investigators.[1,2] However, the reported consistent means of elevating HDLC—alcohol[3] and physical exercise[4]—have some drawbacks and are not applicable to all in need of such measures. Recent reports have indicated that vitamin E may also increase HDLC levels.[5] In the present study, we have investigated the effects of daily vitamin E supplement (800 IU/day) on plasma HDLC levels of 13 women, 13 men, and 19 spinal cord injury (SCI) patients. The latter group has been reported to have very low HDLC levels.[6] After four weeks of treatment, the group of women showed an increase from 66 to 71 mg/dl of plasma HDLC ($p < 0.05$). A group of 8 male athletes with initial HDLC levels of 68 mg/dl did not show any consistent changes, while in the remaining 5 sedentary men, the HDLC rose from 45 to 52 mg/dl ($p < 0.01$). The SCI patients with low initial HDLC demonstrated an increase from 32 to 39 mg/dl ($p < 0.01$). Again, no effect was seen in the 8 SCI patients with the initial levels of 53 mg/dl. A subsequent two-week period without vitamin E supplement led to a slight reduction of HDLC levels in both male groups that responded to the vitamin E treatment.

Interestingly, there were no marked changes in plasma triglyceride levels, except that the subgroup of men with low initial HDLC levels showed a slight rise and men with high initial HDLC levels showed a reduction of the triglycerides. Changes in plasma total cholesterol levels were relatively small, with most groups showing a slight increase during the initial two weeks of vitamin E supplementation, possibly reflecting the rise in HDLC.

Determination of plasma vitamin E levels indicated good compliance with the treatment. Only minimal body weight changes were observed during the four-week experimental period (± 2 pounds); the age of the participants ranged from 22 to 60 years. Our results confirm the previous report that the effect of vitamin E supplement is mainly seen in individuals with initially low HDLC levels.[5]

REFERENCES

1. MILLER, N. E., J. HAMMETT, S. SALTISSI, S. RAO, H. VAN ZELLER, J. COLTART & B. LEWIS. 1981. Br. Med. J. **282:** 1741–1744.
2. BARBORIAK, J. J., A. J. ANDERSON, A. A. RIMM & J. F. KING. 1979. Metabolism **28:** 735–737.
3. BARBORIAK, J. J., A. J. ANDERSON & R. G. HOFFMANN. 1979. J. Lab. Clin. Med. **94:** 348–353.
4. WOOD, P. D. & W. L. HASKEL. 1979. Lipids **14:** 417–427.
5. HERMANN, W. J., K. WARD & J. FAUCETT. 1979. Am. J. Clin. Pathol. **72:** 848–852.
6. HELDENBERG, D., A. RUBINSTEIN & O. LEVTOV. 1981. Atherosclerosis **39:** 163–167.

CLINICAL EVALUATION OF RED BLOOD CELL
TOCOPHEROL*

M. Mino, S. Nakagawa, H. Tamai, and M. Miki

Department of Pediatrics
Osaka Medical College
Takatsuki, 569, Japan

In the course of our study, red blood cells (RBCs) were used as the source of biological membrane.[1-3] This may give us information about a biologically important tocopherol, because RBCs are clinically easy to obtain. To measure RBC tocopherol levels in the clinical situation, the following examinations were performed.

Determination and separation of tocopherol analogues were performed by high-performance liquid chromatography.[1] In this study, tocopherol values are shown only as the α-form unless otherwise designated.

1. The relation of H_2O_2 hemolysis to RBC tocopherol levels was compared with that to plasma tocopherol levels. The H_2O_2 hemolysis test was examined using our slight modification[4] of the original method.[5] Blood was collected from premature and sick infants (96 cases) within six months of birth to obtain specimens with positive hemolysis by this test. All samples were divided into two groups, hemolysis (20% or more; 31 cases) and nonhemolysis (65 cases). As shown in FIGURE 1, there was a large overlap in plasma tocopherol levels between the two groups but the overlap was smaller in RBC levels. This shows that the hemolysis may be more directly related to tocopherol in RBCs than in plasma. We considered the lower limit of normal plasma and RBC tocopherol as 450 μg/dl and 125 μg/dl packed cells, respectively, since more than 85% of infants with hemolysis had less than 450 μg/dl plasma levels, and more than 85% of the hemolysis group and less than 15% of the nonhemolysis group, with respect to RBC levels, had 125 μg/dl packed cells or less. The lower limit of plasma levels in this study was lower than that reported previously, because we determined the α-form alone.

With respect to the discrepancy in correlation of the hemolysis to RBC tocopherol levels (as shown in the overlap area, FIGURE 1), changes in lipid constituents of RBC membranes deficient in vitamin E were examined in rats by the thin-layer chromatography method in combination with flame ionization detection,[6] accompanied by lipid extraction with chloroform-isopropanol 7:11 (v/v) from whole RBCs. Phosphatidylethanolamine and sphingomyelin decreased markedly as tocopherol content became negligible in RBCs after 12 weeks of deficiency. The cholesterol change was minimal, and the changes in phosphatidylcholine and phosphatidylserine were intermediate. The changes in RBC lipids were reversed with recovery from the deficient state. This finding suggests that some of the H_2O_2 hemolysis may result from the constitutional change of membrane lipids caused by underlying diseases, even if tocopherol levels are sufficient in RBCs.

2. During our study, it became clear that plasma in umbilical cord blood and blood of breast-fed infants contained high α- and low γ-tocopherol levels in a ratio resembling that in adults, while that of bottle-fed infants contained

---

*This work was supported by Grant No. 34401 in aid for Scientific Research, Japan.

175

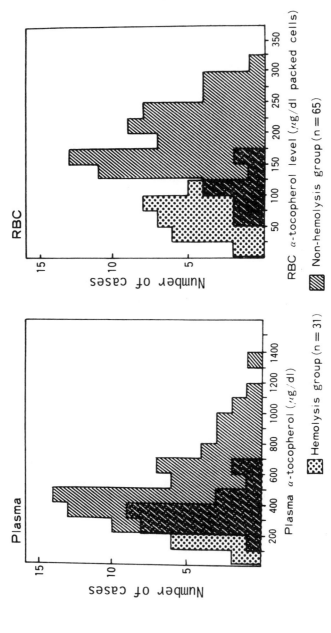

FIGURE 1. Distribution of cases for different plasma and RBC α-tocopherol levels in two groups, nonhemolysis and hemolysis, based on the H_2O_2 hemolysis test.

relatively high γ-tocopherol levels and, additionally, δ-tocopherol (TABLE 1). Because the content of formulas is characterized by large amounts of the γ- and δ-analogue forms, there is no doubt that the plasma tocopherol pattern in bottle-fed infants is due to the intake of large amounts of tocopherol analogues other than the α-form. RBC α-tocopherol levels were lower in bottle-fed infants than in breast-fed infants. This important finding may be explained by the difference in plasma α-tocopherol levels, but the difference was more obvious in RBCs than in plasma. The finding of lower plasma α-tocopherol levels in bottle-fed infants is seemingly contradictory because of the absence of any difference in α-form content between formulas and breast milk. This remains to be explained.

3. The correlation of plasma tocopherol levels to RBC tocopherol levels was studied in nonobese children with a great variety of plasma lipid levels. There was a poor correlation ($r = 0.39$, $p < 0.001$, $n = 195$), but a highly significant correlation was found between the tocopherol content of plasma and the total lipid levels ($r = 0.86$, $p < 0.001$). However, the correlation coefficient increased between RBC tocopherol levels and plasma tocopherol levels based on plasma total lipids ($r = 0.69$, $p < 0.001$), indicating that the transportation of tocopherol from plasma to RBC membranes increases when the tocopherol concentration in plasma lipids increases.

Adiposity may also affect RBC tocopherol. FIGURE 2 shows the relationship between obesity grade and plasma and RBC tocopherol levels. The control group was selected from nonobese children whose plasma lipids were all normal. Plasma tocopherol levels were unrelated to obesity grade, while the RBC tocopherol levels decreased with increased adiposity. Since in the cases examined, no marked differences were detected in plasma lipids among varying adiposity, the decreased RBC tocopherol levels with increased obesity is probably attributable to adiposity. This finding in humans is compatible with the views of Bieri and Machlin.[7,8]

TABLE 1

RELATION OF INFANT FEEDING TO PLASMA AND RBC TOCOPHEROL, AND CONTENT OF TOCOPHEROL ANALOGUES IN MILK AND FORMULA*

Subjects (n)		Tocopherol Levels (μg/dl)			
		α	β	γ	δ
Cord blood (7)	plasma	394.3 ± 21.2	—	60.5 ± 4.7	—
	RBC	162.8 ± 13.4			
Breast fed (17)	plasma	785.7 ± 46.7	—	87.3 ± 9.1	—
	RBC	274.1 ± 21.7			
Bottle fed (18)	plasma	595.9 ± 59.9†	—	233.4 ± 25.7‡	62.6 ± 8.6‡
	RBC	153.6 ± 9.4‡			
Human milk (10)		671.0 ± 74.4	—	77.8 ± 8.1	
Formulas (4)		645.5 ± 95.4	66.0 ± 5.4	1226.5 ± 270.6	774.3 ± 268.2

*Data are indicated as the mean ± standard error of the mean (SEM). RBC tocopherol levels are shown on the basis of packed cell volume. Human milk was obtained 5–7 days after delivery. Each formula was prepared in the concentrations indicated for feeding.

†Difference, breast fed vs. bottle fed, $p < 0.05$.

‡Difference, breast fed vs. bottle fed, $p < 0.01$.

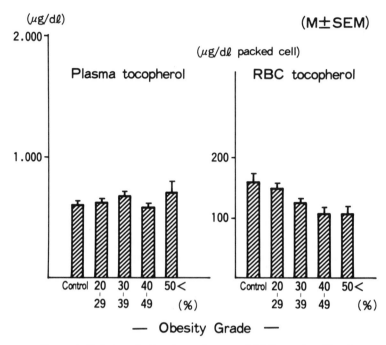

FIGURE 2. Relation of adiposity to plasma and RBC tocopherol levels.

REFERENCES

1. MINO, M., Y. NISHIDA, Y. KIJIMA, M. IWAKOSHI & S. NAKAGAWA. 1979. J. Nutr. Sci. Vitaminol. **25:** 505–516.
2. MINO, M., Y. KIJIMA, Y. NISHIDA & S. NAKAGAWA. 1980. J. Nutr. Sci. Vitaminol. **26:** 103–112.
3. MINO, M., M. KITAGAWA & S. NAKAGAWA. 1981. J. Nutr. Sci. Vitaminol. **27:** 199–207.
4. MINO, M., Y. NISHIDA, K. MURATA, M. TAKEGAWA, G. KATSUI & Y. YUGUCHI. 1978. J. Nutr. Sci. Vitaminol. **24:** 383–395.
5. ISHIBASHI, K., K. ABE, M. OHMAE & G. KATSUI. 1977. Vitamins **51:** 415–422. (In Japanese.)
6. VANDAMME, D., G. VANKERCKHOVEN, R. VERKAEMST, F. SOETEWEY, V. BLATON, H. PEETER & M. ROSSENEU. 1978. Clin. Chim. Acta **89:** 231–237.
7. BIERI, J. G. & R. POUKKA EVARTS. 1975. Proc. Soc. Exp. Biol. Med. **149:** 500–502.
8. MACHLIN, L. J., J. KEATING, J. NELSON, M. BRIN, R. FILIPSKI & O. N. MILLER. 1979. J. Nutr. **109:** 105–109.

SERUM α-TOCOPHEROL, COENZYME Q, AND THIOBARBITURIC ACID-REACTIVE SUBSTANCE IN ACUTE MYOCARDIAL DAMAGE AND STROKE

Masayoshi Kibata and Yoshimi Higuchi

National Sanatorium
Minami Okayama Hospital
Okayama 701-03, Japan

INTRODUCTION

We reported earlier that serum vitamin E level correlates inversely with the serum lipid peroxide level,[1] which in Japan is routinely determined by Yagi's fluorometric method[2] and designated as the thiobarbituric acid (TBA) value. We have also investigated the behaviors of serum TBA and vitamin E in patients with acute myocardial infarction (AMI) and stroke (CVA).[3] Vitamin E dropped rapidly and TBA increased within one to two days from the outbreak of vascular accidents. Oral or cutaneous administration of vitamin E to 54 stroke patients in the acute phase successfully prevented the elevation of TBA, and this was due to the increase of serum vitamin E. The findings led to our assumption that vitamin E migrated to the lesions and was utilized as an extinguisher against the lipid peroxidation process.

Coenzyme Q_{10} is known to be a member of the electron transport system in mitochondria and is receiving attention as a therapeutic agent for cerebral, coronary, or renal artery ischemias in acute stages, as its antioxidative activity is being more and more elucidated.

In this paper, the authors report the results of their observations on the behavior of coenzyme Q_{10} in comparison with that of vitamin E in the acute vascular accidents AMI and CVA. Further, we conducted observations of these factors using, as a model of AMI, rats wherein myocardial necrosis was induced by injection of a large dosage of isoproterenol.

RESULTS

In Humans

In CVA and AMI patients, TBA increased immediately with the attack of CVA or AMI and accompanied the following variations in serum:

1. In acute vascular accidents, vitamin E showed a rapid decrease reaching its minimum in two or three days and coenzyme Q_{10} decreased gradually for one to two weeks until it reached its minimum.
2. Vitamin E and coenzyme Q_{10} decreases were most significant in the high-density lipoprotein (HDL) fraction. In AMI patients, the cholesterol level in HDL attained its minimum within one or two weeks (FIGURE 1).

0077-8923/82/0393-0179 $01.75/0 © 1982, NYAS

In Rats

Administration of isoproterenol, 30 mg/kg, to rats induced myocardial necrosis and, concurrently, an increase in TBA-reactive substance and declines in vitamin E levels as observed in the liver, heart, and serum, most significantly in the liver.

TBA elevation observed with isoproterenol-induced myocardial necrosis (IPMN) was noticeably inhibited by pretreatment with α-tocopheryl nicotinate feeding (for one month) or α-tocopheryl acetate injection (for seven days) (FIGURE 2).

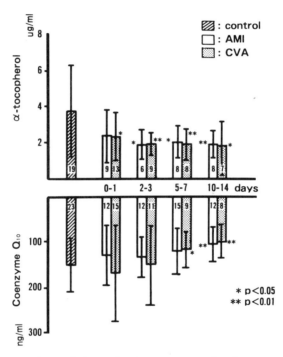

FIGURE 1. Course of HDL cholesterol and coenzyme Q_{10} after the occurrence of CVA and AMI.

Coenzyme Q_9 levels showed a significant decrease in the heart tissue 12 hours after the isoproterenol injection, but were unaffected by the pretreatment with α-tocopherol.

As to lipoprotein fractions in the ordinary state, vitamin E and TBA are distributed in HDL in high percentages and most of the coenzyme Q_9 is located in low-density lipoproteins (LDL). With the occurrence of IPMN, cholesterol, coenzyme Q_9, and TBA increase in LDL and vitamin E decreases in very low-density lipoproteins (VLDL) (FIGURE 3).

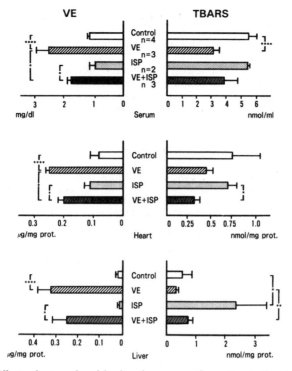

FIGURE 2. Effects of α-tocopherol feeding for one month on vitamin E and TBA-reactive substance (TBARS) in serum, heart, and liver of the control and isoproterenol-injection groups. Control, control diet and placebo solvent injected. VE, vitamin E added to diet. ISP, control diet and isoproterenol injected. VE + ISP, α-tocopherol added to diet and isoproterenol injected. *, $p < 0.05$; **, $p < 0.01$; and ****, $p < 0.001$.

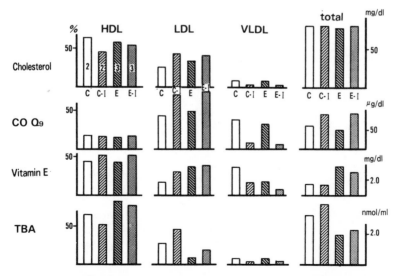

FIGURE 3. Percent distributions of total cholesterol, coenzyme Q_9, vitamin E, and TBA in each lipoprotein under four conditions: C, placebo solvent injected for seven days, then saline injected; C-I, placebo solvent for seven days, then isoproterenol; E, α-tocopheryl acetate 30 mg/kg per day for seven days, then saline; and E-I; α-tocopheryl acetate for seven days, then isoproterenol.

ACKNOWLEDGMENTS

The authors are grateful to Drs. H. Uehara, T. Fuchimoto, K. Shoji, K. Asano, M. Shimono, K. Sakurai, N. Minami, and K. Fukada for their dedicated cooperation in collecting the blood samples and for their technical assistance, and we would like to thank Prof. I. Kimura for his advice on this work.

REFERENCES

1. KIBATA, M., Y. SHIMIZU, K. MIYAKE, M. SHIMONO, K. SHOJI, K. MIYAHARA, T. FUCHIMOTO & Y. NASU. 1977. α-Tocopherol and TBA reactive substance (TBARS) in serum of the stroke at acute stage. Igakunoayumi **101:** 591-592.
2. YAGI, K. 1976. A simple fluorometric assay for lipoperoxide in blood plasma. Biochem. Med. **15:** 212-216.
3. KIBATA, M., Y. SHIMIZU, K. MIYAKE, K. SHOJI, K. MYAHARA, Y. NASU & I. KIMURA. 1978. Studies on vitamin E in lipid metabolism. In Tocopherol, Oxygen and Biomembranes. C. de Duve & O. Hayaisshi. Eds.: 283-295. Elsevier/North-Holland Biomedical Press. Amsterdam & New York.

EFFECT OF TOCOPHEROL ON LOW-DENSITY LIPOPROTEIN CHOLESTEROL ESTER METABOLISM IN THE ARTERIAL WALL

Yasushi Saito, Masaki Shinomiya, and Akira Kumagai

The Second Department of Internal Medicine
School of Medicine
Chiba University
Chiba 280, Japan

INTRODUCTION

Our previous results had suggested that dietary tocopherol plays an important role in both lipid synthesis and degradation in the arterial wall,[1] and the results may account for the accumulation of lipids in atherosclerotic lesions. In order to clarify the mechanisms of derangements of lipid metabolism of tocopherol-deficient rat arterial wall, experiments on binding of enzymes to membrane in which the enzymes were located and metabolism of cholesterol ester of low-density lipoprotein (LDL) were carried out using arterial wall and peritoneal macrophages.

MATERIALS AND METHODS

Reconstituted LDL was prepared by the method of Krieger *et al.*[2] Macrophages were prepared by the method of Goldstein *et al.*[3]

Assay of Hydrolysis of Cholesterol Ester in LDL

The reaction mixture consisted of cholesterol-$[1\text{-}^{14}C]$ oleate, 50 mM acetate buffer (pH 4.5), and enzyme solution. The final volume was 200 μl. The mixture was incubated at 37°C for 120 minutes. The reaction was terminated by the addition of 2 ml of a benzene-chloroform-methanol (10:5:12 v/v) mixture and 0.05 ml of 1 N NaOH. The mixture was vigorously shaken and centrifuged. Radioactivity in the upper layer was counted.

Assay of LDL Cholesterol Ester Hydrolysis–Dependent Cholesterol Ester Synthesis

The initial reaction mixture for LDL cholesterol ester hydrolysis in the lysosome consisted of LDL$[^3H]$cholesterol oleate, 50 mM acetate buffer (pH 4.5), and enzyme solution. The mixture was incubated for 120 minutes. After the incubation, oleoyl-CoA$\cdot^{14}C$ (125 μM) was added to the mixture. The reaction was terminated by the addition of a chloroform-methanol (2:1) mixture. Radioactivity of the cholesterol ester fraction was analyzed by thin-layer chromatography.

Cholesterol ester hydrolysis increased in both conditions in which tocopherol was added to the particulate fraction as an enzyme solution or to the LDL substrate. A slight increase in cholesterol ester hydrolysis in LDL was observed when macrophages were prepared with 10 μg/ml of tocopherol or when tocopherol added to LDL was used.

Effect of Tocopherol on LDL Cholesterol Ester Hydrolysis–Dependent Cholesterol Ester Synthesis in Rat Arterial Wall and Macrophages

Tocopherol increased cholesterol ester synthesis in the arterial wall particulate fraction when the particulate fraction was prepared by the addition of

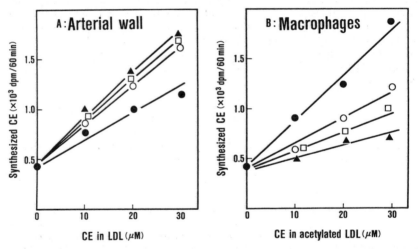

FIGURE 1. Effect of tocopherol on LDL cholesterol ester hydrolysis–dependent cholesterol ester synthesis in rat arterial wall and macrophage particulate fraction. Filled circles, particulate fraction; open circles, particulate fraction with cytosol; filled triangles, particulate fraction added to cytosol fraction with tocopherol; open squares, particulate fraction added to LDL with tocopherol.

tocopherol to homogenate, or when tocopherol was added to the cytosol fraction or added to LDL as shown in FIGURE 1a. However, in the macrophage particulate fraction, tocopherol inhibited cholesterol ester synthesis when the particulate fraction was prepared from macrophages with tocopherol added to the culture medium, to the cytosol fraction, or to LDL as shown in FIGURE 1b.

DISCUSSION

Experiments were carried out using reconstituted LDL[³H]cholesterol oleate in the case of arterial wall particulate fraction or acetylated LDL in the case of rat peritoneal macrophages to examine the effect of tocopherol on cholesterol ester metabolism in LDL.

LDL cholesterol ester hydrolysis was maximal at pH 4.5 and was very small at pH 7.5, although cholesterol esterase has two optima at pH 7.5 and pH 4.5.[4] The same results were obtained in macrophages. These results suggest that LDL cholesterol ester is mainly hydrolyzed in the lysosome both in LDL in the arterial wall and in acetylated LDL in macrophages. Tocopherol increased LDL or acetylated cholesterol ester hydrolysis under some conditions. This result suggests that tocopherol might prevent the deposition of cholesterol ester in the lysosome due to the dysfunction of LDL metabolism.

The effect of tocopherol on esterification of free cholesterol transferred from the lysosome was examined. It was seen that acetylated LDL stimulated the acyl coenzyme A cholesterol acyl transferase (ACAT) reaction, and this caused a net increase in cellular cholesteryl esters. LDL cholesterol ester hydrolysis–dependent cholesterol ester synthesis in the particulate fraction of macrophages was inhibited by the cytosol fraction but stimulated in arterial wall particulate fractions. The difference might be due to the difference of cell function.

Tocopherol stimulated cholesterol ester synthesis in the arterial wall particulate fraction, and inhibited it in macrophages using acetylated LDL. These results suggest that tocopherol might reduce the accumulation of cholesterol ester in macrophages. The mechanisms of action of tocopherol in this reaction are, in part, changes of LDL by binding of tocopherol and interaction between cytosol and tocopherol. Further experiments are now in progress to clarify the mechanism of action of tocopherol and the relationship between lipid accumulation and the action of tocopherol.

ACKNOWLEDGMENTS

The authors gratefully acknowledge the members of the Lipid Research Group in the Second Department of Internal Medicine, Chiba University, Dr. Nobuo Matsuoka, Dr. Kohji Shirai, Dr. Norihiro Sasaki, Dr. Shunichi Murano, and Dr. Masaki Shinomiya for their helpful work and suggestions, and Miss Yoko Fujiyama, Miss Yumi Fujii, and Miss Sayo Izumi for their assistance during the course of this work. Tocopherol was provided by Eisai Co. Ltd.

REFERENCES

1. SHIRAI, K., N. MATSUOKA, N. MORISAKI, S. MURANO, N. SASAKI, M. SHINOMIYA, Y. SAITO, A. KUMAGAI & M. MIZOBUCHI. 1980. Effects of tocopherol deficiency on lipid metabolism in the arterial wall of rats on normal and high cholesterol diets. Artery **6:** 484–506.
2. KRIEGER, M., M. J. McPAUL, J. L. GOLDSTEIN & M. S. BROWN. 1979. Replacement of neutral lipids of low density lipoprotein with ester of long chain unsaturated fatty acids. J. Biol. Chem. **254:** 3845–3853.
3. GOLDSTEIN, J. L., Y. K. HO & M. S. BROWN. 1980. Cholesterol ester accumulation in macrophages resulting from receptor-mediated uptake and degradation of hypercholesterolemic canine β-very low density lipoproteins. J. Biol. Chem. **255:** 1839–1848.
4. SHINOMIYA, M., N. MATSUOKA, K. SHIRAI, Y. SAITO & A. KUMAGAI. 1979. Studies on cholesterol esterase in rat arterial wall. Atherosclerosis **33:** 343–350.

α-TOCOPHEROL AS A POTENTIAL MODIFIER OF DAUNORUBICIN-INDUCED MAMMARY TUMORS IN RATS*

Yeu-Ming Wang and Scott K. Howell

Department of Experimental Pediatrics
The University of Texas Cancer Center
M. D. Anderson Hospital and Tumor Institute
Houston, Texas 77030

The anthracycline antibiotics daunorubicin (daunomycin) and doxorubicin (adriamycin) have been used extensively in the treatment of human neoplastic disease since 1970. The major toxicity of the anthracycline antibiotics is cardiac.[1] In addition, both drugs possess mutagenic and carcinogenic activities.

The incidence of daunorubicin-induced mammary adenocarcinoma increases with dose. More than 50% of female Sprague-Dawley rats will have the tumor in 80 days after a single intravenous injection of the drug (10 mg/kg, or 60 mg/m^2). The mechanism of these activities is not clear. However, free-radical intermediates are formed by the anthracyclines through cellular electron-transport systems, including xanthine oxidase, reduced nicotinamide-adenine dinucleotide phosphate (NADPH) cytochrome P_{450} reductase, and as yet unidentified nuclear electron-transport system(s).[2] The reduction of adriamycin to a semiquinone free radical by NADPH cytochrome P_{450} reductase produced DNA cleavage in a reaction mediated by oxygen *in vitro*; however, the presence of rat liver microsomal or rat liver postmitochondrial preparation reduced the capacity for adriamycin-induced mutagenesis and malignant transformation. Furthermore, the inhibitors of microsomal enzyme activity in mouse cells increased the yield of drug-induced microbial transformants.[3] In addition, from the results obtained by Suojanen et al.[4] and by us (unpublished), we estimated that rat mammary cells have 50% of reduced glutathione level and 10% of glutathione peroxidase activity compared to rat hepatocytes. Rat mammary cells also have relatively less cytochrome P_{450} (3%) and lower activity of NADPH cytochrome P_{450} reductase (10%) compared with rat liver microsomes.[5]

Our preliminary results suggest that pretreatment with vitamin E (*all-rac*-α-tocopheryl acetate 1.8 g/m^2 per day for four days) intraperitoneally can reduce the occurrence or the development of daunorubicin-induced mammary tumors in female Sprague-Dawley rats.[6] However, the drug-induced carcinogenesis appears to be age dependent. The distribution of ^{14}C-α-tocopheryl acetate radioactivity (36 mCi/mole) was significantly different in treated animals with or without daunorubicin. The ^{14}C-α-tocopheryl acetate equivalent was higher in spleen (p < 0.0005) and heart (p < 0.05) in treated animals without daunorubicin as compared with the animals receiving the anthracycline. On the other hand, the radioactivity was higher in erythrocytes (p < 0.05), plasma (p < 0.0025), and mammary fat (p < 0.05) in animals given daunorubicin. Pretreatment with α-tocopheryl acetate also altered the distribution of ^{3}H-daunorubicin. Most significantly, the radioactivity appeared to be retained in the liver.

*Supported in part by a grant from Hoffmann-La Roche, Inc., Nutley, N.J., and a generous donation from Mr. and Mrs. Leland Anderson.

0077-8923/82/0393-0186 $01.75/0 © 1982, NYAS

To test the possibility that the vitamin may alter the intracellular distribution of ^{3}H-daunorubicin, four animals were given either α-tocopheryl acetate (1.8 g/m^2 daily for four days) or a placebo (D-M Pharmaceuticals, Inc., Rockville, Md.) at equal volumes for the same period of time. The animals were killed at day 5. Liver and mammary glands were subjected to single-cell preparation. The cells were then incubated with ^{3}H-daunorubicin for up to two hours, and the intracellular distribution of the daunorubicin radioactivity was analyzed. Preliminary results obtained from the *in vitro* studies suggested a decreased movement of tritium radioactivity into subcellular granules in mammary cells after pretreatment with α-tocopheryl acetate.

To study the metabolic species of daunorubicin further, the radioactivity of the subcellular fraction was extracted and analyzed by high-performance liquid chromatography. A high-performance liquid chromatographic method has also been set up to determine the metabolic species of α-tocopherol.[7] Results obtained in liver cells show that the radioactive profiles of the material eluted have similar patterns in animals treated with placebo and in those treated with α-tocopheryl acetate. The majority of the radioactivity is associated with unchanged carcinogen. However, more tritium radioactivity can be recovered from the subcellular fraction of liver cells, particularly the nuclear fraction, in animals receiving α-tocopheryl acetate. It appears that in those animals treated with placebo, the tritium radioactivity of daunorubicin or its derivatives is more tightly bound to DNA or other macromolecules in the nucleus than in those animals receiving α-tocopheryl acetate treatment.

Our working hypothesis is as follows. In rat tissues other than the mammary gland, such as in liver, daunorubicin is substantially metabolized. The metabolism of daunorubicin decreases carcinogenicity and mutagenicity. In the liver, there are adequate activities of xanthine oxidase, cytochrome P$_{450}$ reductase, and other aldehyde reductases that can metabolize daunorubicin. In these metabolic processes, oxygen radicals and semiquinone radicals of daunorubicin are formed. The oxidative impact of these radicals can be neutralized by the abundant hepatocellular glutathione and glutathione redox enzymes. When comparatively lesser quantities of the parent compound are transported into mitochondria and nuclei, less binding to these cellular macromolecules, including DNA, occurs. Since nuclei possess an electron-transport system(s), formation of radicals from daunorubicin and oxygen can occur that would result in DNA breaks. However, because of decreased availability of the parent compound for transport into the nuclei, there will be no or minimal fragmentation of DNA in the liver. On the other hand, in mammary tissues, there appear to be comparative deficiencies of cytochrome P$_{450}$, cytochrome P$_{450}$ reductase, glutathione, and glutathione peroxidase. Therefore, more parent compound is available to mitochondrial and nuclear DNA. Thus, an increase of DNA fragmentation may occur in the nucleus of mammary gland cells. The function of α-tocopherol in mammary gland cells is to prevent the free-radical oxidation of components in the mammary nucleus. α-Tocopherol will act as a free radical scavenger or inhibitor of the interaction of the anthracycline antibiotics with nuclear macromolecules (FIGURE 1). Furthermore, α-tocopherol decreases the movement of the carcinogen into the nuclear fraction.

A surprising result in animals that received daunorubicin injections was an increase of serum cholesterol.[6] This could be seen as early as 48 hours after intravenous injection of daunorubicin and persisted for over 20 weeks. The role of cholesterol is yet unknown in this model system. Whether the action of daunorubicin free radicals and that of cholesterol epoxide serve as the two hits of

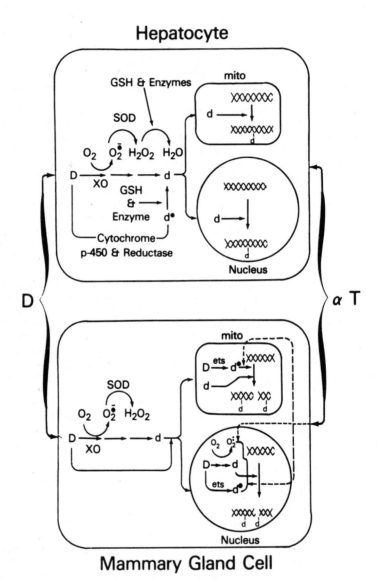

FIGURE 1. Proposed mechanism of action of α-tocopherol in daunorubicin-induced mammary carcinoma in female Sprague-Dawley rats. The abbreviations used are αT, α-tocopherol; D, daunorubicin; d, daunorubicin metabolites; ets, electron transport system(s); GSH, reduced glutathione; SOD, superoxide dismutase; XO, xanthine oxidase.

the Knudson model is unknown. α-Tocopherol may also prevent the formation of cholesterol epoxide.

REFERENCES

1. LEGHA, S. S., Y. M. WANG, B. MACKAY, M. EWER, G. N. HORTOBAGYI, R.S. BENJAMIN & M. K. ALI. Ann. N.Y. Acad. Sci. (This volume.)
2. WANG, Y. M., F. F. MADANAT, J. KIMBALL, C. A. GLISER, M. K. ALI, M. W. KAUFMAN & J. VAN EYS. 1980. Cancer Res. **40:** 1022–1027.
3. MARQUARDT, H. 1979. *In* Chemical Carcinogenesis and DNA. P. L. Grover, Ed. **2:** 159–179. CRC Press. Boca Raton, Fla.
4. SUOJANEN, J. N., R. J. GRAY & R. HIEF. 1980. Biochim. Biophys. Acta **630:** 485–496.
5. RIKANS, L. E., D. D. GIBSON & P. B. MCCAY. 1979. Biochem. Pharmacol. **28:** 3039–3042.
6. WANG, Y. M., S. K. HOWELL, J. C. KIMBALL, C. C. TSAI, J. SATO & C. A. GLEISER. 1982. *In* Molecular Interrelations of Nutrition and Cancer. M. S. Arnott, J. van Eys & Y. M. Wang, Eds.: 369–379. Raven Press. New York, N.Y.
7. HOWELL, S. K. & Y. M. WANG. 1982. J. Chromatogr. **227:** 174–180.

EFFECT OF α-TOCOPHEROL ON SERUM HORMONE AND LIPOPROTEIN CHOLESTEROL LEVELS IN YOUNG AND ADULT FEMALE RATS

G. S. Sundaram, S. Manimekalai, R. S. London, and P. Goldstein

Division of Reproductive Endocrinology
Department of Obstetrics and Gynecology
Sinai Hospital of Baltimore, Inc.
Baltimore, Maryland 21215

Our earlier studies on the effect of α-tocopherol (E) therapy on hormones and lipoproteins in women with fibrocystic disease of the breast showed the following: (a) 67 to 85% remission from disease; (b) urinary levels of 11-desoxy-17-ketosteroids increased and pregnanediol decreased;[1,2] (c) elevated serum levels of luteinizing and follicle-stimulating hormones decreased;[3] and (d) serum high-density lipoproteins increased.[4] Additionally, serum levels of dehydro-epiandrosterone (DHEA) decreased (unpublished observation) with no changes in prolactin,[3] estradiol, estriol, and progesterone.[5] Changes noted after E therapy were statistically significant. These different studies used women ranging in age from 16 to 42 years with varying severity of disease.[1-5] Since blood samples were collected on day 21 of the menstrual cycle, it was conceivable that the midluteal phase might have been missed in some cases. In order to confirm some of the above results in animal experiments under controlled laboratory conditions, female Sprague-Dawley rats at different ages were raised on tocopherol-depleted and -supplemented diets, and the endocrine and lipoprotein status of these animals investigated.

Rats were supplied by Dr. M. Brin of Hoffmann-La Roche, Inc. Two different age groups were studied. The younger rats (100 grams) were raised on normal Purina rat chow (E, 50 IU/kg chow) for the first three weeks of life. For the next three weeks these rats were raised on depleted chow, and then these rats were subdivided into one group that continued on the E-deficient diet for six weeks (D.6) and one group that was maintained on E-supplemented diet (200 IU/kg chow) for six weeks (S.6).

The older rats (225 grams) were raised on normal Purina rat chow for the first 3 weeks of life. For the next 15 weeks, these rats were raised on either E-deficient (D.15) or E-supplemented (S.15) diets. All animals' estrus cycles were monitored twice daily by vaginal cytology during the last 6 weeks of the experiment. When animals maintained at least three regular cycles, they were sacrificed during early diestrous phase between 9 and 10 A.M. and were phlebotomized. Heparinized plasma was isolated.

Plasma E concentration was assayed by a spectrophotometric method. Plasma DHEA, estradiol, and progesterone were assayed by a radioimmunoassay technique. Different lipoproteins were isolated by a sequential preparative ultracentrifugation technique specific for plasma from Sprague-Dawley rats. Total and free cholesterol in plasma and lipoproteins was determined by an enzymatic technique.

All rats raised on vitamin E-deficient chow had no measurable level of plasma E; rats raised on E-supplemented chow increased their plasma E levels to 0.31 ± 0.07 (S.6) and 0.65 ± 0.02 mg/dl (S.15), respectively, the difference in levels

190

probably being due to the length of the supplementation period. Human subjects responding to E therapy in our earlier studies showed similar increases. The older animals in general had higher levels of DHEA and estradiol and lower levels of progesterone when compared with the younger animals, probably due to the difference in age between the two groups.

However, there was no difference in the plasma estradiol and progesterone levels between E-depleted and E-supplemented rats within young and adult groups, with similar findings to those in humans treated with E.[5] Plasma DHEA decreased markedly in the younger group, and a similar but not significant trend was seen with the adult rats (TABLE 1) as a result of E supplementation. In human patients treated with E, DHEA decreased significantly from 5.14 ± 0.19 to 2.06 ± 0.03 ng/ml in those not responding to therapy; in responding patients, a similar but not significant trend was seen with a decrease from 8.31 ± 1.40 to 6.58 ± 1.3 ng/ml. Our earlier studies in humans showed significant increases in the urinary output of DHEA on treatment with E.[1,2] Since plasma levels of DHEA decrease and urinary levels increase, E may only be increasing the catabolism and excretion of DHEA without affecting the synthesis. However, such lowering of

TABLE 1

HORMONE AND LIPOPROTEIN CHOLESTEROL LEVELS

	DHEA (ng/dl)	LDL (mg/dl)	HDL$_3$ (mg/dl)	HDL$_2$ (mg/dl)
D.15 (n = 8)	4.42 ± 1.9	17 ± 0.9	8 ± 0.6	26 ± 1.9
S.15 (n = 6)	2.99 ± 1.4	12 ± 1.5*	10 ± 1.1	20 ± 3.1
D.6 (n = 9)	2.04 ± 0.2	32 ± 3.2	29 ± 2.0	44 ± 9.9
S.6 (n = 8)	1.21 ± 0.1*	24 ± 1.5*	18 ± 2.1*	53 ± 4.4

*Statistically different from corresponding D.15 or D.6 value at $p < 0.05$.

plasma levels of DHEA by E in human subjects with fibrocystic disease and in rats has some important significance. Based on a 10-year prospective study, it has been shown that low plasma levels of DHEA were associated with an increased risk of breast cancer.[6,7] Schwartz showed that supplementation with DHEA to mice delayed and reduced mammary cancer incidence.[8] Our results suggest that the implications of lowering the plasma levels of DHEA with E therapy are to be evaluated carefully, especially in light of the recently reported adverse results associated with E therapy at megadoses.[9]

After E supplementation, low-density lipoprotein (LDL) cholesterol in both groups of rats was significantly lowered. High-density lipoprotein (HDL) did not change significantly in either group. However, in the younger group, HDL$_3$ decreased and HDL$_2$ increased. HDL$_3$ serves as a substrate for lecithin cholesterol acyl transferase (LCAT) enzyme, which converts free cholesterol into ester cholesterol that is deposited in arterial lesions. HDL$_2$ has been shown to afford protection against cardiovascular disease. By decreasing the HDL$_3$ substrate for LCAT and thus the formation of ester cholesterol and by increasing the HDL$_2$ levels, E therapy may be affording a twofold protection against cardiovascular disease in the younger animals. Similar changes were not observed in the adult rats. In humans, although LDL did not change, LDL ester cholesterol decreased and free cholesterol increased significantly. HDL cholesterol significantly increased from 44.14 ± 3.16 to 53.03 ± 4.00 mg/dl in patients responding to E therapy but not in nonresponders. However, HDL_2 as well as HDL_3 increased, suggesting decreased protection against cardiovascular disease as in adult rats.

In summary, the results observed in rats and humans suggest that E supplementation initiated early in life may have marked beneficial effects on lipoproteins implicated in atherosclerosis while supplementation later in life may have less effect.

REFERENCES

1. SOLOMON, D., D. STRUMMER & P. P. NAIR. 1972. Relationship between vitamin E and urinary excretion of ketosteroid fractions in cystic mastitis. Ann. N.Y. Acad. Sci. **203:** 103.
2. LONDON, R. S., D. SOLOMON, E. D. LONDON, D. STRUMMER, J. BANKOWSKI & P. P. NAIR. 1978. Mammary dysplasia: clinical response and urinary excretion of 11-desoxy-17-ketosteroids and pregnanediol following alpha tocopherol therapy. Breast **4:** 19.
3. SUNDARAM, G. S., R. LONDON, S. MARGOLIS, R. WENK, J. LUSTGARDEN, P. P. NAIR & P. GOLDSTEIN. 1981. Serum hormones and lipoproteins in benign breast disease. Cancer Res. **41:** 3814.
4. SUNDARAM, G. S., R. LONDON, S. MANIMEKALAI, P. P. NAIR & P. GOLDSTEIN. 1981. Alpha tocopherol and serum lipoproteins. Lipids **16:** 223.
5. LONDON, R. S., G. S. SUNDARAM, M. SCHULTZ, P. P. NAIR & P. GOLDSTEIN. 1981. Endocrine parameters and alpha tocopherol therapy of patients with mammary dysplasia. Cancer Res. **41:** 3811.
6. BULBROOK, P. D., J. L. HAYWARD & C. SPICER. 1971. Relationship between urinary androgen and corticoid excretion and subsequent breast cancer. Lancet **2:** 395.
7. WANG D. Y. & M. HERRIAN. 1973. Plasma dehydroepiandrosterone SO_4 and breast cancer. Acta Endocrinol. Suppl. **177:** 30.
8. SCHWARTZ, A. G. 1979. Inhibition of spontaneous breast cancer formation in female C3H-AVY/A mice by long-term treatment with dehydroepiandrosterone. Cancer Res. **39:** 1129.
9. ROBERTS, H. J. 1981. Perspective on vitamin E as therapy. J. Am. Med. Assoc. **246:** 129.

EVIDENCE FOR A POSSIBLE PROTEIN-DEPENDENT REGENERATION OF VITAMIN E IN RAT LIVER MICROSOMES

C. C. Reddy, R. W. Scholz, C. E. Thomas, and E. J. Massaro

Center for Air Environment Studies
and
Department of Veterinary Science
Pennsylvania State University
University Park, Pennsylvania 16802

It is generally believed that vitamin E and selenium function synergistically to constitute an important antioxidant defense mechanism(s) to protect biological membranes from peroxidative damage.[1,2] Selenium, as an essential component of Se-dependent glutathione peroxidase (Se GSH-Px), has been proposed to reduce the hydroperoxides formed to less-reactive alcohols. Recently another GSH peroxidase, an Se-independent enzyme, has been implicated in the protection of membranes from peroxidation.[3] However, the hypothesis that either enzyme might play a vital role in the degradation of membrane-bound hydroperoxides has been recently disputed.[4] Vitamin E, as an integral part of cell membrane structure, has long been visualized as a biological antioxidant preventing the formation of lipid hydroperoxides by sequestering free radicals that initiate lipid peroxidation.[5] Thus, Se and E act to control lipid hydroperoxide levels in tissues by interrelated, but independent, mechanisms. Little information is available, however, regarding the exact mechanism of action of E. More recently GSH has been implicated in the protection against membrane lipid peroxidation both *in vivo* and *in vitro*;[4,6] however, the nature of the protection afforded by GSH is not clearly understood. Accordingly these studies were undertaken to elucidate the interrelationships among GSH, Se, and E in the protection of biological membranes against oxidative damage.

These experiments were carried out with liver microsomes obtained from Long-Evans hooded rats fed chemically defined, purified diets containing adequate or documented deficiencies of E, Se, or both (diets: $+E$, $+Se$; $-E$, $+Se$; $+E$, $-Se$; $-E$, $-Se$). It is clear from TABLE 1 that GSH effectively inhibited the formation of thiobarbituric acid (TBA)-reactive products in liver microsomes obtained from E-supplemented rats. There was no effect on the lipid peroxidation of microsomes obtained from E-deficient animals. The inhibitory effect of GSH was observed in both NADPH-Fe^{++}-dependent enzymatic and ascorbate-$ADP \cdot Fe^{++}$-dependent nonenzymatic lipid-peroxidation systems.* However, when the microsomes were denatured by heat treatment, GSH did not cause any inhibition. A possibility that the lack of inhibition in heat-denatured microsomes might be partly due to destruction of E was considered. Vitamin E levels were determined in heat-denatured microsomes and compared to the E concentrations of native microsomes. There were no differences between treatments in the E levels. This suggests that a heat-labile factor is essential for the mediation of the inhibitory effect of GSH on lipid peroxidation. The time course of inhibition

---

*NADPH is nicotinamide-adenine dinucleotide phosphate, reduced; ADP is adenosine diphosphate.

TABLE 1

EFFECT OF REDUCED GLUTATHIONE ON *In Vitro* LIPID PEROXIDATION OF RAT LIVER MICROSOMES

Assay System		Diet Treatment (nmoles TBA products/mg protein per 15 minutes)			
		+E, +Se	−E, +Se	+E, −Se	−E, −Se
NADPH-Fe^{++}-dependent enzymatic assay*	−GSH:	30.8 ± 5.5‡	23.0 ± 6.3	27.6 ± 5.2	20.6 ± 4.8
	+GSH:	2.5 ± 0.7	24.4 ± 5.7	3.42 ± 1.0	13.2 ± 2.3
Ascorbate-ADP·Fe^{++}-dependent nonenzymatic assay†	−GSH:	41.6 ± 7.2	44.6 ± 4.7	42.9 ± 9.7	42.0 ± 2.6
	+GSH:	1.45 ± 0.85	36.4 ± 7.8	9.7 ± 6.1	33.3 ± 7.3
Ascorbate-ADP·Fe^{++}-dependent nonenzymatic assay with heat-denatured microsomes†	−GSH:	39.2 ± 1.2	38.7 ± 7.5	36.5 ± 3.2	32.3 ± 9.2
	+GSH:	38.3 ± 3.5	39.9 ± 7.1	33.0 ± 5.9	29.7 ± 15.1

*NADPH-Fe^{++}-dependent enzymatic assay: The standard assay mixture (1.5 ml) contained: 0.05 M tris-HCl, pH 7.4; 0.25 mM NADPH; 12 µM FeSO$_4$; microsomes (0.5–1.0 mg protein); and 5 mM GSH (where necessary). The reactions were initiated by the addition of microsomes and incubated at 37°C under atmospheric air with continuous shaking. At the end of the incubation period, the reactions were terminated by the addition of 0.4 ml of 20% trichloroacetic acid solution containing 0.05% butylated hydroxytoluene. After termination, 0.6 ml of 50 mM thiobarbituric acid and 0.1 ml of bovine serum albumin (0.5 mg) were added, mixed, and centrifuged at 7,000 × g for 15 minutes. The supernatants were decanted into screw cap test tubes and heated at 95°C for exactly 8 minutes. They were cooled to room temperature, and the TBA-reactive products formed were determined by measuring the pink color at 535 nm. A molar extinction coefficient of 1.56 × 10⁵ M⁻¹ × cm⁻¹ was used in these calculations.

†*Ascorbate-ADP·Fe^{++}-dependent nonenzymatic assay:* Assay conditions were identical to those described for NADPH-Fe^{++}-dependent enzymatic assay except that NADPH was replaced by 0.5 mM ascorbate and 4 mM ADP. In ascorbate-ADP·Fe^{++}-dependent nonenzymatic assays with heat-denatured microsomes, the microsomal fractions heated at 95°C for 20 minutes were used in place of undenatured microsomes.

‡Values are expressed as mean ± standard deviation for six animals.

against peroxidation by GSH in both enzymatic and nonenzymatic lipid-peroxidation systems indicated that GSH could afford protection for up to 20 minutes under the assay conditions utilized in these studies.

Several sulfhydryl compounds, β-mercaptoethanol, dithiothreitol, and cysteine, were used in place of GSH in the *in vitro* test system. Interestingly, β-mercaptoethanol had no effect whereas cysteine and dithiothreitol caused complete inhibition of lipid peroxidation. However, unlike the inhibition pattern observed with GSH, these sulfhydryl compounds exhibited inhibition independent of E. This could be due to their ability to complex with Fe^{++} and thus prevent initiation of lipid peroxidation. We have also tested the effects of homogeneous preparations of Se GSH-Px and non-Se GSH-Px on the formation of TBA-reactive products in the ascorbate-ADP$\cdot$$Fe^{++}$-dependent lipid-peroxidation system using heat-denatured microsomes. Purified forms of both enzymes had no effect on lipid peroxidation, suggesting a questionable involvement in their proposed protective roles in the reduction of membrane-bound lipid hydroperoxides. However, these enzymes may play an important role in the control of cytosolic hydrogen peroxide and lipid hydroperoxide levels and thus prevent the formation of highly reactive oxygen radicals. The data presented here suggest the possibility that E is regenerated by a heat-labile factor(s) in the presence of GSH. Nevertheless, more information is needed to support this hypothesis.

REFERENCES

1. HOEKSTRA, W. G. 1975. Biochemical function of selenium and its relation to vitamin E. Fed. Proc. **34**: 2083–2089.
2. TAPPEL, A. L. 1980. Vitamin E and selenium protection from *in vivo* lipid peroxidation. Ann. N.Y. Acad. Sci. **355**: 18–31.
3. BURK, R. F., M. J. TRUMBLE & R. A. LAWRENCE. 1980. Rat hepatic cytosolic glutathione-dependent enzyme protection against lipid peroxidation in the NADPH-microsomal lipid peroxidation system. Biochim. Biophys. Acta **618**: 35–41.
4. McCAY, P. B., D. D. GIBSON & K. R. HORNBROOK. 1981. Glutathione-dependent inhibition of lipid peroxidation by a soluble, heat-labile factor not glutathione peroxidase. Fed. Proc. **40**: 199–205.
5. McCAY, P. B. & M. M. KING. 1980. Vitamin E as a biological free radical scavenger. *In* Vitamin E. L. J. Machlin, Ed.: 289–317. Marcel Dekker. New York, N.Y.
6. YOUNES, M. & C.-P. SIEGERS. 1980. Lipid peroxidation as a consequence of gluthathione depletion in rat and mouse liver. Res. Commun. Chem. Pathol. Pharmacol. **27**: 119–128.

STRUCTURAL AND BIOCHEMICAL EFFECTS OF ANTIOXIDANT NUTRIENT DEFICIENCY ON THE RAT RETINA AND RETINAL PIGMENT EPITHELIUM

Martin L. Katz,* Kenton R. Parker, Garry J. Handelman,
Christopher C. Farnsworth, and Edward A. Dratz

Division of Natural Sciences
University of California
Santa Cruz, California 95064

We have studied the effects of antioxidant deficiency on the retina and retinal pigment epithelium (RPE) in rats.[1-4] Both albino and pigmented animals fed a diet deficient in vitamin E, selenium, sulfur amino acids, and chromium (−E−Se−S−Cr) from weaning showed a dramatic accumulation of a yellow autofluorescent pigment in the RPE. Slightly less of this pigment accumulated in the RPE of rats deficient only in vitamin E and selenium (−E−Se), while very little pigment was seen in the RPE of +E+Se+S+Cr controls.

In the albino rats, ultrastructural examination showed that the amount of RPE autofluorescence was correlated with the numbers of electron-dense inclusion bodies present in the RPE. Accompanying the pigment buildup in the RPE was the development of an irregularity and an overall increase in RPE cell height. There was also an increase in the number of lipid droplets in the RPE, particularly in the periphery of the eye. In the eyes of deficient animals, cells were occasionally seen which appeared to be RPE cells that had detached from the basal lamina and migrated into the region of the photoreceptor outer segments. Photoreceptor outer segment phagocytosis by the retinal pigment epithelium appeared to be decreased as a consequence of dietary antioxidant deficiency; a great reduction in the number of phagosomes per unit RPE cell volume was seen in the eyes of both deficient groups.

These changes in the RPE of albino rats were accompanied by a pronounced loss of photoreceptor cells, particularly from the central retina. The disk membranes of the photoreceptor outer segments of deficient animals were often swollen, disoriented, and vesiculated, and areas were frequently seen where outer segment debris had accumulated at the interface between photoreceptors and RPE.

Many of the changes in the retina and RPE were more severe in the −E−Se−S−Cr group than in the group deficient only in vitamin E and selenium.

Biochemical studies were carried out in pigmented rats to evaluate the relative importance of vitamin E and selenium to the functional integrity of the retina and RPE. These pigmented rats were maintained on +E+Se, +E−Se, −E+Se, or −E−Se diets. Animals on the −E−Se diet showed a 28% drop in the amount of visual pigment (rhodopsin) per eye relative to the +E+Se controls. The loss of rhodopsin was much less in both the +E−Se and −E+Se groups, suggesting that both vitamin E and selenium are important in maintaining retinal integrity. Vitamin A palmitate levels in the RPE of the dark-adapted rats were reduced to

---

*Present affiliation: Laboratory of Vision Research, National Eye Institute, Bethesda, Md. 20205.

64%, 47%, and 39% of controls in the $+E-Se$, $-E+Se$, and $-E-Se$ groups respectively. Both selenium and vitamin E appear to be important in maintaining normal vitamin A levels in the RPE. Lysosomal enzyme activity was also affected by deficiencies of antioxidant nutrients; acid lipase activity was elevated almost twofold in the RPE of $-E-Se$ rats when compared to $+E+Se$ controls. The $-E+Se$ and $+E-Se$ groups showed lesser elevations in RPE acid lipase activity.

Our findings indicate that both vitamin E and selenium, and probably chromium and sulfur amino acids as well, play important roles in maintaining normal physiological functions of the retina and RPE. Deficiencies in these nutrients appear to accelerate many of the changes that occur normally during aging in the retina and RPE, suggesting that autoxidation may play a significant role in senescence.

REFERENCES

1. KATZ, M. L., W. L. STONE & E. A. DRATZ. 1978. Fluorescent pigment accumulation in retinal pigment epithelium of antioxidant-deficient rats. Invest. Ophthalmol. Vis. Sci. **17:** 1049–1058.
2. FARNSWORTH, C. C., W. L. STONE & E. A. DRATZ. 1979. Effects of vitamin E and selenium deficiency on the fatty acid composition of rat retinal tissue. Biochim. Biophys. Acta **552:** 281–293.
3. STONE, W. L., M. L. KATZ, M. LURIE, M. F. MARMOR & E. A. DRATZ. 1979. Effects of dietary vitamin E and selenium on light damage to the rat retina. Photochem. Photobiol. **29:** 725–730.
4. KATZ, M. L., K. R. PARKER, G. J. HANDELMAN, T. L. BRAMEL & E. A. DRATZ. 1982. Effects of antioxidant nutrient deficiency on the retina and retinal pigment epithelium of albino rats: a light and electron microscopic study. Exp. Eye Res. **34:** 339–369.

ROLE OF VITAMIN E IN THE PREVENTION OF HEPATOCELLULAR DAMAGE: CLINICAL AND EXPERIMENTAL APPROACH

Toshikazu Yoshikawa and Motoharu Kondo

First Department of Medicine
Kyoto Prefectural University of Medicine
Kyoto 602, Japan

INTRODUCTION

Many reports have been published concerning the relationship between liver disease and vitamin E. Much work has also been done in animal experiments with vitamin E. In vitamin E deficiency, various kinds of liver diseases become aggravated, and vitamin E produces a protective effect in the liver. As the actions of vitamin E are diverse, it is of interest to know which action is beneficial against liver disease.

MATERIALS AND METHODS

The subjects of this study consisted of 22 patients with acute hepatitis, 33 patients with chronic hepatitis, 26 patients with liver cirrhosis, 14 patients with liver cancer, 6 patients with fulminant hepatitis, and 9 patients with alcoholic hepatitis.

Wistar strain female rats at four weeks of age were maintained on vitamin E–deficient or -supplemented diet (Oriental Yeast Co. Ltd., Tokyo, Japan) for three months. Serum and liver levels of α-tocopherol,[1,2] β-glucuronidase,[3] acid phosphatase,[4] and thiobarbituric acid (TBA)-reactive substances[5,6] were measured.

RESULTS AND DISCUSSION

Serum levels of vitamin E were significantly depressed in acute hepatitis ($p < 0.01$), fulminant hepatitis ($p < 0.001$), and alcoholic hepatitis ($p < 0.001$), compared with the levels of normal persons as shown in FIGURE 1. Serum levels of vitamin E seem to be much lower during acme than during convalescence. There was no correlation between serum levels of vitamin E and liver function tests—such as alkaline phosphatase, thymol turbidity test, zinc sulfate turbidity test, bilirubin, albumin-globulin ratio, glutamic oxaloacetic transaminase, glutamic pyruvic transaminase (GPT), leucine aminopeptidase, lactate dehydrogenase, and cholinesterase—but a significant correlation existed between serum levels of vitamin E and β-lipoprotein ($r = 0.92$, $p < 0.001$, $n = 17$). Serum vitamin E also showed a significant correlation to cholesterol ($r = 0.57$, $p < 0.01$, $n = 21$) and phospholipid ($r = 0.49$, $p < 0.05$, $n = 18$). These facts suggest that the diminished serum vitamin E in patients with liver disease is ascribable to the depression in the serum level of β-lipoprotein, a vitamin E carrier, because the liver is the major supply source of endogenous β-lipoprotein.

Experimental liver disorders were induced by a single intraperitoneal injection of 0.5 ml/kg of carbon tetrachloride or 750 mg/kg of D-galactosamine-HCl (D-GalN) in rats maintained on a diet deficient in or supplemented with vitamin E. Liver damage by CCl_4 is attributed to the lipid peroxidation that results from the formation of free radicals in the liver microsome.[7] In this experimental study, serum levels of lysosomal enzymes and transaminases as well as serum and tissue levels of TBA-reactive substances were elevated in rats exposed to CCl_4, but the change was marked in vitamin E–deficient rats and only slight in those supplemented with vitamin E. The findings obtained in this study seem to bear out the

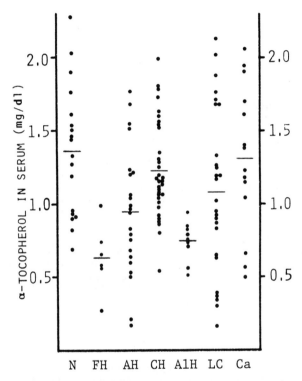

FIGURE 1. Serum α-tocopherol levels in liver diseases. N, normal; FH, fulminant hepatitis; AH, acute hepatitis; CH, chronic hepatitis; AlH, alcoholic hepatitis; LC, liver cirrhosis; Ca, liver cancer.

theory that vitamin E diminishes lysosomal membrane destruction by CCl_4 and protects the liver through its inhibitory action on lipid peroxidation.

D-GalN–induced hepatitis, which resembles viral hepatitis in humans, is believed to impair liver cell function by inhibiting the synthesis of glycogen and glucuronide via uridine-diphosphoglucose.[8] The effect of vitamin E on D-GalN–induced liver impairment was comparable to the results obtained in CCl_4-induced liver disorders; liver disorders were marked in vitamin E–deficient rats and slight in those supplemented with vitamin E (FIGURE 2), and the same was the case with lysosomal enzymes and TBA-reactive products resulting from lipid

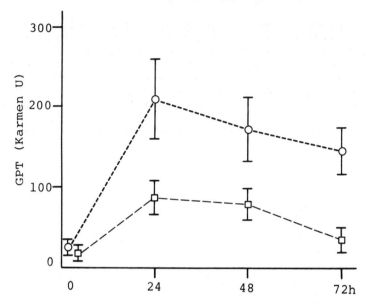

FIGURE 2. Serum levels of GPT before and after injection of 750 mg/kg of D-GalN. In vitamin E-deficient rats, serum GPT levels were markedly elevated after exposure to D-GalN. Circles, vitamin E-deficient rats; squares, vitamin E-supplemented rats. Mean values ± standard deviations are shown for 10 rats.

peroxidation. These findings suggest that vitamin E mitigates the effects of liver disorders. The free radical reaction is not the primary cause of liver impairment in D-GalN hepatitis. Even in this type of hepatitis, once the liver is impaired by a toxic substance, lipid peroxidation can occur, giving rise to secondary and tertiary damage to the liver. It is of interest to note that vitamin E produces a protective effect on the liver even in this type of liver disorder.

REFERENCES

1. ABE, K. & G. KATSUI. 1975. Jpn. J. Food Nutr. **28:** 277–280.
2. TAYLOR, S. L., M. P. LAMDEN & A. L. TAPPEL. 1976. Lipids **11:** 530–538.
3. KATO, K., K. YOSHIDA, H. TSUKAMOTO, M. NOBUNAGA, T. MASUYA & T. SAWADA. 1960. Chem. Pharm. Bull. **8:** 239–242.
4. SHIBKO, S. & A. L. TAPPEL. 1963. Biochim. Biophys. Acta **73:** 76–86.
5. YAGI, K. 1976. Biochem. Med. **15:** 212–216.
6. OHKAWA, H., N. OHISHI & K. YAGI. 1979. Anal. Biochem. **95:** 351–358.
7. RECKNAGEL, R. O. 1967. Pharmacol. Rev. **19:** 145–208.
8. DECKER, K. & D. KEPPLER. 1974. Rev. Physiol. Biochem. Pharmacol. **71:** 77–106.

THE EFFECTS OF VITAMIN E AND CORN OIL ON PROSTACYCLIN AND THROMBOXANE B_2 SYNTHESIS IN RATS*

A. C. Chan† and S. St-J. Hamelin

Department of Foods and Nutrition
University of Manitoba
Winnipeg, Manitoba, Canada R3T 2N2

Recent evidence suggests that dietary antioxidants have the potential to regulate the metabolic turnover of arachidonic acid (AA). Although the quantities of these AA metabolites *in vivo* are small, they have profound and often opposing physiological and pharmacological actions. For example, prostacyclin (PGI_2) is a powerful vasodilator and inhibitor of platelet aggregation whereas thromboxane A_2 (TxA_2) possesses the opposite properties. The balance between platelet TxA_2 and vascular PGI_2 production is important in controlling thrombus formation. Previous studies in this laboratory have shown that PGI_2 release by rabbit aorta can be regulated by dietary vitamin E.[1] In the present study, the relationship between dietary vitamin E (VE) and corn oil (CO) on the synthesis of PGI_2 and TxA_2 in rats was investigated.

Six groups of young male Sprague-Dawley rats were fed purified diets containing 5 and 15% CO with either 0, 100, or 1,000 ppm of *all-rac-α*-tocopheryl acetate for 23 weeks. Body weight, plasma pyruvate kinase, and spontaneous red blood cell (RBC) hemolysis were used to monitor VE status. Aortic PGI_2 production, detected as the stable metabolite 6-keto-$PGF_1α$, and thrombin-stimulated platelet TxB_2 synthesis were quantified by radioimmunoassay (RIA). Platelet malondialdehyde (MDA) production, measured by the thiobarbituric acid (TBA) test, and liver microsomal reduced nicotinamide-adenine dinucleotide phosphate (NADPH)-dependent oxidase were also determined.

Each group of animals showed a different rate of weight gain over time. For the VE-deficient groups, body weights became significantly lower after 10 weeks (5% CO) and 12 weeks (15% CO) of feeding. Plasma pyruvate kinase activity, RBC hemolysis, and platelet protein were significantly greater in VE-deficient rats at both CO levels.

PGI_2 release, while invariably greater in animals fed 15% CO, was increased at the highest dietary VE level (1,000 ppm). On the other hand, platelet TxB_2 production was inversely related to dietary VE levels at 5% CO. Accordingly, the highest PGI_2/TxA_2 molar ratio was found in the 5% CO–1,000 ppm VE group.

Platelet MDA production was also negatively correlated with dietary VE levels. The molar ratio of MDA to TxB_2 was close to 3 in all groups studied, suggesting that MDA production in stimulated platelets was not solely derived from the TxA_2 synthetic pathway.

Liver microsomal NADPH-dependent oxidase was significantly elevated in

*Supported by National Sciences and Engineering Research Council of Canada—A7286.

†Present affiliation: Department of Biochemistry, University of Ottowa, Ottawa, Ontario, Canada K1N 9B4.

rats fed VE-deficient diets. However, this increase was also demonstrated in rats receiving 100 ppm VE and 15% CO.

These findings show a stimulatory effect by high levels of dietary VE on PGI_2 synthesis in the rat aorta concomitant with a decreased platelet TxB_2 production. Further work is presently under way to explain these phenomena.

ACKNOWLEDGMENTS

Prostaglandin (PG) standards and antibodies for 6-keto-$PGF_1\alpha$ and TxB_2 were gifts from Drs. J. Pike, J. A. Salmon, and L. K. Steel respectively.

REFERENCES

1. CHAN, A. C. & M. K. LEITH. 1981. Am. J. Clin. Nutr. **34**(11): 2341–2347.

VITAMIN E-RESPONSIVE HEMOLYTIC ANEMIA
IN OWL MONKEYS*

Simin N. Meydani, Robert J. Nicolosi, Paul S. Brady,
and K. C. Hayes

Nutrition Division
Harvard Medical School
New England Regional Primate Research Center
Southboro, Massachusetts 01772

The owl monkey (*Aotus trivirgatus*) (Aot), a new-world monkey represented by several karyotypes, develops a vitamin E and selenium (E/Se)-responsive spontaneous hemolytic anemia in captivity.[1] Susceptibility to anemia varies as a function of karyotype.[2] Clinical and pathological features of the anemia are consistent with vitamin E deficiency, and preliminary studies demonstrated that intramuscular injection of vitamin E and Se, but not their oral supplementation, was effective in correcting the anemia.[1] Injection of Se alone did not improve the anemia. Dietary vitamin E was adequate, and the serum vitamin E level was within the normal range for most species.

It was hypothesized that vitamin E might act pharmacologically to protect the membrane against lipid peroxidation or to stabilize it against G-6-P dehydrogenase (G6PD) or glutathione synthetase deficiencies. Accordingly, measures were made of lipid peroxidation in red blood cells (RBCs), osmotic fragility, and both H_2O_2-induced hemolysis and time-dependent spontaneous hemolysis as well as the RBC glutathione peroxidase system components. These Aot values also were compared to those of other primates.[3] Anemic Aot tended to have higher ($p < 0.1$) RBC thiobarbituric acid–reactive substance (TBARS) values (an indicator of RBC lipid peroxidation) than did nonanemic Aot. In addition, all Aot TBARS values were twofold greater than either cebus or squirrel monkeys. The RBC osmotic fragility curves in both anemic and nonanemic Aot were similar to that of human RBC. Anemic Aot had increased H_2O_2-induced ($40.0 \pm 15.9\%$ vs. $3.2 \pm 0.4\%$ in nonanemic) and time-dependent ($52.8 \pm 13.1\%$ vs. $1.8 \pm 0.6\%$ in nonanemic) spontaneous hemolysis. Addition of glucose to the system did not provide protection against hemolysis, indicating that the glutathione peroxidase system was intact in anemic Aot. This was confirmed by the lack of differences in reduced glutathione level, glutathione peroxide, total and active glutathione reductase, and G6PD and 6-P-gluconate dehydrogenase (6PGD) activity between anemic and nonanemic Aot or between Aot and other primate species.

From these results and the stabilizing effect of vitamin E on polyunsaturated fatty acids (PUFA) of phospholipids (PL), it was hypothesized that hereditary or environmental factors had altered lipid composition of the RBC membrane in susceptible karyotypes, rendering them vulnerable to oxidative hemolysis. Therefore, the RBC PL profile, fatty acid composition, and free cholesterol to PL (FC/PL) ratio of anemic and nonanemic Aot were compared with those of other primate species.[4] The RBCs from Aot (as a species) had the lowest percentage of phosphatidylserine (PS) (2.1 ± 1.7 in Aot vs. 12.9 ± 2.5 in others) and phosphati-

*Supported in part by U.S. Public Health Service NIH Grant No. AM-26429 and NIH Grant No. PR00168 from the Division of Research Resources.

203

dylethanolamine (PE) (19.3 ± 3.4 vs. 33.2 ± 1.9) and more phosphatidylcholine (PC) (45.6 ± 4.3 vs. 36.5 ± 5.2) and sphingomyelin (Sph) (31.0 ± 4.8 vs. 15.3 ± 2.3) than did those from other primate species. Susceptible Aot had an elevated FC/PL ratio (1.31 ± 0.14), which tended to be even higher (1.48 ± 0.05) in overtly anemic Aot. The FC/PL ratio in anemia-resistant Aot was similar to that of rhesus monkeys. Surprisingly, marmosets and squirrel monkeys, which do not develop the anemia, also had elevated FC/PL ratios (1.39 ± 0.14). Susceptible Aot had a strikingly low percentage of PUFA (especially 18:2w6 and 20:4w6) in their PL compared to anemia-resistant Aot and other primate species, specifically, 1.2 ± 0.6% 20:4w6 and 7.0 ± 1.7% 18:2w6 in anemia-susceptible Aot vs. 15.5 ± 4.1% 20:4w6 and 18.1 ± 1.7% 18:2w6 in anemia-resistant Aot.

To determine whether the altered RBC profile reflected generalized changes in lipid metabolism, the plasma lipoproteins were characterized.[5] The susceptible Aot had depressed total plasma and high-density lipoprotein cholesterol (HDLC) and a higher plasma and HDL free cholesterol to esterified cholesterol ratio (FC/EC) than did anemia-resistant Aot and rhesus monkeys. Aot also had a higher low-density lipoprotein cholesterol to HDL cholesterol (LDLC/HDLC) ratio than did rhesus monkeys; in anemic Aot this ratio was almost double that of the nonanemic Aot. Corn oil supplementation of anemia-susceptible Aot diet changed their plasma and HDL lipid profile to that of anemia-resistant Aot and rhesus monkeys.

The hemolysis thus appears to be associated with peroxidative loss of PUFA in RBC membranes, an altered RBC PL profile, and an increased membrane FC/PL ratio that reflects an altered lipoprotein metabolism. Dietary supplementation with PUFA or protection of PUFA by vitamin E is beneficial, though not remedial. The underlying peroxidative insult remains unresolved.

REFERENCES

1. SEHGAL, P. K., R. T. BRONSON, P. S. BRADY, K. W. MCINTYRE & M. W. ELLIOTT. 1980. Therapeutic efficacy of vitamin E and selenium in treating hemolytic anemia of owl monkeys. Lab. Anim. Sci. **30**(1): 92–98.
2. BELAND, M. T., R. T. BRONSON, N. S. F. MA, K. W. MCINTYRE, P. K. SEHGAL & T. L. KEADLE. 1981. Karyotypic variation in susceptibility to hemolytic anemia and idiopathic eosinophilia of owl monkeys, *Aotus trivirgatus*. Primates **22**(4): 551–556.
3. BRADY, P. S., P. K. SEHGAL & K. C. HAYES. 1982. Erythrocyte characteristics in vitamin E-responsive anemia of the owl monkey (*Aotus trivirgatus*). Am. J. Vet. Res. **43**. (In press.)
4. WALSH, F. X., R. J. NICOLOSI, S. N. MEYDANI, P. K. SEHGAL & K. C. HAYES. 1982. Hemolytic anemia of owl monkeys: red blood cell lipid alterations. Proc. Soc. Exp. Biol. Med. **169**(2): 253–259.
5. MEYDANI, S. N., R. J. NICOLOSI, K. C. HAYES & P. K. SEHGAL. Plasma lipid and lipoprotein characterization in owl monkeys (*Aotus trivirgatus*): possible role in vitamin E-responsive hemolytic anemia. (Submitted for publication.)

CELLULAR IMMUNE RESPONSES, CORTICOSTEROID LEVELS, AND RESISTANCE TO *LISTERIA MONOCYTOGENES* AND MURINE LEUKEMIA IN MICE FED A HIGH VITAMIN E DIET*

Ronald R. Watson and Thomas M. Petro

Department of Foods and Nutrition
Purdue University
West Lafayette, Indiana 47907

Severe deficiencies of dietary vitamin E,[1] like those of many other nutrients,[2] can cause suppression of host defenses. High levels of dietary vitamin E have been reported to alter some immune responses, delay aging, and alter susceptibility to cancer initiation and growth.[3] One of the host cellular immune responses, antibody-dependent cell-mediated cytotoxicity (ADCC), important in resistance to growth of neoplasias, is enhanced by high dietary vitamin E.[4] We measured the growth of a plasmacytoma cell line *in vivo* and a pathogen, *Listeria monocytogenes*, which is destroyed by the cellular immune system, as well as cell-mediated cytotoxicity and serum corticosterone in mice fed a high vitamin E diet.

TABLE 1

Viable *L. monocytogenes* (LOG$_{10}$) per Liver and Spleen Three Days after Infection of Mice Fed Either the Control or High Vitamin E Diets*

Dietary Group	Diet Consumption after Weaning (weeks)	
	2	4
Control	5.38 ± 0.27	5.56 ± 0.22
High vitamin E	4.95 ± 0.27	5.81 ± 0.28

*Mice injected with 4.09 log$_{10}$ *L. monocytogenes* on day 0. No mice died between injection and day 3. Figures are means ± standard error.

The high vitamin E diet had a 20-fold increase in α-tocopherol (400 mg/100 g diet) over the concentration of α-tocopherol found in the control diet.[4] Isolation of splenic lymphocytes, serum corticosterone measurement, and phytohemagglutinin (PHA)-induced mitogenesis have been described previously.[4,5] Cell-mediated cytotoxicity (CMC) after intraperitoneal challenge of mice with L1210 cells, was determined by measuring ^{51}Cr release from labeled L1210 plasmacytoma cells incubated with splenocytes. Resistance against *L. monocytogenes* was determined by measuring the number of bacterial cells infecting the liver and spleen after intraperitoneal infection. No significant differences were observed in the resistance at day 3 after infection compared to mice fed the high vitamin E diet (TABLE 1). Resistance was reduced at day 7 after infection in mice fed the high

*Research support by Phi Beta Psi sorority and Wallace Genetics, Inc., is greatly appreciated.

0077-8923/82/0393-0205 $01.75/0 © 1982, NYAS

TABLE 2

VIABLE *L. monocytogenes* (LOG_{10}) PER LIVER AND SPLEEN SEVEN DAYS AFTER INFECTION
OF MICE FED EITHER THE CONTROL OR HIGH VITAMIN E DIET*

Dietary Group	Diet Consumption after Weaning (weeks)		
	2	4	14
Control	3.43 ± 0.25 (0)	2.87 ± 0.56 (0)	4.03 ± 0.77 (25)
High vitamin E	3.94 ± 0.58 (17)	4.17 ± 0.73 (0)†	3.93 ± 1.07 (28)

*Mice injected with 4.09 log_{10} *L. monocytogenes*. Numbers in parentheses indicate percentage of mice injected with *L. monocytogenes* that died by seven days.
†Significantly different from controls ($p < 0.05$).

TABLE 3

PROLIFERATION OF L1210 LEUKEMIA CELLS INJECTED INTRAPERITONEALLY IN FEMALE
BALB/c MICE FED EITHER A CONTROL OR HIGH VITAMIN E DIET

Dietary Group	Diet Consumption (weeks)	Peritoneal Exudate cells ($\times 10^{-6}$)* (day after injection of L1210 cells)		
		0	7	14
Control	2	1.05 ± 0.05	490.86 ± 36.80	7.55 ± 1.22
High vitamin E		0.70 ± 0.04	507.84 ± 40.93	8.00 ± 1.23
Control	4	1.06 ± 0.19	693.87 ± 57.58	11.60 ± 1.78
High vitamin E		1.36 ± 0.33	424.90 ± 88.80†	9.52 ± 1.94
Control	14	ND	571.90 ± 133.9	28.75 ± 1.88
High vitamin E			768.0 ± 63.40	15.25 ± 2.46†

*Challenged with 1×10^7 L1210 mouse leukemia cells on day 0. Mice sacrificed on day 0 were not injected with L1210 cells. ND means not done.
†Significantly different from controls ($p < 0.05$).

TABLE 4

CELL-MEDIATED CYTOTOXICITY AGAINST L1210 LEUKEMIA CELLS IN MICE
FED THE CONTROL OR HIGH VITAMIN E DIET*

Dietary Group	Diet Consumption (weeks)	CMC Percent Lysis* (days after injection of L1210 cells)		
		0	7	14
Control	2	3.18 ± 0.44	29.60 ± 6.20	42.25 ± 10.0
High vitamin E		3.39 ± 0.36	27.50 ± 4.92	63.45 ± 4.18†
Control	4	9.13 ± 0.73	15.36 ± 3.40	51.78 ± 8.67
High vitamin E		9.51 ± 1.12	15.56 ± 2.29	43.23 ± 2.50
Control	14	ND	35.35 ± 12.50	71.40 ± 8.80
High vitamin E		ND	26.06 ± 8.77	56.96 ± 3.09

*Cell-mediated cytotoxicity (percent lysis) ± standard error of the mean (SEM) using spleen cells from mice challenged with 1×10^7 L1210 mouse leukemia cells. Mice sacrificed on day 0 not challenged; ^{51}Cr-labeled effector cell:target cell was 200:1.
†Significantly different from controls ($p < 0.05$).

TABLE 5

EFFECT OF A HIGH VITAMIN E DIET UPON THE MITOGENIC RESPONSIVENESS
OF SPLEEN CELLS TO PHA IN BALB/c MICE

Dietary Group	Measurement	Diet Consumed after Weaning (weeks)*		
		2	4	14
Control	spleen	8.92 ± 0.49	7.77 ± 0.83	ND
High vitamin E	lymphocytes† (10⁻⁷)	7.08 ± 0.37	9.52 ± 1.19	
Control	mitogenesis	10994 ± 1289	25233 ± 2949	
High vitamin E	to PHA‡	15841 ± 2774	31757 ± 6116	ND
Control	spontaneous	1029 ± 190	2647 ± 682	ND
High vitamin E	mitogenesis‡	1589 ± 576	1194 ± 339§	
Control	stimulation	12.08 ± 2.47	12.28 ± 3.25	ND
High vitamin E	units¶	13.85 ± 3.06	33.76 ± 7.70§	

*Female mice were weaned at 3 weeks of age. Then they were fed *ad libidum* the American Institute of Nutrition (AIN) synthetic diet or the same diet with a 20-fold increase in vitamin E.

†Total lymphocyte number/spleen ± SEM.

‡Counts per minute (cpm) ± SEM of ³H-thymidine 72-hour culture of PHA-stimulated or non-PHA-stimulated (spontaneous) spleen cells (2.5×10^5 cells/culture). Each point represents a minimum of three cultures from each of five mice.

§Significantly different from mice fed the control diet ($p < 0.05$).

¶Stimulation units = cpm of PHA-stimulated cultures ÷ cpm unstimulated cultures.

vitamin E diet for 4 weeks, but not for the longer 14 weeks (TABLE 2). The numbers of L1210 cells isolated 7 days after intraperitoneal challenge were not significantly different between the two dietary groups 2 and 14 weeks after diet initiation (TABLE 3). By 4 weeks after dietary treatment, there was a significant reduction in L1210 cells isolated from the peritoneal cavity of the mice fed the high vitamin E diet. Previous results suggest that increased ADCC, which was normal after prolonged diet consumption, may be the reason for increased leukemia cell resistance in mice fed the high vitamin E diet.[4] Enhanced CMC against L1210 cells was not generally observed above that found in mice fed the control diet (TABLE 4). However PHA-induced T lymphocyte mitogenesis was enhanced by high dietary vitamin E (TABLE 5). Serum corticosterone levels were

TABLE 6

EFFECT OF A HIGH VITAMIN E DIET ON THE SERUM CORTICOSTEROID
LEVEL IN BALB/c MICE*

Dietary Group	Diet Consumed after Weaning (weeks)†		
	2	4	14
Control	40.8 ± 5.4	59.3 ± 1.7	ND
High vitamin E	28.3 ± 1.9‡	38.0 ± 1.9‡	ND

*Numbers are µg corticosterone/100 ml serum. Unconjugated corticosterone concentrations were determined using a spectrofluorometric assay.[4]

†Female mice weaned at 3 weeks of age. Then they were fed *ad libidum* the AIN synthetic diet or the same diet with a 20-fold increase in vitamin E. None of the mice were infected with *L. monocytogenes* or injected with murine leukemia cells.

‡Significantly different from control ($p < 0.01$).

depressed by high dietary vitamin E (TABLE 6). Lower serum corticosterone levels may explain some of the observations of enhanced T lymphocyte activity. Further study is needed to understand the mechanism of resistance, including the regulatory role of corticosteroids on cellular cytotoxicity and resistance to leukemia cell growth.[4,6]

REFERENCES

1. SHEFFY, B. E. & R. D. SCHULTZ. 1978. Nutrition and the immune responses. Cornell Vet. 68(Suppl. 7): 48–61.
2. WATSON, R. R. & D. N. MCMURRAY. 1979. The effects of malnutrition on secretory and cellular immune processes. Crit. Rev. Food Sci. Nutr. 12: 113–159.
3. SCOTT, M. 1979. Studies on vitamin E and related factors in nutrition and metabolism. In The Fat Soluble Vitamins. H. DeLuca & J. Suttie, Eds.: 355. University of Wisconsin Press. Madison, Wis.
4. LIM, T. S., N. PUTT, D. SAFRANSKI, C. CHUNG & R. R. WATSON. 1981. Effect of vitamin E on cell-mediated immune responses and serum corticosterone in young and maturing mice. Immunology 44: 289–294.
5. LIM, T. S., N. MESSIHA & R. R. WATSON. 1980. Immune components of the intestinal mucosae of aging and protein deficient mice. Immunology 43: 401–407.
6. WATSON, R. R. & N. MESSIHA. Enhancement of IgA in intestinal secretions and antibody dependent cytotoxicity in intestinal mucosal cells of mice fed a high vitamin E diet. (Submitted for publication.)

ENDOGENOUS PROSTACYCLIN AND THROMBOXANE BIOSYNTHESIS DURING CHRONIC VITAMIN E THERAPY IN MAN

Garret A. FitzGerald and Alan R. Brash

Division of Clinical Pharmacology
Department of Pharmacology
Vanderbilt University
Nashville, Tennessee 37232

INTRODUCTION

Several groups have shown that preincubation with α-tocopherol inhibits platelet aggregation induced by arachidonic acid and, to a lesser extent, collagen and adenosine diphosphate (ADP) *in vitro*.[1-3] Although α-tocopherol results in a dose-dependent inhibition of platelet thromboxane B_2 (TxB$_2$) formation *in vitro*,[4] complete inhibition of arachidonic acid–induced aggregation occurs at concentrations of α-tocopherol that only minimally inhibit oxidative metabolism of this acid, suggesting an action, at least in part, independent of the cyclooxygenase.[5] Despite the multiplicity of studies on the effect of α-tocopherol on platelet function *in vitro*, studies on *in vivo* indices of platelet function are lacking. This is of importance, as many of the studies *in vitro* were performed in aqueous media at concentrations difficult to attain *in vivo*. However, due to its high lipid solubility, it is possible that much lower concentrations of α-tocopherol might influence prostaglandin (PG) biosynthesis, as suggested by some animal experiments.[6] In addition to its effects on thromboxane formation, α-tocopherol might be expected to modulate prostacyclin biosynthesis. Lipid peroxides may inhibit prostacyclin synthesis,[7] and atherosclerotic blood vessels appear to generate less prostacyclin than do healthy vessels.[8] Thus, α-tocopherol might ameliorate such inhibition of prostacyclin generation by way of its antioxidant properties. We have sought to explore the effects of vitamin E on endogenous prostacyclin and thromboxane biosynthesis in man.

METHODS

Six healthy male volunteers took vitamin E, 1,600 IU per day in four divided doses, for seven days. Urine and blood collections were performed prior to and on the seventh day of vitamin E therapy. Platelet aggregation ex vivo was measured in response to arachidonic acid (0.4, 0.6, 0.8, and 1.0 mM) and ADP (1.0, 2.5, 5.0, and 10.0 μM). Bleeding time was performed by the template technique. Thromboxane B_2 formation by platelets exposed to 5 units thrombin ex vivo was measured by radioimmunoassay. 2,3-Dinor-6-keto-PGF$_{1\alpha}$ (PGI-M) and 2,3-dinor-thromboxane B_2 (Tx-M), major urinary metabolites of prostacyclin and thromboxane, were measured by stable isotope ratio methods, employing gas chromatography–mass spectrometry in the selected ion monitoring mode.

209

RESULTS

The threshold concentration of arachidonic acid necessary to induce platelet aggregation ex vivo increased during vitamin E therapy. The ADP aggregation threshold did not alter. Bleeding time (4.6 ± 0.3 minutes) was not significantly prolonged by vitamin E (5.7 ± 0.5 minutes). Thrombin-stimulated thromboxane generation was measured in four subjects and was significantly depressed from control values (5-25 ng/ml) in all subjects while taking vitamin E. Tx-M was measured in two individuals and fell from 367 and 250 pg/mg creatinine to below 50 pg/mg creatinine on vitamin E. Despite the apparent inhibition of thromboxane biosynthesis, PGI-M excretion was not significantly depressed from control values (137 ± 28 pg/mg creatinine) by chronic therapy with vitamin E (186 ± 49.2 pg/mg creatinine; p, not significant).

DISCUSSION

Platelet tocopherol increases linearly with vitamin E dosage in man up to 1,600 IU per day, above which no further increases occur.[9] Chronic administration of this dose of vitamin E substantially depressed thromboxane biosynthesis in normal volunteers. Chronic therapy of normal volunteers with aspirin at 2,600 mg/day depressed mean Tx-M excretion by 97% and thrombin-stimulated platelet TxB_2 by 99%.[10] However, in contrast to the present study, this was associated with an average 60% decline in PGI-M excretion.[11] Despite thromboxane synthesis inhibition during vitamin E therapy, prostacyclin biosynthesis remained intact and may be enhanced in some individuals. Indirect studies of the effects of vitamin E on arachidonic acid metabolism have provided conflicting results. Thus, Dorman and Panganamala found enhanced prostacyclin biosynthesis by aortae obtained from vitamin E–deficient rabbits,[12] and Okuma et al. found generation of prostacyclinlike activity depressed in rats maintained on a vitamin E–deficient diet.[13] Forster found that vitamin E supplementation depressed thromboxane B_2 formation by rabbit platelets but had no effect on prostacyclin formation by rabbit hearts or aortae.[14] The results of the present study suggest controlled evaluation of the effects of vitamin E on prostaglandin biosynthesis in man, particularly in conditions where prostacyclin synthesis inhibition by lipid peroxides may occur.

REFERENCES

1. FONG, J. S. C. 1976. Alpha-tocopherol: its inhibition of human platelet aggregation. Experientia 32L: 639-641.
2. PANGANAMALA, R. V., J. S. G. MILLER, E. T. WEBER, H. M. SHARMA & D. G. CORNWELL. 1977. Differential inhibitory effects of vitamin E and other antioxidants on prostaglandin synthatase, platelet aggregation and lipoxidase. Prostaglandins 14: 261-270.
3. STEINER, M. & J. ANASTASI. 1976. Vitamin E: an inhibitor of the platelet release reaction. J. Clin. Invest. 57: 732-737.
4. ALI, M., G. GUDBRANSON & J. McDONALD. 1980. Inhibition of human platelet cyclooxygenase by alpha-tocopherol. Prostaglandins Med. 4: 79-85.
5. AGRADI, E., A. PETRONI, GA. SOCINI & C. GALLI. 1981. In vitro effects of synthetic antioxidants and vitamin E on arachidonic acid metabolism and thromboxane

formation in human platelets and on platelet aggregation. Prostaglandins 22(2): 255–265.

6. CHAN, A. C., C. E. ALLEN & P. V. J. HEGARTY. 1980. The effects of vitamin E depletion and repletion on prostaglandin synthesis in semitendinosus muscle of young rabbits. J. Nutr. 110(1): 66–73.

7. MONCADA, S., R. GRYGLEWSKI, S. BUNTING & J. R. VANE. 1976. A lipid peroxide inhibits the enzyme in blood vessel microsomes that generates from prostaglandin endoperoxides the substance (prostaglandin X) which prevents platelet aggregation. Prostaglandins 12: 715–737.

8. SINZINGER, H., W. FEIGL & K. SILBERBAUER. 1979. Prostacyclin generation in atherosclerotic arteries. Lancet 2: 469.

9. STEINER, M. 1978. Inhibition of platelet aggregation by alpha-tocopherol. In Tocopherol, Oxygen and Biomembranes. C. deDuve & O. Hayaishi, Eds.: 142–163. Elsevier/North-Holland Biomedical Press. Amsterdam, the Netherlands.

10. FITZGERALD, G. A., J. A. OATES & J. HAWIGER. 1982. Thromboxane dependent and independent mechanisms of platelet aggregation during chronic aspirin therapy. Clin. Res. 30: 502A.

11. FITZGERALD, G. A., A. R. BRASH, R. L. MAAS, J. A. OATES & L. J. ROBERTS. 1981. Endogenous production of prostacyclin and thromboxane during chronic aspirin therapy. Circulation 64: 55.

12. DORMAN, N. J. & R. V. PANGANAMALA. 1980. The effect of dietary vitamin E on aggregation and thromboxane production in rabbit platelets. Fed. Proc. 38: 1896.

13. OKUMA, M., H. TAKAYAMA & H. UCHINO. 1980. Generation of prostacyclin-like substance and lipid peroxidation in vitamin E-deficient rats. Prostaglandins 19(4): 527.

14. FORSTER, W. 1980. In vivo and ex vivo studies of the effect of vitamin E pretreatment on PGI_2 and TXA_2 synthesis. Acta Med. Scand. 642: 47–48.

PARTIAL RECOVERY OF THE ELECTRORETINOGRAM IN VITAMIN E-REPLETED DOGS

Ellis R. Loew,* Ronald C. Riis,† and Ben E. Sheffy‡

New York State College of Veterinary Medicine
and
Division of Biological Sciences
Cornell University
Ithaca, New York 14853

Beagle dogs weaned onto a purified diet deficient in vitamin E develop, within three months, a retinopathy including disruption and swelling of the photoreceptor cell outer segments and a buildup of autofluorescent lipopigment granules within the cells of the pigment epithelium. The lesions appear to progress from the central retina toward the periphery with the tapetal area more fully involved.

Electroretinography done on dogs three to four months after weaning and having ophthalmoscopic signs of retinopathy gave no detectable electroretinogram (ERG) at any stimulus intensity or duration. Was our inability to detect an ERG due to the simple shunting of the light-induced currents by low-resistance retinal lesions, or does a lack of vitamin E directly affect the production of the ERG?

To examine this question as well as to see if the retinopathy could be halted or reversed, dogs lacking an ERG and having retinal lesions were placed on purified diet repleted with vitamin E. Electroretinography and fundus examination were performed at regular intervals.

Of the five dogs on study all had some sign of an electrical response by three months on the repleted diet. Ophthalmoscopically there was no evidence for recovery, although no increase in lesioning could be seen. The eyes from four of the dogs were removed at this time and examined histologically. No difference could be seen between these dogs and vitamin E-deficient dogs.

One dog was kept on the repleted diet for over a year, with the finding that there was a slow increase in ERG amplitude and the eventual appearance of an a-wave after 9 months. By 13 months there was an almost normal ERG waveform, although the amplitude was reduced and the implicit times were increased. Histological examination of the retina at 13 months still showed many retinal lesions centrally and peripherally with many peripheral areas of reasonably normal retina.

It should be mentioned that while an ERG returned in the repleted dogs and the retinopathy was halted, there was no evidence from behavioral testing that the dogs could see any better than they could before being placed on the repleted diet.

The fact that there is a return of the ERG in vitamin E-repleted animals shows that some recovery from the effects of vitamin E deficiency on the retina is possible. However, this recovery would appear to be limited to the ERG

*Department of Physiology.
†Department of Clinical Sciences.
‡Department of Veterinary Microbiology.

generators, as there was no decrease in retinal lesioning, no change in the amount or distribution of lipopigment in the pigment epithelium, and no improvement in the visual capacity of the test animals.

The simplest explanation for the loss and recovery of the ERG is a shunting model where the slow increase in ERG amplitude with time is related to a "healing" (i.e., a resistance increase) of the retinal lesions present. Although attractive, this model fails to account for the changes in waveform with time, nor is the extremely slow progress of the recovery consistent with a healing or scarring mechanism. In simple shunting the waveform should be normal although reduced in amplitude in proportion to the shunting resistance. The fact that at three months postrepletion, only a positive wave can be seen clearly speaks against simple shunting as the sole cause of the ERG loss.

Another possibility is that vitamin E is necessary for ERG generation. It has been shown that the receptor potential *in vivo* and in isolated outer segments is lost following the induction of lipid peroxidation and that this loss is prevented by treatment with vitamin E. If true for dogs, the loss of the ERG could be due to membrane damage resulting from an increase in lipid peroxidation affecting all retinal photoreceptors. Recovery would then represent regeneration and replacement of peroxidized photoreceptor membrane in the presence of normal vitamin E levels. The first wave to recover might be expected to be the positive b-wave, due to convergence effects. As for the long time required for even partial ERG recovery, it must be remembered that in addition to photoreceptor changes, the pigment epithelium is also markedly affected by vitamin E deficiency.

It is probable that both shunting and a direct effect of vitamin E deficiency are responsible for the ERG loss. Whether repletion before ophthalmoscopic signs of lesioning might lead to a faster, more complete recovery of the ERG is under study.

THE ROLE OF VITAMIN E IN THE ETIOLOGY AND TREATMENT OF PANCREATITIS

Hiroshi Tanimura, Hitoshi Kato, and Yorinori Hikasa

Second Department of Surgery
Faculty of Medicine
Kyoto University
Kyoto 606, Japan

We have already reported that a deficiency of polyunsaturated fatty acids or essential fatty acids (EFA) is one of the diatheses of pancreatitis, especially gallstone pancreatitis. It is thought that vitamin E is closely related to EFA and membrane stability. Thus, in this study, we examined the role of vitamin E in the etiology and treatment of pancreatitis experimentally and clinically.

High-performance liquid chromatography was used to determine all the analogues of vitamin E, that is, α-, β-, γ-, and δ-tocopherol. Serum levels of α-tocopherol in patients with pancreatitis (mean $\pm$ standard deviation, 5.7 $\pm$ 1.2 μg/ml) were significantly lower than those of healthy subjects (9.1 $\pm$ 1.7 μg/ml, p < 0.001).

Vitamin E and Experimental Pancreatitis in Hamsters

Hamsters were weaned at three weeks and, as shown in FIGURE 1, fed the following diets: vitamin E sufficient (*all-rac-α*-tocopheryl nicotinate, 23.4 mg/100 g diet) and stripped corn oil added (group 1); vitamin E deficient with stripped corn oil (group 2); and vitamin E deficient without stripped corn oil (group 3).

A saline solution containing 1.5% taurocholate, 2% trypsin, and 2% cephalothin was adjusted to pH 8.0 by $NaHCO_3$, and 0.2 ml of this solution was infused into the pancreatic duct. Nigrosine was also mixed to confirm the complete regurgitation of this infusate into the tail of the pancreas under 25 cm H_2O pressure. After 24 hours, the clinical response of the hamster was observed, and the abdominal cavity was reopened.

Serum and pancreatic tissue levels of α-tocopherol after four weeks feeding were respectively as follows: group 1, 20.3 $\pm$ 1.4 μg/ml in serum and 15.6 $\pm$ 2.4 μg/g wet weight in the pancreatic tissue; group 2, 0.7 $\pm$ 0.1 μg/ml and 0.6 $\pm$ 0.4 μg/g wet weight; and group 3, 1.1 $\pm$ 0.2 μg/ml and 0.9 $\pm$ 0.4 μg/g wet weight. The values of lipid peroxide in serum and the pancreatic tissues of hamsters after four weeks feeding were respectively as follows: group 1, 3.2 $\pm$ 0.3 nmol/ml in serum and 46.7 $\pm$ 12.2 nmol/g wet weight in the pancreatic tissue; group 2, 3.7 $\pm$ 0.8 nmol/ml and 72.8 $\pm$ 20.6 nmol/g wet weight; and group 3, 2.1 $\pm$ 0.3 nmol/ml and 33.9 $\pm$ 0.7 nmol/g wet weight. The severity of pancreatitis in each diet group of hamsters is summarized in FIGURE 1. Under our criteria, hamsters showing scores of seven or more were classified as severe pancreatitis, and those with scores less than six were classified as mild pancreatitis. Severe pancreatitis, as defined above, was observed in 2 out of 11 (18%) in group 1, 10 out of 11 (91%) in group 2, and 13 out of 14 animals (93%) in group 3. Therefore, severe pancreatitis can be said to occur more frequently in the vitamin E–deficient diet group (groups 2 and 3) than in the vitamin E–sufficient diet group (group 1). The histological findings were almost the same as the macroscopic observations.

214

CLINICAL USE OF VITAMIN E FOR THE TREATMENT OF PANCREATITIS

In a 44-year-old male patient with acute alcoholic pancreatitis, before treatment with fat emulsion, the serum total tocopherol and α-tocopherol levels were 3.6 and 3.4 μg/ml respectively. Serum and urinary amylase levels decreased immediately upon fat emulsion therapy, and the clinical symptoms subsided simultaneously. Serum total and α-tocopherol increased to 10.7 μg/ml and 10.1 μg/ml respectively.

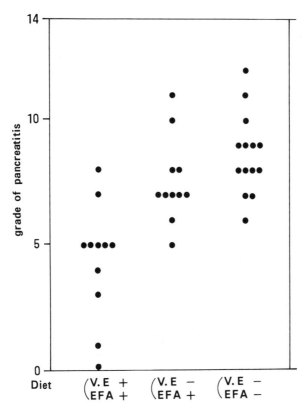

FIGURE 1. Effects of vitamin E and EFA on experimental pancreatitis.

In case 2, a patient with pancreatitis for more than three years and complaining of back pain, the serum level of α-tocopherol before treatment was 5.8 μg/ml. Though *all-rac-α*-tocopheryl acetate was administered at 400 mg per day, hardly any improvement in the clinical symptoms or laboratory findings was seen. But after administration of *all-rac-α*-tocopheryl nicotinate at 600 mg per day, the serum level of α-tocopherol increased up to 25.2 μg/ml. The urinary amylase level decreased markedly, and back pain disappeared almost completely.

Then preliminary products were prepared containing 100 mg of *RRR*-

α-tocopherol in a capsule for the oral treatment of chronic pancreatitis. But the average recovery of α-tocopherol showed 86 mg per capsule.

Case 3 had chronic relapsing pancreatitis with symptoms of persistent epigastric and back pain, and steatorrhea two or three times a day, for three years. Elevated serum and urinary amylase was observed during the acute attack. The intake of six RRR-α-tocopherol capsules caused an increase in serum α-tocopherol to 21.3 μg/ml on the eleventh day. Back pain and repeated steatorrhea subsided.

TABLE 1

SERUM α-TOCOPHEROL LEVELS AND CLINICAL EFFECTS IN PATIENTS WITH PANCREATITIS

Case Number	Initials	Age	Sex	Pancreatitis	Vitamin E	Serum α-Tocopherol (μg/ml) Before	After	Clinical Effect
1	MA	44	M	acute	fat emulsion	3.4	10.1	good
2	ME	39	M	chronic	oral	5.8	25.2	good
3	KK	43	M	chronic	oral	—	21.3	good
4	DH	59	M	chronic	oral	—	15.1*	good
5	SK	40	F	chronic	oral	7.2	19.1	good

*Two days after start.

Case 4 had chronic pancreatitis with steady severe pain, usually radiating into the back. Having heard about the effects of vitamin E, the patient had taken all-rac-α-tocopheryl nicotinate, but his symptoms hardly improved. Upon intake of six RRR-α-tocopherol capsules, his serum α-tocopherol levels increased to 15.2 μg/ml in only two days, he recovered well, and his back pain subsided within one month.

Case 5 suffered from acute epigastric pain; laboratory findings revealed chronic relapsing pancreatitis. Three RRR-α-tocopherol capsules per day were administered. Serum level of α-tocopherol increased from 7.2 μg/ml to 19.1 μg/ml within two weeks. In order to obtain rapid results, six capsules were administered, and the recurrent episodes of epigastric pain disappeared.

A list of patients with pancreatitis treated with vitamin E is shown in TABLE 1. The results were satisfactory.

DEVELOPMENT OF GLUTATHIONE PEROXIDASE ACTIVITY IN MUSCLE AND LIVER OF NORMAL AND VITAMIN E-DEFICIENT DUCKLINGS IN RELATION TO DIETARY SELENIUM CONTENT

C. E. Hulstaert, J. Vos, A. M. Kroon,* and I. Molenaar

Center for Medical Electron Microscopy
University of Groningen
9713 EZ Groningen, the Netherlands

Vitamin E and selenium are active in protecting cells against peroxidative damage. Vitamin E is supposed to stabilize cellular membranes by forming a complex with their polyunsaturated fatty acid (PUFA) moiety,[1,2] while its chromanol ring may scavenge free radicals and thus also protect the membrane PUFA.[3] Selenium forms part of the active center of at least one of the glutathione (GSH) peroxidases,[4,5] which eliminate lipid hydroperoxides and H_2O_2.[6]

Given a combination of vitamin E deficiency and low selenium intake, lipid hydroperoxides accumulate to a critical concentration. This could lead to cell or tissue peroxidosis, which was proposed to be the underlying mechanism in nutritional myopathy in vitamin E-deficient ducklings by Vos et al.[7] These authors showed that the extremely high growth rate during the first 2 weeks of age in E-deprived ducklings was primarily responsible for the drastic decrease of E concentration in various tissues. It also appeared that the nutritional myopathy in these animals was dependent on a low dietary selenium content. We now report on the development of GSH peroxidase activity from shortly before hatching until 10 weeks after hatching in skeletal muscle and liver of normal and E-deficient ducklings in relation to dietary selenium content.

MATERIALS AND METHODS

One-day-old, male Pekin ducklings were raised as described before[7] and fed a semisynthetic diet (Unilever Research Laboratories, Vlaardingen, the Netherlands) described previously.[8] Experimental groups were (a) vitamin E-sufficient diet containing 130 ppb Se (normal Se); (b) E-sufficient diet, 60 ppb Se (low Se); (c) E-sufficient diet, 33 ppb Se (liver study only); and (d) E-deficient diet, 60 ppb Se. The selenium content of the diets of the ducklings' mothers was not known. The E-sufficient diet contained 53.0 mg all-rac-α-tocopheryl acetate/kg food; and the E-deficient diet, 1.5 mg all-rac-α-tocopheryl acetate/kg.[8] The dietary content of selenium mainly depends on the region of origin of the casein component.[9] Special batches of casein were used to prepare the diets with the Se contents described above. Se determinations were carried out in the Unilever Research Laboratories by a method based on hydride evolution combined with atomic absorption spectrometry.[10] The standard deviation of the determinations was 10%.

In all experiments, 12-hour fasted ducklings were used. After decapitation,

*Laboratory of Physiological Chemistry.

0077-8923/82/0393-0217 $01.75/0 © 1982, NYAS

the musculus sartorius and liver were removed, the muscles homogenized in a blender-type homogenizer (Ultra-Turrax), and the livers homogenized in a glass Teflon Potter-Elvehjem homogenizer in 0.15 M KCl at 0–4°C. GSH peroxidase activity was determined according to Hafeman et al.,[11] except that instead of H_2O_2, the organic substrate tert-butyl-hydroperoxide was used in the same concentration. Protein was determined according to Cleland and Slater.[12] The degree of myopathy in the deficient animals was assessed by light microscopy as described by Jager and Vles.[8]

RESULTS

Muscle. After hatching, GSH peroxidase activity in skeletal muscle decreased in all three dietary groups, then remained about the same until seven weeks

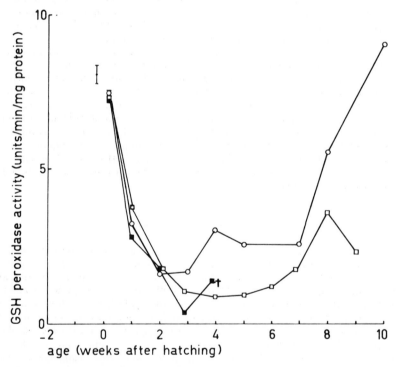

FIGURE 1. Development of activity of GSH peroxidase in the skeletal muscle of the duckling expressed as units/minute per mg protein from 2 days before hatching until 10 weeks after hatching. A unit of activity was defined as a decrease in the log (GSH) of 0.001 per minute after the decrease in log (GSH) per minute of the nonenzymatic reaction was subtracted. Circles, group a; open squares, group b; filled squares, group d. The standard error of the determinations at 2 days before hatching and at 1 day after hatching is represented by bars. The other determination points of the curve consist of the mean of two values. The mean deviation was 12.1%; the maximal deviation was 29.4%. Until 1 week after hatching, muscles of several ducklings were pooled to obtain one value. The myopathy scores[8] in the vitamin E–deficient group (d) at 2 weeks, 5 days were 20 and 8; at 6 weeks, 6 days, 17 and 20.

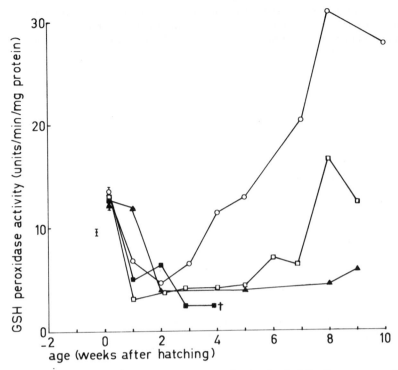

FIGURE 2. Development of activity in GSH peroxidase in the duckling liver, expressed as units/minute per mg protein from 2 days before hatching until 10 weeks after hatching. Symbols as in FIGURE 1; triangles, group c. The mean deviation of the determination points was 8.2%; the maximal deviation was 17.6%. Until 1 day after hatching, livers of several ducklings were pooled to obtain one value.

(FIGURE 1). The level of activity in the embryos two days before hatching was the same as in the ducklings one day after hatching. After seven weeks, groups a and b showed an increase in activity. For two weeks, there was no difference in activity between groups a and b; then they diverged, group b having a markedly lower activity than did group a. This difference remained for the rest of the experimental period. There was no difference in enzyme activities between groups b and d. It therefore appears that vitamin E deficiency has no influence on the level of GSH peroxidase activity at a dietary selenium content of 60 ppb. Group d showed severe signs of myopathy after three weeks, confirmed by light microscopic examination. These animals all died within four weeks.

Liver. In the liver, GSH peroxidase activity decreased after hatching in all four experimental groups until 2 weeks (FIGURE 2). The level of activity in the embryos two days before hatching was in the same range as in the ducklings one day after hatching. After 2 weeks, the activity level remained more or less constant for a variable period of time for each of the groups. After three weeks, activity strongly increased in group a. In group b, activity increased after five weeks, but much less than in group a. In group c, only a slight increase in activity was observed. The large spread in GSH peroxidase activity at one day after hatching between the different groups cannot be attributed to dietary Se content, as these ducklings had not yet been fed. It appears that in the liver also, E deficiency has no influence on GSH peroxidase activity level at a dietary Se content of 60 ppb, as no differences were found between groups b and d.

DISCUSSION

The experiments showed that there is a considerable decrease in GSH peroxidase activity in skeletal muscle and liver from the day of hatching up to two weeks after hatching in all experimental groups (FIGURES 1 and 2). We presume that the low activity level after two weeks causes a critical phase in the development of the duckling, especially when such other factors as vitamin E deprivation during the first two weeks of excessive growth aggravate peroxidative stress.[7] Further, it was shown that GSH peroxidase activity is much lower in muscle than in liver, as also found by others.[6,13,14]

After three weeks, GSH peroxidase level in muscle in group b (60 ppb Se) was about half that of group a (130 ppb Se). Nevertheless, no myopathy occurred. A dietary content of 130 ppb Se is considered normal,[15,16] whereas 60 ppb Se is regarded as a low level that, in combination with E deprivation, would lead to nutritional myopathy.[15,16] And indeed, in group d, myopathy occurred after three weeks: the very low GSH peroxidase level apparently cannot cope with the higher level of lipid hydroperoxides. This leads to cell or tissue peroxidosis. In this situation massive oxidative destruction of cellular membranes takes place in muscle, as was found in rabbits by light and electron microscopy.[17] On the other hand, the liver of ducklings fed a low Se and E-deficient diet has a higher GSH peroxidase level than does muscle and morphologically shows only mild signs of peroxidative stress.[18]

The increase in GSH peroxidase activity in group a ducklings after seven weeks in muscle and 3 weeks in liver should be regarded as a normal developmental process. It is not surprising that this increase is retarded in muscle and liver of ducklings fed the low-Se diet (group b). The observation that in group c (33 ppb Se), there is only a slight increase in GSH peroxidase activity in the liver would mean that the increase in activity in group a after three weeks and group b after five weeks is due to an increase of the Se-dependent GSH peroxidase.

In vitamin E deficiency, symptoms vary widely between species and between organs.[19] GSH peroxidase levels also vary,[14] and this may well be responsible for the many different symptoms reported in E deficiency. We propose that a nutritional shortage of E + selenium leads to symptoms of tissue peroxidosis in those organs where the activity of GSH peroxidase is already low by nature.

REFERENCES

1. LUCY, J. A. 1972. Ann. N.Y. Acad. Sci. **203:** 4.
2. DIPLOCK, A. T. & J. A. LUCY. 1973. FEBS Lett. **29:** 205.
3. MOLENAAR, I., C. E. HULSTAERT & M. J. HARDONK. 1980. In Vitamin E, A Comprehensive Treatise. L. J. Machlin, Ed.: 372–389. Marcel Dekker, Inc. New York, N.Y.
4. ROTRUCK, J. T., W. G. HOEKSTRA & A. L. POPE. 1971. Nature London New Biol. **231:** 223.
5. LAWRENCE, R. A., L. K. PARKHILL & R. F. BURK. 1978. J. Nutr. **108:** 981.
6. HOEKSTRA, W. G. 1975. Fed. Proc. **34:** 2083.
7. VOS, J., C. E. HULSTAERT & I. MOLENAAR. 1981. Ann. Nutr. Metab. **25:** 299.

8. JAGER, F. C. & R. O. VLES. 1970. Int. J. Vitam. Res. **40:** 592.
9. DIPLOCK, A. T. 1976. CRC Crit. Rev. Toxicol. **4:** 271.
10. ELLEN, G. & F. F. DOUMA. 1978. De Waren-Chemicus **8:** 154.
11. HAFEMAN, D. G., R. A. SUNDE & W. G. HOEKSTRA. 1974. J. Nutr. **104:** 1974.
12. CLELAND, K. W. & E. C. SLATER. 1953. Biochem. J. **53:** 547.
13. OMAYE, S. T. & A. L. TAPPEL. 1974. J. Nutr. **104:** 747.
14. SCHOLTZ, R. W., L. S. LOOK & D. A. TODHUNTER. 1981. Am. J. Vet. Res. **42:** 1724.
15. SCOTT, M. L., G. OLSON, L. KROOK & W. R. BROWN. 1967. J. Nutr. **91:** 573.
16. HULSTAERT, C. E., I. MOLENAAR, J. J. M. DE GOEIJ, C. ZEGERS & P. L. VAN PIJPEN. 1976.
    Nutr. Metab. **20:** 91.
17. VAN VLEET, J. F., B. V. HALL & J. SIMON. 1968. Am. J. Pathol. **52:** 1067.
18. MOLENAAR, I., J. VOS & F. A. HOMMES. 1972. Effect of vitamin E deficiency on cellular
    membranes. Vitam. Horm. **30:** 45.
19. SCOTT, M. L. 1970. *In* The Fat-Soluble Vitamins. H. F. DeLuca & J. W. SUTTIE, Eds.:
    355–368. University of Wisconsin Press. Madison, Wis.

TOCOPHEROL LEVELS IN NEEDLE ASPIRATION BIOPSIES OF ADIPOSE TISSUE: NORMAL SUBJECTS AND ABETALIPOPROTEINEMIC PATIENTS*

Lynda Hatam and Herbert J. Kayden

Department of Medicine
New York University School of Medicine
New York, New York 10016

The measurement of tocopherol in plasma and in red blood cells of normal subjects and in patients with abetalipoproteinemia (ABL) has documented strikingly low levels of tocopherol in ABL patients.[1] There is evidence, however, that dietary supplementation with high doses of tocopherol can ameliorate the neurological and muscular abnormalities in these patients, despite minimal increases in plasma levels and only modest changes in the levels of tocopherol in the red blood cells.[2] The low level of plasma tocopherol in these patients is ascribed to the absence of circulating β-lipoproteins, and also to the patients' inability to form chylomicrons necessary for the absorption of dietary tocopherol.[3]

It was apparent, therefore, that the measurement of tissue levels of tocopherol would be essential to the understanding of the effects of tocopherol in patients with an evident plasma E deficiency. Adipose tissue biopsies have been carried out with minimal trauma for many years in ambulatory subjects to evaluate fatty acid distribution and composition.[4] We therefore adapted our previously described, extremely sensitive, high-performance liquid chromatographic (HPLC) system with fluorescence spectroscopy[1] to the analysis of tocopherol in adipose tissue samples obtained during surgery and by needle aspiration biopsy.

The method of analysis was carried out similarly for adipose tissue samples obtained either at surgery or by biopsy. The technique for needle aspiration was performed essentially as described by Hirsch et al.[4] and yielded between 0.7 and 15 mg of adipose tissue per aspirate. Briefly, the samples were saponified in alcoholic potassium hydroxide in the presence of ascorbic acid for 30 minutes at 70°C; following cooling, the samples were extracted with hexane. An aliquot of the hexane was taken for the measurement of tocopherol by HPLC, as previously described; another aliquot was used to determine the total cholesterol content by gas-liquid chromatography using OV 17 as the column support. The aqueous layer was acidified and then extracted with heptane; following methylation of the fatty acids, the total fatty acid content was quantitated by the method of Stern and Shapiro.[5]

The range of adipose tissue tocopherol values in surgically obtained adipose tissue was from 245–335 ng tocopherol per mg triglyceride in normal subjects who did not supplement their diet with additional vitamin E. Surgically obtained specimens from normal subjects who did take supplemental daily doses of vitamin E ranged from 590 to 905 ng tocopherol per mg triglyceride. The validation of the analysis of adipose tissue obtained by needle aspiration was carried out in one subject whose surgically obtained adipose tissue level from

*Supported in part by a grant from Hoffmann-La Roche, Inc., Nutley, N.J.

four separate samples was 594 ± 56 ng tocopherol/mg triglyceride and whose tocopherol value for aspirated adipose tissue was 503 ng/mg triglyceride.

In patients with abetalipoproteinemia who were taking 800 to 1,200 mg of vitamin E daily, the adipose tissue level defined by needle aspiration ranged between 30 and 144 ng E per mg triglyceride, almost reaching 50% of the level observed in our unsupplemented normal control group. (Plasma levels in the ABL patients ranged from 0.2 to 2.4 μg tocopherol per ml of plasma.) In one ABL patient supplemented with 9 g of vitamin E for many years, the adipose tissue level of tocopherol was normal, 242 ng E/mg triglyceride, with a plasma level of only 0.8 μg tocopherol per ml.

We have had the opportunity of measuring the plasma and adipose tissue level (needle aspiration technique) of a normotriglyceridemic ABL patient (absent B 100 component)—described by Malloy et al.—in whom normal chylomicron formation apparently occurs.[6] In this patient receiving supplemental vitamin E at a level of 400 mg/day, the plasma level was 5.85 μg tocopherol per ml plasma. The adipose tissue level was 560 ng tocopherol per mg triglyceride, documenting normal absorption of dietary vitamin E.

These findings demonstrate the usefulness of measurement of adipose tissue concentration of tocopherol in patients with low levels of circulating plasma tocopherol. We have further substantiated the value of this technique in patients with intrahepatic cholestasis, with neurologic abnormalities ascribed to tocopherol deficiency, where the adipose tissue levels were virtually absent. The measurement of tissue levels of tocopherol is therefore of importance in evaluating the metabolism of tocopherol in many pathologic conditions.

REFERENCES

1. HATAM, L. & H. J. KAYDEN. 1979. J. Lipid Res. **20:** 639–645.
2. KAYDEN, H. J., C. K. CHOW & L. BJORNSON. 1973. J. Lipid Res. **14:** 533–540.
3. KAYDEN, H. J. 1972. Annu. Rev. Med. **22:** 285–296.
4. HIRSCH, J., J. FARQUHAR, E. AHRENS, JR., M. PETERSON & W. STOFFEL. 1960. Am. J. Clin. Nutr. **8:** 499–511.
5. STERN, I. & B. SHAPIRO. 1953. J. Clin. Pathol. **6:** 158–160.
6. MALLOY, M. J., J. P. KANE, D. A. HARDMAN, R. L. HAMILTON & K. B. DALAL. 1981. J. Clin. Invest. **67:** 1441–1450.

SELENIUM AND KESHAN DISEASE

Xiao Shu Chen

Keshan Disease Research Group
Institute of Health
Chinese Academy of Medical Sciences
Beijing, The People's Republic of China

Keshan disease is an endemic cardiomyopathy prevailing throughout a wide belt from the northeast to the southwest of China.[1,2] The most susceptible populations are children and women of child-bearing age. The disease has a high rate of fatality. Clinically, it can be divided into four types, i.e., acute, subacute, chronic, and latent.[3] The primary pathological change is multifocal necrosis of the myocardium.

Two facts indicate that selenium deficiency plays an important role in the occurrence of this disease. First, populations in all the endemic areas are in very poor selenium status as compared to those in the nonendemic areas. The Se levels in staple cereals, blood, and hair of populations in the endemic areas are much lower than those in the nonendemic areas. The average blood glutathione peroxidase activities of people in endemic areas are slightly but significantly ($p < 0.05$) lower than those in nonendemic areas. Second, selenium supplementation protects people against this disease. A prophylactic trial was conducted in 12,000 children 1-9 years old in 1974-75. Half of the children were given sodium selenite tablets once a week (ages 1-4 years, 0.5 mg; ages 6-9, 1.0 mg) and the other half were given a placebo. The incidence rate and number of fatal cases were far less in the Se-supplemented group than in the control group. Recently, similar trials with 500,000 subjects were carried out in other provinces, and the results were consistent with previous results.

The etiology of Keshan disease is not clear yet. There are still some epidemiological characteristics that cannot be explained solely by the Se-deficiency hypothesis. Results from epidemiological surveys suggest that viral infection might be another factor. Therefore, the combined effect of Se deficiency and viral infection was studied in mice and their offspring.[4] Weanling mice were divided into a control group (stock diet), two low-Se groups (including grains produced in a Keshan disease area and a semisynthetic diet), and a group supplemented with sodium selenite. Animals in similar groups were mated after six weeks of feeding. The offspring on their seventh day of life were injected intraperitoneally with 0.07 ml of either a virus culture or a virus-free tissue culture. The suckling mice and the adults were sacrificed on the seventh day after injection. Blood selenium content was determined, and pathological examination of viscera was performed. The virus used in these experiments was isolated from the blood of a child who suffered from subacute Keshan disease in 1974. This strain was identified serologically as Coxsackie virus B_4. The results indicated that the offspring of all Se-deficient groups, no matter whether they consumed a natural or a semisynthetic low-Se diet, were much more sensitive to the virus injury. Both the frequency and severity of the heart lesions in the Se-deficient animals were significantly higher than those of the Se-adequate group. Se supplementation depressed virus-induced myocardial necrosis in Se-deficient suckling mice.

REFERENCES

1. Keshan Disease Research Group of the Chinese Academy of Medical Sciences. 1979. Observations on effect of sodium selenite in prevention of Keshan disease. Chin. Med. J. **92**(7): 471–476.
2. Keshan Disease Research Group of the Chinese Academy of Medical Sciences. 1979. Epidemiologic studies on the etiologic relationship of selenium and Keshan disease. Chin. Med. J. **92**(7): 477–482.
3. CHEN, X. S., G. Q. YANG, J. S. CHEN, X. C. CHEN, Z. M. WEN & K. Y. GE. 1980. Studies on the relations of selenium and Keshan disease. Biol. Trace Element Res. **2**: 91–107.
4. BAI, J., S. Q. WU, K. Y. GE, X. J. DENG & C. Q. SU. 1980. The combined effect of selenium deficiency and viral infection on the myocardium of mice. (abst.). Acta Acad. Med. Sinicae **2**(1): 31.

VITAMIN E AND NEUROBLASTOMA

L. Helson, M. Verma, and C. Helson

Pediatric Cancer Research Laboratory
Memorial Sloan-Kettering Cancer Center
New York, New York 10021

The relation of vitamin E to cancer has been relegated to its antioxidant properties. This translates into its potential for preventing toxic effects of free radicals or conversion of precarcinogens to carcinogens in the digestive tract. To date there are no definitive published studies demonstrating a direct effect on human cancer. Recently, K. Prasad observed that mouse neuroblastoma and melanoma cells were sensitive to vitamin E.[1] Based upon this, we tested three vitamin preparations for antitumor effects on human neuroblastoma cells *in vitro* using a microtiter assay technique. In other studies measuring uptake of ³H-thymidine and ³H-uridine, the tumor cells were grown to subconfluence and refed with fresh media containing the vitamin. After 24 hours and 1 hour exposure to radiolabeled thymidine or uridine, the cells were harvested and the amount of radioactivity incorporated into DNA or RNA was determined. The vitamin preparations included (1) Aquasol E (*RRR*-α-tocopheryl acetate), which is solubilized in a Tween 80 vehicle; (2) Ephynal® (*all-rac*-α-tocopherol), which is in a vehicle containing a mixture of alcohols, and Emulphor EL-620; and (3) *RRR*-α-tocopheryl acid succinate, which is soluble in ethyl alcohol. When each complete preparation, i.e., the vitamin and its vehicle, was added to culture medium with final α-tocopheryl or α-tocopherol concentrations of (1) 380 μg/ml, (2) 550 μg/ml, and (3) 50 μg/ml respectively and the cells exposed continuously for 48 hours or more, all three preparations had significant antitumor activity. Cells either lysed or slowed their proliferative activity. Control studies showed that the effect of the vehicle alone of preparation 1 or 2 was indistinguishable from preparations containing the vitamin. In contrast, a 1.0% concentration of ethyl alcohol used to solubilize *RRR*-α-tocopheryl acid succinate had no antitumor effect. We concluded that antitumor activity can be ascribed to *RRR*-α-tocopheryl acid succinate. In contrast with murine tumors, no morphological effects were noted after exposure to preparations 1, 2, or 3.

Uptake of ³H-thymidine into tumor cell DNA of SK-N-DZ was 95% inhibited by exposure to preparation 1 at 500 μg/ml, 75% by exposure to preparation 2 at 500 μg/ml, and 50% by exposure to preparation 3 at 45 μg/ml. ³H-Uridine incorporation into RNA was not affected. Three neuroblastoma patients taking up to 1,600 IU/day of Aquasol E orally as a dietary supplement had serum levels 10–55 μg/ml above normal without clinical antitumoral effects. These data suggest that the form of vitamin E and the route of administration may be important factors in clinical studies undertaken to demonstrate the potential antitumor effects of vitamin E preparations.

REFERENCES

1. PRASAD, K. N. & J. EDWARDS-PRASAD. 1982. Effects of tocopherol acid succinate on morphological alterations and growth inhibition in melanoma cells in culture. Cancer Res. **42:** 550–555.

ETHANE EXHALATION BY VITAMIN E-DEFICIENT RATS

Glen Lawrence and Gerald Cohen

Department of Neurology
Mount Sinai School of Medicine
New York, New York 10029

L. J. Machlin

Vitamins and Clinical Nutrition
Hoffmann-La Roche, Inc.
Nutley, New Jersey 07110

Short-chain hydrocarbon products, such as ethane and n-pentane, are exhaled when lipid peroxidation occurs *in vivo*.[1-3] These volatile hydrocarbons are derived from the breakdown of unsaturated lipids (e.g., linoleate, linolenate, arachidonate) during the free radical-mediated lipid peroxidative process.

The fate of ethane in the body is uncertain. Most researchers agree that it is relatively stable. Longer-chain hydrocarbons appear to undergo metabolic transformation mediated by the cytochrome P_{450} system of the liver.[4,5]

A limitation in current technology for processing breath lies in the quantity of gas that can be injected directly into a gas chromatograph. Some investigators have utilized binding to suitable columns in order to concentrate the hydrocarbons from breath. Ethane presents special problems due to its very low boiling point and its relative unreactivity. We have devised technology employing mainly charcoal at ambient temperature to strip and concentrate ethane from relatively large volumes (e.g., 1 liter) of gas.[6] The concentrated ethane is then injected directly into the gas chromatograph with a flash heater. With this methodology, we looked anew at the exhalation of ethane and pentane by vitamin E-deficient rats. Results are shown in TABLE 1.

The table shows that ethane, but not pentane, was significantly elevated in the chamber air from the vitamin E-deficient rats. Under the experimental conditions, exogenous pentane present in the chamber air was taken up by the rats. Levels of ethane were not significantly different for rats on a standard lab chow diet and rats receiving intraperitoneal tocopherol while on the vitamin E-deficient diet.

Other investigators have studied the exhalation of ethane and pentane by vitamin E-deficient rats: Hafeman and Hoekstra reported increased exhalation of ethane;[2] pentane was not studied. These investigators used a closed rebreathing chamber. Dillard, Dumelin, and Tappel observed increased exhalation of pentane, but not ethane.[3] They used a trapping method in which the air passing by the isolated head of the animal was collected.

Space limitations prevent a full discussion of reasons why results should vary in studies of this type. However, our own experiences and the published literature[1-8] indicate that observed differences between ethane and pentane can depend upon a number of factors:

1. The extremely volatile and nonreactive character of ethane requires special precautions to achieve effective trapping of this hydrocarbon from breath, even when cryogenic techniques are used.
2. The availability of unsaturated fatty acid precursors in the diet may play a

TABLE 1

EXHALATION OF ETHANE AND PENTANE BY MALE SPRAGUE-DAWLEY RATS*

Condition	Ethane†	Pentane†
E-deficient diet (n = 5)	6.80 ± 1.34	0.39 ± 1.16
E-deficient diet with tocopherol injection (n = 5)	1.13 ± 0.17	(−) 1.07 ± 0.38‡
Lab chow diet (n = 7)	1.42 ± 0.25	

*Animals were on the vitamin E-deficient diet [Hoffmann-La Roche diet no. 826: 4% Menhaden oil, 4% stripped lard (stabilized with 0.02% tert-butyl hydroquinone)] for 9 weeks prior to the study. Vitamin E (all-rac-α-tocopherol) was not administered with the diet but, rather, by means of an intraperitoneal injection (50 mg/kg) five times weekly. Animals were starved for 24–30 hours prior to study, except those on a standard lab chow diet, which were fed ad libitum. A rebreathing chamber[2] was used with an oxygen inlet and a carbon dioxide trap. Fifty milliliters of chamber air were assayed at zero time and at 60 minutes.

†nmol/kg body weight per hour, mean ± standard error of the mean.

‡Negative values reflect loss of pentane already present in the chamber air (commercial air, zero grade, Linde, South Plainfield, N.J.).

role. Diets rich in linoleate provide the precursor for pentane, while diets rich in linolenate provide the precursor for ethane.

3. The collection system for breath plays an important role. Rebreathing systems subject exhaled pentane to continuous metabolism.

4. Precautions must be taken to eliminate contributions from either rancification or bacterial action on foodstuffs in the gut. Starvation prior to assay plays a helpful role here.

Our overall assessment is that measurement of hydrocarbons can provide a valuable guide to lipid peroxidation in vivo. In toxicological studies (e.g., the hepatotoxicity of chlorinated hydrocarbons), elevations above baseline levels can be safely followed as a component of cellular toxicity mechanisms. In dietary studies, such as evaluation of endogenous processes in vitamin E deficiency, special considerations are required to avoid contributions from dietary sources.

REFERENCES

1. RIELY, C. A., G. COHEN & M. LIEBERMAN. 1974. Ethane evolution: a new index of lipid peroxidation. Science 183: 208.
2. HAFEMAN, D. G. & W. G. HOEKSTRA. 1977. Lipid peroxidation in vivo during vitamin E and selenium deficiency in the rat as monitored by ethane evolution. J. Nutr. 107: 666.
3. DILLARD, C., E. E. DUMELIN & A. L. TAPPEL. 1977. Effect of dietary vitamin E on expiration of pentane and ethane by the rat. Lipids 12: 109.
4. FRANK, H., T. HINTZE, D. BIMBOES & H. REMMER. 1980. Monitoring lipid peroxidation by breath analysis: endogenous hydrocarbons and their metabolic elimination. Toxicol. Appl. Pharmacol. 56: 337.
5. FROMMER, U., V. ULLRICH & H. STAUDINGER. 1970. Hydroxylation of aliphatic compounds by liver microsomes. I. The distribution pattern of isomeric alcohols. Hoppe-Seyler's Z. Physiol. Chem. 351: 903.
6. LAWRENCE, G. & G. COHEN. Ethane exhalation as an index of in vivo lipid peroxidation: concentrating ethane from a breath collection chamber. Anal. Biochem. (In press.)
7. GELMONT, D., R. A. STEIN & J. F. MEAD. 1981. The bacterial origin of rat breath pentane. Biochem. Biophys. Res. Commun. 102: 932.

PART III. VITAMIN E AND THE FUNCTION OF BLOOD CELLS

INTRODUCTION:
VITAMIN E AND BLOOD CELL FUNCTION*

Stephen B. Shohet and Sushil K. Jain

Cancer Research Institute
University of California
San Francisco, California 94143

First, I would like to thank the organizers, Dr. Lubin, Dr. Macklin, and Dr. Brin, for making this meeting possible. For some years, a large number of separate groups have been working on vitamin E from many different points of view. I cannot recall an opportunity where so many of us have been able to get together to exchange our findings and our views at one time. Already, from the previous sessions, it is clear that the organizers' efforts have been very well spent, and I would like to thank them in advance for the further benefits that I am sure will come to us all in the next couple of days.

This session will concentrate primarily on the role of vitamin E in the function of blood cells. Perhaps imitating the function of a well-balanced bone marrow, the organizers have prepared a program that will include comments on the role of vitamin E in white cells, red cells, and platelets. Reflecting the broad influence of this omnipresent vitamin's biologic processes, these comments will cover subjects as disparate as Dr. Baehner's remarks concerning the ability of the vitamin to modulate the bacterial killing capacity of granulocytes and Dr. Stuart's and Steiner's comments on the possibly fundamental role of the vitamin in the platelet's contribution to coagulation systems. Of course, my old friend the red cell will not be left out of this action either, and Dr. Shapiro and Dr. Sayare will consider the influence of the vitamin on the all-important membrane (and even perhaps that ancillary protein that is occasionally associated with the membrane—hemoglobin.)

Finally, to provide a very brief background for some of these hematologic effects, I am going to present a novel biochemical finding in the red cell membrane that strongly suggests the presence of in vivo membrane lipid peroxidation in at least one hemolytic disorder with reduced vitamin E levels. I hope that these brief comments will serve as a further introduction to the several studies that expand on the hemolytic consequences of vitamin E deficiency.

The first figure, FIGURE 1, indicates that very little is known about what happens to the membrane after the series of complex reactions that occur in the center. Although the generation of Heinz bodies, as indicated on the left arrow, is important, it cannot be the whole story since hemolytic conditions due to membrane defects following peroxidation certainly occur when Heinz bodies are not present. Hence, some direct effects on the membrane, simply indicated here without any comments on mechanism, seem to be likely.

FIGURE 2 shows one biochemical consequence of membrane peroxidation, which Dr. Jain has recently been able to demonstrate in our laboratory and which may be at least a part of the mechanism of the direct effects on the membrane I

*This is publication no. 28 of the MacMillan Cargill Hematology Laboratory of the University of California in San Francisco. It is supported in part by grants from the National Institutes of Health (AM16095) and the Hoffmann–La Roche Company.

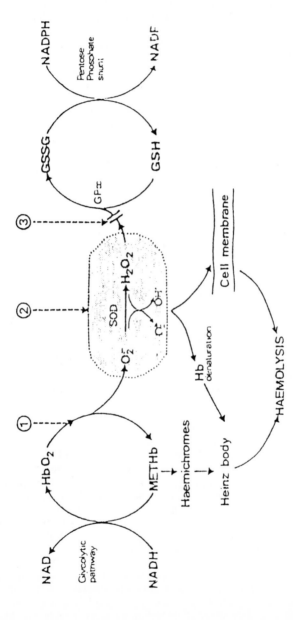

FIGURE 1. Schematic representation of reactions involved in the detoxification and effect of intracellular hydrogen peroxide in red blood cells. (Taken from Reference 7.)

have just mentioned. In this schema, hemoglobin, in this case sickle hemoglobin, is autoxidized to produce various oxidation products that affect membrane fatty acids and, among many other things, produce malonyldialdehyde (MDA), a final product of membrane lipid peroxidation. I would like to summarize a large number of *in vitro* chemical studies now to tell you that Dr. Jain has shown that malonyldialdehyde is capable of a further reaction with the amino groups of positively charged membrane phospholipids to form a Schiff base adduct, which, in effect, cross-links those phospholipids within the membrane. In this case, the heterologous adduct linking phosphatidylserine and phosphatidylethanolamine is demonstrated. Probably the homologous adducts also occur, but because of their similarities in migration in comparison to the parent compounds in most thin-layer systems, they are technically difficult to demonstrate. Without taking time to give you Dr. Jain's evidence for the presence of this adduct,[1] I will only say now that it can be generated with small amounts of malonyldialdehyde, which

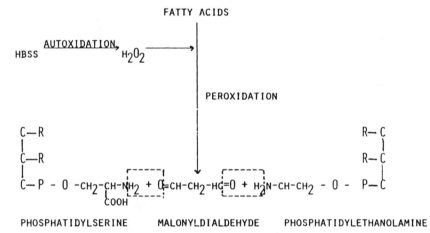

FIGURE 2. Schema showing Schiff's base adduct formation between phosphatidylserine, phosphatidylethanolamine, and malonyldialdehyde.

seem similar to those calculated to be present in the red cell under physiologic conditions.[2] Moreover, since vitamin E has such a preeminent role in moderating peroxidation reactions in biologic systems, one would expect that more of this adduct would be found in conditions with reduced red cell vitamin E. At least with regard to sickle-cell anemia and iron-deficiency anemia, we have found this to be the case.

FIGURE 3 shows the thin-layer analyses of normal red cell membrane lipids obtained from cells treated with malonyldialdehyde *in vitro*. As you can see, with increasing concentrations of malonyldialdehyde, a new spot intermediary between phosphatidylserine and phosphatidylethanolamine is found in this analysis. Moreover, when these lipids were quantitated, it was shown that the phosphatidylserine and phosphatidylethanolamine were nearly stoichiometrically reduced as the new compound was generated. Experiments with pure phosphatidylethanolamine and phosphatidylserine, as well as the hydrolysis of

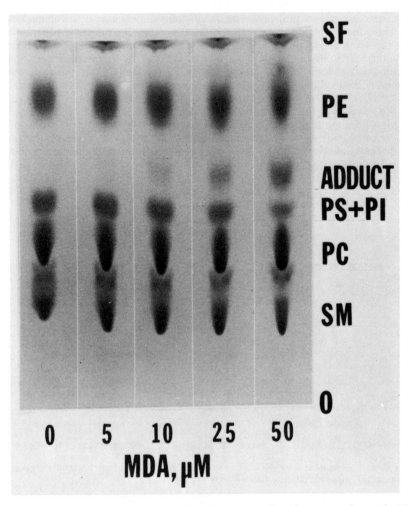

FIGURE 3. Thin-layer chromatogram of lipids from normal erythrocytes and treated with malonyldialdehyde (MDA) for 24 hours.

the novel phospholipid, which shows only phosphatidylethanolamine and phosphatidylserine, confirm that this is indeed the expected Schiff base product. It should be noted that small amounts of the adduct are visible at starting levels of MDA of only 5 μM and that it is clearly apparent at 10 μM starting levels. In the literature it appears that such levels might well be anticipated to be present in red cells, especially those with vitamin E deficiency or unstable hemoglobins.[3]

FIGURE 4 shows that in sickle-cell disease, we found the same adduct in untreated red cells *in vivo*. To be sure, we were only able to demonstrate this in the most dense fractions of irreversibly sickled cell–enriched red cells in sickle-cell patients. However, this does suggest that cross-linked lipid may have some role in the physiologic abnormalities of those highly abnormal cells.

To study this possibility, we then conducted some experiments with malonyl-dialdehyde to see if it had a direct role on cell membrane properties. Briefly, we found that two very important functions of the membrane, the maintenance of cation gradients and the maintenance of normal red cell deformability, could be significantly influenced by modest levels of malonyldialdehyde, which were in the same range as those that generate significant amounts of this novel peroxidation product *in vitro*.

FIGURE 5 very briefly shows that the potassium leak in both normal and discoid sickle cells was appreciably augmented by prior exposure of these cells to malonyldialdehyde—in this case for only one hour.

FIGURE 6 shows that cell deformability as measured in the laser diffraction

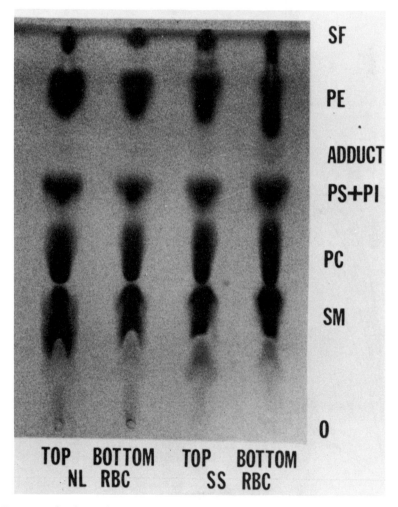

FIGURE 4. Thin-layer chromatogram of lipids of top and bottom fractions of erythrocytes from normal and sickle-cell patients. NL, normal; SS, sickle cell.

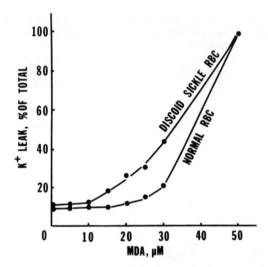

FIGURE 5. K$^+$ leak in normal and sickle cells treated with malonyldialdehyde (MDA) for two hours.

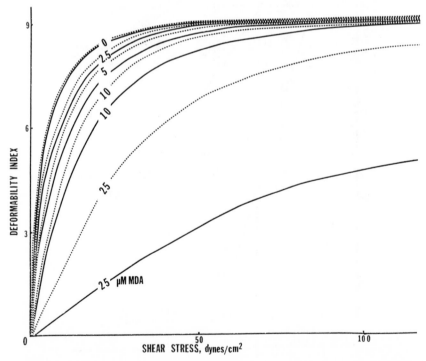

FIGURE 6. The effect of one hour malonyldialdehyde treatment on deformability of normal erythrocytes at various shear stresses. Solid line is MDA in saline buffer. Dashed line is MDA in high K$^+$ buffer.

ellipsometric viscometer, developed by my colleague Dr. Mohandas,[4] was markedly reduced after similar exposures to malonyldialdehyde. These data, which
will be presented in more detail elsewhere,[5] are somewhat complex in that they
reflect an overall membrane effect that may represent both a direct change in the
shear modulus of the membrane itself, and an indirect effect of potassium loss
producing an increase in the mean cell hemoglobin concentration and a global
reduction in cell deformability. Both of these effects are present here, and both
occur at comparatively low, although differing, concentrations of malonyldialdehyde exposure. I should immediately emphasize that we have not shown that the

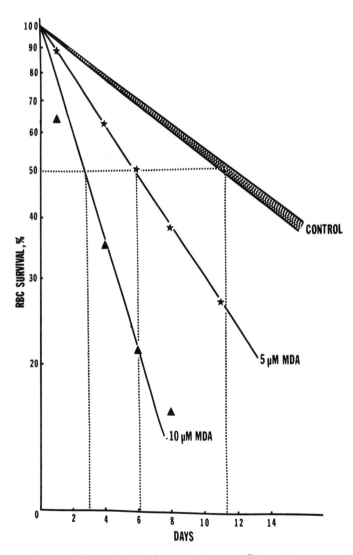

FIGURE 7. The survival rate of malonyldialdehyde-treated ^{51}Cr-erythrocytes in rabbits.

phospholipid adduct itself is directly responsible for these effects. Certainly, secondary effects on membrane proteins are also likely, and in fact we find some membrane protein aggregation under similar conditions.[6] However, we are willing to hypothesize that some of these physical and chemical changes in membrane properties may be due, at least in part, to reactions in the lipid phase.

Finally, FIGURE 7 shows some *in vivo* consequences of these events, which up to now I have described only *in vitro*. As you can see, in this chromium survival study performed with rabbit red cells treated with malonyldialdehyde for only one hour, there was a profound effect of the MDA exposure on red cell survival. The conditions of treatment are known to generate the novel phospholipid that Dr. Jain has described and, again, might well be present in certain red cells that have low vitamin E levels, unstable hemoglobin, or, as is often the case, a combination of both of these factors.

REFERENCES

1. JAIN, S. K. & S. B. SHOHET. 1981. A novel phospholipid in irreversibly sickled erythrocytes: evidence for a possible role of *in vivo* peroxidation for membrane damage. Clin. Res. **29:** 519.
2. JAIN, S. K., N. MOHANDAS, R. M. HOESCH, A. K. PRAMANIK & S. B. SHOHET. 1982. The effect of malonyldialdehyde, a product of lipid peroxidation, on red blood cell deformability, cellular dehydration, ^{51}Cr survival, and formation of irreversibly sickled cells. Clin. Res. **30:** 540A.
3. DODGE, J. T., G. COHEN, H. J. KAYDEN & G. B. PHILLIPS. 1967. Peroxidative hemolysis of red blood cells from patients with abetalipoproteinemia (acanthocytosis). J. Clin. Invest. **46:** 357.
4. MOHANDAS, N., M. R. CLARK, M. S. JACOBS & S. B. SHOHET. 1980. Analysis of factors regulating red cell deformability. J. Clin. Invest. **66:** 563.
5. JAIN, S. K., N. MOHANDAS, R. HOESCH & S. B. SHOHET. The effect of malonyldialdehyde, a product of lipid peroxidation, on deformability, dehydration and ^{51}Cr-survival of erythrocytes. (In press.)
6. JAIN, S. K. & P. HOCHSTEIN. 1980. Polymerization of membrane components in aging red blood cells. Biochem. Biophys. Res. Commun. **92:** 247.
7. CARRELL, R. W., C. C. WINTERBOURN & E. A. RACHMILEWITZ. 1975. Activated oxygen and haemolysis. Br. J. Haematol. **30:** 259.

THE INFLUENCE OF VITAMIN E ON HUMAN POLYMORPHONUCLEAR CELL METABOLISM AND FUNCTION*

Robert L. Baehner, Laurence A. Boxer, Leah M. Ingraham,†
Charles Butterick,‡ and Richard A. Haak§

Department of Pediatrics
Indiana University School of Medicine
Indianapolis, Indiana 46223

INTRODUCTION

Polymorphonuclear leukocytes (PMNs) and monocytes comprise the blood phagocytes. These cells in contrast to the other cellular elements of the blood are capable of leaving the circulation and migrating to extravascular sites of infection and inflammation where they recognize and ingest microbes and other particulate material. Similar to platelets and lymphocytes but distinct from red cells, PMNs and monocytes are capable of achieving a heightened state of functional and metabolic activation in response by their plasma membranes to immunochemical and particulate signals. Metabolic activation of the PMN includes activation of one or more cyanide-insensitive oxidases and related enzyme systems, which oxidize substrate NADH and NADPH,¶ leading to increased oxygen utilization and the subsequent reduction of oxygen to superoxide anion, hydrogen peroxide, hydroxyl radical, and other free radicals.[1] It is well known that these reduced oxygen by-products and free radicals, especially hydrogen peroxide, are utilized for intracellular microbicidal reactions linked to the myeloperoxidase halide system present in PMNs and monocytes.[2]

We have previously reported on the effects of vitamin E deficiency on PMN and monocyte function in the rat model.[3] In this report we discuss our studies on the effect of antioxidants on several phagocytic, oxidative, and membrane-related responses of the human PMN. The daily administration of large amounts of vitamin E resulted in alterations of the ability of human PMNs to ingest and kill bacteria, to utilize oxygen and release the oxygen by-products superoxide anion and hydrogen peroxide, as well as to release arachidonic acid presumably through activation of membrane phospholipase A_2. Changes in membrane fluidity of normal and vitamin E cells at rest and during phagocytosis also occurred. The NADH and NADPH oxidase activities in normal and vitamin E cells could be localized to plasma membranes and phagocytic vesicles. Vitamin E provided a probe to differentiate the metabolic and biologic roles of each oxidase.

*This work was supported by Grant AI-10892, AM-719035 from the National Institutes of Health and a grant from the James Whitcomb Riley Memorial Association. This work was done during the tenure of Dr. Boxer as an Established Investigator of the American Heart Association.
†Department of Biochemistry.
‡Department of Anatomy.
§Department of Microbiology/Immunology.
¶NAD is nicotinamide-adenine dinucleotide.

237

Preparation of Polymorphonuclear Leukocytes

Heparinized venous blood was obtained from normal adult volunteers before and after two to three weeks of administration of 1,600 units of vitamin E in accordance with this institution's Human Investigation Committee. PMNs were separated by dextran sedimentation and Ficoll gradient[4] and freed of contaminating erythrocytes by hypotonic lysis. Final suspension of cells (95–99% PMN) was in phosphate-buffered saline (PBS) or Kreb's Ringer phosphate (KRP). In some instances, 5.5 mM glucose was added to the suspending medium (PBSG or KRPG). Zymosan opsonized with 10% v/v fresh human serum was used as the stimulant for all studies except where otherwise indicated.

Determination of Serum Vitamin E

Serum vitamin E was determined spectrophotometrically by the method of Quaife et al.[5] Briefly, 1 ml serum and 1 ml absolute alcohol were mixed, 1 ml xylene was added, and the mixture was shaken vigorously then centrifuged at $400 \times g$ at 4°C for 10 minutes and 0.7 ml of the upper phase was removed. This sample was mixed with 0.7 ml of a solution containing a,a'-dipyridyl (120 mg/100 ml) in n-propanol, and the optical density at 460 nm was determined. Then 0.2 ml ferric chloride hexahydrate (120 mg/100 ml) in absolute alcohol was added, and the optical density at 520 nm was determined after 1.5 minutes. Absorption readings were compared to standards of α-tocopherol, and corrections for β-carotene were made by use of a standard curve for this substance.

Metabolic Studies

Oxygen Utilization

The oxygen consumption by PMNs was measured by use of an oxygen electrode (Model 53, Yellow Springs Instrument Co., Yellow Springs, Ohio) with an expanded scale Varian recorder (Varian Associates, Palo Alto, Calif.). A suspension of 1×10^7 cells in KRPG was placed in the reaction vessel. After 5 minutes of incubation at 37°C, sodium azide (1 mM) and other agents to be tested were added to give a final volume of 3 ml. Baseline oxygen consumption was measured for 5 minutes, and then 100 μl stimulant was added. Oxygen consumption was recorded for an additional 5 to 12 minutes during the period when the decrease of P_{O_2} was linear. Results of replicate samples were averaged and expressed as nmoles O_2 used/5 minutes per 10^7 cells.

Superoxide Production

Superoxide ion was measured as the superoxide dismutase (SOD)-sensitive reduction of cytochrome C as described by Babior et al.[6] Each tube had a final volume of 0.9 ml:0.75 ml of KRPG containing 3×10^6 cells, 119 μM cytochrome C, and 1 mM sodium azide. In some instances, SOD (60 μg) and/or cytochalasin B (5 μg) was added. After 5 minutes equilibration at 37°C, the reaction was initiated by addition of 100 μl stimulant. At the end of the reaction time (1, 2, 5, or 10 minutes), the tube was placed in ice and 1.0 ml of ice-cold 1 mM N-ethylmaleimide (NEM) was added. The tubes were centrifuged (400 $\times$ g, for 5 minutes, 4°C) and the supernatant absorptions were read at 550 nm on a Gilford spectrophotometer (Model 250, Gilford Instruments Co., Oberlin, Ohio). The results of replicate samples were averaged and converted to nmoles reduced cytochrome C by use of the extinction coefficient of 19.1 $\times$ 10^3 M^{-1} cm^{-1}.

Hydrogen Peroxide Production

The extracellular release of H_2O_2 was quantified by the method of Root *et al.* by measuring the decrease in fluorescence intensity of scopoletin during oxidation by horseradish peroxidase.[7] PMNs, 2.5 $\times$ 10^6, were preincubated at 37°C for 5 minutes in KRPG and 1 mM sodium azide, then stimulated for 5 minutes with opsonized zymosan. The cells were pelleted by centrifugation (250 $\times$ g for 10 minutes). To 0.8 ml of the supernatant was added 0.4 ml KRPG, 0.4 ml of 50 μM scopoletin (Sigma) in PBS, and 0.4 ml of horseradish peroxidase (1 mg/ml). After 30 minutes incubation at room temperature, the decrease in percent fluorescence of the sample mixtures was measured in the Perkin Elmer Model MPF 44B spectrofluorimeter set at an excitation wavelength of 350 nm and an emission wavelength of 460 nm and presented with an H_2O_2 standard curve of 0–100% fluorescence (20–0 nmole H_2O_2). Calculations of the amount of H_2O_2 generated by each sample were determined by their decrease in a percent fluorescence as compared to the H_2O_2 standard curve prepared daily, based on an extinction coefficient of 81 M^{-1} cm^{-1} at an optical density (OD) of 230 nm.

Hexose Monophosphate Shunt Activity

PMNs were suspended in KRPG in 10-ml Erlenmeyer flasks equipped with center wells and vaccine ports. Incubations were carried out at 37°C for 45 minutes after addition of the stimulant. Total cell protein[8] per flask varied between 2.9 mg and 5.5 mg, which represented a cell population of between 2.8 $\times$ 10^7 and 6.0 $\times$ 10^7 in 1.0 ml. $^{14}CO_2$ evolved from the oxidation of glucose-1-^{14}C was trapped in wells containing 0.1 ml 5 N NaOH. The contents of the wells were transferred to vials containing 15 ml scintillation cocktail, and the radioactivity of suitable standards and sample was determined in a Packard Model 460D liquid scintillation counter. The specific activity of the substrates was determined so that radioactivity measurements could be converted to nmoles mg^{-1} protein $hour^{-1}$.[9]

Arachidonic Acid Release

PMNs were suspended in PBSGB [PBS with 100 mg% glucose and 1% fatty acid-free bovine serum albumin (BSA)] at a concentration of 1 $\times$ 10^7 cells/ml. ^{14}C-Sodium arachidonate (1–2 μCi/2 $\times$ 10^7 cells) was added. The cells were incubated in a shaking water bath at 37°C for 30 minutes. Ten volumes of PBSGB were added, and the cells were pelleted by centrifugation (150 $\times$ g, 7 minutes, 20°C). Cells were resuspended in PBSGB to give a cell density of 1 $\times$ 10^7 cells/ml, and additions of stock solutions of calcium chloride and magnesium sulfate were made to give a final concentration of 1.2 mM of each of the divalent cations. After

5 minutes incubation in a shaking water bath at 37°C, stimulating agent was added and the incubation continued for 5 additional minutes. Ice-cold citric acid (final concentration, 15 mM) was added to stop the reaction. The acidified suspension was extracted with chloroform and methanol by a modified Bligh and Dyer extraction.[10] The chloroform phase was dried under nitrogen and redissolved in 100 μl volume of chloroform:methanol (2:1, v/v). Forty-five-microliter samples of the extracts were spotted on silica gel G plates (Uniplate, Analtech, Newark, Del.) for analysis by thin-layer chromatography. The plates were developed in one of two solvents: (I) chloroform:methanol:glacial acetic acid:water (90:8:1:0.8, v/v); or (II) hexane:diethyl ether:glacial acetic acid (50:50:1, v/v). R_f values for phosphatidylcholine, prostaglandin E_2 (PGE$_2$), 5-hydroxyeicosatetraenoic acid (5-HETE), and arachidonic acid are respectively for solvent I, 0.02, 0.37, 0.53, and 0.76; and for II, 0.01, 0.03, 0.28, and 0.65. Location of standards was visualized in iodine vapor, and the lanes for each sample were scraped in 0.5-cm sections. The radioactivity associated with sections corresponding to arachidonic acid was determined in a Packard Model 460D liquid scintillation spectrometer (Packard Instruments, Downey Grove, Ill.). Results of replicate samples were averaged and expressed as disintegrations per minute (dpm)/10^7 cells.

Functional Studies

Ingestion

Rates of ingestion were quantitated by exposure of PMNs to lipopolysaccharide containing oil red O paraffin oil particles.[11] Briefly, 5×10^7 PMNs in 0.8 ml KRPG were incubated with 200 μl lipopolysaccharide-coated oil red O mineral oil droplets. After 5 minutes, 1.0 ml 1 mM NEM was added and the suspension was centrifuged (200 $\times$ g, 5 minutes, 4°C). The cell pellet was washed in NEM, and the cell-associated oil red O was extracted in dioxane. The optical density of the extract at 525 nm was determined.

Bactericidal Activity

Bacterial killing by PMNs was performed using the method of Quie et al.[12] Staphylococcus aureus 502A was used at a bacteria to PMN ratio of 1:1.

Electron Spin Resonance

The spin label 2-(3-carboxy-propyl)-4,4-dimethyl-2-tridecyl-3-oxazolidinyloxyl (5DS) was purchased from Syva (Palo Alto, Calif.). Stock solutions at 5 mM were made up in ethanol and stored at −20°C.

For spin labeling, tubes were prepared by addition of 8 μl 5DS stock solution; the solvent was evaporated under a stream of N_2 gas to provide a thin film of label in the bottom of each tube.[13] The PMN suspension, 1×10^{-8} ml, was transferred to a tube containing the 5DS. After 5 minutes at 20°C, PMNs were centrifuged (400 $\times$ g for 1 minute at 20°C) into the sealed tip of a Pasteur pipette and the electron spin resonance (ESR) spectrum of the pellet was recorded. Effects of spin labeling on viability of PMNs were determined by trypan blue exclusion. Cell suspensions labeled with 5DS were 95% viable.

ESR spectra were obtained on a standard balanced-bridge spectrometer with diode detection operating at 9.1 GHz. Phase-sensitive detection with 50 kHz magnetic field modulation frequency was used. Sample heating and broadening of spectral lines were avoided by recording all spectra at low microwave power (12 mW) incident on the Varian V4535 large access cavity (Varian Associates, Palo Alto, Calif.). A peak-to-peak modulation amplitude of 1.5 gauss (G) was used for 5DS-labeled PMNs. All instrument settings were identical for a particular set of samples being compared. First derivative absorption spectra were recorded with a 100-G field sweep, a scan time of 5 minutes, and a time constant of 0.2 second. The magnetic field sweep was calibrated with a nuclear magnetic resonance (NMR) gaussmeter (Varian Associates, Palo Alto, Calif.). Sample temperature was monitored with a thermocouple and was maintained to within $\pm 0.5\,°C$ of the desired temperature (usually 25 °C) through use of a chilled or heated N_2 gas-flow system.

Ultrastructural Localization of NADH and NADPH Oxidase

The localization of hydrogen peroxide generated by NADH or NADPH oxidase by phagocytosing PMNs was performed by a modification of the method of Briggs et al.[14] PMNs were suspended in autologous serum (1.5×10^7 PMNs/ml) and allowed to adhere to 35-mm petri dishes.

Opsonized zymosan particles at a ratio of 20 particles per cell were added to the adhering PMNs and incubated with the cells at 37 °C for 10 minutes. The supernatant was then discarded, and 0.1 M tris-maleate buffer pH 7.6 containing 7% sucrose (tris-mal-suc) and 1 mM 3-amino-1,2,4,triazole (AT) (Aldridge Chemical Co., Milwaukee, Wis.) was added for 10 minutes to inhibit granule myeloperoxidase. The supernatant was then decanted, and the final incubation medium consisting of 0.1 M tris-mal-suc, 10 mM AT, 1 mM $CeCl_3$, and 0.71 mM NADH or NADPH (Sigma Chemical Co., St. Louis, Mo.) was added for a period of 20 minutes at 37 °C. The final incubation medium was prepared within 10 minutes of use. After incubation, the PMNs were washed briefly in 0.1 M tris-maleate buffer in 7% sucrose, 25 °C. The cells were then removed from petri dishes by rubber policemen and suspended in the 0.1 M tris-mal-suc. The cells were fixed in 3% glutaraldehyde in 0.05 M sodium cacodyalate buffer pH 7.4 and then washed with 0.05 M cacodyalate buffer pH 7.4 with 7% sucrose at room temperature for 10 minutes. Cells were postfixed in 1% osmium tetroxide in 0.05 M tris-mal-suc for an additional 60 minutes at room temperature, en bloc stained in 0.5% aqueous uranyl acetate overnight at 4 °C, then dehydrated in a graded series of alcohol and embedded in Spurr resin and examined on a Philips 400 transmission electron microscope. The reaction product, cerium perhydroxide, was verified by use of the Edax x-ray microanalyzer. Counts of 200 seconds were made on unstained sections mounted on copper grids.

RESULTS AND DISCUSSION

Serum Vitamin E Levels

The total serum vitamin E levels of the 12 volunteers not receiving vitamin E varied from 0.93 to 1.22 mg/dl (mean = 1.12 ± 0.20), whereas levels for the 4

TABLE 1

Effect of Daily Administration of Vitamin E on Oxidative
Responses of Human PMNs*

Oxidative Response†	Control‡	Vitamin E‡	p Value
Oxygen utilization§	61 ± 4	66 ± 2	0.12
Superoxide production¶	5 ± 2	7 ± 2	0.29
Hydrogen peroxide release‖	3 ± 1	0.1 ± 0.3	0.015

*Vitamin E given at 1,600 U/day for at least two weeks.
†Procedures are detailed in Materials and Methods.
‡Nanomoles/minute per 10^7 PMNs. Values are the means and standard deviations of replicate samples.
§Based on 5-minute value.
¶Based on 25-minute value.
‖Based on 5-minute value.

volunteers receiving 1,600 units/day for two or more weeks varied from 1.77 to 1.85 mg/dl (mean = 1.80 ± 0.30, p < 0.01).

Metabolic Studies

TABLE 1 shows data for oxygen utilization, superoxide production, and H_2O_2 generation. There was a slight increase in oxygen use for PMNs from subjects receiving vitamin E and a similar small enhancement of superoxide production. In contrast, there was a significant inhibition in H_2O_2 release (p = 0.015). Thus the vitamin E PMN displays a brisk respiratory burst leading to the release of superoxide, but H_2O_2 release is markedly impaired.

To assess the availability of H_2O_2 inside of the cell, hexose monophosphate shunt (HMPS)—which depends upon generation of intracellular H_2O_2—was determined. The pyridine nucleotide $NADP^+$ is reduced in the first step of the glutathione pathway and is regenerated by reactions utilizing H_2O_2.

$$2\,GSH + H_2O_2 \rightarrow GSSG + 2\,H_2O \tag{1}$$

$$GSSG + NADPH_2 \rightarrow 2\,GSH + NADP^+ \tag{2}$$

Accordingly, we examined the PMNs from subjects taking vitamin E for

TABLE 2

Effect of Daily Administration of Vitamin E on Hexose
Monophosphate Shunt Activity of PMNs*

HMPS†	Control‡	Vitamin E‡	p Value
Resting	67 ± 19	38 ± 10	0.20
Phagocytosing§	299 ± 42	113 ± 8	0.025

*Vitamin E given at 1,600 U/day for at least two weeks.
†Procedures are detailed in Materials and Methods.
‡Micromoles $^{14}CO_2$/30 minutes per 10^6 PMNs. Values are means and standard errors of the means of five separate experiments with samples run in duplicate.
§Particles were opsonized zymosan.

evolution of $^{14}CO_2$ derived from the reaction:

$$^{14}\text{C-1-glucose-6-PO}_4 + \text{NADP}^+ \rightarrow {}^{14}\text{CO}_2 + \text{ribulose-5-PO}_4 + \text{NADPH}^+ \quad (3)$$

The results of these determinations are shown in TABLE 2. Compared to control PMNs, vitamin E cells had significantly decreased oxidation of glucose-1-^{14}C during phagocytosis of opsonized zymosan but not under resting conditions.

Membrane-associated enzymes might be especially vulnerable to oxidative attack, not only because of the possibility of direct damage, but also because of the potential disruption of their lipid milieu through lipid peroxidation. The data for superoxide production suggest that the membrane-associated NAD(P)H oxidase activated during phagocytic stimulation of PMNs is not especially vulnerable to oxidative attack, since cells from normal controls show nearly the same values as PMNs from subjects taking vitamin E (TABLE 1). We decided to examine another membrane-associated enzyme, phospholipase A_2, which is activated during phagocytic challenge and which preferentially releases arachidonic acid from membrane phospholipids. PMNs were labeled with ^{14}C-arachidonate and subsequently exposed to opsonized zymosan. The amount of ^{14}C-arachidonate, as determined by thin-layer chromatographic analysis of chloroform-methanol

TABLE 3

EFFECT OF DAILY ADMINISTRATION OF VITAMIN E ON RELEASE
OF ^{14}C-ARACHIDONIC ACID*

Condition†	Control‡	Vitamin E‡	p Value
Resting	271 ± 38	424 ± 25	0.02
+ 0.7 mg zymosan	950 ± 180	1462 ± 320	0.02
+ 1.4 mg zymosan	1943 ± 230	2370 ± 811	0.50

*Vitamin E given at 1,600 U/day for at least two weeks.
†Procedures are detailed in Materials and Methods.
‡Dpm/5 minutes per 10^7 PMNs. Values are means and standard deviations for replicate samples.

extracts, was slightly higher in vitamin E PMNs compared to normal cells; however, the difference was not significant (TABLE 3).

Functional Studies

We have compared normal and vitamin E PMNs for their abilities to ingest particles and to kill staphylococci. Rate of ingestion of oil red O paraffin oil droplets coated with lipopolysaccharide of *Escherichia coli* and opsonized with fresh serum was enhanced in vitamin E cells (TABLE 4). On the other hand, despite greater ability to phagocytose, vitamin E PMNs show a mildly reduced ability to kill bacteria (TABLE 4). The extent of this acquired abnormality was far less than that observed for PMNs of patients with defects of oxidase and peroxidase activities. These results suggest that the decreased release of H_2O_2 (TABLE 1) by vitamin E PMNs may result in less oxidative damage to their membranes so that they are more efficient in ingestion, but that the failure to produce this reactive species also serves to protect the ingested microorganisms from the peroxide-mediated attack[2] that results in their demise.

TABLE 4

EFFECT OF DAILY ADMINISTRATION OF VITAMIN E ON FUNCTIONAL ABILITIES OF PMNs*

Function†	Control‡	Vitamin E‡
Ingested oil red O§	0.060 ± 0.001	0.070 ± 0.002
Bacterial count (× 10⁷)¶	0.60 ± 0.10	1.30 ± 0.30

*Vitamin E given at 1,600 U/day for at least two weeks.
†Procedures are detailed in Materials and Methods.
‡Values are means and standard deviations for replicate samples.
§Values are expressed as mg paraffin oil/10^7 per minute.
¶Viable *Staphylococcus aureus* 502A after 100 minutes incubation with PMNs. Bacteria incubated alone for the same time period had a count of 2.3×10^8.

Electron Spin Resonance Spectrometry

To assess the possible effects of vitamin E on membrane fluidity changes that accompany phagocytosis,[15] PMNs were spin labeled with 5DS, an analogue of stearic acid. PMNs were then incubated with or without opsonized zymosan for 15 minutes, and the electron spin resonance spectrum determined. Order parameter (S) was calculated from spectral parameters.[13] TABLE 5 shows data from PMNs of normal subjects, volunteers receiving vitamin E, and children with chronic granulomatous disease (CGD), a condition in which no oxidative burst accompanies phagocytosis. PMNs at rest from the various subjects showed similar order parameters; however, upon exposure to opsonized zymosan, all but the cells from CGD patients showed a marked increase in order parameter (TABLE 5). Since S varies inversely to fluidity, the changes suggest that both normal and vitamin E PMNs have membrane changes during phagocytosis that lead to lessened fluidity (i.e., greater rigidity). One effect of membrane lipid peroxidation is increased rigidity.[16] We postulated that reduced oxygen by-products evolved during the phagocytosis-induced respiratory burst might cause oxidative attack upon the membrane lipids, and that the failure of the CGD PMNs to show changes in S might be a reflection of their lack of oxidative activity. In support of this hypothesis is the finding that inclusion of catalase (1,600 units/ml), an enzyme that scavenges H_2O_2, in the incubation medium diminished the order parameter increase in normal PMNs phagocytosing opsonized zymosan (zymosan, 0.657 ± 0.004; zymosan + catalase, 0.649 ± 0.006, p = 0.04). Addition of superoxide dismutase (100 μg/ml) and sodium benzoate (1 mM), scavengers respectively of superoxide ion and hydroxyl radical, does not further diminish the change in S (data not shown). These results suggest that H_2O_2 may be responsible for alterations of order parameter in phagocytosing PMNs. The vitamin E PMNs, however, despite their lessened production of H_2O_2 (TABLE 1) still show the same

TABLE 5

ORDER PARAMETERS OF 5DS-LABELED HUMAN PMNs*

Condition	Control	Vitamin E	CGD
Resting	0.64 ± 0.003†	0.639 ± 0.002	0.638 ± 0.002
+ zymosan	0.656 ± 0.004	0.654 ± 0.003	0.643 ± 0.002

*S was calculated from electron spin resonance spectral parameters.
†Mean and standard error of the mean for replicate determinations.

FIGURE 1. X-ray microanalysis of reaction product generated in phagocytic vesicles of PMNs incubated with opsonized zymosan, CeCl₃, NAD(P)H. Panel A indicates the characteristic L-alpha and L-Beta peaks of Ce at 4.84 and 5.26 keV respectively, whereas panel B indicates a spectrum of a vesicle without Ce. Scale factor is 1135 and 1075 respectively.

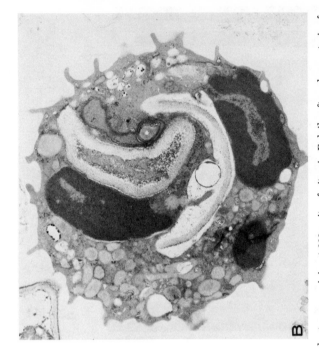

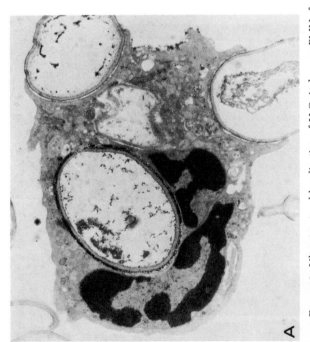

FIGURE 2. Ultrastructural localization of H_2O_2 in human PMNs from volunteers receiving 1,600 units of vitamin E daily after phagocytosis of opsonized zymosan. Panel A indicates results obtained with 0.71 mM NADH. Note the presence of reaction product in the phagocytic vesicles and on the plasma membrane. Panel B indicates results obtained with 0.71 mM NADPH. There is marked attenuation of the reaction product. Magnification ×8000.

increase in S, suggesting that vitamin E is unable to prevent the changes that 5DS detects. Since 5DS has its nitroxide reporter group at the fifth carbon, it probes relatively near the surface of the phospholipid bilayer. Vitamin E inclusion in the membrane may be at locations different from this region, or alternatively, the vitamin may scavenge H_2O_2 at a location not probed by the spin label.

Localization of NADH and NADPH Oxidase in Normal and Vitamin E PMNs

The site of H_2O_2 produced by NADH and NADPH oxidase was determined in PMNs obtained from the blood of normals and volunteers receiving 1,600 units of vitamin E daily. For these studies, PMNs were incubated in the presence of either NADH or NADPH and cerious chloride and allowed to generate H_2O_2 by phagocytosing opsonized zymosan particles. The H_2O_2 formed from NADH and/or NADPH reacts with the cerium to form an electron-dense reaction

TABLE 6

EFFECT OF 1,600 UNITS VITAMIN E PER DAY ON HUMAN PMN RESPONSES

	Response
Phagocytic Functions	
Ingestion	↑
Bacterial killing	↓
Metabolic Functions	
O_2 utilization	↑
O_2^- release	↑
H_2O_2 release	↓
HMPS stimulation	↓
Membrane Functions	
Order parameter	normal
Phospholipase A_2	normal to ↑
NADH oxidase	no effect
NADPH oxidase	↓

product, cerium perhydroxide, detected either visually or by x-ray microanalysis (FIGURE 1).

$$NAD(P)H + O_2 + H^+ \text{ oxidase} \rightarrow NAD(P) + H_2O_2 \qquad (4)$$

$$2 H_2O_2 + CeCl_3 \rightarrow Ce(OH)_2OOH + H^+ \qquad (5)$$

Reaction product was identified on the plasma membrane as well as within phagocytic vesicle membranes surrounding ingested zymosan when either NADH or NADPH was employed as the substrate with normal PMNs. When PMNs obtained from volunteers receiving vitamin E were incubated with NADH, a similar reaction was noted. However, when vitamin E PMNs were incubated with NADPH, no reaction product developed either within the phagocytic vesicles or on the plasma membrane, suggesting that the two oxidases are geographically separate within the cell and that vitamin E is capable of scavenging H_2O_2 generated by NADPH oxidase (FIGURE 2).

SUMMARY

These studies on the effect of administration of 1,600 units of vitamin E to humans indicated the following responses to the PMNs (TABLE 6). Functional alterations occur with an increased ability to ingest particles but a mild decrease in bactericidal potency of the PMN. Although the respiratory burst is slightly enhanced as is superoxide anion release, H_2O_2 release from the PMN is markedly impaired. The hexose monophosphate shunt activity, which is dependent on intracellular H_2O_2, is decreased during phagocytosis. Membrane responses such as changes in order parameter during phagocytosis as reported by the stearic acid analogue probe 5DS are similar to those of normal PMNs. The release of arachidonic acid from membranes of vitamin E PMNs during phagocytosis of opsonized zymosan is slightly enhanced, indicating normal phospholipase A_2 activation. NADH oxidase-derived H_2O_2 is not impaired within phagocytic vesicles of vitamin E PMNs. However, vitamin E selectively depletes H_2O_2 generated by NADPH oxidase in phagocytic vesicles, accounting for impairment in HMPS activity and bactericidal activity in these cells.

REFERENCES

1. BAEHNER, R. L., L. A. BOXER & L. M. INGRAHAM. 1982. Reduced oxygen byproducts and white blood cells. In Free Radicals in Biology. W. A. Pryor, Ed.: 91–113. Academic Press, Inc. New York, N.Y.

2. KLEBANOFF, S. J. & R. H. CLARK. 1978. Myeloperoxidase-H_2O_2-halide system antimicrobial activity. In The Neutrophil Function and Clinical Disorders: 410–434. Elsevier/North-Holland Biomedical Press. Amsterdam, the Netherlands.

3. HARRIS, R. E., L. A. BOXER & R. L. BAEHNER. 1980. Consequences of vitamin E deficiency on the phagocytic and oxidative function of the rat polymorphonuclear leukocyte. Blood 55: 338–343.

4. BOYUM, A. 1968. Introduction. Separation of leukocytes from blood and bone marrow. Scand. J. Clin. Lab. Invest. Suppl. 21: 7.

5. QUAIFE, M. L., N. S. SCRIMSHAW & O. H. LOWRY. 1949. A micromethod for assay of total tocopherols in blood serum. J. Biol. Chem. 180: 1229–1235.

6. BABIOR, B. M., R. S. KIPNES & J. T. CURNUTTE. 1973. Biological defense mechanisms. The production by leukocytes of superoxide, a potent bactericidal agent. J. Clin. Invest. 52: 741–944.

7. ROOT, R. K., J. METCALF, N. OSHINO & B. CHANCE. 1975. H_2O_2 release from human granulocytes during phagocytosis. J. Clin. Invest. 55: 945–955.

8. LOWRY, O. H., N. J. ROSENBROUGH, A. L. FARR & R. J. RANDALL. 1951. Protein measurement with the Folin phenol reagent. J. Biol. Chem. 193: 265–275.

9. BAEHNER, R. L., D. G. NATHAN & M. L. KARNOVSKY. 1970. Correction of metabolic deficiences in the leukocytes of patients with chronic granulomatous disease. J. Lab. Clin. Invest. 49: 865–870.

10. MARCUS, A. J., B. B. WEKSLER, E. A. JAFFE & M. J. BROEKMAN. 1980. Synthesis of prostacyclin from platelet-derived endoperoxides by cultured human epithelial cells. J. Clin. Invest. 66: 979–986.

11. STOSSEL, T. P. 1973. Evaluation of opsonic and leukocyte function with spectrophotometric test in patients with infection and with phagocytic disorders. Blood 42: 121–130.

12. QUIE, P. G., J. G. WHITE, B. HOLMES & R. A. GOOD. 1967. In vitro bactericidal capacity of human polymorphonuclear leukocytes: diminished activity in chronic granulomatous disease of childhood. J. Clin. Invest. 46: 688.

13. HAAK, R. A., L. M. INGRAHAM, R. L. BAEHNER & L. A. BOXER. 1979. Membrane fluidity in human and mouse Chediak-Higashi leukocytes. J. Clin. Invest. 64: 138–144.

14. BRIGGS, R. T., D. B. DRATH, M. L. KARNOVSKY & M. J. KARNOVSKY. 1975. Localization of NADH oxidase on the surface of polymorphonuclear leukocytes by a new cytochemical method. J. Cell. Biol. **67:** 566–586.
15. INGRAHAM, L. M., L. A. BOXER, R. A. HAAK & R. L. BAEHNER. 1982. Membrane fluidity changes accompanying phagocytosis in normal and in chronic granulomatous disease polymorphonuclear leukocytes. Blood **58:** 830–835.
16. DOBRETSOZ, C. E., T. A. BORSCHEVSKAYA, V. A. PETROV & Y. A. VLADIMIROV. 1977. The increase of phospholipid bilayer rigidity after lipid peroxidation. FEBS Lett. **84:** 125.

DISCUSSION

B. LUBIN (*Children's Hospital Medical Center, Oakland, Calif.*): How do white cells from deficient animals function? Secondly, from a clinical standpoint, do you see this as a potential problem for the safety of vitamin E?

R. L. BAEHNER: In some of our studies, the rats were placed on a vitamin E-deficient diet and PMNs were obtained from the peritoneal cavity. This is a little different from the system where cells are derived from the human peripheral blood system. In the rat, the cells had a marked impairment in their ability to move in response to chemotactic signals. The cells appeared to have increased adherent qualities to nylon wool fibers or endothelial cells. The cells were also impaired in their ability to take up oil red particles. The results with E-deficient rat cells appear to be the corollary to the increased responses that we saw in the human system in the presence of excess vitamin E.

Whether megadoses of vitamin E would pose a potential toxicity to the human system I think is unlikely. The changes that we see here in the bactericidal impairment are very minimal changes, and certainly none of the volunteers who were on the vitamin E experienced any increased susceptibility to infection. I think vitamin E has been useful mainly as a probe to understand some of the molecular events that occur within the PMN.

G. R. BUETTNER (*Wabash College, Crawfordsville, Ind.*): As I understand it, these cells could be considered to be on a suicide mission. Do the cells last longer as they go about their work?

R. L. BAEHNER: We don't have any data on whether they will last longer or remain more viable after the phagocytic event and the bacterial killing. But *in vivo*, the cells are on a "suicide mission," since they leave the circulation and never return again. They are turning over quite rapidly in the circulation, with a half-life of something like six hours. We would expect that even if they did have a slight increase in their survival, it would probably be for only a few hours.

P. B. McCAY (*Oklahoma Medical Research Foundation, Oklahoma City, Okla.*): You found that vitamin E had a rather small effect on bacterial killing, although the production of hydrogen peroxide was reduced to one-fifth of what it was without vitamin E supplementation. Do you think that this means that the amount of hydrogen peroxide normally produced is in great excess to that actually needed to effect bacterial killing?

R. L. BAEHNER: Yes, I think so.

H. W. SEEGER (*Justus-Liebig University, Giessen, Federal Republic of Germany*): Did you measure the incorporation of arachidonate into phospholipids? Phospholipase activity is very much influenced by the form of the substrate. Did you find any correlation between the slight differences in membrane fluidity and any possible alteration in phospholipase activity?

R. L. BAEHNER: Following the incubation with ^{14}C-arachidonate, there was about an equivalent amount of uptake of the label into the cells. The starting point was approximately the same. We don't have data yet on the total phospholipid content of the membranes under the influence of vitamin E.

The relationship between the fluidity changes and release of free arachidonic acid can only be speculative at this point. Some of the early studies performed by Dr. Shohet showed a change in the polyunsaturated fatty acid content of the phospholipids with phagocytosis. With phagocytosis I believe there is less polyunsaturate, which might explain the changes in membrane fluidity.

F. A. OSKI (State University of New York, Syracuse, N.Y.): Would you speculate on the role of vitamin E deficiency in the newborn as related to the variable incidence and magnitude of a number of leukocyte functional defects that have been described and have been ascribed to developmental phenomena. Perhaps they are not developmental phenomena at all but may be of nutritional origin.

R. L. BAEHNER: The vitamin E-deficient state results in a change in the adherent qualities of the vitamin E-deficient PMNs, and they appear to be more able to aggregate together in response to a challenge with chemoattractants or any immunochemical signal.

In addition to their adherent qualities, the changes in membrane potential may be altered as well. We heard yesterday that in membranes from vitamin E-deficient systems, there was an increase in electronegativity on the surface membrane. Some of these aspects may be important in terms of responses in the newborn, where it has been shown that the PMNs are less able to move in and evacuate from the circulation in response to chemoattractants.

It is conceivable that these cells are impaired either through oxidative assault or because of the fact that their levels of vitamin E are lowered in the membrane. This in turn could lead to a variety of conditions, some of which could lead to aggregation of the cells with each other in the circulation, with deposition of these aggregates in the lung to produce perhaps a transient respiratory distress syndrome. I think we have to consider that in the newborn—in some aspects of respiratory distress as well as some of the other conditions—there may be a real role for a modification of the PMN response by the vitamin E-deficient state that occurs in newborns and especially in prematures.

EFFECT OF VITAMIN E ON THE BINDING OF
HEMOGLOBIN TO THE RED CELL MEMBRANE*

Mitchel Sayare, Marina Fikiet, and Jeanne Paulus

Biochemistry and Biophysics Section
Biological Sciences Group
The University of Connecticut
Storrs, Connecticut 06268

Little is known about the effects of vitamin E deficiency on the protein architecture of the erythrocyte membrane. No apparent structural differences between the membrane proteins of vitamin E–deficient and nondeficient cells are revealed by comparison of their Coomassie Blue staining patterns following sodium dodecyl sulfate polyacrylamide gel electrophoresis (SDS PAGE). However, a number of experimental observations have led us to believe that reduced levels of dietary vitamin E increase the ability of the erythrocyte membrane to serve as a substrate for the oxidative formation of disulfide bonds between proteins not normally covalently linked.

One such observation is that erythrocytes from vitamin E–deficient animals are unusually sensitive to Cu^{2+}-induced hemolysis.[1] When incubated in the presence of 100 μM Cu_2SO_4, vitamin E–deficient erythrocytes lyse, with only 20–30% of the cell population remaining after two hours at 37°C. In our laboratory, we have used Cu^{2+}-mediated oxidation to examine the putative hemoglobin binding sites on the cytoplasmic surface of the erythrocyte membrane,[2,3] and it seemed reasonable to apply this technique to monitor the circumstances surrounding the Cu^{2+} sensitivity of vitamin E–deficient red blood cells.

It has been shown by several investigators that normal human red blood cell membranes are capable of binding hemoglobin.[4-10] The amounts of hemoglobin bound[11,12] and the ability of glyceraldehyde-3-P dehydrogenase (G3PD) to compete for the binding site[11,13] suggested that membrane protein band 3 might serve as the binding site. Indeed, we have established by SH-group oxidation that hemoglobin can be cross-linked to band 3, presumably the membrane component to which it is bound, with a stoichiometry of 1:1 (hemoglobin monomer to band 3 monomer).[2]

The addition of hemoglobin A to normal human erythrocyte ghosts at concentrations such that stoichiometric binding of hemoglobin prevails (see Reference 11), followed by catalytic oxidation with Cu^{2+}-o-phenanthroline, results in the disappearance of band 3 upon gel electrophoresis and the appearance of a new band at a position corresponding to a molecular weight of 106,000 (FIGURE 1, tracks III and IV). If no hemoglobin is added to these ghosts (FIGURE 1, track II), or if hemoglobin is added to whole cells or resealed right-side-out ghosts (data not shown), the 106,000-dalton band does not appear upon oxidation.

Cross-linking of membrane-free solutions containing hemoglobin at concentrations used in the experiments above yields no bands other than the 16,000-dalton material at the bottom of the gel. At concentrations of hemoglobin

*This research was supported by grants from the United States Public Health Service (HL-25646) and Hoffmann-La Roche to M.S.

251

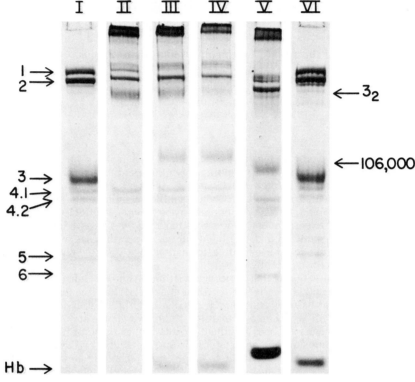

FIGURE 1. Cross-linking of membrane ghosts in the presence and absence of hemoglobin. Fresh ghosts (3.5 × 10⁷ ghosts/ml), with and without added hemoglobin A, were cross-linked and, with the exception of track V, washed with PBS, pH 8.0, and subjected to electrophoresis on 4.5% polyacrylamide gels. Samples containing 15–20 μg of membrane protein were applied to the gel. The numbers to the left of the figure indicate the band notation according to Steck,[15] while those on the right refer to cross-linked products observable in tracks II, III, IV, and V. Track I, membrane ghosts, no cross-linking. Track II, membrane ghosts, cross-linked. Track III, membrane ghosts + 2.3 × 10¹³ molecules hemoglobin A tetramer per ml, cross-linked. Track IV, membrane ghosts + 4.6 × 10¹³ molecules hemoglobin A tetramer per ml, cross-linked. Track V, membrane ghosts + 4.6 × 10¹³ molecules hemoglobin A tetramer per ml, cross-linked, but not PBS washed. Track VI, sample from track IV reduced with 2.5% 2-mercaptoethanol prior to electrophoresis.

approximately 100-fold higher, however, some globin dimer (molecular weight, approximately 32,000) is seen to occur (data not shown). No higher order globin polymer is detectable. In all cases of hemoglobin and/or membrane cross-linking, the normal gel profile is restored if prior to loading the gel, the sample is treated with 2-mercaptoethanol (FIGURE 1, track VI).

The molecular weight of band 3 is reported to be between 90,000 and 96,000.[14] Since the globin subunit molecular weight is between 15,000 and 16,000, the molecular weight of the 106,000-dalton band suggests it is composed of a single subunit of hemoglobin covalently bound to a band 3 monomer. This was tested using ^{14}C-hemoglobin in experiments similar to those in FIGURE 1. Gels were prepared in duplicate for Coomassie Blue staining and for fluorography. The top of FIGURE 2B shows the pattern of radioactive material from a membrane sample cross-linked with ^{14}C-hemoglobin and run in SDS PAGE. Note that the label is distributed in four regions of the gel. Small amounts of radioactivity can be seen at the top of the gel and in the region of band 3 dimer. The bulk of the label, however, is found both in the region of the 106,000-dalton species and in the region of the 16,000-dalton globin subunit near the bottom of the gel.

The identity of the 106,000-dalton species was confirmed by two-dimensional SDS PAGE, exploiting the reversibility of the disulfide bond formation catalyzed by Cu^{2+}. A sample of ghosts cross-linked with ^{14}C-hemoglobin was run on a tube gel. The gel was placed horizontally on a slab gel, atop a layer of agarose containing 2.5% 2-mercaptoethanol (FIGURE 2A). In the second dimension, the 106,000-dalton band, which is reduced by the 2-mercaptoethanol, runs with a mobility equivalent to band 3. This position is significantly below the diagonal formed by peptides that were not affected by the catalytic oxidation. An identical 2D gel was prepared for fluorography. The resulting autoradiogram is shown in FIGURE 2B (bottom), which compares it with an autoradiogram of the same sample run only in one dimension (without 2-mercaptoethanol). Note that there are four radioactive globin bands at the bottom of the 2D gel corresponding to the four positions seen in autoradiography of the first dimension (top of FIGURE 2B).

It is noteworthy that nearly all of the labeled globin can be accounted for in association with band 3 (either as band 3 monomer or dimer), or as free globin running at a molecular weight of 16,000, or at the top of the gel. Globin at the top of the gel is associated with a high molecular weight complex that, upon reduction and electrophoresis in the second dimension (as shown in FIGURE 2A), yields a number of peptides as well as globin. One of these peptides is band 3, whose presence in this complex is consistent with results from other laboratories.[3,16] The complete absence of label from regions of the gel where one would expect to recover cross-linked products of globin and bands 1, 2, 4.1, 4.2, 5, or 6 suggests that hemoglobin cross-links rather specifically to band 3.

In an effort to determine the stoichiometry of the association of band 3 and hemoglobin, samples similar to that shown in FIGURE 2 were run on one-dimensional gels and scanned densitometrically to determine the protein content of each of the bands. The four bands that were shown to contain over 90% of the ^{14}C-globin (by autoradiography of replicate gels) were then sliced out of the gels, solubilized, and counted. The results of eight such experiments are shown in TABLE 1. The values indicate that the stoichiometry between band 3 and globin found in the 106,000-dalton peptide is essentially 1:1 (globin monomer to band 3 monomer). No such stoichiometric relationship between globin and the band 3 dimer is evident.

It has recently been shown that membranes prepared from erythrocytes of animals deficient in dietary vitamin E contain significantly reduced amounts of glyceraldehyde-3-P dehydrogenase.[17] Since G3PD has been shown to compete with hemoglobin binding to the inner surface of human erythrocyte membranes,[11-13] two experiments were designed to test this competition in the cross-linking system described above. In the first, ghosts were stripped of glyceraldehyde-3-P dehydrogenase (band 6), hemoglobin was added, and cross-linking was carried out as described. The results in the form of densitometry scans of gels of glyceraldehyde-3-P dehydrogenase–depleted and nondepleted ghosts are shown in FIGURE 3 and suggest that the depleted ghosts have a greater amount

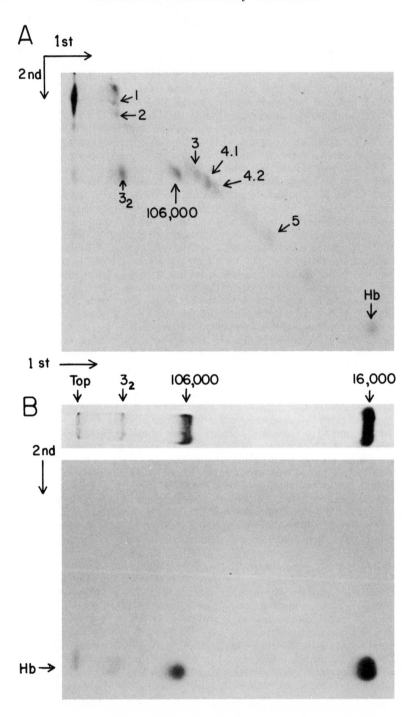

TABLE 1

STOICHIOMETRY OF BAND 3 AND HEMOGLOBIN UPON CROSS-LINKING*

Gel Slice	Protein (picomoles)	^{14}C-Globin (picomoles)
106,000-dalton peptide	13.0 ± 0.3	12.9 ± 0.7
band 3 dimer	11.3 ± 0.2	4.4 ± 0.8

*Membranes (3.5×10^7/ml) were cross-linked with ^{14}C-hemoglobin at a concentration (4.6×10^{13} molecules tetramer/ml) sufficient to saturate the putative binding sites. Membrane pellets (20 μg membrane protein) were applied to 4.5% SDS PAGE, and the gels were stained and scanned densitometrically to determine protein concentrations in selected bands. The indicated concentrations are based on a band 3 monomer molecular weight of 90,000. The radioactive bands, as determined by fluorography, were sliced out of the gels, solubilized, and counted. Dpm were converted to picomoles of 16,000-dalton subunit based on the specific activity of ^{14}C-hemoglobin. The calculated protein values in each band were reduced by the amount contributed by globin, based on radioactivity recovered from the gel slice. The numbers given are averages of eight different experiments ± standard deviation.

of cross-linked product in the region of 106,000 daltons (3-Hb in FIGURES 3 and 4). In a second series of experiments, rabbit muscle glyceraldehyde-3-P dehydrogenase was added to normal ghosts in 2:1 and 5:1 molar ratios with hemoglobin. Cross-linking was carried out, and the results of gels scanned densitometrically are shown in FIGURE 4. In this case it seems that exogenously added glyceraldehyde-3-P dehydrogenase reduces the amount of cross-linked product in the 106,000-dalton region (3-Hb) and a new product appears with an electrophoretic mobility equivalent to 115,000 daltons (G_3 in FIGURE 4). In two-dimensional gels using the sample from FIGURE 4B, the 115,000-dalton fragment as well as G_2, G_4, and G_5 were all shown to be cross-linked homopolymers of glyceraldehyde-3-P dehydrogenase. No hemoglobin was found associated with these products, nor is there evidence that glyceraldehyde-3-P dehydrogenase is cross-linked to band 3 in this system. Thus, glyceraldehyde-3-P dehydrogenase has competed with hemoglobin for accessibility to the band 3 cross-linking site. Coupled with the previous experiment, these results suggest that both endogenous glyceraldehyde-3-P dehydrogenase and exogenously added rabbit muscle glyceraldehyde-3-P dehydrogenase compete with hemoglobin for binding to band 3.

The importance of this observation rests on the data of Shapiro and coworkers,[17] reported at this conference. They have shown that in vitamin E–deficient cells, and in membranes derived from such cells, there is a significant reduction in the amount of G3PD associated with the membrane. This might therefore permit more extensive cross-linking of hemoglobin to band 3. This suggestion, in

FIGURE 2. Two-dimensional gel electrophoresis of erythrocyte ghosts cross-linked with ^{14}C-hemoglobin. The experiment was carried out essentially as described for FIGURE 1, track III, except that ^{14}C-hemoglobin was used and 30 μg of membrane protein was applied to the gel. Following electrophoresis in the first dimension, the gel was transferred to a slab overlaid with agarose containing 2-mercaptoethanol, and electrophoresis was again carried out. The orientation of the first dimension is left to right; and the second dimension, top to bottom. A. Coomassie Blue staining pattern. B. Autoradiogram of a replicate gel prepared for fluorography, above which is an autoradiogram of an identical sample run in one dimension.

addition to the observation of increased sensitivity of vitamin E–deficient cells to Cu^{2+}, forms the basis of the following series of experiments.

Erythrocytes from vitamin E–deficient and nondeficient rats were isolated, washed, and exposed to 100 μM Cu_2SO_4 in phosphate-buffered saline (PBS), pH 8.0. After two hours incubation at 37°C, low-speed centrifugation of the suspensions yielded a cell pellet containing 40% and 100% of the cell populations of the vitamin E–deficient and nondeficient cells, respectively. The pellets of both sets of cells were washed extensively in the presence of 0.1 M ethylenediamine-tetraacetic acid (EDTA) and then lysed osmotically. The resulting membranes

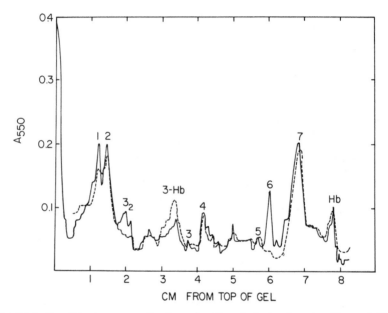

FIGURE 3. Densitometry scans of polyacrylamide gel electrophoresis of hemoglobin A cross-linking to normal and glyceraldehyde-3-P dehydrogenase–depleted ghosts. Experimental design as in FIGURE 1, except that one set of ghosts was depleted of glyceraldehyde-3-P dehydrogenase (band 6) by incubation in 150 mM sodium phosphate buffer (pH 8.0) prior to cross-linking. 3-Hb is the 106,000-dalton cross-linked product of band 3 and hemoglobin. Hemoglobin A concentration, 3.5×10^{13} molecules tetramer/ml. Both samples were placed on the same slab gel with 4.5% acrylamide. Solid line, normal ghosts; dashed line, glyceraldehyde-3-P dehydrogenase–depleted ghosts.

were then further washed to yield, in the case of the vitamin E–deficient membranes, a pink ghost pellet. The nondeficient membranes yielded a white pellet. The supernatant fraction obtained by low-speed centrifugation of the vitamin E–deficient cells was centrifuged at high speed and yielded, after extensive washing, a pellet of pink ghosts. All membrane pellets were then solubilized in SDS and run on SDS PAGE. The results are shown in FIGURE 5. The gel patterns shown in the first two tracks are of membranes orginating from nondeficient and vitamin E–deficient cells, respectively, that were not treated with Cu^{2+}. A Coomassie Blue staining pattern very similar to human erythrocyte

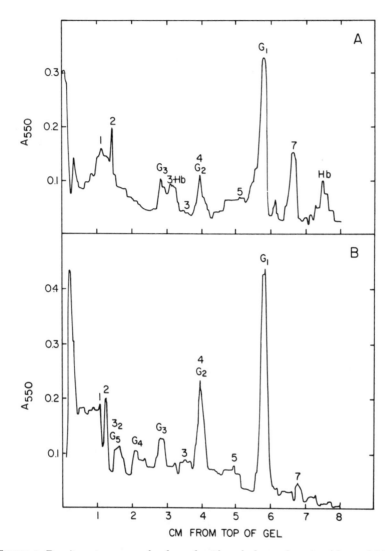

FIGURE 4. Densitometry scans of polyacrylamide gel electrophoresis of hemoglobin A cross-linking to normal ghosts in the presence of added glyceraldehyde-3-P dehydrogenase. Experimental design as in FIGURE 1, except that rabbit muscle glyceraldehyde-3-P dehydrogenase was added at the same time as hemoglobin A. Hemoglobin concentration, 3.5×10^{13} molecules tetramer/ml. G_2–G_5 refer to cross-linked homopolymers of glyceraldehyde-3-P dehydrogenase, dimer to pentamer, determined by two-dimensional gels of sample B. G_1 is glyceraldehyde-3-P dehydrogenase monomer. A, 7×10^{13} molecules glyceraldehyde-3-P dehydrogenase tetramer/ml. B, 17.5×10^{13} molecules glyceraldehyde-3-P dehydrogenase tetramer/ml.

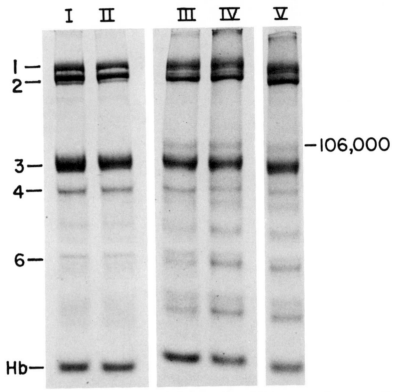

FIGURE 5. Sensitivity of vitamin E–deficient and nondeficient rat erythrocytes to Cu^{2+}. Erythrocytes isolated from rats fed on a diet deficient in vitamin E or on a vitamin E–supplemented diet were washed and resuspended in PBS, pH 8.0, containing 100 μM Cu_2SO_4. At the end of two hours incubation at 37°C, low-speed centrifugation (3,500 × g) was used to collect whole cells. This was followed by centrifugation of the supernatant fraction at 20,000 × g to pellet ghosts resulting from Cu^{2+}-induced lysis. Those cells that resisted Cu^{2+}-induced lysis were lysed osmotically and washed by standard procedures. These ghosts, as well as those isolated directly from the initial cell suspension, were solubilized in SDS and electrophoresis was carried out. Track I, membranes isolated by osmotic lysis of control cells; track II, membranes isolated by osmotic lysis of vitamin E–deficient cells; track III, membranes isolated by osmotic lysis of control cells treated with Cu^{2+}; track IV, membranes isolated by osmotic lysis of vitamin E–deficient cells treated with Cu^{2+}; track V, membranes isolated by high-speed centrifugation of the low-speed supernatant fraction of a vitamin E–deficient cell suspension treated with Cu^{2+}.

membranes is seen. Membranes obtained from the Cu^{2+}-induced lysis of vitamin E–deficient cells provided the sample for track V. Several changes in the gel pattern can be identified. One of these is the formation of a 106,000-dalton band, corresponding to the position of the hemoglobin–band 3 product seen in FIGURE 1 with human erythrocyte membranes. Additionally, there is material at the top of the gel and at locations with mobilities greater than band 3, none of which are present in membranes from cells not treated with Cu^{2+}. The remaining two tracks show the staining patterns of membranes prepared by osmotic lysis of those vitamin E-deficient cells that resisted Cu^{2+}-induced lysis and of nondeficient cells. Both sets of membranes seem to have approximately the same amount of 106,000-dalton material, but there are differences in the intensities of the new bands distributed on the gel below the band 4 complex. The membranes originating from vitamin E-deficient cells have significantly more of this material.

Identification of this new material was made utilizing the two-dimensional gel techniques described in FIGURE 2. A portion of the sample used in FIGURE 5, track V, was run in two dimensions, the second dimension in the presence of 2-mercaptoethanol, and the results are shown in FIGURE 6. Apparent are numerous bands running with the mobility of hemoglobin in the second dimension, which were distributed in the first dimension in a manner identical to the new material described in FIGURE 5, tracks III–V. This material, in the nonreduced state, is almost certainly pure hemoglobin. The bands are distributed in the typical exponential pattern of increasing order of homopolymer, beginning with the 16,000-dalton hemoglobin monomer and increasing detectably to 64,000 daltons. Were we to try to explain the increased size of the hemoglobin bands in the first dimension as products of hemoglobin and membrane components, we would not see the simple exponential distribution shown. In addition, we would expect to

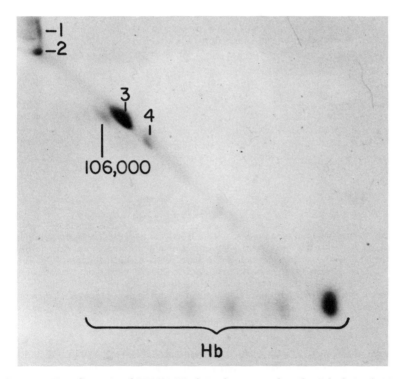

FIGURE 6. Two-dimensional SDS PAGE of membranes resulting from the lysis of vitamin E-deficient erythrocytes treated with Cu^{2+}. An identical sample to that used in FIGURE 5, track V, was run in two dimensions. The gel technique employed is the same as in FIGURE 2.

see off-diagonal membrane components. With the exception of band 3, none are visible. The off-diagonal band 3, combined with hemoglobin, results in the new 106,000-dalton product, and seems to be the only membrane component to which hemoglobin is covalently bound.

The hemoglobin that cross-linked to itself and not to membrane components must nevertheless be bound to the membrane in order to be present in these gels.

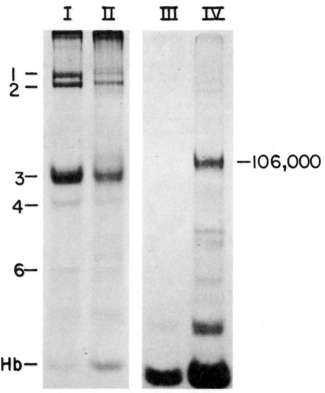

FIGURE 7. Incubation of membranes isolated from vitamin E–deficient and nondeficient rat erythrocytes with ^{14}C-hemoglobin. Membranes obtained from vitamin E–deficient and nondeficient cells by osmotic lysis were incubated with ^{14}C-hemoglobin at 37°C for one hour. Membranes were then washed, solubilized in SDS, and electrophoresis carried out as in FIGURE 1. In all cases the hemoglobin concentration was 4.6×10^{13} molecules tetramer/ ml. Track I, membranes from control cells incubated with hemoglobin; track II, membranes from vitamin E–deficient cells incubated with hemoglobin. Tracks III and IV, autoradiogram of an identical gel prepared for fluorography.

Although no strong evidence exists, we assume that this hemoglobin is also bound to band 3, but not covalently. Perhaps, upon oxidation, the SH-groups available on hemoglobin were quickly used up in forming homopolymer, essentially blocking disulfide bond formation with band 3 (or other membrane components).

Thus, we have shown that Cu^{2+} asserts an oxidizing potential on whole cells, such that when the membranes of these cells are isolated by osmotic lysis in the absence of Cu^{2+}, changes in membrane protein architecture can be found. The major change seems to be the covalent cross-linking of hemoglobin to band 3 and formation of hemoglobin homopolymer.

The preceding experiments relied on the presence of large amounts of Cu^{2+} to detect differences in the sensitivity of vitamin E-deficient and nondeficient membranes to oxidation. It is pertinent to also examine possible differences in membrane sensitivity in the absence of Cu^{2+}. Thus, membranes isolated by osmotic lysis of vitamin E-deficient and nondeficient cells were incubated in the presence of ^{14}C-hemoglobin at 37°C for one hour.

FIGURE 7 shows that in the absence of all but the trace amounts of Cu^{2+} or other cations present in double-distilled water or dry buffer components, the membranes from vitamin E-deficient cells covalently cross-linked significantly more ^{14}C-hemoglobin than did the nondeficient membranes. Autoradiography gives a reasonable indication of where the ^{14}C-hemoglobin is distributed on the gel, and as can be seen in track IV, most of the cross-linked hemoglobin is associated with the 106,000-dalton band discussed above.

These results suggest that membranes from vitamin E-deficient cells have a greater propensity to cross-link hemoglobin to band 3 than do membranes from nondeficient cells. Whether this is a direct result of the reduced levels of the antioxidant power of vitamin E or is a secondary effect of reduced amounts of G3PD (band 6) on the inner surface of the membrane is currently being investigated.

REFERENCES

1. SHEETZ, M. 1981. Personal communication.
2. SAYARE, M. & M. FIKIET. 1981. J. Biol. Chem. (In press.)
3. SAYARE, M. & T. M. SCHUSTER. 1980. Fed. Proc. **39:** 1916.
4. DODGE, J. T., C. MITCHELL, & D. J. HANAHAN. 1963. Arch. Biochem. Biophys. **100:** 119–130.
5. BANK, A., G. MEARS, R. WEISS, J. V. O'DONNELL & C. NATTA. 1974. J. Clin. Invest. **54:** 805–809.
6. FISCHER, S., R. L. NAGEL, R. M. BOOKCHIN, E. F. ROTH, JR. & I. TELLEZ-NAGEL. 1975. Biochim. Biophys. Acta **375:** 422–433.
7. LESSIN, L. S. & C. WALLAS. 1973. (Abst.). Blood **42:** 978.
8. SCHNEIDER, R. G., I. TAKEDA, L. GUSTAVSON & J. B. ALPERIN. 1972. Nature London New Biol. **235:** 88–90.
9. HANAHAN, D. J., J. E. EKHOLM & G. HILDENBRANDT. 1973. Biochemistry **12:** 1374–1387.
10. MITCHELL, C. D., W. B. MITCHELL & D. J. HANAHAN. 1965. Biochim. Biophys. Acta **104:** 348–358.
11. SHAKLAI, N., J. YGUERABIDE & H. M. RANNEY. 1977. Biochemistry **16:** 5585–5592.
12. SALHANY, J. M. & N. SHAKLAI. 1979. Biochemistry **18:** 893–899.
13. SHAKLAI, N., J. YGUERABIDE & H. M. RANNEY. 1977. Biochemistry **16:** 5593–5597.
14. STECK, T. L. 1978. J. Supramol. Struct. **8:** 311–324.
15. STECK, T. L. 1974. J. Cell Biol. **62:** 1–19.
16. SALHANY, J. M., K. A. CORDES, E. D. GAINES & P. B. RAUENBUEHELER. 1981. *In* Proceedings of the International Conference on the Interaction between Iron and Proteins in Oxygen and Electron Transport. C. Ho, Ed. Elsevier/North-Holland Biomedical Press. New York, N.Y. (In press.)
17. SHAPIRO, S. S. & D. J. MOTT. Ann. N.Y. Acad. Sci. (This volume.)

DISCUSSION

L. BOWIE (*Evanston Hospital, Evanston, Ill.*): I'd like to know if you had considered whether or not the interaction between hemoglobin and band 3 was dependent upon either the oxidative state or the conformational state of the hemoglobin. Did you do the experiment with the deoxyhemoglobin as well?

M. SAYARE: Yes the experiment does work with deoxyhemoglobin. You can get some disulfide cross-linking, although it's reduced.

L. BOWIE: Do you attribute that to conformational aspects or do you attribute that to the requirements for oxygen?

M. SAYARE: I attribute that exclusively to the presence or absence of oxygen simply because you can do the same experiment with CO-hemoglobin, which retains the oxy conformation. In the absence of oxygen, you get approximately the same amount of cross-linking as you do with deoxyhemoglobin.

E. A. RACHMILEWITZ (*Hadassah University Hospital, Jerusalem, Israel*): We did some studies on the pattern of red cell membrane proteins in thalassemia, and there was some indication that there is some cross-linking. We stressed the cells with hydrogen peroxide rather than copper. We believe the changes that are causing the proteins to oxidize in the membrane are from the intracellular milieu. When vitamin E was administered, we were not able to correct this defect. I wonder if your elegant work could also be done with some pathological red cells.

M. SAYARE: That's a very good idea.

L. PACKER (*University of California, Berkeley, Calif.*): Is it possible that the older cells might be the ones that have a greater propensity for the hemoglobin binding?

M. SAYARE: We haven't done that yet, but we're aware of the differences in the population in terms of age of red blood cells. For example in the case of sickle-cell anemia with irreversibly sickled cells, there are differences in sensitivity to oxidation of band 3 and hemoglobin. So I do assume that with age or with other differences in the population, you may find differences in the gel patterns.

ALTERATIONS OF ENZYMES IN THE RED BLOOD
CELL MEMBRANE IN VITAMIN E DEFICIENCY

Stanley S. Shapiro and Dante J. Mott

Vitamins and Clinical Nutrition
Hoffmann-La Roche, Inc.
Nutley, New Jersey 07110

The importance of vitamin E as an antioxidant, providing protection against free radical–induced membrane damage, has been well documented.[1-3] However, at this time it is not known if all the physiological roles of vitamin E relate to its antioxidant properties. Vitamin E is localized in the membrane components of the cell, and certainly a major role for vitamin E is to terminate free radical-generated chain reactions, particularly in membranes that are rich in polyunsaturated lipids. This is consistent with numerous reports that the primary site for the observed pathology in vitamin E deficiency is the cellular membrane.

Investigations were initiated to identify the biochemical lesions at the membrane level resulting from low vitamin E status. Initially we have studied the red blood cell (RBC) membrane. It is an ideal model for studying the antioxidant role of vitamin E in membranes. Hemoglobin is known to catalyze lipid peroxidation as well as enhance the decomposition of lipid hydroperoxides to the corresponding free radicals.[4,5] Autoxidation of oxyhemoglobin to methemoglobin results in the generation of superoxide radical.[6,7] The reaction of superoxide radical with peroxides in the RBC produces highly reactive intermediates, such as the hydroxyl radical ($OH \cdot$). These radicals in turn react with the lipid and protein components of the membrane, damaging its integrity and leading to eventual hemolysis of the cell.[4] However, little is known concerning the specific alterations in either the lipid or protein components of the membrane during this process. Any disruption of the native membrane structure may in turn modulate any of the numerous functions of the membrane, and have a secondary effect on processes in the cell. In addition to lipid peroxidation, proteins interspaced in the bilayer may possibly be altered by free radicals originating in the lipid phase of the membrane. Furthermore, there are structural proteins arranged in a filamentous network on the cytoplasmic face of the membrane. This network is responsible for supporting and maintaining the intactness of the bilayer. Because of the proximity of these structural proteins to the membrane, these proteins may also be modified by free radicals emanating in the phospholipid bilayer.

A number of functional proteins associated with the plasma membrane have been studied in RBCs obtained from vitamin E–deficient rhesus monkeys. It has been observed that the activity of some specific membrane-associated enzymes is indeed modified in vitamin E deficiency. Our observations are consistent with the concept that membrane modification resulting from vitamin E deficiency resides on the cytoplasmic side of the membrane.

Glyceraldehyde-3-phosphate Dehydrogenase

The effects of vitamin E deficiency on the activity of the membrane-bound enzyme glyceraldehyde-3-phosphate dehydrogenase (GAPDH; EC 1.2.1.12) was

0077-8923/82/0393-0263 $01.75/0 © 1982, NYAS

studied. This is a peripheral protein located on the cytoplasmic side of the cell membrane and is believed to be associated with the integral membrane protein designated as band 3.[8-11] The enzyme is readily dissociated from the membrane by extraction with high ionic strength solution.[8,12-14] GAPDH plays a major role in glycolysis, which is the principal means by which the red blood cell obtains its adenosine triphosphate (ATP) and reduced nicotinamide-adenine dinucleotide (NADH). The enzyme is present in extraordinary amounts and constitutes approximately 6% of the total membrane protein. Because band 3 is the anion transport protein, a participative role for GAPDH in the regulation of phosphate transport has been postulated.

TABLE 1

COMPARISON OF GAPDH ACTIVITY IN VITAMIN E-SUPPLEMENTED AND DEFICIENT
CYTOPLASM, GHOSTS, AND GHOST EXTRACT*

Experiment	E Status	Cyto-plasm	E−/E+ (%)	Ghosts	E−/E+ (%)	Extract	E−/E+ (%)
1	+	5.74	90.0	4.00	67.5	3.20	65.9
	−	5.18		2.70		2.11	
2	+			4.41	65.9	3.60	67.5
	−			2.91		2.43	
3	+			4.05	64.2	2.97	57.6
	−			2.60		1.71	

*Values represent a sample derived by mixing equal volumes of blood from three deficient or supplemented monkeys. Activity = μmoles NADH $\times 10^{-10}$/minute per vesicle. All animals were fed a semipurified diet containing 25% casein, 46% sucrose, 11% cellulose, 11% "stripped" lard, 1% menhaden oil, 4% salts, 2% vitamin mixture. E− monkeys had plasma levels of less than 0.1 mg/dl. E+ monkeys were fed the diet with 500 mg/kg all-rac-α-tocopheryl acetate added. Their plasma levels were well over 1.2 mg/dl.

Effect of Low Vitamin E Status on GAPDH Activity

It is evident that E− animals show a lower GAPDH activity in salt extract of ghosts compared to E+ animals (TABLE 1). This difference can also be seen when unsealed ghosts are assayed prior to extraction. In representative experiments, it was found that GAPDH extract preparations from E− animals have 34 to 42% lower activity than do those of supplemented animals (TABLE 1). In the unsealed ghosts prior to extraction, activity in E− animals was reduced by approximately 35% as compared with E+ animals (TABLE 1). Thus, there was a clear reduction in membrane GAPDH activity in E− animals. There is relatively little (if any) change in the soluble GAPDH. The reduced levels of bound GAPDH cannot be accounted for by higher levels in the soluble state (TABLE 1). Extracted GAPDH stored overnight at 4°C resulted in a 10-25% loss of activity (TABLE 2), while a membrane preparation stored overnight at 4°C with bound GAPDH showed no significant loss of the enzyme (TABLE 2). The ghosts contain approximately 20% more enzyme activity than does the zero time extract. This cannot be explained in terms of only partial removal of the enzyme. Subsequent detergent treatment or repeated salt extraction did not account for the difference in enzyme activity. It is possible that GAPDH has a higher specific activity in the bound state relative to the soluble state.

TABLE 2

STABILITY OF EXTRACTED AND MEMBRANE-BOUND GAPDH

Experiment	E Status	GAPDH Activity*			Extract 18 Hr./ Extract 0 Hr. (%)	E − Extract 0 Hr./ E + Extract 0 Hr. (%)
		Extract 0 Hr.	Extract 18 Hr.	Bound 18 Hr.		
1†	+	714 ± 167 [3]	583 ± 147 [3]		81.7	55.7
	−	398 ± 91 [3]	330 ± 72 [3]		82.9	
2†	+	459	412	559	89.8	41.8
	−	192	144	239	75.2	

*Activity = μmoles NADH × 10^{-3}/minute per mg ghost protein.
†Values represent a pooled sample derived by mixing equal volumes of blood from three deficient or supplemented monkeys.

Reconstitution of RBC Membranes with Extracted GAPDH

We attempted to explain this observation by one of three alternative hypotheses: (1) vitamin E has an obligatory role in the enzyme reaction; (2) the absence of vitamin E results in modification of the enzyme (reduced activity, or affinity for the membrane); or (3) a modification of the band 3 binding site for the enzyme. To test these alternative hypotheses, we prepared solubilized GAPDH and stripped ghosts from RBCs of deficient and supplemented animals. The stripped ghosts and eluted enzyme were reconstituted with all possible pair combinations of ghost and enzyme from deficient and supplemented animals. To a fixed amount of enzyme, varying amounts of ghosts were added, and the degree of reassociation was determined. Dialyzed GAPDH was added to both E+ and E− ghosts as follows: ghosts (5 µl to 200 µl) from both E+ and E− RBCs were added to small test tubes. GAPDH obtained from E+ and E− membranes was incubated with either extracted E+ or E− membranes. In all incubations, unless otherwise stated, 0.21 unit/ml of GAPDH was present. A unit is equal to one µmole of NADH formed per minute. Additional 5 mM phosphate buffer pH 8.0 (5P8) was

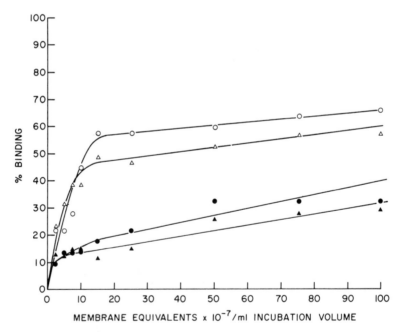

FIGURE 1. Reconstitution of RBC membranes with extracted GAPDH. E+ = GAPDH extracted from animals on vitamin E-supplemented diets. E− = GAPDH extracted from animals on vitamin E-deficient diets. V+ = unsealed membrane ghosts from animals on vitamin E-supplemented diets. V− = unsealed membrane ghosts from animals on vitamin E-deficient diets. Unsealed ghosts and extract were combined as follows: O = E+V+; △ = E−V+; ▲ = E+V−; ● = E−V−. Both + and − ghost suspensions contained 5.03×10^9 membrane equivalents/ml. Aliquots of 5 to 200 µl of unsealed ghosts were added to test tubes containing 5P8. An enzyme activity of 0.24 unit (a unit is equivalent to one µmole of NADH formed per minute from NAD) of extracted GAPDH, E+ or E−, was added in a volume of 0.19 ml. The total incubation volume was 1.0 ml.

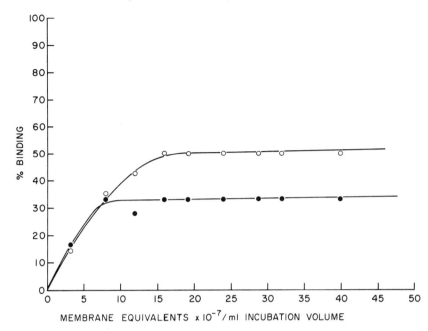

FIGURE 2. Reconstitution of vitamin E-supplemented and deficient RBC membranes with crystalline GAPDH. V+ = unsealed membrane ghosts from animals on vitamin E-supplemented diets. V− = unsealed membrane ghosts from animals on vitamin E-deficient diets. V+ and V− ghost suspensions contained 3.2×10^9 membrane equivalents/ml. Aliquots of ghost suspensions (5 to 150 µl) were added to test tubes with 5P8; 0.164 unit of crystalline GAPDH was added in a volume of 0.1 ml. The total incubation volume was 1.0 ml. O = V+; ● = V−.

added to give a total volume of 1.0 ml. Samples in duplicate were incubated on ice with shaking for 1.5 to 2 hours. It is apparent (FIGURE 1) that the vitamin E status of the animals from which the ghosts were obtained was the determining factor in the level of membrane-bound enzyme. In any given set of ghosts, solubilized GAPDH from deficient and supplemented RBCs bound with approximately equal affinity (FIGURE 1).

Additionally, this was confirmed by reconstituting deficient and supplemented ghosts with crystalline rabbit muscle GAPDH (FIGURE 2). In this case, rabbit muscle GAPDH bound to a greater extent with the supplemented ghosts than with the deficient ghosts. Thus, we concluded that GAPDH, per se, is not altered with low vitamin E status, and the modification occurs on the membrane binding site (band 3).

Exogenous Addition of all-rac-α-Tocopherol to Whole Blood

In order to assess the possibility that modification of the GAPDH binding site occurred in vitro as a result of laboratory manipulation, or that all-rac-α-tocopherol played an obligatory role in the association process, all-rac-α-tocopherol was added to freshly drawn blood. After incubation of whole blood with

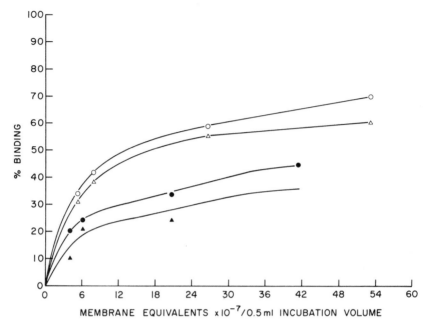

FIGURE 3. Reconstitution of vitamin E–supplemented and deficient RBC membranes with crystalline GAPDH after incubation of whole blood with *all-rac-α*-tocopherol. V+ = unsealed membrane ghosts from animals on vitamin E–supplemented diets. V− = unsealed membrane ghosts from animals on vitamin E–deficient diets. *all-rac-α*-Tocopherol was added *in vitro* to whole red blood cells to give a concentration of 0.2 mg/ml, and cells were incubated 1.0 hour at room temperature. Membranes were prepared, and aliquots of ghosts (10 to 100 μl) from the V+ suspension containing 5.33×10^9 membrane equivalents/ml and from the V− suspension containing 4.16×10^9 membrane equivalents/ml were added to test tubes with 5P8. Crystalline GAPDH, 0.086 unit, was added in a volume of 0.05 ml. The total incubation volume was 0.5 ml. This gives an enzyme concentration of 0.172 unit/ml in each incubation; $\triangle$ = V+ without added tocopherol; O = V+ with added tocopherol; $\blacktriangle$ = V− without added tocopherol; $\bullet$ = V− with added tocopherol.

tocopherol for one hour at room temperature, aliquots were withdrawn and RBC tocopherol levels were determined. As anticipated based on the observations of Bieri *et al.* and Bjornson *et al.*,[15,16] exogenously added tocopherol was rapidly taken up by the RBCs. The tocopherol level in vitamin E–deficient RBCs increased from 0.4 μg/ml to 26.67 μg/ml. For any given concentration of membranes, those membranes prepared from supplemented animals had a greater association for GADPH than did membranes prepared from deficient animals (FIGURE 3). In addition, it can be seen that the presence of high levels of *all-rac-α*-tocopherol *in vitro* resulted in a modest enhancement of enzyme association in both E+ and E− membranes (FIGURE 3).

External Membrane Markers

Since band 3 is a transmembrane protein and responsible for anion transport, it was of interest to ascertain if the external side of band 3 was also modified by vitamin E deficiency. The interaction of 4,4'-diisothiocyano-2,2'-stilbenedisul-fonic acid (DIDS) with band 3 was investigated. DIDS is among the most potent of the specific anion transport inhibitors and is known to bind with the transport site.[17] Interaction of DIDS with RBCs was followed by inhibition of $^{35}SO_4^{2-}$ efflux. Washed cells at a 50% hematocrit were incubated at 4°C overnight with 10 μCi $^{35}SO_4^{2-}$. DIDS was added to a 10% hematocrit for 30 minutes at 5°C, and then the cells were washed three times at 4°C. The cells were diluted to 2.5% hematocrit. Cells were then incubated at 30°C, and at the indicated time (FIGURE 4), the cells were centrifuged and an aliquot of supernatant was counted in a liquid scintillation counter to determine the release of $^{35}SO_4^{2-}$. As monitored by inhibition of $^{35}SO_4^{2-}$ transport, DIDS reacts identically with E-deficient and E-supplemented RBCs (FIGURE 4). Thus it was concluded that the DIDS binding site was not modified in vitamin E-deficient RBCs.

Acetylcholinesterase Activity

Acetylcholinesterase is known to face the external side of the RBC plasma membrane. Its activity was compared in vitamin E-deficient and supplemented RBCs. This assay was adapted from Steck and Kant[10] with the following modification: acetylthiocholine iodide was used as the substrate. As shown in

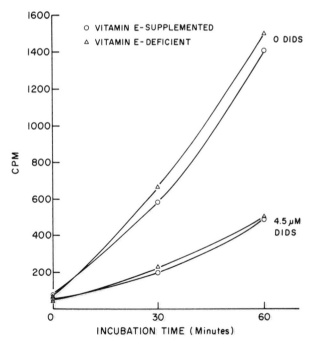

FIGURE 4. $^{35}SO_4^{2-}$ transport in vitamin E-deficient and supplemented RBCs. Washed cells (50% hematocrit) were incubated at 4°C overnight with 10 μCi of $^{35}SO_4^{2-}$. DIDS was added to a 10% hematocrit of the cells for 30 minutes at 5°C. Cells were washed, diluted to a 2.5% hematocrit, and incubated at 30°C. Cells were then centrifuged, and the supernatant was counted in Aquasol. O = vitamin E-supplemented; Δ = vitamin E-deficient.

TABLE 3

ACETYLCHOLINESTERASE ACTIVITY IN VITAMIN E-SUPPLEMENTED AND
VITAMIN E-DEFICIENT RBCs AND RBC GHOSTS

| | | Acetylcholinesterase Activity | |
		Supplemented	Deficient
RBC	EXP I†	1.21	1.21
	EXP II†	0.95	1.00
	EXP II†	1.14	1.07
RBC Ghost‡		6.31 ± 0.21 (3)	6.34 ± 0.47 (3)

*Acetylcholinesterase activity in moles/l per minute $\times$ 10^{-12} of acetyl thiocholine iodide hydrolyzed.

†Each value represents a pooled sample derived by mixing equal volumes of blood from three deficient or supplemented monkeys.

‡Acetylcholinesterase activity in moles/l per minute $\times$ 10^{-3} in 1.0 ml of suspension. The suspension represents 4.5 ml of lysed whole blood and the unsealed ghosts resuspended in 3.0 ml of 5P8.

TABLE 3, there was no apparent difference in the RBC acetylcholinesterase activity in vitamin E-deficient or supplemented RBCs.

β-Adrenergic Receptor

The effect of vitamin E deficiency on the ability of the β-adrenergic receptor to bind to specific ligands was determined. For this series of experiments, rat RBCs were used. Washed ghosts from rat vitamin E-deficient and supplemented RBCs were incubated with ^{3}H-dihydroalprenolol (DHA) alone and with various amounts of L-isoproterenol. The membranes were filtered and counted in a liquid scintillation counter.[18,19] There was no difference in the binding of ^{3}H-DHA to E-deficient or supplemented membranes in the absence or presence of L-isoproterenol. Thus it was concluded that vitamin E deficiency does not alter the RBC β-adrenergic receptor.

METHYLATION PATHWAYS

We have studied two types of methylation reactions that take place in the membranes and compared these reactions in the vitamin E-deficient state to the supplemented state. One set of reactions involve the membrane lipid component, and the other reactions involve methylation of specific membrane proteins. Both reactions require S-adenosylmethionine (SAM) as a cosubstrate.

Phosphatidyltransmethylase Activity

S-Adenosylmethionine:phosphatidylethanolamine methyltransferase (EC.2.1.1.17) (transferase I) and S-adenosylmethionine:phosphatidylmonomethylethanolamine and phosphatidyldimethylethanolamine methyltransferase (transferase II) are involved in the biosynthesis of phosphatidylcholine from phosphatidylethanolamine. This enzyme system represents an alternative to the cytidine diphosphate (CDP)-choline pathway. The first enzyme (transferase I) converts phosphatidylethanolamine (PE) to monomethyl PE (MMPE). This enzyme is located on the cytoplasmic side of the membrane. The second enzyme converts MMPE to the dimethyl derivative DMPE and ultimately to phosphatidylcholine (PC). Transferase II is located on the external face of the membrane. Thus the asymmetrical distribution of these methyltransferases causes the movement of PE from the cytoplasmic face, resulting in the formation and localization of PC on the external face of the membrane.[20]

Recent reports from Axelrod's laboratory[20] implicate the methyltransferases in the mediation of transmembrane signals from messages such as neurotransmitters, peptide hormones, lectins, and immunoglobulins. They have suggested that these messages activate transferase I, which results in an increase in PC, which leads to increased fluidity and initiation of a cascade of events such as increased Ca^{2+} and adenosine 3',5'-cyclic monophosphate (cAMP), and release of arachidonic acid and histamine.[20]

Transmethylase I enzyme activity was compared in vitamin E-deficient and vitamin E-supplemented ghosts. Membranes were prepared by following the established procedures.[21,22] The ghosts were suspended in 25 mM tris-glycylglycine, 5 mM $MgCl_2$, and 0.5 M ethylenediaminetetraacetic acid (EDTA) at pH 8.0 (1.4 ml buffer for 2.0 of cells lysed). The methylation was carried out according to the procedure of Hirata and Axelrod.[21] Fifty microliters of the membrane suspension were incubated with 4 μM SAM (specific activity = 11.1 Ci/mmole) in a final volume of 112 μl. Extraction of phospholipids with $CHCl_3$:CH_3OH:HCl (2:1:0.02) was carried out according to the procedure of Appel.[22] Identification of PL was done on silica gel thin-layer chromatography (TLC) with n-propanol:propionic acid:$CHCl_3$:H_2O (3:2:2:1) as previously described.[22] Intact RBCs were also incubated with L-[methyl^{3}H] methionine (s.a. = 12 Ci/mmole) as follows: 25 μl of packed RBCs were incubated with phosphate buffer pH 7.2 and 3.2 nmoles (40 μCi) of labeled methionine in a final volume of 100 μl. The cells were then lysed in cold 5 mM phosphate pH 6.8, and membranes were collected, washed, and extracted as described above. As shown in TABLE 4, vitamin E-deficient ghosts synthesize 21–34% less (C^3H_3)-phosphatidyl lipids than do supplemented ghosts. When intact, washed RBCs were incubated with ^{3}H-methionine (TABLE 4, experiment 6), similar results were obtained. Deficient cells incorporated 27% less radiolabel in PL than did supplemented cells. PE was not limiting in the deficient cells. When exogenous PE was added to the incubation, there was no enhancement of the amount of radiolabeled PL synthesized. However, this does not preclude the possibility that the exogenously added PE was not available to

TABLE 4

C^3H_3 INCORPORATION INTO PHOSPHOLIPIDS*

Experiment	Ghosts	RBC	Incubation (minutes)	Vitamin E Status		Difference (%)
				(+)	(−)	
1	Ghosts		35	4.41	3.49	21.0
2	Ghosts		35	4.88	3.76	22.9
3	Ghosts		35	5.48	3.62	34.0
4	Ghosts		35	4.80	3.60	25.1
5	Ghosts		90	9.20	6.71	27.1
6		RBC	75	0.392	0.284	27.5

*Values are expressed as cpm/mg protein $\times 10^4$.

TABLE 5

DISTRIBUTION OF C³H₃-PHOSPHOLIPIDS*

Vitamin E Status	MMPE	DMPE	PC
Deficient	2811 (23.1)	1980 (16.3)	7383 (60.6)
Supplemental	4200 (24.5)	2942 (17.2)	9971 (58.3)

*Values are expressed as cpm/mg ghost protein. Values in parentheses are the relative percentages of radioactivity of each phosphatidyl lipid.

the enzyme. The relative distribution of radiolabeled MMPE, DMPE, and PC was compared in the deficient and supplemented ghosts after incubation with ³H-SAM. Essentially there was no difference in the relative distribution of the intermediates and PC in the deficient or supplemented ghosts (TABLE 5). At higher levels of ³H-SAM (200 μM vs. 4 μM), there was no difference between the deficient or supplemented ghosts. This may indicate that the observed difference in PC formation results from a decreased affinity of the enzyme for SAM, which is compensated for when the reaction is carried out at high levels of SAM.

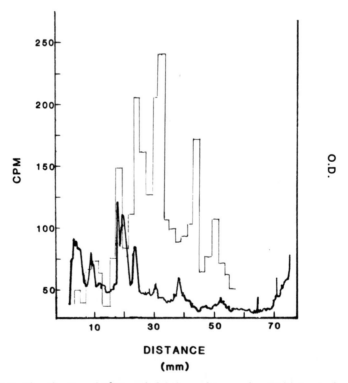

FIGURE 5. Identification of C³H₃ methylated membrane polypeptides in monkey RBCs. The membranes were methylated as described in the text and subjected to SDS PAGE according to Fairbanks and Avruch.[29] The smooth curve represents a protein stain densitometric tracing superimposed on the radioactive profile.

Protein Methylase II

S-Adenosylmethionine:protein-carboxyl-O-methyl transferase (EC 2.1.1.24) methylates (esterifies) free carboxyl groups of aspartic acid in specific protein acceptors.[23-25] The RBC protein methylase is cytoplasmic, but all the acceptors are localized on the cytoplasmic face of the membrane.[26] Esterification of membrane components has the net effect of reducing the overall anionic character of the membrane.[27] The charge change alters membrane properties. There is an esterase that hydrolyzes the methyl ester, and this enzyme system may serve as a subtle regulatory control mechanism. We have monitored the protein methylation in deficient and supplemented RBCs. Protein methylation was carried out essentially unmodified according to the procedure of Terwilliger and Clarke.[28] RBCs were washed, and to 0.1 ml of packed RBCs, 0.01 ml of C^3H_3-SAM was added at a final concentration of 4.6 μM. Samples were frozen, thawed, and incubated at 37°C for 35 minutes. After incubation membranes were washed, collected, and extracted according to the above procedure.[28] The washed membranes were solubilized with 0.5 ml of 10 mM acetic acid and 2.5% sodium dodecyl sulfate (SDS). Acid SDS polyacrylamide gel electrophoresis (PAGE) was carried out

TABLE 6

COMPARISON OF C^3H_3-PROTEINS IN VITAMIN E-DEFICIENT
AND SUPPLEMENTED RBC MEMBRANES

SDS PAGE Peak Number	Assigned Band or Molecular Weight	E−/E+	
		In Vitro	*In Vivo*
I	band 2.1	—	0.64
II	band 3	0.57	0.70
III	band 4.1	0.60	0.73
IV	56K	0.82	0.71
V	32.5K	0.71	0.76
VI	23.2K	0.64	0.62

according to the procedure of Fairbanks and Avruch.[29] Methylation with intact RBCs was carried out as described by Freitag and Clarke,[30] and the molecular weights assigned by comparison with proteins of known molecular weight (FIGURE 5). The amount of label incorporated into proteins is reduced (TABLE 6). When C^3H_3 ghosts are electrophoresed in SDS PAGE, we see that corresponding protein peaks from deficient cells contain less radioactivity than do proteins derived from supplemented cells.

CONCLUSIONS

We have identified biochemical alterations in the membrane of RBCs from vitamin E-deficient rhesus monkeys. (1) Band 3, a transmembrane protein found associated with GAPDH, is modified by vitamin E deficiency. There is less GAPDH bound to band 3 in the deficient state. This decreased association results from modification of band 3 and not GAPDH. (2) In addition, conversion of PE to MMPE is reduced in the vitamin E-deficient RBC. Reduced conversion does not appear to result from reduced PE. (3) The methylation of specific membrane and membrane-associated proteins is also reduced in the E-deficient RBC. The reduced accessibility or availability of the aspartic carboxyls in the specific protein acceptors, the reduced lipid transferase I activity, and the altered band 3-GAPDH interaction may result from conformational changes in these proteins. These might be allosteric changes induced by changes in the surrounding lipid compartments of the membrane. Alternatively, these changes may result from direct modification of the protein molecules such as disulfide formation or other oxidative cross-linkages, or possibly destruction of amino acid residues. The work of Sayare[31] would strongly suggest that in the example of GAPDH-band 3 interaction, oxidative cross-linkage of band 3 with hemoglobin may explain decreased GAPDH binding. At this point it is attractive to speculate on the relationship between the altered properties of the membrane proteins as monitored by altered methyl ester formation and the observed changes in deformability and fragility of the vitamin E-deficient RBC. Perhaps this may represent conformational or structural changes in those proteins that are necessary for maintenance of the native membrane structure. Interestingly, the markers measured on the external face of the membrane are not altered by low vitamin E status (e.g., acetylcholinesterase, DIDS binding). Based on these observations we propose as a working hypothesis that the sites of membrane damage in vitamin E-deficient RBCs are on the cytoplasmic face of the membrane, closer to the source of the reactive radical species.

REFERENCES

1. McCay, P. B. & M. M. King. 1980. In Vitamin E, A Comprehensive Treatise. L. J. Machlin, Ed.: 289–319. Marcel Dekker. New York, N.Y.
2. Menzel, D. B. 1980. In Vitamin E, A Comprehensive Treatise. L. J. Machlin, Ed.: 373–494. Marcel Dekker. New York, N.Y.
3. Walton, J. R. & L. Packer. 1980. In Vitamin E, A Comprehensive Treatise. L. J. Machlin, Ed.: 495–518. Marcel Dekker. New York, N.Y.
4. Chiu, D., B. Lubin & S. B. Shohet. 1981. In Free Radicals in Biology. W. A. Pryor, Ed. 5: 115–154. Academic Press, Inc. New York, N.Y.
5. Tappel, A. L. 1953. Arch. Biochem. Biophys. 44: 378–395.
6. Koppenol, W. H. & J. Butler. 1977. FEBS Lett. 83: 1–6.
7. Weaver, R., B. Owdeeja & B. F. Van Gelder. 1973. Biochim. Biophys. Acta 302: 475–478.
8. Kant, J. A. & T. L. Steck. 1973. J. Biol. Chem. 248: 8457–8464.
9. Liu, S-C., C. Fairbanks & J. Palek. 1977. Biochemistry 16: 4066–4074.
10. Steck, T. L. & J. A. Kant. 1973. Methods Enzymol. 31: 172–180.
11. Steck, T. L., et al. 1978. Biochemistry 17: 1216–1222.
12. Carraway, K. L. & B. C. Shin. 1972. J. Biol. Chem. 247: 2102–2108.
13. McDaniel, C. F. & M. E. Kirtley. 1974. J. Biol. Chem. 249: 6478–6485.
14. Shin, B. C. & K. L. Carraway. 1973. J. Biol. Chem. 248: 1436–1444.
15. Bieri, J. G., R. P. Evarts & S. Thorp. 1977. Am. J. Clin. Nutr. 30: 686–690.
16. Bjornson, L., C. Gniewkorwski & H. J. Kayden. 1975. J. Lipid Res. 16: 39–53.
17. Cabantchick, Z. I., P. A. Knaut & A. Rothstein. 1978. Biochim. Biophys. Acta 515: 239–302.
18. Lefkowitz, R. J. 1976. Life Sci. 18: 461–472.
19. Williams, L. T., L. Jarrett & R. J. Lefkowitz. 1976. J. Biol. Chem. 251: 3096–3104.
20. Hirata, F. & J. Axelrod. 1980. Science 209: 1082–1090.
21. Hirata, F. & J. Axelrod. 1978. Proc. Nat. Acad. Sci. USA 75: 2348–2352.
22. Moore, B. R. & S. H. Appel. 1980. Exp. Neurol. 70: 380–391.
23. DiLiberto, E. J. & J. Axelrod. 1974. Proc. Nat. Acad. Sci. USA 71: 1701–1704.
24. Kim, S. & W. K. Paik. 1970. J. Biol. Chem. 245: 1806–1813.
25. Janson, C. A. & S. Clarke. 1980. J. Biol. Chem. 255: 11640–11643.

26. GALLETH, P., W. K. PAIK & S. KIM. 1979. Eur. J. Biochem. **97:** 221–227.
27. KIM, S. & W. K. PAIK. 1976. Experientia **32:** 982–984.
28. TERWILLIGER, T. C. & S. CLARKE. 1981. J. Biol. Chem. **256:** 3067–3076.
29. FAIRBANKS, G. & J. AVRUCH. 1972. J. Supramol. Struct. **1:** 66–75.
30. FREITAG, C. & S. CLARKE. 1981. J. Biol. Chem. **256:** 6102–6108.
31. SAYARE, M., M. FIKIET & J. PAULUS. Ann. N.Y. Acad. Sci. (This volume.)

DISCUSSION

K. C. HAYES (*Harvard School of Public Health, Boston, Mass.*): Have you tried to explain some of your conformational or enzyme changes based on phospholipid or cholesterol changes in the membrane?

S. S. SHAPIRO: No, we've only looked at the relative distribution of PE and PC, and we do not see a measurable change. The methylase pathway is a minor pathway in terms of the biosynthetic route and is envisioned more as a regulatory pathway controlling fluidity of the membrane.

A. T. QUINTANILHA (*University of California, Berkeley, Calif.*): Your extraction of band 6 from the membranes using high ionic strengths suggests that the interaction between band 6 and band 3 is probably an electrical one. When you do your reconstitutions, have you ever tried to change the ionic strength of the medium or the pH to see whether the reduced binding of band 6 may be due to a change in surface charge of the membrane?

S. S. SHAPIRO: No, that's a good point.

S. B. SHOHET (*University of California, San Francisco, Calif.*): Could you tell us just what percentage you observe in regard to PC synthesis from PE in terms of total economy of the cell.

S. S. SHAPIRO: Since we are using radiolabeled material, the amount of PC we are making under our experimental conditions is in the picomole range. We have not compared the pathways in terms of total output, and it's been reported in the literature that this is a minor pathway. It may be that physiologically, this is not important in terms of affecting total PC, but it is a window to look at what's happening inside the membrane as a result of vitamin E deficiency.

S. B. SHOHET: One might expect that in terms of the fluidity or changes in the physical properties of the membrane that you alluded to, the fatty acids would be even more important than the carbon subchain and the change from PE to PC might be comparatively unimportant.

E. A. RACHMILEWITZ (*Hadassah University Hospital, Jerusalem, Israel*): If you take your E-deficient red cells and add vitamin E, are you able to correct the changes that you had seen?

S. S. SHAPIRO: We've done that for the GAPDH–band 3 interaction, and it doesn't. Apparently, the modification has happened before we ever rupture the cell.

E. A. RACHMILEWITZ: And the other parameters that you have prescribed?

S. S. SHAPIRO: We haven't done it with other parameters.

E. A. RACHMILEWITZ: Do you think that this could be some irreversible damage?

S. S. SHAPIRO: Yes, and that it is happening *in vivo*.

M. McKENNA (*National Institutes of Health, Bethesda, Md.*): Could you comment a little more on the changes in band 2 and whether or not you saw differences in the absolute amount of band 2. I noticed in Dr. Sayare's slide that it looked like there were changes, but he didn't comment on that.

S. S. SHAPIRO: We have not monitored total protein. When we just look at the gel, there are no obvious differences between the deficient and the supplemented groups. Only with the sophisticated two-dimensional technique that Dr. Sayare used were changes apparent.

VITAMIN E DEFICIENCY: ITS EFFECT ON PLATELET-VASCULAR INTERACTION IN VARIOUS PATHOLOGIC STATES*

Marie J. Stuart

Division of Hematology-Oncology
Department of Pediatrics
State University of New York
Upstate Medical Center
Syracuse, New York 13210

Vitamin E is an essential nutrient in man. A deficiency of this vitamin in both animals and man is manifested by a variety of symptoms that are highly variable from species to species. In man, vitamin E deficiency has been associated with the hemolytic anemia of low-birth-weight infants, the shortened red cell life span that occurs as a consequence of prolonged impairment of fat absorption, and the pathological findings in patients with hereditary abetalipoproteinemia.

To place the hemostatic changes induced by vitamin E deficiency in perspective, it is helpful to review platelet and vascular metabolism of arachidonic acid.[1] Arachidonic acid is released from platelet membrane phospholipid in response to various stimuli and can be converted by either the lipoxygenase or cyclooxygenase pathway. The lipoxygenase converts arachidonic acid to 12 L-hydroperoxy-5,8,14-eicosatetraenoic acid (HPETE), which is further reduced to the final product HETE. Fatty acid cyclooxygenase converts arachidonic acid to prostaglandins (PG) and their metabolites. The first recognizable intermediates in this pathway are the cyclic endoperoxides prostaglandins G_2 and H_2. Thromboxane A_2, the most potent proaggregatory metabolite of arachidonic acid identified to date, is formed enzymatically from either of these prostaglandins. Thromboxane A_2 is unstable, undergoing rapid hydrolysis to thromboxane B_2, a stable substance. A major alternative pathway for metabolism of the cyclic endoperoxides is by further degradation to a C_{17} hydroxy fatty acid and malonyldialdehyde (MDA), a three-carbon fragment. Smith and associates have previously shown that platelet MDA may be used as an indicator of platelet prostaglandin synthesis.[2] In the endothelium of the vessel wall, conversion of the cyclic endoperoxides to prostacyclin (PGI_2) occurs. Because thromboxane A_2 is proaggregatory and prothrombotic whereas PGI_2 is antiaggregatory and antithrombotic, a balance between the biosynthesis of these two opposing compounds plays a significant role in normal hemostasis. Besides its potent antiplatelet effect, PGI_2 is also a strong relaxant of vascular smooth muscle *in vitro* and a potent vasodilator *in vivo*. These effects of PGI_2 have important implications in maintaining normal vascular patency, and have formed the basis for the therapeutic administration of PGI_2 in various pathological conditions associated with vascular insufficiency. In addition, Remuzzi and coworkers have suggested that pathologic states associated with microthrombosis and microvascular insufficiency may be related to a deficiency or total lack of plasma constituents necessary for normal PGI_2 synthesis by vascular tissue.[3] The effects of vitamin E deficiency on platelet and

*Supported by a grant from The National Foundation March of Dimes.

vascular arachidonic acid metabolism in certain physiologic and pathologic states associated with the neonate and child form the basis of this report.

MATERIALS AND METHODS

Assay for Plasma PGI$_2$-Regenerating Activity in the Neonate and Adult

Blood samples were collected after informed consent from 11 normal adult controls aged 24 to 36 years who had not ingested any medication for 10 days before evaluation, and from 11 normal full-term neonates. All infants weighed more than 2,500 g and were born of healthy mothers after full-term pregnancies and uneventful deliveries. Immediately after delivery, clamps were placed on the umbilical cord, a 19-gauge needle was inserted into the umbilical vein, and blood was drawn into a plastic syringe. Blood samples were also obtained on 8 infants aged 3 to 5 months.

Blood samples were mixed with 0.126 M trisodium citrate. The adult blood was anticoagulated by using 9 parts of blood to 1 part citrate. To adjust for the higher hematocrit of cord blood, the blood-citrate ratio in the latter experiments was 11:1. Platelet-free plasma was obtained by centrifugation of the citrated blood for 15 minutes at 1,800 × g.

The capacity of plasma (control adult versus neonate) to stimulate the generation of PGI$_2$-like activity was performed by the method of Remuzzi,[3] using "exhausted" human umbilical arterial rings obtained from normal, full-term deliveries. The umbilical arteries were thoroughly cleaned, cut into fine rings, and kept in Hanks balanced salt solution (HBSS) without calcium (pH 7.4) at 0°C. Rings (30 to 45 mg) were incubated with 120 μl of HBSS with calcium (pH 8.1) for 3 minutes at 22°C. Aliquots (30 μl) of the supernatant were added to 70-μl samples of normal platelet-rich plasma (300,000 platelets/μl), and the mixture was incubated for 1 minute before the addition of adenosine diphosphate (ADP) at a final concentration of 3.0 μM. Prostacyclinlike activity was evaluated in a Payton dual-channel aggregometer by the bioassay described by Moncada.[4] Antiaggregatory activity was detected in all umbilical vessels evaluated. The umbilical arterial rings were then washed several times with HBSS (pH 7.4) until no antiaggregatory activity could be detected as evaluated by the above method. The exhausted vascular rings were then incubated for 30 minutes at 37°C with 120 μl plasma (control adult versus neonate) in each of 11 sets of experiments, with incubations being performed in duplicate. Under these conditions, plasma from the normal control adults stimulated the exhausted vascular rings to generate PGI$_2$-like, or antiaggregatory, activity. The amount of antiaggregatory activity of both the adult control and neonatal plasma was expressed as ng of PGI$_2$ per mg wet tissue by extrapolation from a dose-response standard curve obtained concomitantly with PGI$_2$ (The Upjohn Co., Kalamazoo, Mich.). PGI$_2$ activity was further characterized according to previous criteria.[4] Mixing experiments were also performed in which 1 part neonatal plasma was incubated with 1 part adult control plasma, and the plasma PGI$_2$-regenerating activity of the resultant mixture was determined and contrasted to control plasmas diluted 1:1 with HBSS.

In six further paired experiments, vitamin E was evaluated *in vitro* for its ability to potentiate the effect of normal neonatal plasma to regenerate PGI$_2$-like activity. Vitamin E (all-rac-α-tocopherol in vehicle; Hoffmann-La Roche, Nutley, N.J.) at a final concentration of 0.2 mg/ml, or the E vehicle alone, was added to neonatal plasma before incubation with exhausted umbilical arterial rings. After the incubation procedure previously outlined, the ability of neonatal plasma in the presence of either vitamin E or E vehicle to generate PGI_2-like activity in the exhausted vascular tissue was evaluated. PGI_2-regenerating ability was also assayed in duplicate from blood samples obtained from eight infants aged 3 to 5 months.

Plasma vitamin E was assayed by the method of Quaife.[5] Statistical comparison of results was made using the paired and unpaired Student t-tests.

Hemostasis in the Diabetic Mother and the Infant of the Diabetic Mother (IDM)

Blood samples were obtained from 19 control mother-neonate pairs (group 1) and 22 pairs where maternal diabetes mellitus was present (groups 2 and 3). Classification of maternal diabetes mellitus was established according to the standard criteria and included class A ($n = 5$), class B ($n = 5$), class C ($n = 6$), class D ($n = 3$), class F ($n = 1$), and class R ($n = 2$). Maternal ages ranged between 18 and 36 years in the control group and 18 and 35 years in the patient groups. All infants weighed more than 2,500 grams and were delivered by elective cesarean section. Mean gestational ages of both controls and IDM were similar at 38.2 ± 1.3 and 37.6 ± 1.9 weeks respectively. No control or diabetic mother had ingested aspirin within 2 weeks of delivery, nor received any drug recognized to affect platelet function.

Immediately after delivery, clamps were placed on the umbilical cord. A 19-gauge needle was inserted into the umbilical vein, and blood was drawn into a plastic syringe with a two-syringe technique. At the same time, maternal blood was drawn from the antecubital vein. All blood samples were anticoagulated with 0.1 M buffered citrate anticoagulant in a ratio of 9 parts of blood to 1 part of citrate in the adult, and 11:1 in the neonate. Hemoglobin estimation and platelet counts were performed by Coulter counter. Platelet lipid peroxide formation induced by N-ethyl maleimide (NEM) (1 mM) was determined by means of a modification of the method of Okuma et al.,[6] where the products of lipid peroxidation were measured as MDA after its reaction with 2-thiobarbituric acid.[7] Platelet aggregation studies were performed as previously described,[8] with platelet-rich plasma (PRP) prepared by centrifuging the citrated blood at $150 \times g$ (800 rpm) at $22°C$ for 8 minutes and adjusting the platelet count to approximately 200,000 to 300,000/ mm^3. Besides evaluating the PRP for spontaneous aggregation, the aggregating agents employed to induce platelet aggregation in the adult included ADP (0.05, 0.2, 0.8, and 1.6 μM final concentrations) and epinephrine (0.005, 0.01, 0.04, and 6.2 μM final concentrations). The PRP obtained from the neonate was evaluated for spontaneous aggregation and also for aggregation induced by ADP (3, 6, and 9 μM final concentrations). All aggregation experiments were performed with a Payton dual-channel aggregometer, and the PRP was kept in full, tightly capped plastic test tubes prior to use. All aggregation studies were performed within 120 minutes of platelet harvesting. Platelet hyperfunction or hyperaggregability was said to occur in the maternal PRP if either spontaneous aggregation (i.e., an increase in light transmission of $<25\%$ over baseline, in the presence of microscopic gross platelet aggregates, that occurred within 10 minutes of stirring) or increased sensitivity to the aggregating agents ADP and epinephrine was present. Increased sensitivity to ADP or epinephrine was defined as irreversible platelet aggregation at ADP concentrations of <0.8 μM and at epinephrine concentrations of <0.4 μM. Platelet hyperfunction or hyperaggregability was said

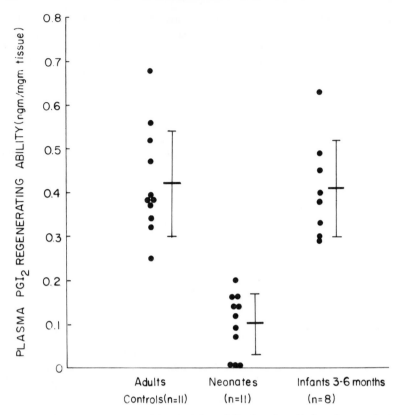

FIGURE 1. PGI$_2$-regenerating activity of adult, umbilical cord, and infant plasmas. Activity is expressed as ng/mg wet weight of "exhausted" human umbilical arteries. Mean ±1 SD. (Reproduced from Reference 26 by permission of The Williams and Wilkins Company.)

to occur in the PRP from the neonate if either spontaneous aggregation occurred (as previously defined) or irreversible platelet aggregation occurred at ADP concentrations of <9 μM. These concentrations of aggregating agents were chosen since previous evaluation of adult and neonatal populations in our laboratory had shown that normal control subjects did not demonstrate irreversible platelet aggregation at concentrations below these threshold levels.

Assessment of the coagulation and fibrinolytic system included routine determination of the prothrombin and partial thromboplastin times, fibrinogen, factor VIII levels, and assays for fibrin-degradation products (FDP).[9] Plasminogen levels were performed by radial immunodiffusion, and plasma vitamin E by the method of Quaife and associates.[5] Blood glucose and cholesterol were performed by means of standard assay techniques.

Platelet Function and Survival in Vitamin E Deficiency

The studies were performed on four children with cystic fibrosis and exocrine pancreatic insufficiency. The patients were aged 1.5, 2, 8, and 17 years respectively. The patients were on no medications at the time of evaluation except for pancreatic enzyme supplements. They were restudied following periods of vitamin E supplementation (100 units orally) that ranged from 1 month to 5 months.

Initial and follow-up evaluations included standard techniques for the measurement of hemoglobin concentration, and platelet counts. Standard techniques were also used for the measurement of platelet aggregation with ADP, epinephrine, and collagen. Platelet MDA formation was evaluated by the method of Okuma,[6] platelet life span was determined by the nonradioisotopic method of Stuart and associates,[7] and plasma vitamin E levels were assayed by the method of Quaife.[5]

RESULTS

PGI$_2$-Regenerating Activity of Neonatal and Adult Plasma

As depicted in FIGURE 1, adult platelet-poor plasma stimulated exhausted human umbilical arterial rings to produce 0.42 ± 0.12 [±1 standard deviation (SD)]

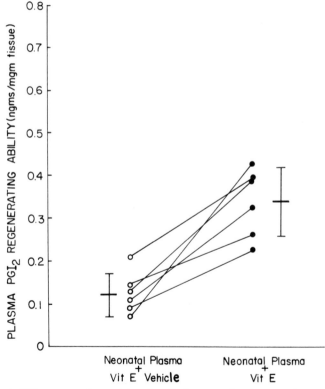

FIGURE 2. PGI$_2$-regenerating activity of cord plasma in the absence of vitamin E (open circles) and in the presence of 0.2 mg/ml of vitamin E (filled circles). Results of six paired experiments are depicted. Activity is expressed as ng/mg wet weight of "exhausted" human umbilical arteries. Mean ±1 SD. (Reproduced from Reference 26 by permission of The Williams and Wilkins Company.)

ng of PGI_2-like activity per mg wet weight of tissue. This value was significantly greater (p < 0.001) than the PGI_2-like generating ability of normal neonatal plasma (0.10 ± 0.07 ng/mg). The deficiency in plasma PGI_2-regenerating activity did not appear to be due to the presence of an inhibitor in neonatal plasma because appropriate correction (0.24 ± 0.06) was observed in the 1:1 mixing experiments. By three to five months of life, the PGI_2-regenerating ability of plasma had normalized (0.41 ± 0.11 ng/mg) and was similar to the values present in adult control plasma.

FIGURE 2 depicts the results of the six further paired experiments in which vitamin E was evaluated in vitro for its ability to potentiate the PGI_2-regenerating capacity of normal neonatal plasma. In the presence of the vitamin E vehicle, cord blood regenerating activity was similar to that of cord blood alone (0.12 ± 0.05 ng/mg). However, the addition of vitamin E in vitro to neonatal plasma significantly (p < 0.01) increased its ability to regenerate PGI_2-like activity (0.34 ± 0.08 ng/mg). Mean plasma vitamin E level in the 11 adult controls was 1.26 ± 0.56 mg/dl, which was significantly higher than the value obtained in the neonates (0.28 ± 0.15 mg/dl).

Evaluation of Hemostasis in the Diabetic Mother and the IDM

No control group 1 mother demonstrated either spontaneous aggregation or platelet hyperaggregability as previously defined. Using platelet malonyldialdehyde production (following exposure to N-ethyl maleimide) as an indicator of platelet prostaglandin endoperoxide formation, control group 1 mothers demonstrated a value of 3.18 ± 0.33 (1 SD) nmoles per 10^9 platelets (TABLE 1), which is similar to the normal adult control values we have established previously.[9] The 22 mothers with diabetes were subdivided into groups 2 and 3, depending on the results of the platelet aggregation studies. Group 2 consisted of 15 diabetic mothers in whom either spontaneous platelet aggregation or platelet hyperaggregability was present and included diabetic patients of the following classes: A (n = 3), B (n = 3), C (n = 4), D (n = 2), F (n = 1), and R (n = 2). As depicted in TABLE 1, when platelet malonyldialdehyde was used as an indicator of endoperoxide

TABLE 1

HEMOSTATIC VALUES FOR THE THREE MATERNAL GROUPS*

Test Performed	Group 1	Group 2	Group 3
Hemoglobin (g/dl)	11.9 ± 0.9 (19)	12.1 ± 0.9 (15)	12.2 ± 1.1 (7)
Platelet count (per mm³)	266 ± 60 (19)	252 ± 42 (15)	239 ± 51 (7)
Platelet MDA (nmol/10⁹ plts)	3.18 ± 0.33 (19)	†3.88 ± 0.23 (15)	3.14 ± 0.18 (7)
Fibrinogen (mg/dl)	349 ± 70 (13)	417 ± 125 (10)	365 ± 117 (6)
Factor VIII (%)	190 ± 98 (13)	228 ± 147 (10)	243 ± 68 (5)
Plasminogen (mg/dl)	14.6 ± 3.2 (13)	15.4 ± 3.5 (10)	15.1 ± 4.6 (5)
FDP (µg/ml)	4.7 ± 3.7 (10)	6.3 ± 6.9 (12)	5.4 ± 8.5 (5)
Vitamin E (mg/dl)	1.6 ± 0.6 (15)	1.5 ± 0.7 (13)	1.3 ± 0.3 (7)
Blood glucose (mg/dl)	132 ± 24 (19)	207 ± 71 (13)	188 ± 99 (7)
Serum cholesterol (mg/dl)	186 ± 37 (13)	207 ± 57 (10)	185 ± 37 (6)

*Values are means ± standard deviations. Numbers in parentheses equal number of patients evaluated for each assay performed. Group 1, normal control subjects; group 2, diabetics with platelet hyperfunction; group 3, diabetics with normal platelet function.

†Difference statistically significant by the unpaired t-test when compared to group 1.

TABLE 2

HEMOSTATIC VALUES FOR THE THREE INFANT GROUPS*

Test Performed	Group 1	Group 2	Group 3
Hemoglobin (g/dl)	16.0 ± 1.6 (19)	16.5 ± 1.0 (15)	15.6 ± 1.3 (7)
Platelet count (per mm³)	276 ± 68 (19)	248 ± 94 (14)	312 ± 32 (7)
Platelet MDA (nmol/10⁹ plts)	2.49 ± 0.6 (19)	†3.49 ± 0.57 (15)	2.6 ± 0.61 (7)
Fibrinogen (mg/dl)	182 ± 32 (13)	172 ± 21 (8)	165 ± 46 (5)
Factor VIII (%)	51 ± 20 (13)	56 ± 37 (8)	51 ± 15 (5)
Plasminogen (mg/dl)	8.2 ± 2.4 (15)	†4.4 ± 2.1 (8)	†5.3 ± 0.5 (5)
FDP (μg/ml)	3.0 ± 3.2 (10)	2.1 ± 1.6 (10)	3.1 ± 4.6 (5)
Vitamin E (mg/dl)	0.29 ± 0.12 (11)	†0.18 ± 0.13 (10)	0.22 ± 0.09 (6)
Blood glucose (mg/dl)	143 ± 76 (10)	126 ± 66 (14)	132 ± 63 (7)
Serum cholesterol (mg/dl)	69 ± 9 (13)	70 ± 25 (10)	88 ± 30 (5)

*Values are means ± SD. Numbers in parentheses equal number of patients evaluated for each assay performed. Group 1, control neonates; group 2, IDM with platelet hyperfunction; group 3, IDM with normal platelet function.

†Differences statistically significant by the unpaired t-test when compared to group 1.

formation, values were markedly increased in group 2 mothers, when compared to group 1 controls (3.88 ± 0.23; p < 0.001). Group 3 consisted of the remaining 7 mothers with diabetes mellitus in whom platelet aggregation was similar to that of group 1 controls without evidence for either spontaneous aggregation or platelet hyperaggregability. This group included the following diabetic classes: A (n = 2), B (n = 2), C (n = 2), and D (n = 1). Malonyldialdehyde production was normal in this group (3.14 ± 0.18 nmoles per 10⁹ platelets). Apart from the presence of platelet hyperaggregability and increased prostaglandin endoperoxide formation in group 2 mothers, there appeared to be no differences in any of the other hemostatic parameters evaluated. Since hypercholesterolemia and vitamin E deficiency can lead to platelet hyperfunction and a prothrombotic tendency, serum cholesterols and plasma vitamin E levels were obtained in all groups evaluated. As shown in TABLE 1, no evidence of significant differences in values was seen in group 2 diabetic mothers who evinced platelet hyperfunction when compared to maternal groups 1 and 3.

Results of the hemostatic evaluations of the infants born to groups 1, 2, and 3 mothers are depicted in TABLE 2. Although no evidence for platelet hyperaggregability (as defined under Methods) was present in group 1 and 3 neonates, platelet hyperaggregability and increased production of malonyldialdehyde was seen in group 2 neonates (p < 0.01). The finding of platelet hyperfunction in group 3 neonates was associated with a significant decrease (p < 0.05) in plasma vitamin E levels in group 2 when compared to control group 1 neonates. Cholesterol levels remained similar in all groups evaluated. Among the coagulation factors evaluated, although no differences in factors I and VIII and FDP were found, plasminogen values were significantly decreased in groups 2 and 3 neonates when compared to group 1 controls.

Platelet Function and Survival in Vitamin E Deficiency

TABLE 3 depicts the platelet function studies in all four patients with vitamin E deficiency prior to therapy. Plasma vitamin E levels during the period of E deficiency were markedly decreased (0.1 to 0.3 mg/dl). Besides thrombocytosis, which is a hallmark of the E-deficient state, platelet hyperaggregability to ADP, epinephrine, and collagen was present, and N-ethyl maleimide–induced platelet MDA formation was increased in three out of four patients. Platelet life span measurements revealed a normal half-life of 5 and 4.5 days in the two children aged 1.5 and 2 years respectively (cases 1 and 2). However, in the 8- and 17-year-old patients with vitamin E deficiency (cases 3 and 4), platelet survival was decreased with a half-life of 2.4 days and 2.0 days respectively. No abnormalities were detected in the other hematologic measurements monitored. Following E repletion, when plasma E levels were in the normal range, platelet counts and platelet aggregation studies had returned to normal. In the two children with E deficiency and shortened platelet life span, platelet survivals were repeated following therapy with vitamin E. At five months following E repletion, platelet survivals were completely normal at 4.7 and 4.2 days respectively. The normalization in platelet survival following vitamin E repletion in both these patients occurred without any other changes in their primary disease status.

TABLE 3

PLATELET FUNCTION STUDIES IN FOUR CHILDREN WITH VITAMIN E DEFICIENCY

Measurement	Normal Value	Case 1	Case 2	Case 3	Case 4
Sex		M	F	M	M
Age (years)		1.5	2	8	17
Plasma vitamin E (mg/dl)	0.5–1.5	0.3	0.3	0.1	0.1
Platelet count ($10^3 \times mm^3$)	150–350	720	690	455	540
Lowest ADP concentration inducing biphasic aggregation (μM)	1.6	0.1	0.2	0.05	0.1
Lowest epinephrine concentration inducing biphasic aggregation (μM)	0.4	0.05	0.05	0.01	0.01
Lowest collagen concentration inducing 50% aggregation	1:16	1:64	1:128	1:256	1:256
Total NEM-induced lipid peroxides (nmoles MDA/10^9 plts)	2.6–3.6	3.6	4.5	3.9	4.0
Platelet half-life (days)	2.9–5.9	5	4.5	2.4	2.0

DISCUSSION

Abnormalities in platelet function or platelet-vascular interaction have thus been demonstrated to occur in three conditions associated with low plasma levels of vitamin E. We have shown that patients with an impairment in fat absorption (i.e., cystic fibrosis) who have not been supplemented with vitamin E demonstrated enhanced platelet aggregation and malonyldialdehyde (MDA) formation, and in some cases a decrease in platelet life span (TABLE 3). Following E repletion when plasma vitamin E levels were in the normal range, platelet aggregation studies and survival measurements had returned to normal, suggesting a cause-

and-effect relationship. In the hemostatic evaluations performed on maternal diabetics and their offspring, an interesting and potentially important finding was the significantly lower level of plasma vitamin E in the IDM (group 2) who demonstrated platelet hyperaggregability and increased platelet MDA formation, when compared to group 1 control neonates with normal platelet function (TABLE 2). The third finding is that neonatal plasma has a decreased ability to stimulate PGI$_2$-like activity in vascular tissue that has been "exhausted," i.e., washed free of all endogenous bioassayable PGI$_2$. This deficiency appears in part to be due to the decreased antioxidant potential of neonatal plasma, since vitamin E *in vitro* enhanced the ability of neonatal plasma to regenerate PGI$_2$-like activity (FIGURE 2).

Khurshid and associates have described an infant with vitamin E deficiency and a platelet functional defect.[10] At 16 months of age, this infant with hepatic fibrosis and cholestatic jaundice demonstrated defective prothrombin consumption, thrombocytosis, and abnormal ristocetin-induced platelet aggregation. Aggregation with ADP, thrombin, epinephrine, and collagen was normal, although no effort was made to titrate the concentrations used to demonstrate a possible hyperaggregability to these agents. Following E supplementation, correction of the initially abnormal ristocetin aggregation and prothrombin consumption was observed, although the serum vitamin E level was still abnormal. In 1977, we first described the presence of platelet hyperaggregability to ADP, epinephrine, and collagen in two infants with vitamin E deficiency.[11] Complete reversal of the platelet abnormalities occurred following the attainment of normal plasma vitamin E levels. This report confirms our previous data, and demonstrates two additional findings. When platelet MDA formation was used as an indicator of platelet prostaglandin endoperoxide formation, increased production of this product was found, suggesting enhanced activity of the platelet cyclooxygenase pathway in vitamin E deficiency. These findings are consistent with the data of Machlin and Hope, who demonstrated that in experimentally induced E deficiency in an animal model, collagen-induced platelet aggregation was increased and serum levels of PGE$_2$ and PGF$_{2\alpha}$ were elevated.[12,13] Although our *in vitro* findings are of interest, they cannot be assumed to be synonymous with a hypercoagulable state, since *in vivo* hypercoagulability implies that prothrombotic changes detected in blood *in vitro* are pathogenically important for the development of thrombosis *in vivo*. We, therefore, further determined platelet life span measurements in our four subjects with vitamin E deficiency in an attempt to determine whether the presence of *in vitro* platelet hyperaggregability is associated with an *in vivo* hypercoagulable state.

A number of investigators have evaluated the role of platelet survival and turnover in patients with thromboembolic disorders. A decrease in platelet survival in subgroups of patients with diffuse arterial disease, arterial thrombosis, homocystinuria, vasculitis, valvular heart disease, prosthetic heart valve replacement, recurrent venous thrombosis, and ischemic heart disease has been demonstrated.[14] This reduction in platelet life span is associated with an increased risk of thromboembolism. Although no symptoms or clinical evidence of thrombosis was apparent during the E-deficient state in our patients, thromboses and vascular necrosis have been observed in experimentally induced E deficiency in animals. Nafstad, working with E-deficient piglets, has demonstrated myocardial necrosis accompanied by widespread thrombosis of the myocardial microcirculation.[15] Her studies also suggested the participation of platelet thrombi in the etiology of vascular injury, with the presence of platelets sub- and intraendothelially in the damaged vasculature of the E-deficient animals. A decreased platelet life span was present in two of our study children. These two children possessed the lowest levels of vitamin E, were the most hyperaggregable of the group (TABLE 3), and being the oldest had been vitamin E deficient for the longest period of time. The normalization in platelet survival following E repletion, without any other change in their primary disease status, implicates vitamin E deficiency as the cause of the abnormality in platelet survival. These data support the animal work of Nafstad indicating that platelets participate in the pathological phenomenon accompanying the E-deficient state. Studies of human vitamin E deficiency have so far been limited to premature infants and patients with malabsorptive states. However, relative E deficiency with abnormal tocopherol-to-lipid ratios[16] may also occur in conditions of iron overload or in situations associated with free radical generation. Thus, the finding of platelet hyperaggregability and decreased platelet life span in E deficiency may not be confined to the patient with malabsorption alone, but may have broader implications in the pathogenesis of thromboembolic disease.

In the adult with diabetes mellitus, an increase in platelet proaggregatory thromboxane A_2,[17] together with a decrease in vascular PGI_2 production, has been demonstrated.[18] Evidence from studies in the IDM indicates that similar abnormalities may occur in the offspring of diabetic mothers.[19,20] Using platelet malonyldialdehyde production as an indicator of platelet endoperoxide production, we have shown that a subgroup of maternal diabetics (group 2) demonstrate platelet hyperfunction, i.e., increased platelet aggregability, and increased MDA production. As shown in TABLE 1, we could not demonstrate any differences in fluid phase coagulation factors between these group 2 mothers and either control pregnant women (group 1) or group 3 diabetic mothers who demonstrated normal platelet function. Values for cholesterol and vitamin E were also similar in all maternal groups evaluated. In the evaluation of the neonate (TABLE 2), it was found that group 2 mothers gave birth to offspring with similar evidence of platelet hyperfunction, i.e., platelet hyperaggregability and increased MDA production. An interesting associated finding was the significantly lower levels of vitamin E in the group 2 neonates when compared to group 1 controls. Vitamin E is an antioxidant concerned with the prevention of peroxidative damage to cells and subcellular elements. Since increased peroxidative damage and increased production of lipid peroxides occur in diabetes, the association between the increased production of lipid peroxide platelet products (MDA) and the significant decrease in antioxidant vitamin E in this particular subgroup of infants (group 2) appears relevant. However, since platelet hyperaggregability and increased MDA formation occur in the E-deficiency state per se, it is not possible to separate the cause-and-effect relationship in this study.

Finally, we have shown that the decreased ability of neonatal plasma to regenerate PGI_2-like activity in "exhausted" vascular tissue is in part due to its decreased antioxidant capacity. The only physiologic state associated with hypercoagulability and an increased susceptibility to thrombotic complications occurs in the neonatal period.[21] Various components of the hemostatic mechanism have been previously evaluated in the neonate in an attempt to elucidate the cause of this hypercoagulable state. Fluid phase coagulation factors are either normal (I, V, and VIII) or decreased (II, VII, IX, X, XI, and XII), and platelet function is well recognized to be impaired[22] such that the hypercoagulable state cannot be ascribed to these changes. A deficiency of antithrombin III, the most important of the zymogen inhibitors, is present in the neonate.[23] Inasmuch as familial antithrombin III deficiency predisposes affected individuals to thrombosis, neonatal hypercoagulability has been ascribed to the decrease in the level of antithrombin III that occurs neonatally.

In the hemolytic uremic syndrome and in thrombotic thrombocytopenic purpura, the thrombotic tendency and hypercoagulable state appear to be related to a deficiency in or absence of the ability of plasma to regenerate PGI_2 in exhausted vascular tissue.[3] We have demonstrated a similar abnormality in neonatal plasma. This finding of a decrease in the ability of neonatal plasma to regenerate vascular PGI_2 may provide an explanation for the presence of a normal bleeding time in the newborn and, together with the previously described antithrombin III deficiency, explains the newborn's susceptibility to thrombosis. The nature of the plasma factor regulating prostacyclin or PGI_2 activity has not been characterized at the present time. Our findings suggest that the decrease in activity is not due to a plasma inhibitory factor. The deficiency, however, appears related to the markedly decreased antioxidant potential of neonatal plasma, which in part appears due to the low levels of plasma vitamin E seen in the neonate. Most recently, Okuma has demonstrated that the vessels from vitamin E-deficient rats produced markedly decreased amounts of PGI_2, with a concomitant increase in lipid-peroxidation products.[24] After E repletion, vascular lipid peroxidation decreased and PGI_2 activity returned to normal. Although we did not evaluate vascular thiobarbituric acid–reactive material as an indicator of lipid peroxidation, it is possible that the state of relative E depletion seen in the neonate causes increased lipid peroxidation of vascular tissue, with the net result being a decrease in PGI_2 synthesis. The free-radical scavenger vitamin E, by inhibiting lipid peroxidation, would enhance PGI_2 synthesis. Thus, the results of Okuma et al. are complementary to our findings.

Moncada and associates have previously demonstrated that the generation of PGI_2 is strongly inhibited by 15 hydroperoxy-arachidonic acid.[25] This observation has led them to suggest that inhibition of vascular PGI_2 by lipid peroxides could contribute to those diseases in which excessive lipid peroxidation occurs, such as atherosclerosis. Our finding that vitamin E when added to neonatal plasma in vitro increased its potential for vascular PGI_2 regeneration, together with the previous data, provides a rationale for the use of antioxidants in the prevention and treatment of atherothrombotic disorders.

REFERENCES

1. MONCADA, S. & J. R. VANE. 1979. N. Engl. J. Med. **300:** 1142–1147.
2. SMITH, J. B., C. M. INGERMAN & M. J. SILVER. 1976. J. Lab. Clin. Med. **88:** 167–172.
3. REMUZZI, G., R. MISIANI, D. MARCHESI, M. LIVIO, G. MECCA, G. DEGAETANO & M. B. DONATI. 1978. Lancet **2:** 871–872.
4. MONCADA, S., E. A. HIGGS & J. R. VANE. 1977. Lancet **1:** 18–20.
5. QUAIFE, M. L., N. S. SCRIMSHAW & O. H. LOWRY. 1949. J. Biol. Chem. **180:** 1229–1235.
6. OKUMA, M., M. STEINER & M. BLADINI. 1970. J. Lab. Clin. Med. **75:** 283–296.
7. STUART, M. J., S. MURPHY & F. A. OSKI. 1975. N. Engl. J. Med. **292:** 1310–1313.
8. BORN, G. V. R. 1962. Nature **194:** 927–928.
9. MERSKEY, C., G. J. KLEINER & A. J. JOHNSON. 1966. Blood **28:** 1–18.
10. KHURSHID, M., T. J. LEE, I. R. PEAKE & A. L. BLOOM. 1975. Br. Med. J. **4:** 19–21.
11. LAKE, A. M., M. J. STUART & F. A. OSKI. 1977. J. Pediatr. **90:** 722–725.
12. MACHLIN, L. J., R. FILIPSKI, A. L. WILLIS, D. C. KUHN & M. BRIN. 1975. Proc. Soc. Exp. Biol. Med. **149:** 275–277.
13. HOPE, W. C., C. DALTON, L. J. MACHLIN, R. J. FILIPSKI & F. M. VANE. 1975. Prostaglandins **10:** 557–571.
14. DIDISHEIM, P. & V. FUSTER. 1978. Semin. Hematol. **15:** 55–72.
15. NAFSTAD, I. 1974. Thromb. Res. **5:** 25–28.
16. FARRELL, P. M., J. G. BIERI, J. F. FRATANTONI, R. E. WOOD & P. A. DI SANT'AGNESE. 1977. J. Clin. Invest. **60:** 233–241.

17. HALUSHKA, P. V., R. C. ROGERS, C. B. LOADHOLT & J. A. COLWELL. 1981. J. Lab. Clin. Med. **97:** 87–96.
18. JOHNSON, M., H. E. HARRISON, A. T. RAFTERY & J. B. ELDER. 1979. Lancet **1:** 325. (Letter.)
19. STUART, M. J., H. ELRAD, J. E. GRAEBER, D. O. HAKANSON & S. G. SUNDERJI. 1979. J. Lab. Clin. Med. **94:** 12–17.
20. STUART, M. J., S. G. SUNDERJI & J. B. ALLEN. 1981. J. Lab. Clin. Med. **98:** 412–416.
21. HATHAWAY, W. E. 1975. Semin. Hematol **12:** 175–188.
22. STUART, M. J. 1979. Am. J. Pediatr. Hematol. Oncol. **1:** 227–234.
23. MAHASANDANA, C. & W. E. HATHAWAY. 1973. Pediatr. Res. **7:** 670–673.
24. OKUMA, M., H. TAKAYAMA & H. UCHINO. 1980. Prostaglandins **19:** 527–536.
25. MONCADA, S., R. GRYGLEWSKI, S. BUNTING & J. R. VANE. 1976. Prostaglandins **12:** 715–737.
26. STUART, M. J. 1981. Pediatr. Res. **15:** 971–973.

DISCUSSION

L. A. BOXER (*Indiana University, Indianapolis, Ind.*): Thrombin will induce the release of PGI_2 from endothelium. Have you attempted to add normal thrombin constituents to the neonatal plasma to see if you can augment PGI_2 release? Secondly, do you have any information as to whether the lipoxygenase pathway is also altered in the neonatal situation?

M. J. STUART: We have looked at neonatal platelets, and there's a slight increase in lipoxygenase products.

M. L. BIERENBAUM (*New Jersey College of Medicine, Newark, N.J.*): Would you speculate as to why the mothers of the children with low vitamin E levels and increased aggregability did not show low vitamin E levels themselves.

M. J. STUART: Vitamin E levels in the neonate are decreased to start off with. The safety margin is much lower in the infant than in the mothers. Perhaps the increased lipid-peroxidation products in vascular tissue in the neonates result in a greater rate of destruction of tocopherol than in the adult.

P. M. THURLOW (*Duke University Medical Center, Durham, N.C.*): We've had difficulty in performing platelet studies in the most extremely vitamin E–deficient patients, simply because platelets did not survive the trip from the patient's vein to the test tube. Have you observed this?

M. J. STUART: We haven't.

P. M. THURLOW: Can you exclude artifacts of platelet loss in performing the biochemical tests for platelet release of various compounds you've described?

M. J. STUART: We haven't done any differential separation of these products. When we looked at the return of platelet survival versus the return of MDA to normal in those two children that we described, we found that the platelet MDA came back to normal long before the platelet survival was corrected. So it appears from that observation that it's not just due to the young platelet population with a decrease in platelet life span.

D. P. R. MULLER (*Institute of Child Health, London, United Kingdom*): Did I understand correctly that the infants from the diabetic mothers were divided into two groups depending on whether they had increased platelet aggregation?

M. J. STUART: We divided them into two groups depending on the characterization of the maternal studies, not the infant studies. It was observed that for those mothers who had hyperfunctioning platelets, those infants had hyperfunctioning platelets too.

MECHANISM OF ACTION OF VITAMIN E ON PLATELET FUNCTION*

Manfred Steiner and Richard Mower

Division of Hematologic Research
The Memorial Hospital
Pawtucket, Rhode Island 02860

and

Department of Medicine
Brown University
Providence, Rhode Island 02912

INTRODUCTION

Platelet aggregation is an oxygen-requiring process. Induced by certain agents, it is associated with a burst in oxygen consumption needed principally for the metabolism of arachidonic acid liberated from membrane phospholipid.[1-4] Lipid peroxidation, a by-product of this process, was early recognized as an essential feature of aggregation.[5] This aspect prompted the investigation of α-tocopherol as a potential antiaggregating agent. Although its activity was found to be rather moderate in strength,[6-10] interest in vitamin E has continued as it represents one of the few natural substances with aggregation-inhibiting activity. The mechanism of action of α-tocopherol proved difficult to define. The premise on which its use as an antiplatelet agent was initially based was demonstrably incorrect, since it was shown that fully oxidized vitamin E was equally effective in reducing platelet aggregability.[11]

We have performed a series of experiments designed to elucidate the effect of this vitamin on platelet function. Our efforts have concentrated on two biochemical pathways that are intimately associated with platelet aggregation and release, i.e., the oxidative conversion sequence of arachidonic acid and the synthesis and degradation of adenosine 3',5'-cyclic monophosphate (cAMP). Investigation of the former was made possible by the utilization of platelets prelabeled with nonaggregating doses of ^{14}C-arachidonic acid rather than the pulse-labeling method commonly used for studies of oxidative conversion of arachidonic acid. Our studies give solid evidence that vitamin E and its quinone inhibit cyclooxygenase over the lipoxygenase pathway and inhibit cAMP phosphodiesterase but leave cAMP synthesis essentially unchanged. These findings together with previous results of the effect of vitamin E on membrane fluidity form the basis of a hypothesis of α-tocopherol action in platelets.

RESULTS AND DISCUSSION

Vitamin E and Arachidonate Metabolism in Platelets

α-Tocopherol is an inhibitor of the platelet-release reaction. A direct demonstration of this effect can be obtained by measuring aggregation and adenosine

*Supported in part by Research Grant HL 22951 from the National Heart and Lung Institute.

0077-8923/82/0393-0289 $01.75/0 © 1982, NYAS

triphosphate (ATP) release simultaneously (FIGURE 1). In previous studies, we have shown that platelet secretory release is inhibited in a dose-dependent manner by α-tocopherol.[8] Although this *in vitro* effect was not as potent as that of aspirin, definite proof that cyclooxygenase activity was reduced in vitamin E-treated platelets was not found. At least two groups of investigators have studied this problem and have obtained results that either showed an inhibition of the lipoxygenase reaction[12] or else no significant effect on arachidonate metabolism.[10,13]

In view of our observation that arachidonic acid–induced platelet aggregation was also reduced by vitamin E,[11] we felt that an inhibition of cyclooxygenase or an interference with arachidonic acid utilization was to be expected in α-tocopherol-

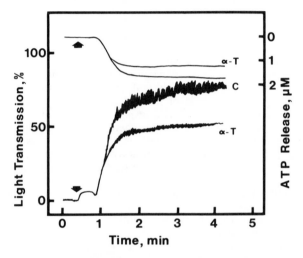

FIGURE 1. Platelet aggregation and release induced by epinephrine was compared in control (C) and vitamin E-pretreated (α-T) platelets. Platelet-rich plasma obtained from citrated blood was incubated for 30 minutes at 37°C with or without a colloidal suspension induced by sonication of α-tocopherol in 0.05 M tris-HCl in 0.145 M NaCl pH 7.4 (TBS) at a final concentration of 1 mM. The arrow indicates addition of epinephrine, 10 μM. Release was measured by the amount of ATP reacting with luciferase (right ordinate and upper curves), while aggregation was recorded by the change in optical transmission through the stirred platelet suspension.

treated platelets. Failure to find such evidence could be due to the methods usually applied in investigations of this type. One method is the preparation of α-tocopherol as an ethanolic solution. Its denaturant effect and its inhibition of platelet aggregation, which becomes manifest at concentrations of $\geq 0.5\%$ alcohol, are definite disadvantages. These concentrations are readily exceeded by levels of vitamin E > 0.5 mM. Also, the transfer of vitamin E to platelets is not optimal under these conditions (unpublished observations). This problem could be resolved by preparing α-tocopherol as a colloidal suspension in an aqueous medium. Another method that presents distinct problems is the pulse labeling of platelets with ^{14}C-arachidonic acid. Although widely used to assess the oxidative

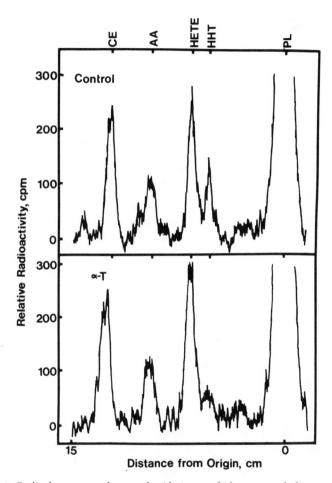

FIGURE 2. Radiochromatograph scan of oxidative arachidonate metabolites produced by control and vitamin E (α-T)-treated platelets. Platelets were isolated by gel filtration. After a 5-minute preincubation with or without vitamin E (see legend to FIGURE 1), platelets suspended in TBS were incubated with 1.0–1.5 μCi ^{14}C-arachidonic acid (specific activity, 55.8 mCi/mmol), which was added in a solution of 0.5% bovine serum albumin. After 40 minutes at 25°C, the suspensions were gel filtered. Aggregation was induced either by addition of 1 U bovine thrombin/ml and 2.5 mM $CaCl_2$ (shown in this figure) or by addition of 1/10 volume platelet-poor plasma and 20 μg collagen. The platelet suspensions were continuously stirred at 35°C. After 3 minutes the reactions were stopped by addition of an equal volume of 1 N HCl and rapid extraction/partition with 10 volumes of chloroform containing 2 mg% butylated hydroxytoluene. The extracts were flash evaporated and applied to thin-layer plates coated with silica gel 60F 254 (E. Merck, Federal Republic of Germany). The plates were then developed in isooctane–ethyl acetate–acetic acid (75:100:1), and radioactivity scanned.

TABLE 1

EFFECT OF α-TOCOPHEROL ON HETE:HHT RATIOS IN PLATELETS

α-Tocopherol (mM)	Experiment 1	Experiment 2	Experiment 3
0	2.4	3.8	3.9
0.1	2.0	3.8	3.2
0.5	3.0	4.6	3.7
1.0	3.6	4.5	6.3

conversion of arachidonic acid, this technique makes it virtually impossible to analyze the effect of less potent antiplatelet agents. To circumvent this difficulty, we have prelabeled platelets with nonaggregating doses of ^{14}C-arachidonic acid. The distribution of radioactivity in the lipid extracts of such platelets differs in important aspects from that seen in platelets that were pulsed with arachidonic acid. The radiochromatograph scan (FIGURE 2) reveals a distinct peak that cannot be seen in extracts of pulse-labeled platelets. On thin-layer chromatograph plates and by high-performance liquid chromatography (HPLC), this band comigrated with cholesterol esters. Confirmation of the identity of this material was obtained by analysis of the products of hydrolysis, which yielded cholesterol and free fatty acid. Platelets prelabeled with nonaggregating doses of ^{14}C-arachidonic acid show a completely normal aggregation response when stimulated with collagen, ADP, epinephrine, or thrombin. The ability to titrate the amount of such agents to the lowest concentration capable of inducing aggregation enhanced the sensitivity of this method of labeling oxidative arachidonate metabolites so that it could reveal smaller changes in the activity of lipoxygenase or cyclooxygenase pathways.

Applying this method to vitamin E–treated platelets, we were able to show changes in the activity of cyclooxygenase. The inhibition of this enzyme ranged from 8–14% when 0.25 mM α-tocopherol was used.[14] The effect of vitamin E was best shown by estimating the ratio of 12-L-hydroxy-5,8,10,14-eicosatetraenoic acid (HETE) to 12-L-hydroxy-5,8,10-heptadecatrienoic acid (HHT) in platelets. This ratio of the two principal determinants of lipoxygenase and cyclooxygenase pathways showed a dose-dependent increase up to 1 mM vitamin E tested (TABLE 1). At low concentrations of α-tocopherol, 0.1 mM, a moderate decrease of this ratio was a constant finding. These results thus suggest that vitamin E inhibits cyclooxygenase, channeling more arachidonic acid though the lipoxygenase pathway.

The Effect of Vitamin E Quinone on Oxidative Conversion of Arachidonic Acid in Platelets

α-Tocopheryl quinone, tested in the concentration range usually utilized for treating platelets with vitamin E, also inhibited platelet aggregation, the secretory release reaction, and cyclooxygenase. Its action was approximately equivalent to that of α-tocopherol. None of the experiments with the quinone resulted in the marked inhibition described by Cox et al.[15] These authors reported a far greater reduction of platelet aggregation and release than with vitamin E. Furthermore, they reported that the effect of cyclooxygenase, barely noticeable with α-tocopherol, was markedly enhanced when vitamin E quinone was used. This surprising result prompted us to investigate the problem further. We were able to show that the method of nitric acid oxidation used by Cox et al.[15] was responsible for the unusually high degree of inhibition. The actual quinone was about as efficient as vitamin E itself in suppressing platelet aggregation and cyclooxygenase activity.[16]

These findings clearly cast serious doubt on the antioxidant theory as the basic mechanism responsible for the action of vitamin E in platelets. Unless tocopheryl quinone can be readily reduced in platelets—a supposition for which we have found no evidence whatsoever so far—vitamin E must be assumed to act in other ways than by supplying reducing potential. The hypothesis of a physicochemical interaction between the phytyl side chain of α-tocopherol and polyunsaturated fatty acyl residues of membrane phospholipids[17] was attractive in that it could offer an explanation for the effectiveness of both the oxidized and reduced forms of vitamin E. Based on this hypothesis, reduction of the available arachidonic acid should be expected. However, our experiments gave no sign of a curtailment of substrate flow via the oxidative metabolic pathways in platelets. As yet, we cannot refute the hypothesis outright. Higher doses of α-tocopherol may be needed to accomplish inhibition of arachidonate availability. The abundance of polyunsaturated fatty acids in general and arachidonic acid in particular[18] would make high concentrations of vitamin E essential to achieve the necessary stoichiometry for inhibition. Further studies are in progress to clarify this point.

cAMP Metabolism in α-Tocopherol-Treated Platelets

Adenylate Cyclase

The above hypothesis has stimulated our interest in membrane-associated platelet activities. Adenylate cyclase and cAMP phosphodiesterase were examined in vitamin E-treated platelets. These two enzymes fulfill a critical role in regulating the sensitivity of platelets toward aggregating agents. cAMP is known to be a potent inhibitor of platelet aggregation,[19] and several of the physiologic antiplatelet agents exert their inhibition by effecting stimulation in cAMP production.[20-22] The basal activity of adenylate cyclase (TABLE 2) showed a slight increase in platelets that were pretreated with vitamin E. However, the difference between control and preincubated platelets did not reach statistical significance. Stimulation of adenylate cyclase by prostaglandin E_1 (PGE_1) (1 mM) increased cAMP production 6.3-fold in control platelets, while in platelets

TABLE 2

EFFECT OF α-TOCOPHEROL ON ADENYLATE CYCLASE ACTIVITY

	cAMP* (pmol/minute per mg protein)
Control	
Basal activity	7.4 ± 0.9
+ PGE_1	59.1 ± 8.5
α-Tocopherol (0.4 mM)	
Basal activity	10.4 ± 1.0
+ PGE_1	54.8 ± 5.8

*Mean $\pm$ standard deviation (SD) of 12 experiments.

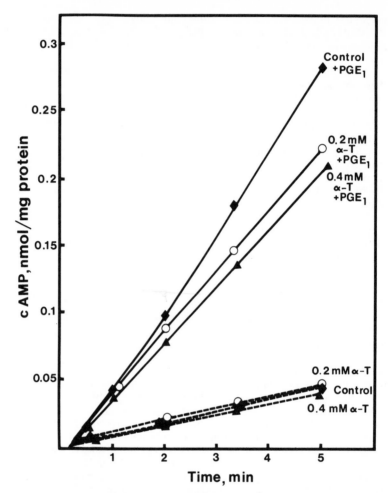

FIGURE 3. Time course of adenylate cyclase activity in control and vitamin E–pretreated platelets (see legend to FIGURE 1). Basal activity and PGE$_1$-stimulated (1 μM) activity were measured over a 5-minute interval. The preincubated platelets were washed two times with TBS, sonicated for 20 seconds at low-power output setting, and then incubated at a concentration of 120–150 μg protein in a mixture containing 5 mM MgCl$_2$, 20 mM creatine phosphate, 25 mM tris, pH 7.5, 1 mM cAMP, 6 mM theophylline, 1 mM ^{32}P-ATP (2 μCi/sample), and 100 U/ml creatine phosphokinase with or without 1 μM PGE$_1$. The enzyme reactions were stopped by addition of 2% sodium dodecyl sulfate, 40 mM ATP, and 1.4 mM cAMP. cAMP was determined by the method of Salomon et al.[34]

preincubated with 0.4 mM α-tocopherol, the prostaglandin-induced stimulation was always lower, rising on average only 5.3-fold (TABLE 2 and FIGURE 3). The production rate of cAMP in such platelets was slightly lower than in the corresponding controls, but again failed to reach statistically significant levels. In this, as in all other experiments, we have tried to confine our studies to a range of

TABLE 3

INHIBITION OF cAMP PHOSPHODIESTERASE BY α-TOCOPHEROL

α-Tocopherol (mM)	Enzyme Activity [% of control (nmol/mg protein per minute)]
0 (control)	100 (5.6 ± 0.6)*
0.1	85.5
0.5	66.4
1.0	60.0

*Mean ± SD of four experiments.

α-tocopherol concentrations that could be obtained by dietary intake. It is therefore possible that prolonged exposure of platelets to α-tocopherol at higher concentrations might have brought the difference between normal and vitamin E-treated platelets into a statistically significant range.

It is interesting that increases in cholesterol or membrane acyl chain ordering have been found to raise the basal adenylate cyclase activity, but were shown to prevent the usual PGE$_1$- or fluoride-induced stimulation of the enzyme.[23] Cholesterol is well known for its enhancement of membrane microviscosity.[24-30] Vitamin E, on the other hand, decreased apparent membrane viscosity at temperatures greater than 27°C, but produced an increase at temperatures lower than 24–27°C.[31] The absence of a significant change in adenylate cyclase activity of vitamin E-treated platelets may thus reflect the fluidity behavior of α-tocopherol-enriched platelet membranes.

cAMP Phosphodiesterase

The degradation of cAMP by cyclic nucleotide phosphodiesterase was also examined. Evaluation of this enzyme activity in α-tocopherol-preincubated platelets gave definite evidence of a rather marked reduction (TABLE 3). A multitude of enzyme forms appear to be present in most tissues. In the platelet, at least two different cAMP phosphodiesterases have been described, one with high and one with low K_m.[23] α-Tocopherol treatment of platelets changed the affinity of the high-K_m enzyme for its substrate, causing a two- to threefold increase in the K_m (TABLE 4 and FIGURE 4). Low-K_m enzyme was not affected by vitamin E. The net result of the changes incurred by loading platelets with α-tocopherol can thus be

TABLE 4

KINETIC CONSTANTS FOR PLATELET cAMP PHOSPHODIESTERASE

	K_m (μM)	V_{max} (nmol/mg protein per minute)
Low K_m		
Control platelets	45	1.3
Vitamin E-treated platelets	42	1.2
High K_m		
Control platelets	235	6.0
Vitamin E-treated platelets	588	10.0

expected to lead to an increased level of cAMP. This will affect platelet function by decreasing aggregability and increasing the threshold concentrations of aggregating agents needed to induce a shape change.

How Does Vitamin E Act in Platelets?

The question of how vitamin E acts in platelets remains a difficult one. The fact that the fully oxidized form of the vitamin is equally effective as α-tocopherol

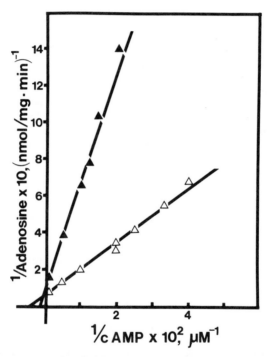

FIGURE 4. Lineweaver-Burke plot of cAMP phosphodiesterase activity of control (open triangles) and vitamin E-treated (closed triangles) platelets. Sonicates of washed platelets that had been pretreated with or without 1 mM α-tocopherol (see legend to FIGURE 1) were incubated in 50-μg aliquots in 50 mM tris buffer, pH 8.0, with 4 mM MgCl$_2$ and 0.5 mM mercaptoethanol. After a 5-minute preincubation at 30°C, ^{3}H-cAMP was added in concentrations ranging from 10–1,000 μM. Incubations were carried out at 30°C for 10 minutes. The amount of cAMP hydrolyzed was estimated after conversion to adenosine by 5-nucleotidase.[35]

in human platelets makes it necessary to look for alternative explanations to those rooted in the antioxidant theory. One of the first problems to be addressed is to determine which part of the molecule is essential for the observed effect. Two types of experiments have shed some light. If the hypothesis of Diplock and Lucy were correct,[17,32] the phytyl side chain would be essential. We have tried to investigate this point by using changes in membrane microviscosity as a parameter. The free alcohol phytol proved to be without effect when added to intact platelets or platelet membranes in concentrations up to 2 mM. On the other hand, vitamin K_1 showed similarity to vitamin E in decreasing apparent membrane microviscosity at high temperatures (> 20 °C). In view of the structural similarities between vitamin E and the group of bioflavinoids, we have recently tested a number of these substances and found several of them quite potent in their inhibition of platelet cyclooxygenase and of aggregation induced by the common physiological aggregating agents. Among the compounds that were examined, inhibitory action was limited to the aglycones. The corresponding glycones were uniformly noninhibitory.

The peculiar effect of α-tocopherol on the apparent membrane microviscosity alluded to above, and demonstrated by a tilt of the monophasic relation of fluorescence anisotropy of diphenyl-hexatriene-labeled platelets and temperature, seemed to be predicated on the presence of protein.[31] Liposomes prepared from platelet lipids failed to share this behavior of platelets or platelet membranes. When treated with α-tocopherol, their anisotropy conformed to that expected of a lipid matrix enriched with a substance that aligns itself with the prevailing direction of phospholipid acyl chains. We are inclined to speculate that there exists a close association of α-tocopherol with certain proteins and their coordinated lipids. This could lead to a partitioning of the vitamin into distinct lipid domains. This is further supported by the observation that α-tocopherol is selectively lost during extraction of lipids from vitamin E–prelabeled platelets (unpublished observations). We like to stress that more direct evidence is needed in support of this hypothesis. Lipid interactions, asymmetry and sidedness of phospholipids, and angle of curvature of the lipids in the bilayer could all affect the results obtained with liposomes. Nevertheless, the findings of the present study are compatible with such a hypothesis, which can form the basis for future experiments.

CONCLUDING REMARKS

Although the changes in platelet metabolism and function induced by vitamin E loading are generally of moderate degree, they should not be considered insignificant. Unlike pharmacological agents, α-tocopherol preexists at a fairly high concentration in platelets.[8,33] Expressions of its function should be evaluated in comparison to vitamin E–deficient states. These to our knowledge are quite rare in adult humans, however. Does vitamin E have a role in platelets beyond its physiological action? We believe that its effect on platelets, based on a different mode of action from most pharmacological agents, could make platelets more sensitive to the latter. Furthermore, it should be pointed out that most aggregation-inducing stimuli in vivo are less potent than when used in vitro. Therefore, inhibitors of platelet function can be effective in vivo even though their in vitro action does not completely block such function.

ACKNOWLEDGMENTS

We wish to express our thanks to Miss Carolyn Vieira for expert technical assistance.

REFERENCES

1. HUSSAIN, Q. Z. & T. F. NEWCOMB. 1964. J. Appl. Physiol. **19:** 297–300.
2. MURER, E. H. 1968. Biochim. Biophys. Acta **162:** 320–326.
3. MUENZER, J., E. WEINBACH & S. WOLFE. 1975. Biochim. Biophys. Acta **376:** 243–248.
4. PICKETT, W. C. & P. COHEN. 1976. J. Biol. Chem. **251:** 2536–2538.
5. OKUMA, M., M. STEINER & M. BALDINI. 1971. J. Lab. Clin. Med. **77:** 728–742.
6. HIGASHI, O. & Y. KIKUCHI. 1974. Tohoku J. Exp. Med. **112:** 271–278.
7. MACHLIN, L. J., R. FILIPSKI, A. L. WILLIS & D. C. KUHN. 1975. Proc. Soc. Exp. Biol. Med. **149:** 275–277.
8. STEINER, M. & J. ANASTASI. 1976. J. Clin. Invest. **57:** 732–737.
9. FONG, J. S. C. 1976. Experientia **32:** 639–641.
10. RAO, G. H. R., J. M. GERRARD, S. W. EATON & J. G. WHITE. 1978. Photochem. Photobiol. **28:** 845–850.
11. STEINER, M. 1978. *In* Tocopherol, Oxygen and Biomembranes. C. de Duve & O. Hayaishi, Eds.: 143–163. Elsevier/North-Holland Biomedical Press. New York, N.Y.
12. GWEBU, E. T., R. W. TREWYN, D. G. CORNWELL & R. V. PANGANAMALA. 1980. Res. Commun. Chem. Pathol. Pharmacol. **28:** 361–367.
13. RAO, G. H. R., S. M. BURRIS, J. M. GERRARD & J. G. WHITE. 1979. Prostaglandins Med. **2:** 111–120.
14. MOWER, R. & M. STEINER. 1982. Biochim. Biophys. Acta. (In press.)
15. COX, A. C., G. H. R. RAO, J. M. GERRARD & J. G. WHITE. 1980. Blood **55:** 907–914.
16. MOWER, R. & M. STEINER. 1982. Prostaglandins. (In press.)
17. LUCY, J. A. 1972. Ann. N.Y. Acad. Sci. **203:** 4–11.
18. MARCUS A. J., L. B. SAPIER & H. L. ULLMAN. 1972. *In* Blood Lipids and Lipoproteins. Quantitation, Composition and Metabolism. G. J. Nelson, Ed.: 417–439. John Wiley & Sons, Inc. New York, N.Y.
19. SALZMAN, E. W. & L. LEVINE. 1971. J. Clin. Invest. **50:** 131–141.
20. ROBISON, G. A., A. ARNOLD & R. C. HARTMAN. 1969. Pharmacol. Res. Commun. **1:** 325–332.
21. GORMAN, R. R., S. BUNTING & O. V. MILLER. 1977. Prostaglandins **13:** 377–388.
22. MILLS, D. C. B. & D. E. MACFARLANE. 1974. Thromb. Res. **5:** 401–412.
23. SINHA, A. K., S. J. SHATTIL & R. W. COLMAN. 1977. J. Biol. Chem. **252:** 3310–3314.
24. CHAPMAN, D. & S. A. PENKETT. 1966. Nature **211:** 1304–1305.
25. LADBROOKE, B. D., R. H. WILLIAMS & D. CHAPMAN. 1968. Biochim. Biophys. Acta **150:** 333–340.
26. PAPAHADJOPOULOS, D., M. COWDEN & H. KIMELBERG. 1973. Biochim. Biophys. Acta **330:** 8–26.
27. COGAN, U., M. SHINITZKY, G. WEBER & T. NISHIDA. 1973. Biochemistry **12:** 521–528.
28. SHINITZKY, M. & M. INBAR. 1976. Biochim. Biophys. Acta **433:** 133–149.
29. DEMEL, R. A. & B. DE KRUIJFF. 1976. Biochim. Biophys. Acta **457:** 109–132.
30. SHATTIL, S. J. & R. A. COOPER. 1976. Biochemistry **15:** 4832–4837.
31. STEINER, M. 1981. Biochim. Biophys. Acta **640:** 100–105.
32. DIPLOCK, A. T. & J. A. LUCY. 1973. FEBS Lett. **29:** 205–208.
33. STROM, E. & A. NORDOY. 1974. Thromb. Res. 4(Suppl. 1): 73–74.
34. SALOMON, Y., C. LONDOS & M. RODBELL. 1974. Anal. Biochem. **58:** 541–548.
35. BUBLITZ, C. 1978. Anal. Biochem. **88:** 109–113.

———————◆———————

DISCUSSION

E. R. SIMONS (*Boston University School of Medicine, Boston, Mass.*): I think on the whole, the picture with blood cells and vitamin E is becoming somewhat clearer. I was interested in what Dr. Steiner has found with the depolarization of fluorescence, since we measure things the same way. When one supplements rat diets with vitamin E, rather than doing incubation *in vitro*, then as you just reported, one does not find a difference in the depolarization of fluorescence. There's a little change, but it is not statistically significant. There is in fact no change in either the platelets or the red cells, nor is there a change in the degree of unsaturation of the lipids. So that clearly the *in vivo* system, at least in the rat, has some way of compensating.

M. STEINER: I agree with this comment wholeheartedly.

R. BRYANT (*George Washington University Medical School, Washington, D.C.*): Your changes in the ratios of HETE to HHT with the addition of tocopherol were quite interesting, but I am somewhat concerned about identification of the HHT band. We have done quite a bit of work on identification of arachidonic acid products in platelets and have found lipoxygenase products that are rather like HHT. Have you shown that your HHT band in prelabeled platelets disappears with aspirin, that is, is it a cyclooxygenase product?

M. STEINER: We have done what you suggested. Furthermore, we identified each band that we got on the carbon-labeled radiochromatograph scan by mass spectrometry to be absolutely certain that what we label as HHT or HETE is in fact the real product.

V. SRINIVASAN (*National Naval Medical Center, Bethesda, Md.*): Are α-tocopherol and the quinone comparable in terms of penetration into the platelet? Also, when you mention the changes in the membrane, are these enzymes located on the inner side or the outside of the membrane?

M. STEINER: As far as the penetration of the vitamin E quinone is concerned, I think we know that it distributes itself in the platelet membrane. I'm not sure if it can reach membranous structures within the platelet. We tried to determine the distribution of vitamin E and vitamin E quinone in the various structures of the platelets. It is very difficult to be absolutely certain that one doesn't have significant contamination with plasma membranes. I would say at this time that at least tocopheryl quinone can get into the plasma membrane.

As far as the orientation of the enzymes, certainly for cAMP, the receptor site for the hormones is directed toward the outside. The catalytic unit of the enzyme seems to be directed toward the inside of the cell. As far as phosphodiesterase is concerned, I'm not certain whether it's on the outside or the inside of the membrane.

J. NIXON (*Linus Pauling Institute, Palo Alto, Calif.*): Do you show any increases in cAMP or changes in phosphorylation in the presence of vitamin E?

M. STEINER: We didn't do those experiments.

DEMONSTRATION OF SPECIFIC BINDING SITES FOR ^{3}H-RRR-α-TOCOPHEROL ON HUMAN ERYTHROCYTES*

Abbas E. Kitabchi† and Jay Wimalasena

*Departments of Medicine and Biochemistry
and Clinical Research Center
University of Tennessee Center for Health Sciences
Memphis, Tennessee 38163*

INTRODUCTION

RRR-α-Tocopherol (vitamin E) not only acts as a biological antioxidant but has been shown to have a wide variety of roles in membrane-related activities.[1-3] These include adrenocorticotropin (ACTH)–activated membrane-bound adenyl-cyclase in steroidogenic activity of isolated adrenal cells of rats[4-7] as well as a function in prevention of erythrocyte fragility demonstrated by increased hemolysis to hemolytic agents.[8-9] Recent work from our laboratory has demonstrated the presence of specific binding sites for ^{3}H-RRR-α-tocopherol (^{3}H-dαT) on cell membranes of isolated adrenocortical cells of rat adrenal that show saturability and specificity of binding as well as reversibility with unlabeled tocopherol.[10] Quantitative studies of ^{3}H-dαT binding to these membranes were analyzed by Scatchard plot, and a saturation plot evolved that demonstrated two classes of binding sites. The higher-affinity site had an apparent equilibrium association constant (K_a) of 7×10^6 M^{-1}, and the lower-affinity site exhibited a K_a of 0.4×10^6 M^{-1} (FIGURE 1). The binding capacities were 12 and 120 pmol/mg for the higher- and lower-affinity sites respectively.

As tocopherol deficiency is associated with increased susceptibility of red blood cells (RBCs) to hemolysis,[8-9] we investigated tocopherol binding sites in human RBCs. These studies suggested that human red blood cells, similar to our finding in cell membranes of rat adrenal, contain two specific sites for RRR-α-tocopherol—one with high affinity, low capacity and the second with low affinity, high capacity. The details of these data are presented elsewhere[11-13] and are summarized below.

MATERIALS AND METHODS

^{3}H-RRR-α-Tocopherol (specific activity, 13 Ci/mmol; purity, 98%) was purchased from Amersham-Searle Radiochemicals. RRR-α-Tocopherol, RRR-γ-tocopherol, and RRR-α-tocopheryl acetate were purchased from Eastman Kodak. The following tocopherol analogs were gifts from Hoffmann-La Roche: RRR-α-tocopheryl acid succinate, *all-rac*-α-tocopheryl nicotinate, *rac*-6-hydroxy-2,5,7,8-tetramethyl-chroman-2-carboxylic acid (Trolox), and RRR-α-tocopheryl

*This work was supported by U.S. Public Health Service Grants RR00211, AM07088, and AM19717.

†Please address all correspondence to 951 Court Avenue, Room 327B, Memphis, Tenn. 38163.

quinone. Trypsin and lima bean trypsin inhibitor were obtained from Millipore Laboratories. All other chemicals used were of reagent grade and were obtained from Sigma Chemicals. ^{3}H-dαT stock solution was aliquoted and kept at $-60°$C under nitrogen. Specific binding of ^{3}H-dαT did not change during storage under these conditions for two to three months.

Blood was withdrawn from normal volunteers, and RBCs were obtained by the modified procedure described by us previously.[14] Erythrocytes were separated using Ficoll/Hypaque solution by the method of Boyum.[15] RBCs were washed once in saline and resuspended at 4°C to the original volume of blood. These erythrocytes were used in the assay within one hour of the preparation. In

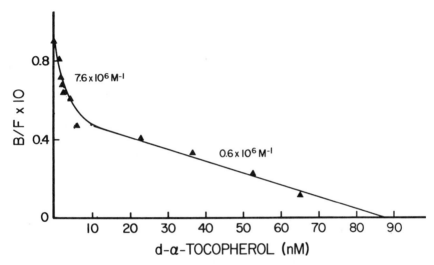

FIGURE 1. Quantitative analysis of binding of ^{3}H-RRR-α-tocopherol to rat adrenal membrane in the presence of increasing concentrations of unlabeled RRR-α-tocopherol. Reaction mixture consisted of 5–25 μg protein membrane, 0.9 ml of tris-Ringer buffer with 1% BSA, pH 7.1, and the amount of unlabeled tocopherol as specified. ^{3}H-RRR-α-Tocopherol (13 Ci/mmol) was diluted in absolute ethanol. Each tube contained 200,000 cpm of ^{3}H-dαT in 5 μl of absolute ethanol. Incubation was carried out for 4 hours at 37°C. Assay was terminated by addition of 0.5 ml tris-Ringer BSA (4°C) to the polypropylene tube, followed by transferring the contents to Eppendorf microfuge tubes. The latter were centrifuged for 30 minutes at 4°C at full speed. After aspiration of the supernatant, the bottoms of the tubes containing the pellets were cut and collected in a vial and counted as described in Methods. (Data from Reference 10.)

the routine binding assay, an aliquot of RBC suspension (4–5 × 10^9 cells/ml) was incubated for 4 hours at 37°C in a total volume of 1.0 ml of tris-Ringer [0.025 M tris, 0.120 M NaCl, 0.0012 M MgSO$_4$, 0.0025 M KCl, 0.01 M glucose, 0.001 M ethylenediaminetetraacetic acid (EDTA)] bovine serum albumin (BSA) (1%) pH 7.1 in 12 × 75 mm plastic tubes. dαT or other vitamin E analogs were added in ethanol, with a final ethanol concentration of 0.5%. Routinely, 220,000–280,000 cpm of ^{3}H-dαT were used per tube. At the end of incubation, the mixture was carefully placed on a layer of 1 ml dibutyl phthalate (bottom) and 1 ml of tris-Ringer buffer (middle), and the tubes were centrifuged at 800 × g in a

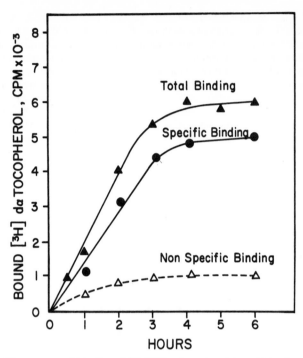

FIGURE 2. Time course of binding of ^{3}H-RRR-α-tocopherol to red blood cells at 12 nM concentration was measured at several time intervals. Binding was measured as in Methods. (Data from Reference 11.)

Beckman TJ-R centrifuge for 15 minutes at 4°C. The red cell pellets were solubilized in 15 ml of Scinti-Verse (Fisher-Scientific) and counted in a Nuclear Chicago scintillation spectrometer at an efficiency of 40%. Correction for quenching was made as described previously.[11] Binding was measured in triplicate, and the individual values were within 10% of the mean. Red blood cells were counted in a Hi Cell counter.

Specific tocopherol binding was defined as total ^{3}H-dαT binding minus nonspecific binding, which was the binding in the presence of 110 μM of dαT. Nonspecific binding was found to be routinely 10–20% of total bound ^{3}H-dαT. Binding data were analyzed by Scatchard plot,[16] and average affinity profile by the method of De Meyts and Roth.[17] The affinity constant (K_a) was also calculated by the method of Thakur et al.[18] for nonlinear Scatchard plots. For statistical analysis, Student's t-test was used. All data were expressed as mean ± standard error of the mean (SEM).

For preparation of human red blood cell membranes, RBC ghosts were first prepared according to the method of Fairbanks et al.[19] These RBC ghost pellets were then homogenized in 5 mM phosphate buffer (pH 8.0) in an all-glass homogenizer, and the suspension was centrifuged at 39,000 × g for 20 minutes in a Beckman J2-21 centrifuge, using a JA-20 rotor at 4°C. The details of this method have been described elsewhere.[11,12] The incubation mixture was the same as discussed above except that the RBCs were replaced by 0.2 ml of membrane preparation. For the membrane studies, protein was measured by the method of Lowry et al.,[20] using bovine serum albumin as standard.

Dissociation of specifically bound ^{3}H-dαT was studied as follows. After incubation of ^{3}H-dαT with RBCs of 0.8 × 10^9 cells, the cells were separated from the incubation medium and resuspended at a 100-fold dilution with buffer. To one incubation mixture, unlabeled dαT was added at a concentration of 110 μM, while an equivalent volume of absolute alcohol was added to a second incubation mixture without unlabeled tocopherol. Samples were removed at different intervals during the dissociation reaction at 37°C, and specific binding was measured.

RESULTS

Time Course and the Effects of Different Concentrations of Ligand

The time course of binding at 12 nM of ^{3}H-dαT to RBCs at 37°C is depicted in FIGURE 2. This figure shows that equilibrium was reached by three hours at 37°C. The amount bound was concentration dependent up to 24 nM and was optimum at 37°C[11] (data not shown).

Effect of Cell Number

The quantity of ^{3}H-dαT bound increased linearly with number of RBCs up to 70 × 10^7 cells/ml of incubation (FIGURE 3). Routine assays were performed with

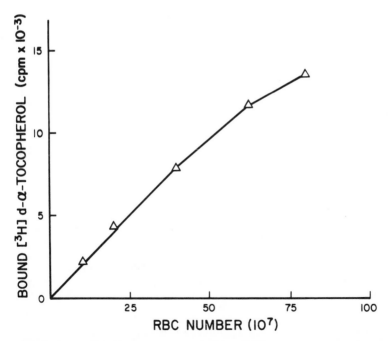

FIGURE 3. Binding of ^{3}H-*RRR*-α-tocopherol to human RBCs as a function of cell number. Binding of ^{3}H-dαT was measured at several concentrations of erythrocytes as described in Methods. (Data from Reference 11.)

50×10^7 cells/ml, which was within linear range of the curve. As cell numbers were increased over 70×10^7, fractional increase of specifically bound ^{3}H-dαT decreased; and over 100×10^7 cells/ml, the fractional increase was substantially less than that in the linear part of the curve (data not shown).

Acidity Profile

The binding reaction demonstrated a pH optimum of 7.0–7.2 (FIGURE 4). The decrease of binding on the alkaline side of the profile was more pronounced than on the acid side.

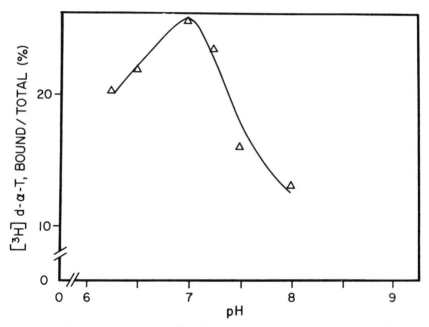

FIGURE 4. Effect of pH. Binding of ^{3}H-RRR-α-tocopherol was measured as in Methods at several pH values of the reaction mixture. (Data from Reference 11.)

Kinetics of Association and Dissociation

Dissociation of bound ^{3}H-dαT was studied after the binding reaction reached equilibrium. Cells were separated by centrifugation, washed once, and reincubated in the presence of an excess of unlabeled dαT or only tris-Ringer BSA (FIGURE 5). As can be seen, addition of unlabeled dαT did not enhance the rate of dissociation of ^{3}H-dαT and dissociation of the ligand receptor complex was curvilinear.

Quantitative Data

By measurement of ^{3}H-dαT bound at several concentrations of unlabeled RRR-α-tocopherol, data for the Scatchard plot were generated. FIGURE 6 depicts

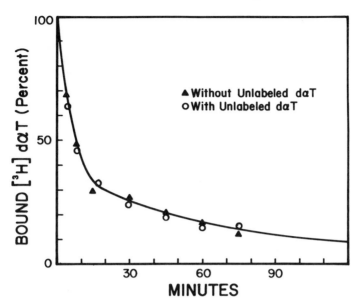

FIGURE 5. Time course of dissociation reaction of bound ^{3}H-RRR-α-tocopherol in the presence and absence of unlabeled tocopherol. See text for details. (Data from Reference 11.)

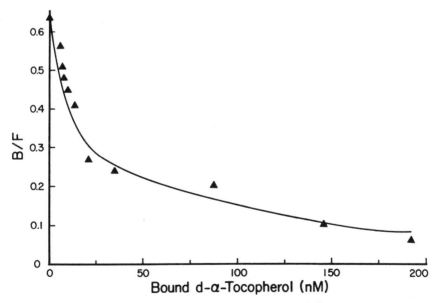

FIGURE 6. Scatchard plot for ^{3}H-RRR-α-tocopherol binding to human RBCs. Quantity of ^{3}H-dαT bound at equilibrium to RBCs in the presence of several concentrations of unlabeled dαT was measured. Binding and equilibrium association constant (K_a) were measured as in Methods. (Reproduced from Reference 11 with the permission of the publisher.)

the presence of two classes of binding sites—a high-affinity, low-capacity site and a low-affinity, high-capacity site. The equilibrium association constant (K_a) for site 1 was approximately 50-fold that of site 2. TABLE 1 presents additional data on the number of sites per cell for low-capacity and high-capacity sites as well as rate constants for the forward reaction (k_1) and the reverse reaction (k_2).

Specificity of the Binding Reaction

Comparative displacement of ^{3}H-dαT in the presence of several concentrations of various tocopherol analogs demonstrated no displacement of ^{3}H-dαT by *RRR*-α-tocopheryl acetate, *all-rac*-α-tocopheryl nicotinate, *RRR*-α-tocopheryl quinone, or the inactive vitamin E analog Trolox.[11] However, *RRR*-γ-tocopherol exhibited some competition for binding.

TABLE 1

QUANTITATIVE MEASUREMENTS OF ^{3}H-*RRR*-α-TOCOPHEROL BINDING
TO HUMAN ERYTHROCYTES

Parameter	First Site	Second Site
K_a*	$2.64 \pm 0.4\dagger \times 10^7$ M^{-1}	$1.2 \pm 0.3\dagger \times 10^6$ M^{-1}
n	7,000–8,000 sites/cell	140,000–160,000 sites/cell
k_1	1.2×10^4 mol^{-1} minute^{-1}	
k_2	1.6×10^{-3} minute^{-1}	
$k_1/k_2\ddagger$	7.5×10^6 M^{-1}	

*Calculated from data in FIGURE 6.
†SEM.
‡k_1 was calculated from data analogous to FIGURE 2. k_2 was calculated from data in FIGURE 5.

FIGURE 7 demonstrates the competition curve for binding of ^{3}H-dαT to erythrocytes with unlabeled *RRR*-α-tocopherol or *RRR*-γ-tocopherol at various concentrations. As can be seen, *RRR*-γ-tocopherol demonstrated competition for ^{3}H-dαT binding, which was most pronounced at high concentrations of 44 μM, but even at this concentration, *RRR*-γ-tocopherol was only 50% as effective as *RRR*-α-tocopherol, which reached its maximum competition for ^{3}H-dαT at about 4 μM. These experiments demonstrate that the binding of dαT is a highly specific reaction.

Nature of the Binding Sites

We tested a number of agents that are known to interact with RBC membranes (TABLE 2). Hydrogen peroxide almost totally inhibited binding at 1%. This concentration also produced hemolysis, as evidenced by leakage of hemoglobin (data not shown). Selenium dioxide, an antioxidant, was partially effective in blocking the inhibition by H_2O_2, although by itself selenium dioxide had no effect.

Binding of ^{3}H-dαT was markedly inhibited by preincubation of RBCs at 65°C for one hour, at which time there was considerable hemolysis. Preincubation with

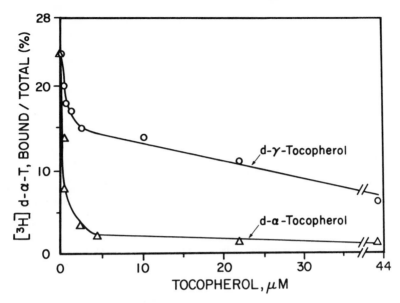

FIGURE 7. Competition for binding of ³H-dαT to erythrocytes. Bound ³H-dαT in the presence of several concentrations of RRR-γ-tocopherol and RRR-α-tocopherol as described in Methods. These results are expressed as percent of added ³H-RRR-α-tocopherol that was specifically bound to 1 × 10⁹ RBCs.

TABLE 2

EFFECTS OF VARIOUS AGENTS ON ³H-dαT ERYTHROCYTE BINDING*

Additions	Binding as Percent of Control
Control	100
Sodium ascorbate (1 mM)	94
Calcium chloride (1 mM)	98
Hydrogen peroxide (1%)	14
+ Selenium dioxide (1 mM)	34
Selenium dioxide (1 mM)	97
Trypsin (45 minutes, 37°C)	27
+ Trypsin inhibitor	82
Trypsin (1 hour, 37°C) subsequent to binding†	66
Dithiothreitol (DTT) (10 mM)	100
N-Ethylmaleimide (NEM) (10 mM)	46
DTT + NEM	126

*Red blood cells were preincubated for 1 hour as indicated, centrifuged, resuspended, and assayed for binding as described under Methods. The control that is taken as 100% consists of value of 20% binding of ³H-dαT per 1 × 10⁹ cells. (Reproduced from Reference 11 with permission from the publisher.)

†Cells were incubated with ³H-dαT for 3 hours and treated with trypsin (1.25 mg/ml) before measurement of bound ³H-dαT. Results are the mean of two experiments with three measurements per each experiment.

TABLE 3

EFFECT OF PREINCUBATION OF HUMAN ERYTHROCYTES WITH TOCOPHEROLS
ON H_2O_2-INDUCED HEMOLYSIS*

Compound	Concentration (μg/ml)	Percent Hemolysis
Control	—	100
RRR-α-Tocopherol	0.5	37
RRR-α-Tocopherol	5.0	24
RRR-γ-Tocopherol	0.5	62
RRR-γ-Tocopherol	5.0	25
RRR-α-Tocopheryl quinone	5.0	85
all-rac-α-Tocopheryl nicotinate	5.0	110

*0.4×10^9 red blood cells were preincubated ($37°C$) with the tocopherols at the designated concentrations for 3 hours. They were centrifuged, washed ($4°C$), and incubated with 5% H_2O_2 for 45 minutes at $37°C$, and hemolysis was measured.[21] To the control tubes, only C_2H_5OH (vehicle for tocopherol) was added. The hemolysis in the control tubes is taken as 100% and represents 14–16% of total hemoglobin released when the red blood cells were hemolyzed with H_2O_2. The results depicted are the mean of two experiments. (Data from Reference 11.)

trypsin at 1.24 mg/ml decreased binding (assayed after neutralization with trypsin inhibitor, 4 mg/ml, centrifugation, wash, and resuspension), while addition of trypsin inhibitor before trypsin blocked the effects of trypsin (TABLE 2).

Preincubation of red blood cells with N-ethylmaleimide (NEM) for one hour at $37°C$ decreased binding by 50%, while dithiothreitol (DTT) by itself had no effect on binding. DTT completely blocked the inhibition due to NEM. In the presence of DTT and NEM, binding was somewhat greater than the control (TABLE 2); however, this increase was not significant. These results taken together strongly suggest that dαT binding is at least partly due to a thermolabile protein that may have sensitive disulfide bonds.

Tocopherol Binding in Normal Volunteers

Studies in seven normal volunteers (six males, one female) revealed a range of net tocopherol binding from 18.1–24.1% of added ^{3}H-dαT (per 10^9 cells/4 hours), with a mean of 20.4 $\pm$ 0.9%. The day-to-day variability of binding was less than 10% between subjects and between groups (data not shown).

Correlation of Binding and Antihemolytic Effects of Various Tocopherols

Although the significance of RRR-α-tocopherol binding sites in physiologic action of red blood cells is not known, we attempted to evaluate and correlate the binding data with the antihemolytic effect of tocopherol by preincubating red blood cells with 0.5 and 5.0 μg RRR-α-tocopherol or RRR-γ-tocopherol/ml incubation or 5 μg/ml of other tocopherol analogs (tocopheryl quinone or tocopheryl nicotinate) upon hemolysis by H_2O_2. The results are presented in TABLE 3. RRR-α-Tocopherol at 0.5 μg/ml reduced hemolysis by more than 60%, whereas RRR-γ-tocopherol at the same concentration inhibited the hemolysis by about 40%. Neither RRR-α-tocopheryl quinone nor all-rac-α-tocopheryl nicotinate at 5 μg/ml concentration inhibited RBC hemolysis. These results are compatible with the binding displacement data, where RRR-γ-tocopherol and

RRR-α-tocopherol are the only two compounds that compete for binding with labeled tocopherol.

Subcellular Localization of Binding Sites on Red Blood Cell Fractions

In order to localize the site of binding in red blood cells, erythrocytes were hemolyzed and the ghost pellet was homogenized as stated in Methods. The suspension was washed with tris buffer four times by centrifugation (40,000 × g) and resuspension. Binding studies were carried out in the same medium as for the intact red blood cells. Binding of ^{3}H-dαT to these membranes demonstrated that 80-90% of the specific binding sites were recovered in the membranes derived from an equivalent number of cells (0.8 × 10^9 cells bound 20% of added ^{3}H-dαT; membranes from 0.8 × 10^{10} cells bound 17.6% of added ^{3}H-dαT).[12] Binding to membranes had the same time, temperature, cell concentration, and pH dependence as the intact cells.[12] Scatchard plot analysis revealed a curvilinear plot with high affinity (3.3 ± 0.2 × 10^7 M^{-1}), low capacity (4.1 pmol/mg protein) and low affinity (1.50 ± 0.4 × 10^6 M^{-1}), high capacity (66 pmol/mg protein).[12]

As with the intact RBCs, both increased temperature (65°C) and trypsinization of the membrane decreased the ability of the membrane to bind ^{3}H-dαT.[12] Furthermore, these membranes exhibited the same pH optimum as intact RBCs and demonstrated decreased binding by NEM treatment.[12]

Specificity of Binding Sites

Using standard procedure for the tocopherol binding studies on membranes, various tocopherol analogs at 5 μg/ml concentration were used to investigate their competition with ^{3}H-dαT. The results of these studies, which are depicted in FIGURE 8, demonstrate that dαT reduced the binding by more than 75% whereas

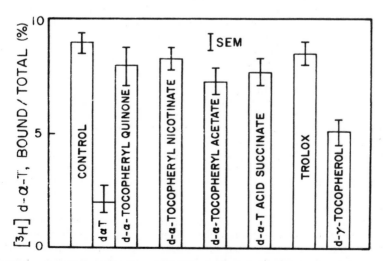

FIGURE 8. Specificity of binding of ^{3}H-RRR-α-tocopherol to membranes from 0.8 × 10^9 red blood cells. Binding was measured for three hours at 37°C using the same buffer as for red blood cells at 200,000 cpm of ^{3}H-RRR-α-tocopherol. Tocopherol concentration, 5 μg/ml. (Reproduced from Reference 11 with the permission of the publisher.)

RRR-γ-tocopherol reduced it by only about 40%. RRR-α-Tocopheryl quinone, all-rac-α-tocopheryl nicotinate, RRR-α-tocopheryl acetate, RRR-α-tocopheryl acid succinate, or Trolox did not significantly inhibit the binding. The dose-response curve for displacement of ^{3}H-dαT with various tocopherol analogs is described in detail elsewhere.[12] These studies suggest that the major tocopherol binding site in the intact RBC is on the membrane with similar specificity for RRR-α-tocopherol as the intact red blood cell.

Solubilization of Tocopherol Binding Sites

Although numerous agents were used to solubilize tocopherol binding sites in RBC membranes, only Triton X-100 proved to give satisfactory results at 1% concentration. The results of these studies are presented elsewhere.[12] Further purification of the solubilized tocopherol binding site complex on Sepharose 6B revealed two peaks with a major band with a molecular weight of 65,000 and a minor component with a molecular weight of 125,000. Both of these peaks were significantly reduced with addition of RRR-α-tocopherol or RRR-γ-tocopherol but not with tocopheryl nicotinate. In addition, the larger component of 125,000 daltons, upon further rechromatography, was converted to 65,000 daltons molecular weight,[12] thus suggesting that the major binding site has a molecular weight of 65,000, with the possibility of existing in a monomer-dimer form.

DISCUSSION

Studies from our laboratory presented here and elsewhere[11,12] suggest that intact human red blood cells have specific binding sites for RRR-α-tocopherol that are saturable and have properties compatible with a biologically significant receptor. These binding sites are at least partly protein in nature. The kinetic parameters appear to be similar to those observed by us on the rat adrenocortical cell membranes.[10] Further evidence presented elsewhere[11,12] and reported here suggests that RBC membrane contains the major portion of the tocopherol binding site of the intact cell and that it shows a specificity similar to that of the intact cell. Both intact cell and membrane data on Scatchard analysis reveal a curvilinear plot with two possible sites—one with high affinity, low capacity and the second with low affinity, high capacity. Tocopherol binding has not been previously reported for the membrane but has been demonstrated in the cytosol portion of rat liver by Catignani and Bieri.[22,23] However, these authors did not report equilibrium binding data. In addition, Nair et al. proposed that the rat liver nucleus may have a binding site for dαT.[24]

Since the normal concentration of vitamin E in serum is about 22 μM, it is likely that both of these sites have an important role in red cell function.

Exhibition of high specificity for RRR-α-tocopherol and lack of response to quinone or nicotinate and Trolox suggest the site is specific for intact chroman ring and requires alcohol side chain (FIGURE 9).

RRR-α-Tocopherol is a well-known antioxidant in vitro[25] and has been demonstrated to decrease the hemolytic damage to RBCs by hemolytic agents (TABLE 3). Such a beneficial effect of RRR-α-tocopherol may be responsible for the clinical effect the agent has in hemolytic anemias of diverse origins.[9] Since the disruption of red blood cell membrane is a likely locus of action of oxidative stress and dαT has been proposed to be important in the maintenance of membrane structure and function,[7,26] it is possible that dαT binding protein or receptors in RBCs may serve a protective function. Our studies show that normal human RBCs have two classes of specific binding sites for dαT. The properties of these sites are compatible with biologically significant sites. However, the detailed nature and purification of the protein have not been demonstrated although the biochemical properties—including heat lability and trypsin and disulfide bond inhibitor susceptibility—suggest a possible protein nature of these binding sites and a

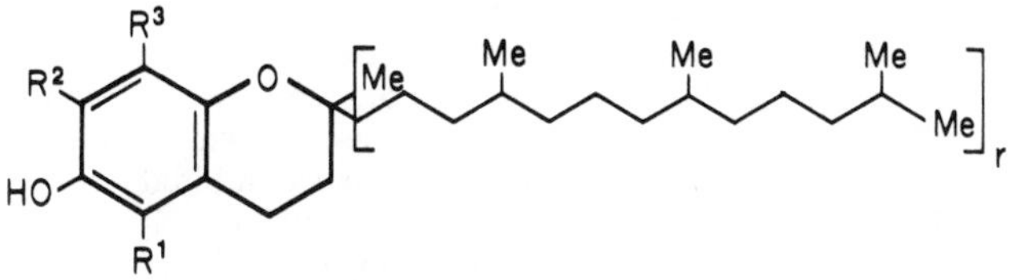

Compound	R^1	R^2	R^3
α-Tocopherol	Me	Me	Me
β-Tocopherol	Me	H	Me
γ-Tocopherol	H	Me	Me
δ-Tocopherol	H	H	Me

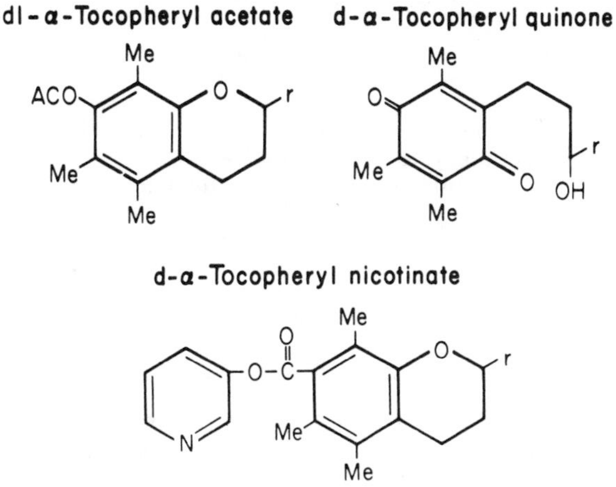

dl-α-Tocopheryl acetate   d-α-Tocopheryl quinone

d-α-Tocopheryl nicotinate

FIGURE 9. Chemical structure of tocopherols and various analogs.

transmembrane location of these proteins in erythrocytes. It is also possible that the high-affinity, low-capacity site plays a restricted role in RBC function, perhaps in specific cellular reaction, or that the low-affinity, high-capacity site has a more generalized structural role in RBC function. Since phagocytosis generates peroxide free radicals[27] that may be damaging to erythrocyte membranes,[28] it is tempting to postulate that tocopherol in RBC membranes confers a certain amount of protection against this potential damage to erythrocytes.

Summary

Previous work from our laboratory demonstrated specific binding sites for ^{3}H-RRR-α-tocopherol (^{3}H-dαT) in membranes of rat adrenal cells.[10] As tocopherol deficiency is associated with increased susceptibility of red blood cells to hemolysis, we investigated tocopherol binding sites in human RBCs. Erythrocytes were found to have specific binding sites for ^{3}H-dαT that exhibited saturability and time and cell-concentration dependence as well as reversibility of binding. Kinetic studies of binding demonstrated two binding sites—one with high affinity (K_a of 2.6×10^7 M^{-1}), low capacity (7,600 sites per cell) and the other with low affinity (1.2×10^6 M^{-1}), high capacity (150,000 sites per cell).

In order to localize the binding sites further, RBCs were fractionated and greater than 90% of the tocopherol binding was located in the membranes. Similar to the finding in intact RBCs, the membranes exhibited two binding sites with a respective K_a of 3.3×10^7 M^{-1} and 1.5×10^6 M^{-1}. Specificity data for binding demonstrated 10% binding for RRR-γ-tocopherol, but no other tocopherol analog exhibited competition for ^{3}H-dαT binding sites. Instability data suggested a protein nature for these binding sites.

Preliminary studies on Triton X-100 solubilized fractions resolved the binding sites to a major component with an M_r of 65,000 and a minor component with an M_r of 125,000.

We conclude that human erythrocyte membranes contain specific binding sites for RRR-α-tocopherol. These sites may be of physiologic significance in the function of tocopherol on the red blood cell membrane.

Acknowledgments

The authors wish to thank Richard Fleming and Michael Davis for technical assistance and Linda Balentine for editorial assistance. They are grateful to Dr. W. E. Scott of Hoffmann-La Roche for the gifts of various tocopherol analogs.

References

1. NELSON, J. S. 1980. In Vitamin E. L. J. Machlin, Ed.: 397–428. Marcel Dekker. New York, N.Y.
2. SLATER, T. F. & B. C. SAWYER. 1971. Biochem. J. **123**: 823–828.
3. KITABCHI, A. E. 1980. In Vitamin E. L. J. Machlin, Ed.: 348–371. Marcel Dekker. New York, N.Y.
4. NATHANS, A. H. & A. E. KITABCHI. 1975. Biochim. Biophys. Acta **399**: 244–253.
5. KITABCHI, A. E., A. H. NATHANS & L. C. KITCHELL. 1973. J. Biol. Chem. **248**: 835–840.
6. CIVEN, M., J. E. LEEB, R. M. WISHNAIN & R. J. MORIN. 1980. Int. J. Vitam. Nutr. Res. **50**: 70–78.
7. KITABCHI, A. E., A. NATHANS, J. BARKER, L. KITCHELL & B. WATSON. 1978. In Tocopherol, Oxygen and Biomembranes. C. de Duve & O. Hayaishi, Eds.: 201–219. Elsevier/North Holland Biomedical Press. Amsterdam, the Netherlands.
8. CORASH, L., S. SPIELBERG, C. BARTSOCAS, L. BOXER, R. STEINHERZ, M. SHEETZ, M. EGAN, J. SCHLESSLEMAN & J. D. SCHULMAN. 1980. N. Engl. J. Med. **303**: 416–420.
9. SCHULMAN, J. D., Moderator. 1980. Ann. Intern. Med. **93**: 330–346.
10. KITABCHI, A. E., J. WIMALASENA & J. BARKER. 1980. Biochem. Biophys. Res. Commun. **96**: 1739–1746.

11. KITABCHI, A. E. & J. WIMALASENA. 1982. Biochim. Biophys. Acta **684**: 200–206.
12. WIMALASENA, J. & A. E. KITABCHI. 1981. (Submitted.)
13. WIMALASENA, J., M. DAVIS & A. E. KITABCHI. 1981. Fed. Proc. **40**: 874.
14. YASUDA, K. & A. E. KITABCHI. 1980. Diabetes **29**: 811–814.
15. BOYUM, A. 1968. Scand. J. Clin. Invest. **21**(Suppl. 97): 77–89.
16. SCATCHARD, G. 1949. Ann. N.Y. Acad. Sci. **51**: 660–672.
17. DE MEYTS, P. & J. ROTH. 1975. Biochem. Biophys. Res. Commun. **66**: 1118–1126.
18. THAKUR, A. K., M. L. JAFFE & D. RODBARD. 1980. Anal. Biochem. **107**: 279–295.
19. FAIRBANKS, G., T. L. STECK & D. F. H. WALLACH. 1971. Biochemistry **10**: 2606–2717.
20. LOWRY, N. J., A. L. ROSEBROUGH, A. L. FARR & R. J. RANDALL. 1951. J. Biol. Chem. **193**: 265–271.
21. FARRELL, P. M., J. G. BIERI, J. F. FRATANTONI, R. F. WOOD & P. A. DI SANT'AGNESE. 1977. J. Clin. Invest. **60**: 233–241.
22. CATIGNANI, G. L. 1975. Biochem. Biophys. Res. Commun. **67**: 66–72.
23. CATIGNANI, G. L. & J. G. BIERI. 1977. Biochim. Biophys. Acta **497**: 349–357.
24. NAIR, P. P., R. N. PATNAIK & J. W. HAUSWIRTH. 1978. In Tocopherol, Oxygen and Biomembranes. C. de Duve & O. Hayaishi, Eds.: 121–130. Elsevier/North Holland Biomedical Press. Amsterdam, the Netherlands.
25. TAPPEL, A. L. 1972. Ann. N.Y. Acad. Sci. **203**: 12–28.
26. MCCAY, P. B. & M. KING. 1980. In Vitamin E. L. J. Machlin, Ed.: 289–317. Marcel Dekker. New York, N.Y.
27. ROOS, D. & R. S. WEENING. 1979. In Oxygen Free Radicals and Tissue Damage: 225–262. Excerpta Medica. Amsterdam, the Netherlands.
28. WILSON, R. L. 1979. In Oxygen Free Radicals and Tissue Damage: 19–42. Excerpta Medica. Amsterdam, the Netherlands.

DISCUSSION

S. S. SHAPIRO (*Hoffmann-La Roche, Inc., Nutley, N.J.*): Have you determined the relationship between the number of binding sites and how much tocopherol is found in the red blood cell membrane?

A. E. KITABCHI: You've touched upon a very important point. These membranes are washed very thoroughly, and there isn't much tocopherol in them by the time we are through washing the red blood cells. If we take what is available in the literature, the tocopherol concentration in the RBC is 11 μM.

S. S. SHAPIRO: I think sometimes we forget that molecules like vitamin A, vitamin E, and corticosteroids are not soluble in the cytoplasm. If we find them in cells, they have to be bound either to proteins or to receptors or exist in the lipid environment of the cells. What you're looking at might be a binding site on the external face to get it into the membrane and not the actual binding site or the storage site in the membrane, if there is one.

A. E. KITABCHI: We never did say storage site.

L. PACKER (*University of California, Berkeley, Calif.*): How thoroughly have you investigated the ability of tritiated tocopherol to exchange with unlabeled tocopherol? If these proteins are going to be important in tocopherol function in erythrocytes, they ought to be able to exchange and move about.

A. E. KITABCHI: No, we have not investigated this, and I think it's a very good suggestion.

R. E. OLSON (*St. Louis University School of Medicine, St. Louis, Mo.*): It isn't clear to me how pure your receptor protein is.

A. E. KITABCHI: Oh, not at all pure.

R. E. OLSON: What can you tell us about it? Does it require detergent for solubility? Does it require phospholipid? If it does, how can you do binding studies?

A. E. KITABCHI: We have tried numerous detergents, and we can't get any reasonably satisfactory result except for Triton at 1%. It looks like it is a micelle and is not a pure protein.

R. E. OLSON: You mean to say a phospholipid-protein micelle?

A. E. KITABCHI: Probably.

R. E. OLSON: But have you done any binding studies with purified protein?

A. E. KITABCHI: No.

R. E. OLSON: So the inference that this is a protein is based upon the effect of trypsin and so forth.

A. E. KITABCHI: Exactly. It's probably a lipid-protein complex.

M. SAYARE (University of Connecticut, Storrs, Conn.): Are the membranes you used leaky (open) ghosts?

A. E. KITABCHI: They are, and they have been washed thoroughly so they are not pink.

G. L. CATIGNANI (North Carolina State University, Raleigh, N.C.): On most of your slides you had 250,000 counts per minute during your incubations and your cells were binding anywhere from 5,000 to 20,000. This represents a pretty small percentage of the total counts in the incubation. Most of us who work with tritiated tocopherol know it as a notoriously unstable compound. Keeping its radiochemical purity above 90% is really an ongoing job. Have you ever extracted any of the membrane radioactivity to prove that it's actually α-tocopherol?

A. E. KITABCHI: With tritiated tocopherol, you have to throw it away after three weeks because of decomposition. We do observe almost 90% reversibility with unlabeled tocopherol.

P. MARFEY (State University of New York, Albany, N.Y.): I'd like to make one suggestion. There is some analogy with ubiquinone binding to certain proteins. To demonstrate specific protein binding, a ubiquinone was made into a reagent. Then the particular protein was covalently attached to the ubiquinone. I think that it is possible to make vitamin E into a reagent as well. One possibility would be to attach a halogen to one of the methyl groups on the aromatic ring. That would effectively alkylate a protein where it lands in a membrane. Then one would be able to have a covalent product that would be stable for isolation and further characterization.

S. B. SHOHET (University of California, San Francisco, Calif.): Is there a possibility that the low-affinity binding that you observed might be a solubility function, that is, just the equilibration solubility of vitamin E in the lipid spaces in the membrane?

A. E. KITABCHI: I can't rule it out.

THE EFFECT OF VITAMIN E ON RED CELL HEMOLYSIS AND BILIRUBINEMIA

Steven J. Gross

Department of Pediatrics
Duke University Medical Center
Durham, North Carolina 27710

Stephen A. Landaw

Department of Medicine
State University of New York
Upstate Medical Center
Syracuse, New York 13210

The life span of the term infant's erythrocytes is approximately two-thirds that of the erythrocytes of normal adults.[1] The red cells of premature infants have an even shorter life span than do the red cells of term infants.[2] The mechanisms responsible for this accelerated senescence are unknown.

Premature infants, at birth, are deficient in vitamin E. Deficiency of vitamin E, a naturally occurring antiperoxidant, can produce a shortening of red cell life span.[3] The purpose of this investigation was to determine if the presence of vitamin E deficiency in the premature infant during the first week of life played a contributory role in the shortened red cell survival. In addition, since hyperbilirubinemia is, in part, secondary to red cell breakdown, we examined the influence of early vitamin E supplementation on bilirubinemia in preterm infants.

MATERIALS AND METHODS

The initial study involved 20 infants, each weighing less than 2,500 grams and born before 36 weeks gestation. All infants were free of major disease, were breathing room air, had a hemoglobin value in excess of 13.0 g/dl on the third day of life, and had no evidence of Rh or ABO isoimmunization. Throughout the study period, all infants were fed Similac (20 calories per ounce) formula without iron (Ross Laboratories, Columbus, Ohio).

Infants were randomly assigned to treatment and control groups. Infants in the treatment group received all-rac-α-tocopherol (Roche Laboratories, Nutley, N.J.) administered intramuscularly. Infants were given a total dose of 125 mg/kg. The vitamin was administered in eight divided doses, an injection in each thigh, on days 4, 5, 6, and 7 of life. This treatment schedule allowed for small volumes to be given in each injection site in order to minimize local reactions.

On days 3 and 8 of life, venous blood samples were obtained for the measurement of blood carboxyhemoglobin (COHb) levels. The level of carboxyhemoglobin was determined by gas chromatography as previously described.[4]

In the second set of experiments, two groups of appropriate-for-gestational-age preterm infants were studied: (1) 20 infants with birth weights between 1,000 and 1,500 g, and (2) 20 infants with birth weights between 1,501 and 2,000 g. Infants with a hemoglobin value less than 13.0 g/dl or with Rh or ABO isoimmunization were excluded from the study. Infants were fed Enfamil (20

315

0077-8923/82/0393-0315 $01.75/0 © 1982, NYAS

TABLE 1

PERCENT CARBOXYHEMOGLOBIN IN THREE GROUPS OF PATIENTS

Adults (n = 20)	Term Infants on Day 3 (n = 20)	Premature Infants on Day 3 (n = 20)
0.34 ± 0.10*	0.56 ± 0.11	1.08 ± 0.20
(0.15–0.47)	(0.34–0.76)	(0.64–1.38)

*Figures represent mean and one standard deviation. Ranges are indicated in parentheses. Significance: adults vs. term infants, $p < 0.001$; adults vs. premature infants, $p < 0.001$; term infants vs. premature infants, $p < 0.001$.

calories per ounce) without iron (Mead-Johnson and Co., Evansville, Ind.) or human milk.

Half the infants in each birth weight group were assigned randomly to a treatment group, and the other half of each group served as controls. Infants in the treatment groups received all-rac-α-tocopherol intramuscularly at a total dose of 50 mg/kg. The vitamin was administered in six divided doses, an injection in each thigh, on days 1, 2, and 3 of life.

Venous blood was obtained from all infants on the day of birth (before tocopherol administration in the treatment groups) and on day 8 of life for determinations of plasma tocopherol levels.[5] Blood was also obtained on day 8 of life for determination of hydrogen peroxide hemolysis, a measure of red cell susceptibility to peroxidation.[6] Serum bilirubin measurements were performed daily during the first week of life on capillary blood samples by modification of the method of Jendrassik and Grof.[7]

Phototherapy was administered using a bank of six Westinghouse special blue fluorescent bulbs (20 W). Phototherapy was instituted for serum bilirubin values >5 mg/dl within the first 24 hours of life, >7.5 mg/dl between 24 and 48 hours of life, and >9.0 mg/dl after 48 hours of life. Phototherapy was discontinued when the serum bilirubin was decreasing and less than 8.0 mg/dl. No infants underwent exchange transfusion.

Student's t-test was used for the statistical interpretation of the data.

TABLE 2

CHARACTERISTICS OF THE STUDY POPULATION

	Control Group (n = 10)	Vitamin E– Supplemented Group (n = 10)
Gestational age (weeks)	33.2 ± 1.4*	33.5 ± 1.7
	(31–36)	(31–36)
Birth weight (g)	1631 ± 397	1717 ± 176
	(1180–2438)	(1590–2010)
Five-minute Apgar score	7.9 ± 0.9	8.7 ± 0.9
	(6–9)	(7–10)

*Figures represent mean and one standard deviation. Ranges are indicated in parentheses.

Effect of Vitamin E Administration on Carboxyhemoglobin Levels

Prior to this study, carboxyhemoglobin determinations were performed on day 3 of life in 20 healthy premature infants and 20 term infants and compared with values in 20 healthy, nonsmoking adults. These analyses demonstrated that the mean percent carboxyhemoglobin level was significantly higher in premature infants than in term infants (TABLE 1). Both groups had values that were significantly higher than those observed in the adults.

The study group was composed of 10 infants who received vitamin E and 10 infants who served as controls. These two groups did not differ with respect to gestational age, birth weight, or five-minute Apgar score (TABLE 2).

On day 3 of life, prior to vitamin E administration, the two groups had similar percent carboxyhemoglobin levels (TABLE 3) and were indistinguishable from the 20 premature infants who had been evaluated prior to the initiation of the study.

TABLE 3

PERCENT CARBOXYHEMOGLOBIN LEVELS IN 10 α-TOCOPHEROL-SUPPLEMENTED
PREMATURE INFANTS AND 10 CONTROLS

Age in Days	Controls	Tocopherol Supplemented
3	0.96 ± 0.19*	1.08 ± 0.17
	(0.80–1.25)	(0.89–1.40)
8	0.96 ± 0.32	0.78 ± 0.16†
	(0.51–1.56)	(0.57–1.07)

*Figures represent mean and one standard deviation. Ranges are indicated in parentheses.
†Change in percent of COHb, day 3 to day 8, $p < 0.005$.

The 10 infants who received vitamin E demonstrated a significant decrease ($p < 0.005$) in their mean carboxyhemoglobin values between day 3 and day 8 of life (1.08% to 0.78%), whereas the mean value remained unchanged at 0.96% in the control group (TABLE 3). In the treatment group, 9 of 10 infants displayed a decrease in carboxyhemoglobin values, whereas a decrease was observed in only 4 of 10 controls.

Effect of Vitamin E Administration on Neonatal Bilirubinemia

Infants with Birth Weight 1,000 to 1,500 Grams

Ten infants received vitamin E, and 10 infants served as controls. The two groups did not differ with respect to gestational age, birth weight, or five-minute Apgar score. (TABLE 4).

The mean plasma tocopherol concentration on day 1 of life was 0.3 ± 0.1 mg/dl in control and treatment groups. The mean level on day 8 of life was 0.5 ± 0.3 mg/dl in the control group and 3.0 ± 1.0 mg/dl in the vitamin E-supplemented group ($p < 0.001$). Hydrogen peroxide hemolysis values on day 8 of life were

TABLE 4

CHARACTERISTICS OF STUDY POPULATIONS

	Infants with Birth Weight 1000–1500 Grams		Infants with Birth Weight 1501–2000 Grams	
	Control Group (n = 10)	Vitamin E– Supplemented Group (n = 10)	Control Group (n = 10)	Vitamin E– Supplemented Group (n = 10)
Gestational age (week)	29.7 ± 1.3* (29–32)	29.1 ± 1.0 (27–30)	32.5 ± 1.1 (31–34)	32.2 ± 1.3 (31–35)
Birth weight (grams)	1232 ± 111 (1040–1425)	1132 ± 120 (1000–1400)	1731 ± 162 (1530–2000)	1726 ± 161 (1510–1970)
Five-minute Apgar score	6.9 ± 2.1 (2–9)	7.7 ± 2.0 (4–9)	8.2 ± 1.1 (6–9)	8.2 ± 1.8 (4–10)

*Figures represent mean and one standard deviation. Ranges are indicated in parentheses.

abnormal (>10%) in six infants in the control group and in none in the treatment group (TABLE 5).

Serum bilirubin values during the first week of life are depicted in FIGURE 1. After day 1, lower serum bilirubin values were consistently observed for the vitamin E-supplemented infants. The mean bilirubin levels on day 3 of life were 8.8 ± 2.2 mg/dl for the control group and 6.5 ± 2.2 mg/dl for the treatment group (p < 0.5). In addition, the highest serum bilirubin value obtained during the first week of life averaged 10.6 ± 2.6 mg/dl for the control group and 8.3 ± 2.2 mg/dl for the treatment group (p < 0.05).

The mean duration of phototherapy during the first week of life was 107 ± 31 hours for the control group compared with 48 ± 18 hours for the vitamin E-supplemented group (p < 0.001).

TABLE 5

PLASMA TOCOPHEROL AND HYDROGEN PEROXIDE HEMOLYSIS IN STUDY POPULATIONS

	Infants with Birth Weight 1000–1500 Grams		Infants with Birth Weight 1501–2000 Grams	
	Control Group (n = 10)	Vitamin E– Supplemented Group (n = 10)	Control Group (n = 10)	Vitamin E– Supplemented Group (n = 10)
Plasma tocopherol				
Day 1	0.3 ± 0.1* (0.1–0.5)	0.3 ± 0.1 (0.1–0.5)	0.5 ± 0.2 (0.3–0.8)	0.6 ± 0.2 (0.2–0.9)
Day 8	0.5 ± 0.3 (0.2–0.9)	3.0 ± 1.0† (1.7–4.8)	0.7 ± 0.3 (0.4–1.4)	3.9 ± 1.1† (2.3–5.0)
Hydrogen peroxide hemolysis (%)				
Day 8	25.5 ± 33.3 (0–91)	0.0 ± 0.0	19.2 ± 24.8 (0–83)	0.0 ± 0.0

*Figures represent mean and one standard deviation. Ranges are indicated in parentheses.

†Change in plasma tocopherol, day 1 to day 8, p < 0.001.

Infants with Birth Weight 1,501 to 2,000 Grams

The 10 infants who received vitamin E and the 10 infants who served as controls did not differ with respect to gestational age, birth weight, or five-minute Apgar score (TABLE 4).

The mean plasma tocopherol concentration on day 1 of life was 0.5 ± 0.2 mg/dl for the control group and 0.6 ± 0.2 mg/dl for the treatment group. The mean level on day 8 of life was 0.7 ± 0.3 mg/dl for the control group and 3.9 ± 1.1 mg/dl for the treatment group (p < 0.001). On day 8 of life, hydrogen peroxide

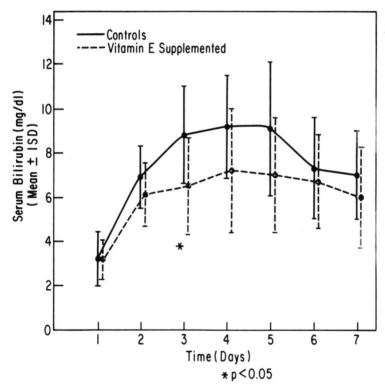

FIGURE 1. Serum bilirubin in vitamin E-supplemented infants and controls with birth weight 1,000 to 1,500 g.

hemolysis values were abnormal (>10%) in seven infants in the control group and in none in the treatment group (TABLE 5).

Serum bilirubin values during the first week of life are depicted in FIGURE 2. Values were not different between groups except on day 7 of life, when the mean serum bilirubin of 6.7 ± 1.3 mg/dl for the vitamin E-treated group was significantly lower than the mean value of 9.0 ± 2.3 mg/dl for the control group. The highest serum bilirubin obtained during the first seven days averaged 11.5 ± 2.3 mg/dl for the control group and 9.8 ± 1.4 mg/dl for the treatment group (0.05 < p < 0.1).

The mean durations of phototherapy during the first week of life for the control group (66 ± 46 hours) and treatment group (60 ± 50 hours) were not different.

No detectable toxicity related to vitamin E administration was noted. Mild, transient erythema and induration at the site of injection were commonly observed.

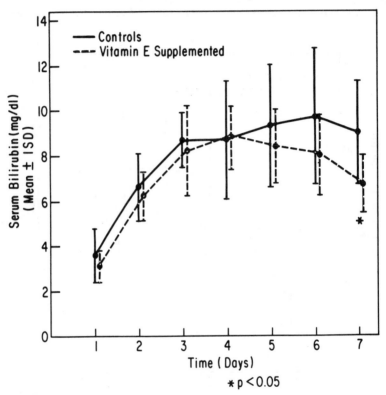

FIGURE 2. Serum bilirubin in vitamin E-supplemented infants and controls with birth weight 1,501 to 2,000 g.

DISCUSSION

The catabolism of heme is accompanied by the equimolar formation of carbon monoxide (CO) and bilirubin. The percent of carboxyhemoglobin in circulating blood has been found to be a good measure of red cell hemolysis and bilirubin production.[8,9] We have found that preterm infants have an elevated percentage of carboxyhemoglobin on day 3 of life, which persists at age 8 days.

At birth, the preterm infant is deficient in vitamin E. Body stores and plasma concentration vary directly with birth weight.[10] All newborns with birth weight ≤1,500 g had plasma tocopherol levels ≤0.5 mg/dl. Neonates with birth weight between 1,500 and 2,000 g demonstrated a wider range of tocopherol values at birth, although all were <1.0 mg/dl. The intramuscular administration of 125 mg/kg of tocopherol, a dose known to produce prompt sufficiency,[11] was followed by a significant decrease in the percent carboxyhemoglobin at the end of the first week of life. Even the lower intramuscular dose of vitamin E (50 mg/kg) uniformly corrected the existing deficiency, as measured by plasma tocopherol level and red cell susceptibility to peroxidation. Further, the administration of 50 mg/kg of the vitamin also resulted in a significant decrease in serum bilirubin concentration as well as a significant reduction in duration of phototherapy during the first week of life for infants with birth weight <1,500 g.[12]

The effect of early vitamin E administration on hematologic parameters has been investigated previously. Dyggve and Probst studied 133 preterm infants with birth weight less than 2,500 g.[13] Half of the infants received 100 mg *all-rac-α*-tocopherol intramuscularly on the day of birth, and half of the infants served as controls. Lower serum bilirubin values were found during the first week of life in the vitamin E–treated infants, although the difference was not statistically significant.[13] The hemoglobin values were significantly higher in the infants who received vitamin E than in the control infants.[13] These findings suggested that vitamin E administered intramuscularly resulted in decreased erythrocyte hemolysis. No measurements of tocopherol sufficiency were reported.

Abrams *et al.* investigated the relationship between vitamin E and early idiopathic hyperbilirubinemia in 40 term newborns.[14] Twenty infants received 10 mg *α*-tocopheryl acetate by mouth daily from birth. Twenty control infants received no added tocopherol. There was no difference in plasma bilirubin or hemoglobin during the first five days of life between the vitamin E–supplemented and control groups.[14] Review of the data suggest, however, that the oral administration of the vitamin was not effective in correcting the existing deficiency. After a week of daily oral tocopherol, red cell susceptibility to autoxidation, as measured by malonyldialdehyde (MDA) production, remained grossly abnormal. Plasma tocopherol levels were below the normal level of 0.80 mg/dl as determined by the authors in four of the five cases studied. Consequently, vitamin E sufficiency was never achieved.

The results of the present study demonstrate that the administration of intramuscular vitamin E appears to reduce, but not eliminate, the accelerated red cell destruction that characterizes the preterm infant. Furthermore, the early administration of tocopherol results in significantly lower serum bilirubin values and decreased duration of requirement for phototherapy during the first week of life in very low birth weight infants.

REFERENCES

1. PEARSON, H. A. 1967. Life-span of the fetal red blood cell. J. Pediatr. **70:** 166.
2. O'BRIEN, R. T. & H. A. PEARSON. 1971. Physiologic anemia of the newborn infant. J. Pediatr. **79:** 132.
3. RITCHIE, J. H., M. B. FISH, V. MCMASTERS & M. GROSSMAN. 1968. Edema and hemolytic anemia in premature infants. N. Engl. J. Med. **279:** 1185.
4. GROSS, S. J., S. A. LANDAW & F. A. OSKI. 1977. Vitamin E and neonatal hemolysis. Pediatrics **59:** 995.
5. QUAIFE, M. L., N. S. SCRIMSHAW & O. H. LOWRY. 1949. A micromethod for assay of total tocopherols in blood serum. J. Biol. Chem. **180:** 1229.
6. ROSE, C. S. & P. GYORGY. 1952. Specificity of hemolytic reaction in vitamin E–deficient erythrocytes. Am. J. Physiol. **168:** 414.
7. JENDRASSIK, L. & P. GROF. 1938. Vereinfachte photometrische Methoden zur Bestimmung des Blutbilirubins. Biochem. Z. **297:** 81.
8. ENGEL, R. R., F. L. RODKEY & C. E. KRILL. 1971. Carboxyhemoglobin levels as an index of hemolysis. Pediatrics **47:** 723.

9. ALDEN, E. R. & S. R. LYNCH. 1974. Carboxyhemoglobin determination in evaluating neonatal jaundice. Am. J. Dis. Child. **127:** 214.
10. DALLMAN, P. R. 1974. Iron, vitamin E, and folate in the preterm infant. J. Pediatr. **85:** 742.
11. GRAEBER, J. E., M. L. WILLIAMS & F. A. OSKI. 1977. The use of intramuscular vitamin E in the premature infant. Optimum dose and iron interaction. J. Pediatr. **90:** 282.
12. GROSS, S. J. 1979. Vitamin E and neonatal bilirubinemia. Pediatrics **64:** 321.
13. DYGGVE, H. V. & J. H. PROBST. 1963. Vitamin E to premature infants. Acta Paediatr. Scand. **146:** 48.
14. ABRAMS, B. A., J. M. C. GUTTERIDGE, J. STOCKS, M. FRIEDMAN & T. L. DORMANDY. 1973. Vitamin E in neonatal hyperbilirubinema. Arch. Dis. Child. **48:** 721.

DISCUSSION

R. S. LONDON (*Sinai Hospital of Baltimore, Inc., Baltimore, Md.*): A few questions. First of all, were your mothers on prenatal supplementation containing tocopherol?

S. J. GROSS: Mothers received standard prenatal vitamins, but did not receive any additional tocopherol.

R. S. LONDON: When you started these babies on formula by nasogastric feeding, did you have tocopherol in the formula in both groups?

S. J. GROSS: In the first set of studies, where we were looking at carboxyhemoglobin, all infants were fed Similac without iron, which did have 10 units of tocopherol per liter. In the second set of studies, infants were fed either Enfamil without iron or human milk. Since we only examined these infants over the first week of life, only small amounts of milk were ingested. There were no differences in hematologic parameters between infants fed formula or human milk.

R. S. LONDON: Do you have any data on the intraventricular hemorrhage rates in the prematures?

S. J. GROSS: These were healthy preterm infants. We did not do routine ultrasound to pick up subtle hemorrhages. However, none of these infants had any significant hemorrhage that was apparent clinically.

P. HOCHSTEIN (*University of Southern California, Los Angeles, Calif.*): Can you comment on the morphology of the cells from the infants. Are there volume changes? Are these bizarre-looking cells?

S. J. GROSS: No, these were normal premature infants and had normal red cell morphology. There were no striking differences between the groups over the first week of life.

P. HOCHSTEIN: May I also ask, Is it possible to do granulocyte function tests in these infants? Do you know whether granulocytes are able to take up bacteria and kill them *in vitro*?

S. J. GROSS: We did not look at any white cell functions.

G. R. BUETTNER (*Wabash College, Crawfordsville, Ind.*): What is the significance of the carboxyhemoglobin studies that you did?

S. J. GROSS: The catabolism of heme, derived primarily from the degradation of hemoglobin, is the sole endogenous source of carbon monoxide. The latter is transported as carboxyhemoglobin eventually to be eliminated through the lungs. In the absence of exposure to exogenous carbon monoxide and provided pulmonary function is normal, blood carboxyhemoglobin levels correlate well with rates of carbon monoxide production.

PEROXIDATION, VITAMIN E, AND
SICKLE-CELL ANEMIA*

Danny Chiu, Elliott Vichinsky, Maggie Yee,
Klara Kleman, and Bertram Lubin

Bruce Lyon Memorial Research Laboratory
Children's Hospital Medical Center
Oakland, California 94609

INTRODUCTION

Sickle-cell anemia (SCA) is a genetic disorder caused by a point mutation in DNA that codes for valine rather than glutamic acid in the sixth position of the β-globin chain of the hemoglobin tetramer. Upon deoxygenation, this amino acid substitution causes sickle hemoglobin to polymerize and form filaments, which eventually distort the red cell into the characteristic sickle-shaped red cells. This process is referred to as sickling and is reversible when the hemoglobin is reoxygenated. However, upon repeated cycles of sickling and unsickling, the red cell membrane becomes damaged and no longer permits the cell to return to a biconcave shape. These irreversibly deformed cells are called irreversibly sickled cells (ISCs). Although ISCs are believed to influence clinical severity in SCA, the precise factors that contribute to formation of ISCs *in vivo* have not been established.

The clinical manifestations of SCA are characterized by chronic hemolytic anemia, recurrent vasoocclusive painful attacks, frequent bacterial infections, and, in some cases, eventual loss of organ function. However, a marked clinical diversity exists in this disease. For instance, some sickle-cell patients have many vasoocclusive crises and require frequent blood transfusions and hospitalizations while others rarely have complications. Although there is little doubt that the molecular defect of SCA resides in the hemoglobin, additional or secondary factors must be considered to explain these diverse clinical manifestations. One of these factors may relate to membrane peroxidative damage and its effects on the pathophysiology of SCA.

Peroxidative reactions have been proposed to be factors that contribute to the degenerative processes eventually resulting in cellular breakdown.[1,2] Circulating red cells are particularly susceptible to peroxidative damage because conditions that favor peroxidation are seemingly optimal in red cells: the membrane of these cells is rich in polyunsaturated fatty acids, the cells are continuously exposed to high oxygen tensions, and the cells contain hemoglobin, one of the most powerful catalysts for the initiation of peroxidative reactions.[3] The fact that normal red cells are protected from peroxidative damage *in vivo* can be attributed to efficient antioxidant mechanisms. This antioxidant protection is, in part, a function of the structural integrity of each cellular constituent and, in part, a reflection of the antioxidant systems within the cell. These include superoxide dismutase, glutathione peroxidase, catalase, and vitamin E. An impairment in any of these defense mechanisms may render the red cells more susceptible to peroxidative damage and eventually lead to its demise.

*This study was supported in part by U.S. Public Health Service Grant No. HL 27059 and in part by a grant-in-aid from Hoffmann-La Roche, Inc.

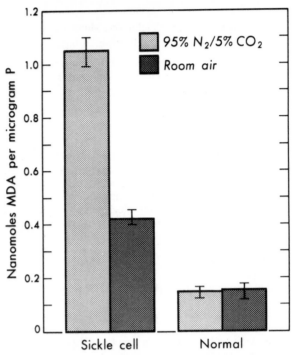

FIGURE 1. Effect of sickling on the susceptibility of sickle erythrocytes to lipid peroxidation. The MDA generated from normal and sickle erythrocytes following two hours incubation under either room air or 95% N_2–5% CO_2 at 37°C was measured. The mean values as well as the ranges are shown. (Data from Reference 4.)

INCREASED SUSCEPTIBILITY OF SICKLE ERYTHROCYTES TO PEROXIDATION

Since there is a major distortion of the red cell shape upon sickling and hence a loss of structural integrity, one might expect an increase in susceptibility of sickled erythrocytes to peroxidation. This is indeed what we have found.[4] In our experiments, normal and sickle red blood cells were incubated under both oxygenated and deoxygenated conditions in the presence of hydrogen peroxide. The susceptibility to peroxidation, as measured by malonyldialdehyde (MDA) generation, of sickle erythrocytes was increased threefold when the cells were sickled under anaerobic conditions (FIGURE 1). In contrast, similar incubations of normal erythrocytes did not change their susceptibility to peroxidation.

Using both chemical and enzymatic probes,[4,5] we demonstrated that membrane phospholipid reorganization occurs during the sickling process, with an increased quantity of phosphatidylethanolamine and phosphatidylserine exposed to the outer lipid bilayer. Since these aminophospholipids contain primary polyunsaturated fatty acids, it is conceivable that such abnormal membrane phospholipid organization induced by sickling is one of the factors that renders sickle erythrocytes more susceptible to lipid peroxidative damage.

Decreased Blood Vitamin E Levels in SCA

The increased susceptibility to peroxidation of sickle erythrocytes is not entirely due to abnormal membrane lipid asymmetry. As shown in Figure 1, even under oxygenated conditions in which most red blood cells (RBCs) containing sickle hemoglobin are biconcave disks, such erythrocytes are still more susceptible to lipid peroxidation than are normal RBCs. This finding suggests an abnormality in the antioxidant system in addition to that induced by abnormal membrane lipid asymmetry. Indeed, an additional abnormality has been identified to be low serum levels of vitamin E.[6,7]

Figure 2 shows the plasma vitamin E levels in 54 sickle-cell patients and 16 normal controls. The majority of sickle-cell patients had vitamin E levels below the mean for the control group. In this patient population, ranging in age from 18 months to 24 years, the vitamin E levels varied from 0.17 to 1.07 mg/dl, with a mean of 0.61 ± 0.19 mg/dl. The mean level for 16 age-matched normal controls was 0.89 ± 0.25 mg/dl ($p < 0.01$). An alternate method of expressing the data showed that 30% of sickle-cell patients had a serum vitamin E level below 0.5 mg%. Further, the molar ratio of vitamin E to red cell membrane phospholipid in sickle erythrocytes was 7.8×10^{-4} compared to 15.1×10^{-4} in normal red cells.

The susceptibility of sickle erythrocytes to peroxidation was drastically reduced by preincubation of sickle erythrocytes with vitamin E.[6] In these experiments, both sickle and normal erythrocytes were separated into two equal

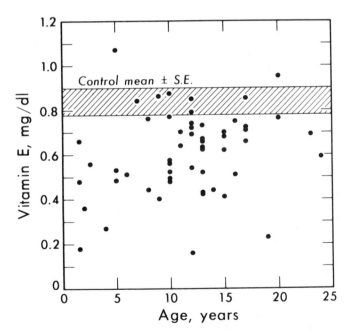

Figure 2. Plasma vitamin E concentrations from sickle-cell anemia patients plotted against age. The mean ± standard error (SE) plasma vitamin E concentrations of age-matched controls are shown in the cross-hatched bar.

portions. One portion was preincubated with 3 mg/ml of vitamin E for 16 hours, washed, and then reincubated with 5 mM hydrogen peroxide. TABLE 1 shows that the susceptibility of sickle erythrocytes to peroxidation was reduced to normal by preincubation with vitamin E. These results provide further evidence that the increased susceptibility to peroxidation of sickle erythrocytes is, in part, due to low plasma and red cell vitamin E levels in patients with SCA.

ABNORMAL GASTROINTESTINAL ABSORPTION OF VITAMIN E IN PATIENTS WITH SCA

In an effort to investigate the etiology of vitamin E deficiency in SCA, we carried out a vitamin E absorption study. The result of our experiment indicates a considerable abnormality in the absorption of vitamin E in SCA. Patients and controls were fasted overnight and then given a vitamin E tablet containing 400 IU of all-rac-α-tocopherol accompanied by a standard breakfast. At intervals of two hours, blood samples were taken from each subject for vitamin E analysis.

TABLE 1

EFFECT OF VITAMIN E ON THE SUSCEPTIBILITY OF SICKLE-CELL AND NORMAL ERYTHROCYTES TO LIPID PEROXIDATION

RBC	n	Incubated without Vitamin E*	Incubated with Vitamin E*
Sickle erythrocytes (SS)	5	177 ± 67	74 ± 20
Normal erythrocytes (AA)	5	74 ± 29	58 ± 10

*Figures are nmol MDA/g hemoglobin, mean ± standard deviation.

FIGURE 3 shows the results of this study. The vitamin E absorption curve in sickle-cell patients was significantly different from that of normal control subjects. The concentration of vitamin E in the blood of sickle-cell patients at all time intervals during our absorption study was less than that in the normal control subjects.

The explanation for decreased gastrointestinal absorption of vitamin E in SCA is unknown. However, we speculate that impaired bile salt secretion in the intestinal lumen might be a factor. Such a defect could be due to bilirubin sludging in bile canaliculi and/or liver parenchyma. Our finding of significantly lower (40–60%) plasma cholesterol levels[8] in SCA patients provides support for our hypothesis that the secretion of bile salts into the intestinal lumen may be impaired in SCA.

PATHOPHYSIOLOGIC SIGNIFICANCE OF ENHANCED RED CELL PEROXIDATION IN SCA

The pathophysiologic significance of red cell peroxidation in SCA has not been well defined. Since Stocks and Dormandy clearly demonstrated that peroxidant injury to red cells can eventually lead to hemolysis in vitro,[9] it is reasonable to speculate that enhanced susceptibility of sickle erythrocytes to peroxidation may contribute to hemolysis in vivo. An enhanced susceptibility to peroxidation secondary to vitamin E deficiency has been correlated with several

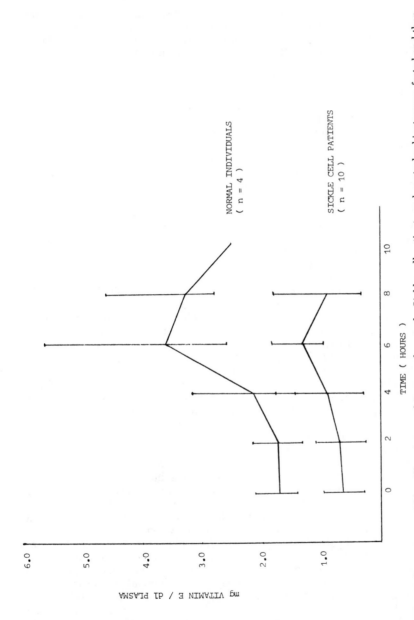

FIGURE 3. Vitamin E absorption in sickle-cell patients and in normal controls. Sickle-cell patients and control subjects were fasted and then were given 400 IU of *all-rac-α*-tocopherol orally accompanied by a standard breakfast. At intervals of two hours, blood samples were taken from each subject for vitamin E analysis.

erythrocyte abnormalities. Structural abnormalities, such as an increased number of distorted and contracted red cells, have been found in vitamin E-deficient premature infants.[10] Shortened red cell survival has been reported in vitamin E-deficient adults,[11] vitamin E-deficient premature infants,[10] and cystic fibrosis patients who have low blood vitamin E levels.[12] The hematological abnormalities observed in these vitamin E-deficient states can be corrected by vitamin E supplementation.[10-12] Taken together, these findings suggest that enhanced susceptibility of sickle erythrocytes to peroxidation may be a factor that contributes to the shortened red cell life span characteristic of SCA.

In addition to accelerated red cell destruction, peroxidative damage may play an important role in the pathogenesis of ISCs. As stated earlier, the ISC is morphologically identified by its failure to return to a biconcave disk when fully oxygenated and is mechanically identified by its entrance fragility and rigidity. Despite the fact that a positive correlation between percent ISC in peripheral blood and vasoocclusive episodes has not been demonstrated,[13] Serjeant et al. have shown a direct relationship between the percentage of circulating ISCs and extent of hemolysis.[14] Since ISCs are highly undeformable,[15] only a few may be required to initiate episodes of capillary obstruction leading to vasoocclusive complications.

The mechanism of ISC formation is presently unknown. Current concepts of ISC formation focus on irreversible deformation of the spectrin-actin lattice—the membrane skeletal proteins of the red cell—and on cellular dehydration secondary to abnormal membrane ion permeability. Studies by Lux et al. indicate irreversible deformation of the spectrin-actin lattice in ISCs and demonstrate that this deformation is not dependent upon the persistent interaction between sickle hemoglobin and the spectrin-actin lattice.[16] These investigators suggest that ISC formation is the result of a permanent alteration in the spectrin-actin lattice.[16] On the other hand, studies by Clark et al. indicate that the reduced deformability of ISCs is mainly due to dehydration of these cells and that the abnormal deformability of ISCs can be returned to normal following cellular rehydration.[15] The findings of Clark et al. imply that the inability of ISCs to return to their original biconcave shape is due to a high internal viscosity, which results from cellular dehydration caused by abnormal membrane ion permeability.[15]

These two theories do not have to be mutually exclusive. We hypothesize that peroxidative damage can lead to a permanent alteration in the spectrin-actin lattice as well as to abnormal membrane permeability. In the case of the spectrin-actin lattice defect, perhaps a structurally normal spectrin-actin network is passively deformed by the oriented microfilaments of hemoglobin S and then becomes fixed in an abnormal configuration. Malonyldialdehyde, a product of lipid peroxidation, is capable of cross-linking between free amino groups in proteins and could potentially contribute to formation of the abnormal spectrin-actin lattice in ISCs. In the case of abnormal membrane permeability, it is possible that peroxidative damage affects membrane components required to maintain normal permeability. Such damage could alter cation transport, create 70-Å holes in the membrane as suggested by Jacob and Lux,[17] and lead to abnormal passive ion transport. A comparison of several properties of vitamin E-deficient red cells following peroxidant injury to those of ISCs may provide some support for our hypothesis that peroxidative damage is involved in ISC formation.

Abnormal cation permeability is a well-documented membrane defect in ISCs.[18-20] The exact cause of this membrane defect has not been defined. It should be noted that H_2O_2 can induce a similar permeability defect in vitamin E-deficient human red cells. FIGURE 4 shows the loss of [42]K from vitamin E–deficient human red cells following peroxidant injury. Loss of potassium precedes hemolysis. This change in membrane permeability may represent a direct toxic effect of peroxidation on membrane integrity. It has long been recognized that changes in fatty acid composition contribute to alteration of membrane permeability in both artificial membrane and intact red cells.[21,22] Changes in membrane permeability are closely associated with changes in cell volume. Immediately following peroxidant injury, vitamin E–deficient red cells shrink due to water loss. Eventually, the defects in the membrane become so great that lysis occurs due to a colloid osmotic effect. Similar changes have been observed in mitochondrial and lysosomal membranes as a consequence of peroxidant injury.[23] Based upon these similarities, we hypothesize that peroxidation may contribute to the cation permeability defect in ISCs.

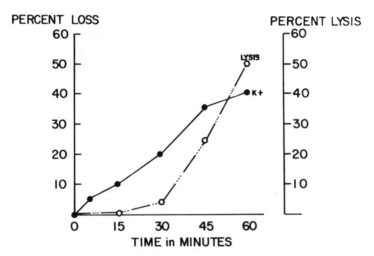

FIGURE 4. Effect of H_2O_2 on potassium permeability and hemolysis of vitamin E–deficient red cells. Potassium leakage of H_2O_2-treated vitamin E–deficient red cells was monitored by measuring the release of [42]K into the incubation medium at different time intervals following the addition of H_2O_2. The [42]K was first incorporated into red cells prior to incubation with H_2O_2. Hemolysis was monitored by the release of hemoglobin from red cells into the incubation medium.

Reduced deformability is another well-documented abnormality in ISCs.[15] Peroxidant injury to vitamin E–deficient human red cells can produce similar reduction in deformability. Red cell deformability, as measured by filtration techniques, was markedly decreased in vitamin E–deficient cells that had previously been incubated for 15 minutes with hydrogen peroxide (TABLE 2). When vitamin E–sufficient red cells were similarly incubated with hydrogen peroxide, they showed no change in filterability. In the absence of hydrogen peroxide, filtration rates for vitamin E–deficient cells were not significantly different from those of normal cells.

A more direct line of evidence to support our hypothesis that peroxidative damage may play a role in the pathogenesis of ISCs is provided by our in vitro experiment showing that oxidants enhance ISC formation whereas vitamin E

TABLE 2

EFFECT OF H_2O_2 ON RED CELL FILTERABILITY

RBC Samples	Rate of Filtration (mm³/second)
Normal	122
H_2O_2-treated normal	149
Vitamin E deficient	142
H_2O_2-treated vitamin E deficient	49

partially inhibits ISC formation. In our experiments, ISC-free sickle red blood cells were incubated under repeated oxygen and nitrogen cycles in the presence of either H_2O_2, MDA, vitamin E, or buffer alone for 24 hours. Upon completion of incubation, all samples were reoxygenated and the percent of ISCs determined. The results (TABLE 3) show that oxidant (H_2O_2) and peroxidation product (MDA) were capable of enhancing ISC formation whereas antioxidant (vitamin E) was able to reduce ISC formation. Similar results were obtained by Bowie et al.[24] The incomplete inhibition of ISC formation by vitamin E implies that peroxidative damage to red cell membrane may not be the only mechanism leading to ISC formation. This implication is consistent with the observation of Palek and Liu that there are several subpopulations of ISCs.[25]

Since vitamin E can partially inhibit ISC formation *in vitro*, vitamin E supplementation to sickle-cell patients should reduce ISC counts in their peripheral blood. This is exactly what Natta et al. have found.[26] In their study, six sickle-cell patients with initial ISC counts ranging from 17% to 35% (mean, 25%) were supplemented with 450 IU of vitamin E per day. ISC counts were rapidly reduced after vitamin E supplementation. After 10 weeks of vitamin E supplementation, most patients had reduced their ISC count by more than 50%. This reduction in ISC counts was accompanied by a significant elevation of blood vitamin E level. No further reduction in ISC counts was observed during the subsequent 24 weeks of vitamin E supplementation. We have been carrying out a similar clinical study, and the results show that the plasma vitamin E levels were significantly elevated following vitamin E supplementation and this was accompanied by reduced susceptibility of sickle red cells to peroxidation. However, there was no significant difference in ISC count between pre- and post–vitamin E supplementation periods.

A closer examination of the two studies indicates differences in the initial ISC counts in the two populations of sickle-cell patients. Our patients had an average initial ISC count of 12%, whereas the patients in Natta et al.'s study had an average initial ISC count of 25%.[26] Following vitamin E supplementation, the average ISC counts of Natta et al.'s patients were reduced to 11% and remained at that level throughout subsequent study. It is possible that patients in Natta et al.'s

TABLE 3

EFFECT OF OXIDANT AND VITAMIN E ON ISC FORMATION *In Vitro*

RBC Samples	Percent of ISC
Control	13
20 mM H_2O_2	19
20 mM MDA	22
3 mg% vitamin E	8

study were clinically distinct from our patients, since they had higher ISC counts to begin with. Since our *in vitro* experiment suggests that vitamin E only partially inhibits ISC formation, we speculate that in addition to peroxidative damage, other mechanisms also contribute to ISC formation. Nevertheless, these results strongly suggest that peroxidative damage is an important factor in the pathogenesis of ISCs.

SUMMARY

In summary, we propose the following scheme (FIGURE 5) to describe the role of peroxidation in the pathophysiology of SCA. Sickle erythrocytes are more susceptible to peroxidation than are normal erythrocytes. This increased susceptibility to peroxidation is, in part, due to decreased blood vitamin E levels and

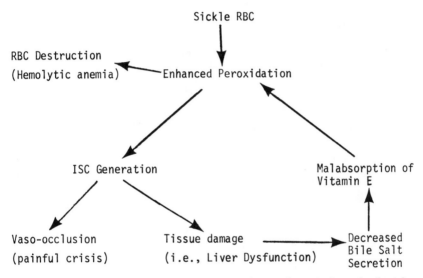

FIGURE 5. A proposed scheme describing the role of peroxidation in the pathophysiology of sickle-cell anemia.

abnormal membrane phospholipid organization induced by sickling. The peroxidative damage of sickle erythrocytes may accelerate or contribute to loss of cell deformability and to chronic hemolysis. Peroxidative damage can produce abnormal cellular properties, such as potassium leak and reduced filterability, and contribute to formation of ISCs. Increased red cell rigidity can initiate episodes of capillary obstruction, leading to vasoocclusive painful crises and to tissue infarction. Liver dysfunction as well as increased production of bilirubin secondary to hemolysis could result in bile sludging and decreased secretion of bile salts into the intestinal lumen. Reduced bile salt secretion leads to partial fat and vitamin E malabsorption. Vitamin E deficiency enhances red cell susceptibility to peroxidation and promotes a vicious cycle in SCA. Although we have not studied factors that might initiate peroxidative damage, sickle hemoglobin and excess body iron should be considered as potential sources. Our studies suggest that vitamin E supplementation to sickle-cell patients could be of clinical benefit.

ACKNOWLEDGMENTS

The authors are grateful to the sickle-cell staff at Children's Hospital Medical Center, Oakland, California, and the sickle-cell staff at Alta Bates Hospital, Berkeley, California. The authors would also like to thank Marion Douglass for an excellent job in typing this manuscript.

REFERENCES

1. TAPPEL, A. L. 1973. Lipid peroxidation damage to cell components. Fed. Proc. **32:** 1870–1874.
2. PRYOR, W. W. 1977. The involvement of radical reactions in aging and carcinogenesis. Med. Chem. **5:** 331–359.
3. CHIU, D., B. LUBIN & S. B. SHOHET. 1982. Peroxidative reactions in red cell biology. In Free Radicals in Biology. W. Pryor, Ed. **5:** 115–160. Academic Press, Inc. New York, N.Y.
4. CHIU, D., B. LUBIN & S. B. SHOHET. 1979. Erythrocyte membrane lipid reorganization during the sickling process. Br. J. Haematol. **41:** 223–234.
5. LUBIN, B., D. CHIU, B. ROELOFSEN & L. L. M. VAN DEENEN. 1981. Abnormalities in membrane phospholipid organization in sickle erythrocytes. J. Clin. Invest. **67:** 1643–1649.
6. CHIU, D. & B. LUBIN. 1979. Abnormal vitamin E and glutathione peroxidase levels in sickle cell anemia. J. Lab. Clin. Med. **94:** 542–548.
7. NATTA, C. & L. MACHLIN. 1979. Plasma levels of tocopherol in sickle cell anemia subjects. Am. J. Clin. Nutr. **32:** 1359–1362.
8. LUBIN, B., R. KRAUSS, K. KLEMAN, E. SIMMONS & D. CHIU. 1979. Reduced total serum cholesterol, high density and low density proteins in patients with sickle cell anemia. Blood **54**(Suppl. 1): 30a.
9. STOCKS, J. & T. L. DORMANDY. 1971. The autoxidation of human red cell lipids induced by hydrogen peroxide. Br. J. Haematol. **20:** 95–110.
10. OSKI, F. A. & L. A. BARNESS. 1967. A previously unrecognized cause of hemolytic anemia in the premature infant. J. Pediatr. **70:** 211–220.
11. LEONARD, P. J. & M. S. LOSOWSKY. 1971. Effect of alpha-tocopherol administration on red cell survival in vitamin E–deficient human subjects. Am. J. Clin. Nutr. **24:** 388–393.
12. FARRELL, P. M., J. G. BIERI, J. F. FRANTANTONI, R. E. WOOD & P. A. DI SANT'AGNESE. 1977. The occurrence and effects of human vitamin E deficiency: a study in patients with cystic fibrosis. J. Clin. Invest. **60:** 233–241.
13. RIEBER, E. E., G. VELIZ & S. POLLACK. 1977. Red cells in sickle cell crisis: observations on the pathophysiology of crisis. Blood **49:** 967–979.
14. SERJEANT, G. R., B. E. SERJEANT & P. F. MILNER. 1969. The irreversibly sickled cell: a determinant of haemolysis in sickle cell anemia. Br. J. Haematol. **17:** 527–533.
15. CLARK, M. L., N. MOHANDAS & S. B. SHOHET. 1980. Deformability of oxygenated irreversibly sickled cells. J. Clin. Invest. **65:** 189–196.
16. LUX, S. E., K. M. JOHN & M. J. KARNOVSKY. 1976. Irreversible deformation of the spectrin-actin lattice in irreversibly sickled cells. J. Clin. Invest. **58:** 955–963.
17. JACOB, H. S. & S. E. LUX. 1968. Degradation of membrane phospholipids and thiols in peroxide hemolysis: studies in vitamin E deficiency. Blood **32:** 549.
18. EATON, J. W., T. D. SKELTON, H. S. SWOFFORD, C. E. KALPIN & H. S. JACOB. 1973. Elevated erythrocyte calcium in sickle cell disease. Nature London **246:** 105–106.

19. GLADER, B. E. & D. G. NATHAN. 1978. Cation permeability alterations during sickling:
     relationship to cation composition and cellular hydration of irreversibly sickled cells.
     Blood **51:** 983–989.
20. CLARK, M. R., C. E. MORRISON & S. B. SHOHET. 1978. Monovalent cation transport in
     irreversibly sickled cells. J. Clin. Invest. **62:** 329–337.
21. MOORE, J. L., T. RICHARDSON & H. F. DeLUCA. 1968. Essential fatty acids and ion
     permeability of lecithin membranes. Chem. Phys. Lipids **3:** 39–45.
22. KOGL, F., J. DeGIER, I. MULDER & L. L. M. VAN DEENEN. 1960. Metabolism and functions
     of phosphatides: specific fatty acid composition of red cell membrane. Biochim.
     Biophys. Acta **43:** 95.
23. WILLS, E. D. & A. E. WILKINSON. 1966. Release of enzymes from lysosomes by
     irradiation and the relationship of lipid peroxide formation to enzyme release.
     Biochem. J. **99:** 657–664.
24. BOWIE, L. J., S. A. CARREATHERS & A. G. WRIGHT. 1979. Lipid membrane peroxidation,
     vitamin E, and the generation of irreversibly sickled cells in sickle cell anemia.
     (abst.). Clin. Chem. **25:** 1076.
25. PALEK, J. & S. C. LIU. 1979. Dependence of spectrin organization in red blood cell
     membranes on cell metabolism: implications for control of red cell shape, deform-
     ability, and surface area. Semin. Hematol. **16:** 75–94.
26. NATTA, C. L., L. J. MACHLIN & M. BRIN. 1980. A decrease in irreversibly sickled
     erythrocytes in sickle cell anemia patients given vitamin E. Am. J. Clin. Nutr.
     33: 968–971.

DISCUSSION

[Portions of this discussion refer back to material presented in Dr. Shohet's
Introduction to Part III (see page 229).—EDITOR]

M. K. HORWITT (*St. Louis Medical Center, St. Louis, Mo.*): Recently, when we
were discussing the ability of tocopherol to prolong the life of irreversibly sickled
cells, it was pointed out to me that this may not be clinically desirable. I wonder if
someone can enlighten me on this.

S. B. SHOHET (*University of California, San Francisco, Calif.*): The question is,
Would the preservation of irreversibly sickled cells be a good thing clinically? I
guess not, if we believe our biases. I think the more important question would be,
Is the prevention of the generation of the irreversibly sickled cell a useful thing? I
believe that's what these data suggest.

R. J. SOKOL (*Children's Hospital Medical Center, Cincinnati, Ohio*): I'm a little
worried about your scheme for malabsorption of vitamin E in sickle-cell disease.
We've done oral tolerance tests similar to yours in patients with glycogen storage
disease, where they've had very high serum lipids—as opposed to your patients
who are hypocholesterolemic—and abnormally high rises in their serum vitamin
E levels and much larger areas of the curve compared to our controls. This would
suggest that perhaps the reason that your patients had poor results on their oral
absorption tests was that they were hypocholesterolemic, as opposed to our
patients who were hypercholesterolemic.

The second thing I wanted to ask was have you done any intraduodenal
intubations and gallbladder stimulations to document the intraluminal bile acid
deficiency that you are proposing?

B. LUBIN: I'll try to help with that question. First, as you know, patients with
sickle-cell disease frequently have gallstones. Bile sludging is also a common

problem, even without the presence of gallstones. We propose that the hypocho-lesterolemia in these patients may be related to abnormal bile metabolism. Just as in Dr. Guggenheim's patients with biliary atresia, where two of the patients had hypocholesterolemia as well. This is very much like the cystic fibrosis patient; in fact, the lipid profiles that we have are identical to cystic fibrosis patients. Also, there is evidence that bile salt and micellar concentration in the gastrointestinal tract is required to stabilize pancreatic exocrine function. Second, we have not studied bile acid excretion, but plan to do so.

R. J. SOKOL: The classic teaching on patients with biliary tract disease is that they have high cholesterols, not low. The patients in Dr. Guggenheim's paper, I believe, were on cholestyromine and were receiving therapy for their original hypercholesterolemia. It would be unusual in patients with biliary tract disease to have low serum cholesterol. I agree with you that sickle-cell disease patients have hypocholesterolemia.

B. LUBIN: And the cystic fibrosis patients?

S. J. SOKOL: That's probably due to nutrition more than to biliary tract disease.

B. LUBIN: Perhaps nutrition is also a problem in sickle-cell disease.

V. P. MANKAD (Mobile, Ala.): Encouraged by initial studies by Dr. Natta and Dr. Machlin, we are conducting a double-blind placebo control study of vitamin E in sickle-cell disease. The code is not broken yet, so I can't report the results, but maybe I can indicate some of the confounding problems that a study of this kind could face. The absorption problems that you documented and the compliance factors of the patients could make it difficult to obtain the desired information. Blood transfusions and changes in the clinical course affect the parameters that we are trying to measure. It might take a long time and large numbers of patients, but I think that your elegant studies give us a further rationale to continue the studies and perhaps expand them with other centers.

A question I have for you is related to calcium metabolism in sickle cells. There is accumulation of calcium in the irreversibly sickled cells, perhaps due to membrane changes, and also there is strong evidence from Dr. Vincenzi's lab that adenosine triphosphatase, calcium ATPase, that is, is not activated by calmodulin to the same extent in sickle-cell disease. I wonder if you could speculate on the relationship between vitamin E and calcium metabolism.

D. CHIU: Phosphatidyl serine may modulate calcium ATPase function in red cells. Perhaps due to the peroxidant injury, phosphatidyl serine is altered and the activity of calcium ATPase decreased, leading to calcium accumulation. Vitamin E may prevent peroxidation of phosphatidyl serine, deterioration of the calcium ATPase, and the accumulation of calcium.

E. A. RACHMILEWITZ (Hadassah University Hospital, Jerusalem, Israel): Did you do any other malabsorption studies, like β-carotene or xylose? Do you base your idea of vitamin E malabsorption in sickle-cell disease solely on the absorption curves that you showed us?

B. LUBIN: We haven't done xylose absorption studies. There have been reports of vitamin A and vitamin E deficiency in sickle-cell patients at Children's Hospital of Philadelphia. The low vitamin E could also be secondary to increased turnover of vitamin E.

E. A. RACHMILEWITZ: Dr. Shohet, did you try to see whether MDA cross-links proteins? Have you tried any of these elegant studies on the lipids?

S. B. SHOHET: The last question is the easiest—no, we haven't. As to the first question, we haven't looked for protein effects in a systematic way, but we certainly think they're there, and I actually alluded to them. We do see some high molecular weight material at the top of our [sodium dodecyl sulfate, SDS] gels. Dr.

Jain strongly feels that this is protein and that this is an effect of MDA, even at low concentrations. You can make a Schiff base with a protein just as well as with a lipid.

W. A. PRYOR (*Louisiana State University, Baton Rouge, La.*): Did you use malonyldialdehyde itself or was it the ethanol adduct, the acetal, that you used?

S. B. SHOHET: We prepared fresh MDA by acid hydrolysis of malonaldehyde-bis-[di methyl acetal] immediately prior to each experiment.

W. A. PRYOR: Let me list a few chemical questions that you all might look at. Malonyldialydehyde probably doesn't have a very long life span, so when you put in five micromolar, I'm not sure how much of it is getting to the membrane. It was shown by Goldstein to be not very mutagenic in the Ames test—although it clearly can cross-link proteins—and probably the reason is that it doesn't live very long. So I think that's a real problem. Now, if it's made by autoxidation *in situ*, that's one thing, but if you are adding it by itself, that's another. A group in Austria about 15 years ago showed that when lipids are oxidized, a large number of unsaturated products, α-β-unsaturated carbonyl products, are formed. When we think of malonyldialdehyde, we have to think about a very complex set of chemical reactions to do with protein cross-linking. Maybe what you ought to do is autoxidize lipid and take a fraction of that and put it in with red cells.

S. B. SHOHET: I couldn't agree more strongly. Malonyldialdehyde is just a model. I believe it represents only about 2% of total peroxidation products. I think that *in situ*, the specialness about malonyldialdehyde is that if it's generated, it's generated in just the right place to cause the trouble.

C. C. REDDY (*Pennsylvania State University, University Park, Pa.*): Dr. Chiu, you said that lipid peroxidation is enhanced in red cells obtained from sickle-cell anemia patients, and you also showed data that selenium glutathione peroxidase is increased in these cells by threefold. If indeed selenium glutathione peroxidase is involved, why did it not prevent lipid peroxidation?

D. CHIU: Glutathione peroxidase activity didn't increase threefold, it increased about 50% from normal. Such an increase probably reflects a response to increased oxidant stress *in vivo*.

VITAMIN E DEFICIENCY DUE TO INCREASED CONSUMPTION IN β-THALASSEMIA AND IN GAUCHER'S DISEASE*

Eliezer A. Rachmilewitz, Abraham Kornberg,
and Mehmet Acker†

*Departments of Hematology and Pediatrics†
Hadassah University Hospital
Hebrew University Hadassah Medical School
il-91120 Jerusalem, Israel*

Introduction

α-Tocopherol (vitamin E) is known to protect from a nonenzymatic attack of molecular oxygen on polyunsaturated fatty acids.[1] Low serum vitamin E levels in humans have been reported in two kinds of disorders: In the first group, i.e., chronic steatorrhea such as cystic fibrosis,[2] or in prematurely delivered infants[3] the cause for vitamin E deficiency is inadequate absorption due to physiological or pathological changes in the gastrointestinal tract. In the second group, i.e., congenital hemolytic anemias such as β-thalassemia,[4] sickle-cell anemia,[5] and glucose-6-phosphate dehydrogenase deficiency,[6] vitamin E deficiency most probably results from its increased consumption while neutralizing oxidative damage in pathological erythrocyte membranes and in other tissues. However the evidence supporting this concept has so far been indirect.[4-7]

In lysosomal lipid storage disorders, the disproportionate expansion of the reticuloendothelial (RE) cell mass in relation to the amount of the accumulating substrate[8] suggests that the storage material is not an inert inclusion and might be acting as a stimulus to phagocytic cell activation. Since activated phagocytes generate oxidative radicals,[9] sustained stimulation of these cells may lead to excessive production of oxidative radicals and consequently to increased utilization and eventual deficiency in vitamin E. This idea was examined in a group of 20 patients with varying degrees of severity of Gaucher's disease. The results demonstrate that increased consumption of vitamin E in its capacity as an antioxidant is not confined only to red cell disorders.

In some disorders where vitamin E deficiency is a result of increased consumption beyond the dietary intake, therapeutic trials have been carried out with oral supplementation of vitamin E. For instance, in patients with β-thalassemia, while the levels in both serum and erythrocytes are significantly increased following vitamin E administration, there seems to be minimal beneficial effect on transfusion requirements and hemoglobin levels.[10]

In the present study an attempt was made to expand the antioxidant potential of vitamin E in patients with thalassemia by supplementation with an additional antioxidant, canthaxanthin (4,4'-diketo-β-carotene), which has been used to treat patients with erythrohepatic protoporphyria.[11] The results in a group of nine patients treated for 4-10 months show that the addition of canthaxanthin did not make any difference compared with the results obtained with vitamin E alone.

*These studies were supported in part by a grant from Hoffmann-La Roche, Inc., to E.A.R.

Thalassemia

Nine patients, seven with β^+-thalassemia major and two with β-thalassemia intermedia, were selected for the present studies. Five were Kurdish Jews, and four local Arabs. Seven patients were regularly transfused every four to eight weeks. The main clinical hematological features of most of these patients have been reported previously.[4,10] Three patients (E.Am., E.Ar., and G.M.) were included in our first report on vitamin E deficiency in β-thalassemia major.[10] Fresh anticoagulated or noncoagulated blood was obtained repeatedly from all patients preceding blood transfusion every four to eight weeks. Routine hematological examinations were carried out using the same method described for the Gaucher's patients.

Gaucher's Disease

Twenty patients with chronic nonneuropathic Gaucher's disease were investigated. Most of them had been followed for many years in the Hematology and Pediatric Departments of Hadassah Hospital. Fourteen were Ashkenazi Jews, five were Sephardic Jews, and one was an Arab. The mean age of the patients was 29.7 years ranging from 14 months to 70 years. The diagnosis in all cases was established by the presence of numerous "Gaucher cells" in the bone marrow, elevated serum tartrate-resistant acid phosphatase, and decreased activity of leukocyte β-glucosidase. All patients had complete blood counts performed on Coulter counter model S-senior (Coulter Electronics, Ltd., Hialeah, Fla.) and underwent careful physical examination, with particular emphasis on the spleen and liver sizes.

CONTROLS

Fifty healthy children and adults served as controls for vitamin E estimations, while undergoing routine blood tests. The general well-being of all these subjects was ascertained by detailed medical history, general physical examination, and complete blood counts. The mean age of the control group was 32 years, ranging from 3 to 56 years.

METHODS

Estimation of Vitamin E

Serum and plasma were immediately separated and kept at 4°C until their determination on the same day. Otherwise, samples were frozen at $-20°C$ and were assayed within 48 hours of their collection. Serum or plasma α-tocopherol (vitamin E) levels were determined according to the method of Hashim and Schuttringer.[12] A standard curve was prepared every few weeks using a pure solution of α-tocopherol (Hoffmann-La Roche, Inc., Nutley, N.J.).

Malonyldialdehyde Determination

Susceptibility of erythrocyte membrane lipids to autoxidation after oxidative stress was based on the generation of malonyldialdehyde (MDA), a secondary breakdown product of lipid peroxidation, following the method of Stocks and Dormandy.[13] The normal levels in our laboratory are between 80–100 μg/g hemoglobin (Hb).

Serum tartrate-resistant acid phosphatase activity was assayed using conventional techniques where the capacity of the acidified test sample to hydrolyze p-nitrophenyl phosphate (Sigma, St. Louis, Mo.) is measured in the presence of tartrate.

Therapeutic Trial with Vitamin E and Canthaxanthin

all-rac-α-Tocopheryl acetate (vitamin E), oil-soluble, and canthaxanthin were prepared specifically for the present studies by Hoffmann-La Roche, Inc., Nutley, N.J., and Basel, Switzerland. Three to four capsules containing 250 mg vitamin E and three capsules containing 25 mg canthaxanthin were given to the patients in divided doses, three times daily for an average period of seven months.

RESULTS

β-Thalassemia

The results of the therapeutic trial with vitamin E and canthaxanthin are summarized in TABLE 1. It can be seen that there were no significant differences in hemoglobin levels, hematocrits, and transfusion requirements in all the patients studied between the period of 5–7 months when they received only vitamin E and the period of 4–10 months when canthaxanthin was added to vitamin E. Earlier observations had already shown that similar results were obtained when a group of patients who received vitamin E were compared to a group who received placebo or nothing at all.[10] The addition of canthaxanthin had no effect on serum vitamin E levels, which remained normal or high throughout the period of both trials.

Normal MDA levels (less than 100 μg/g Hb) were found in five patients during the two periods of treatment. In one patient (Ch.M.) with β-thalassemia intermedia who was not treated before with vitamin E, the high MDA levels were significantly decreased after four months of treatment with both agents. In another patient (K.Al.), MDA levels decreased from an average of 228 to 160 μg/g Hb in the period when canthaxanthin was added to vitamin E. In two patients, L.D. and G.M., MDA levels increased in the period when canthaxanthin was added. In one of them (L.D.), the possible explanation is lack of compliance in taking the recommended doses. In the other patient (G.M.), there is no explanation for the differences in the MDA levels.

Gaucher's Disease

The manifestation of Gaucher's disease in the present group of patients showed a wide spectrum and covered a broad range of clinical expression. Four

TABLE 1

HEMATOLOGICAL AND BIOCHEMICAL PARAMETERS IN PATIENTS WITH β-THALASSEMIA MAJOR TREATED WITH VITAMIN E AND CANTHAXANTHIN*

Name	Age	Sex	Period of Treatment (months)		Hemoglobin† (g/dl)		Hematocrit† (%)		Vitamin E† (mg%)		MDA† (μg/g Hb)		Number of Transfusions per Month†	
			Vitamin E	Vitamin E + Canthaxanthin										
K.Al.	21	M	5	7	8.3	8.5	28.7	28.3	1.3	1.4	228	160	0.8	1
Al.N.	9	F	5	7	9.4	10.2	30.5	31.7	0.8	1.3	93	79	0.8	1
Al.J.	13	F	5	7	7.9	8.5	24.2	6.5	0.8	1.2	90	72	1	1
Ef.Ar.	17	M	6	7	9.1	9.1	30.0	28.0	1.2	1.0	98	95	1.3	1.4
Ef.Am.	15	M	5	6	9.7	9.0	31.4	27.0	0.7	1.2	85	79	1.7	1.5
D.K.	30	M	7	6	9.1	9.4	28.0	30.0	0.5	1.0	103	93	—	—
Ch.M.	30	M	—	4	8.0	7.6	30.3	27.0	0.1	0.6	752	230	—	—
L.Df.	16	F	7	8	7.8	7.1	25.5	23.4	0.5	0.5	223	357	0.8	0.8
G.M.	27	F	7	10	8.2	8.3	26.4	26.5	1.9	1.3	102	235	0.9	0.8

*Vitamin E given at 750–1,000 mg/day; canthaxanthin given at 75 mg/day.
†Each number represents a mean value of 5–10 determinations obtained during treatment with vitamin E (left column) and vitamin E + canthaxanthin (right column).

patients (nos. 12-15) were asymptomatic, with mild organomegaly and close to normal hematological values (TABLE 2). The diagnosis of Gaucher's disease was made in adult life during medical investigation of unrelated complaints. The remaining 16 patients had a more advanced form of the disease. The rate of progression and the severity of their clinical manifestations varied from moderate (nos. 8-11) to very severe (nos. 1-7). Their spleens were palpable 5 cm or more below the costal margin (range, 5-18 cm). Five patients were splenectomized because of massive splenomegaly and pancytopenia (nos. 16-20). All 16 patients had hepatomegaly—4-9 cm and 4-18 cm below costal margin in those who were nonsplenectomized and splenectomized, respectively—and were thrombocyto-penic (prior to splenectomy), with platelet counts below 70,000 per mm^3 (range 23,000-68,000 per mm^3). Seventy-five percent had hemoglobin levels below 12 g/dl. More than 50% of these patients either complained of bone pain or had pathological fractures and/or avascular necrosis of the head of the femur.

Serum tartrate-resistant acid phosphatase activity was elevated in all the patients (range, 0.95-8.4 units/ml; TABLE 1). Patients with the severe form of the disease had significantly higher levels than did those with the more benign form of the disease.

Plasma vitamin E levels showed a wide variation in the different patients and ranged from zero to levels in the normal range (TABLE 2). The mean plasma vitamin E level was low (0.29 mg% ± 0.22 standard deviation) and differed significantly from the levels measured in normal controls (0.73 mg% ± 0.12 SD). The levels in 17 patients were two standard deviations below the normal mean value.

The patients with the most benign form of the disease had higher plasma vitamin levels (0.63 mg% ± 0.13 SD), and in 3 of them the levels were within the normal range. The 16 patients with the progressive course had lower levels (0.21 mg% ± 0.14 SD). The lowest values of vitamin E within this group (0.08 mg% ± 0.05 SD) were found in the 7 patients with a rapidly progressive course manifested by profoundly enlarged spleens and severe "hypersplenism." There was a linear correlation between the degree of thrombocytopenia and plasma vitamin E levels in unsplenectomized patients (p < 0.001). The spleen size showed a linear inverse correlation with plasma vitamin E levels (p < 0.0001). Similar correlation seemed to exist between the degree of hepatomegaly in unsplenectomized patients and serum vitamin E levels. Spleen size, however, did not seem to be the only factor determining vitamin E utilization since low levels were found in both splenectomized and nonsplenectomized patients with the progressive forms of the disease. In one patient (no. 5), vitamin E levels were measured before and two months postsplenectomy. The transiently increased vitamin E levels returned to the preoperative levels associated with concurrent rapid increase in liver size.

DISCUSSION

Several intracellular changes in thalassemic erythrocytes could account for the oxidative damage in their membrane components. These changes, illustrated in FIGURE 1, consist of oxidation of excess α-hemoglobin subunits and intracellular excess of iron, which result in excess formation of free oxygen radicals.[14] Due to the decreased amounts of intracellular hemoglobin that can serve as a substrate for the active oxygen radicals (low mean corpuscular hemoglobin concentration), the potent radicals can have an easier access to the cell membrane and oxidize its

TABLE 2

HEMATOLOGICAL AND LABORATORY DATA IN PATIENTS WITH GAUCHER'S DISEASE

Course	No.	Age (years)	Sex	Liver*	Spleen*	Hemoglobin (g/dl)	WBC† (per mm³)	Platelets (×10³/mm³)	Acid Phosphatase (units/ml)	Vitamin E (mg%)
Rapidly progressive	1	4	F	4	14	9.2	5,400	68	8.00	0.08
	2	11	M	7	17	9.7	5,300	27	5.00	0.10
	3	14	F	7	18	10.7	2,800	23	7.80	0.10
	4	14	M	8	17	9.2	4,400	37	8.00	0.05
	5	4	F	8	16	7.5	3,100	24	8.40	0.01
	6	1.2	M	7	14	9.0	2,700	45	4.14	0.16
	7	3	F	9	16	8.0	2,100	47	3.65	0.07
Progressive	8	41	F	5	6	12.0	4,000	48	1.70	0.24
	9	38	M	8	10	13.2	4,700	67	1.29	0.31
	10	36	F	3	5	11.1	5,800	60	2.70	0.42
	11	50	F	5	8	12.8	4,200	47	2.20	0.42
Benign	12	49	F	3	2	12.0	4,800	106	1.20	0.58
	13	27	F	NP‡	3	13.0	8,000	150	2.40	0.43
	14	70	M	NP	NP	13.0	6,800	110	1.10	0.69
	15	35	F	NP	0.5	13.0	4,400	98	0.95	0.70
Splenectomized	16	43	M	10	—	13.0	11,000	484	—	0.24
	17	50	F	12	—	13.4	12,700	166	3.60	0.11
	18	28	F	7	—	11.1	12,900	103	4.50	0.36
	19	56	M	18	—	9.7	10,000	95	3.75	0.26
	20	20	F	4	—	10.6	12,600	212	2.10	0.35

*Centimeters below costal margin.
†WBC, white blood cells.
‡NP, not palpable.

various components.[14] While the concept of excess free radical formation in the thalassemic erythrocytes is most appealing, these ideas are at present still speculative, since no direct evidence of excess free oxygen radical formation in thalassemic erythrocytes has been reported. Indirect evidence for the deleterious role of the free radicals was obtained from the studies of the lipid membranes of thalassemic erythrocytes, where decreased levels of polyunsaturated fatty acids and increased generated MDA levels have been found.[4,15] Membrane proteins are also oxidized as shown by the decreased number of titratable sulfhydryl groups and by cross-linking of several membrane proteins following exogenous

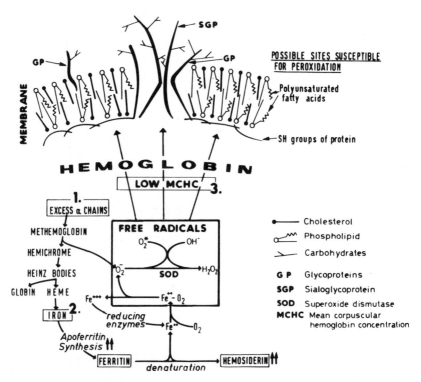

FIGURE 1. Schematic figure of a thalassemic RBC illustrating the possible metabolic pathways resulting in increased production of free oxygen radicals and their deleterious effects on the RBC membrane.

oxidant stress.[16-17] Further support for the concept of oxidative damage to the cell membrane came from several reports from different countries on decreased serum vitamin E levels in thalassemia,[18] particularly in a group of patients with β-thalassemia intermedia who were not regularly transfused in spite of having severe anemia.[10] Since malabsorption was ruled out as a cause for vitamin E deficiency,[4] the most likely explanation for low vitamin E levels in thalassemia is the increased consumption of the vitamin for the neutralization of the free oxygen radicals and their deleterious effects on the erythrocyte membranes. Consequently, a therapeutic trial with vitamin E was initiated. The results, which were summarized in a previous report,[10] were disappointing. Although one could restore both serum and erythrocyte vitamin E to normal or to high levels and the high MDA levels were decreased, indicating partial neutralization of lipid membrane peroxidation, no significant changes were found in the transfusion requirements of eight patients under study, and in only three out of seven patients was the ^{51}Cr-erythrocyte survival prolonged after 12 months of treatment.[10]

In the present study, the antioxidant effect of the carotenoid canthaxanthin, which is a photoprotective agent,[11] was examined in order to see whether it would potentiate the antioxidant effect of vitamin E. The addition of canthaxanthin was based on the fact that tissue mobilization and storage of β-carotene is different when compared to vitamin E[19] and therefore might expand the therapeutic antioxidant potential. Although the trial was carried out on a small group of patients, no major changes occurred in the hematological and biochemical parameters that were examined. The ultimate conclusion from these studies is that additional antioxidants may be required, particularly those that may prevent the oxidation of membrane components other than lipids, which may have been the only intracellular constituents that were protected by vitamin E with or without canthaxanthin.

The available data on the increased consumption of vitamin E due to the resultant imbalance between the antioxidant potential and the oxidative stress due to excessive oxygen radical generation have been limited to date to congenital red cell disorders, such as thalassemia,[4] sickle-cell anemia,[5] and glucose-6-phosphate dehydrogenase deficiency.[6] The results of the present study indicate that the same concept may also apply to lysosomal storage disorders.

Low plasma vitamin E levels were found in a large group of patients with Gaucher's disease and could not be related to changes in plasma levels of total lipids and lipoproteins.[20] The absence of symptoms of steatorrhea in any of the patients studied, and normal xylose tolerance tests and normal fat balance studies in a selected group of three patients with severe serum vitamin E deficiency (TABLE 2, nos. 1, 2, and 4), rule out the possibility of malabsorption as a contributory factor in the observed decrease in serum vitamin E levels. The finding of an inverse correlation between the degree of organomegaly, acid phosphatase activity, and plasma vitamin E levels implies that the decrease in plasma vitamin E levels is proportional to reticuloendothelial cell proliferation and mononuclear phagocyte activation. This assumption was made in light of circumstantial evidence suggesting that both the elevated serum hydrolase (acid phosphatase) activity and the increased organomegaly are most likely in response to activation of the mononuclear phagocytic system by the accumulating substrate.[8] Systemic administration of certain undegradable artificial substrates has been shown to promote RE cell hyperplasia.[21] In vitro endocytosis of these substrates induces morphological modulation typical for activated macrophages with a concomitant increase in lysosomal enzyme activity and selective exocytosis of lysosomal hydrolases.[22]

Unlike the red cell disorders where "hard data" are still required, it has been shown by several investigators that activated macrophages generate free oxygen radicals,[9] and their excess production exerts an increased demand on the protective antioxidant mechanisms including vitamin E, which is limited by dietary intake. Therefore, it is conceivable that the low levels of plasma vitamin E found in Gaucher's disease could be due to its utilization in neutralizing oxygen radicals produced in excessive amounts by the RE system, which is under sustained stimulation by the storage material.

Susceptibility of a given cell to oxidative damage is a function of the overall balance between the magnitude of the oxidative stress and its antioxidant potential. A loss of this potential resulting from vitamin E deficiency may predispose the cell to the deleterious consequences of oxidative injury. In the patients with Gaucher's disease, no gross abnormalities in clinical symptoms and no impaired laboratory data have been found that could result directly from vitamin E deficiency. However, one must keep in mind that deficiency of vitamin E by itself predisposes cell membranes to lipid peroxidation and sulfhydryl oxidation,[23] to shortened erythrocyte survival,[2] and to hemolysis following exogenous oxidant stress.[24] Moreover, white cells derived from vitamin E–deficient rats exhibit a twofold increase in polyunsaturated fatty acid peroxidation, excessive hydrogen peroxide production, and defective function.[25]

In view of widespread deleterious consequences of oxidative injury at cellular or subcellular level, reduced antioxidant potential associated with vitamin E deficiency may lead to occult or overt organ dysfunction, or may predispose to injurious effects of relatively innocuous oxidative agents.

Awareness of vitamin E deficiency in Gaucher's disease may lead to early recognition and proper management of any of these possible complications. Moreover, in view of the positive correlation between the decrease of vitamin E and the severity of manifestation of Gaucher's disease, plasma vitamin E levels may give a quantitative expression of individual severity in any particular patient and may be a useful additional parameter in following the clinical course of this disease. The benefit of replacement therapy in the vitamin E–deficient patients is currently being evaluated.

SUMMARY

Plasma vitamin E levels were found to be decreased (<0.5 mg) in thalassemia and in 17 out of 20 patients with Gaucher's disease, where the levels were two standard deviations below the normal mean value. In the latter, the decrease in vitamin E levels correlated with the severity of the clinical expression of the disease and correlated inversely with the degree of hepatosplenomegaly and serum tartrate-resistant acid phosphatase activity. In both diseases, there was no evidence for intestinal malabsorption of the lipid-soluble vitamin. In spite of the different etiology, pathophysiology, and clinical expression, severe vitamin E deficiency could result in both diseases by a common mechanism. In thalassemia, rapid consumption of vitamin E occurs while neutralizing oxidative damage in the pathological erythrocyte membranes and in other tissues. In Gaucher's disease, lysosomal accumulation of glucocerebroside may stimulate phagocytes into a maintained "respiratory burst" with excessive production of oxygen free radicals, resulting in increased utilization and eventual deficiency of vitamin E. Efficacy of antioxidant therapy was evaluated by administration of vitamin E with and without canthaxanthin, which has similar antioxidant properties to β-carotene, to patients with β-thalassemia. The results showed increased serum vitamin E levels and a decrease in the extent of erythrocyte lipid membrane peroxidation, while no significant changes occurred in hemoglobin levels and in transfusion requirements.

ACKNOWLEDGMENTS

The authors wish to thank Drs. Brin, Machlin, and Bermond from Hoffmann-La Roche, Inc., Nutley, N.J., and Basel, Switzerland, for supplying standard vitamin E solutions and the various preparations of vitamin E and canthaxanthin, and for their fruitful discussions. The technical assistance of Mrs. Olga Fradkin is highly appreciated.

REFERENCES

1. LEHNINGER, A. L. 1970. Biochemistry: 358. Worth Publishers, Inc. New York, N.Y.
2. FARREL, P. M., J. G. BIERI, J. F. FARANTONI, R. E. WOOD & P. A. DI SANT'AGNESE. 1977. The occurrence and effects of human vitamin E deficiency: a study in patients with cystic fibrosis. J. Clin. Invest. **60:** 233.
3. MALHORN, D. K. & S. GROSS. 1971. Vitamin E–dependent anemia in the premature infant. II. Relationship between gestational age and absorption of vitamin E. J. Pediatr. **79:** 581.
4. RACHMILEWITZ, E. A., B. H. LUBIN & S. B. SHOHET. 1976. Lipid membrane peroxidation in β-thalassemia major. Blood **47:** 495.
5. CHIU, D. & B. LUBIN. 1979. Abnormal vitamin E and glutathione peroxidase levels in sickle cell anemia. J. Lab. Clin. Med. **94:** 542.
6. CORASH, L., S. SPIELBERG, C. BARTSOCAS, L. BOXER, R. STEINHERTZ, M. SHEETZ, M. EGAN, J. SCHLESSLEMAN & D. D. SCHULMAN. 1980. Reduced chronic hemolysis during high-dose vitamin E administration in Mediterranean-type glucose-6-phosphate dehydrogenase deficiency. N. Engl. J. Med. **303:** 416.
7. RACHMILEWITZ, E. A. 1976. The role of intracellular hemoglobin precipitation, low MCHC and iron overload on red blood cell membrane peroxidation in thalassemia. Birth Defects Orig. Artic. Ser. **12**(8): 123.
8. BRADY, R. O. 1978. Glucosyl ceramide lipidosis: Gaucher's disease. *In* The Metabolic Basis of Inherited Disease. J. B. Stanbury, J. B. Wyngaarden & D. S. Frederickson, Eds. 4th edit.: 739. McGraw-Hill Book Company. New York, N.Y.
9. DRATH, D. B. & M. L. KARNOVSKY. 1975. Superoxide production by phagocytic leukocytes. J. Exp. Med. **141:** 257.
10. RACHMILEWITZ, E. A., A. SHIFTER & I. KAHANE. 1979. Vitamin E deficiency in β-thalassemia major: changes in hematological and biochemical parameters after a therapeutic trial with α tocopherol. Am. J. Clin. Nutr. **32:** 1850.
11. EALES, L. 1978. The effect of canthaxanthin on the photocutaneous manifestations of porphyria. S. Afr. Med. J. **54:** 1050.
12. HASHIM, S. A. & G. R. SCHUTTRINGER. 1966. Rapid determination of tocopherol in macro and microquantities of plasma. Am. J. Clin. Nutr. **19:** 137.
13. STOCKS, J. & T. L. DORMANDY. 1971. The autoxidation of human red cell lipids induced by hydrogen peroxide. Br. J. Haematol. **20:** 11.
14. RACHMILEWITZ, E. A. & I. KAHANE. 1980. The red blood cell membrane in thalassemia. Br. J. Haematol. **46:** 1. (Annotation.)
15. STOCKS, J., E. L. OFFERMAN, C. B. MODELL & T. L. DORMANDY. 1972. The susceptibility to antioxidation of human red cell lipids in health and disease. Br. J. Haematol. **23:** 713.
16. KAHANE, I. & E. A. RACHMILEWITZ. 1976. Alterations in the red blood cell membrane and the effect of vitamin E on osmotic fragility in thalassemia major. Isr. J. Med. Sci. **12:** 11.
17. KAHANE, I., A. SCHIFTER & E. A. RACHMILEWITZ. 1976. Cross-linking of red blood cell membrane proteins induced by oxidative stress in thalassemia. FEBS Lett. **85:** 267.
18. ZANNOS-MARIOLEA, L. F., K. TZORTZATAKU, CH. KATERELLOS, M. KAVALLARI & N. MASTONIOTIS. 1974. Serum vitamin E levels with β thalassemia major: a preliminary report. Br. J. Haematol. **26:** 193.
19. BJORNSON, L. K., H. J. KAYDEN, E. MILLER & A. MOSHELL. 1976. The transport of α-tocopherol and β-carotene in human blood. J. Lipid Res. **17:** 343.
20. ACKER, M., *et al.* (In preparation.)
21. RIGGI, S. J. & N. R. DILUZIO. 1961. Identification of a reticuloendothelial stimulating agent in zymosan. Am. J. Physiol. **200:** 297.

22. PAGE, R. C., P. DAVIES & A. C. ALLISON. 1974. Participation of mononuclear phagocytes in chronic inflammatory disease. J. Reticuloendothelial Soc. **15:** 415.
23. BROWNLESS, N. R., J. J. HUTTNER, R. V. PANGANAMALA & D. G. CORNWELL. 1977. The role of vitamin E in glutathione induced oxidant stress: methemoglobin oxidation, lipid peroxidation and hemolysis. J. Lipid Res. **18:** 635.
24. MELHORN, D. K. & S. GROSS. 1971. Vitamin E dependent anemia—premature infant. Effect of large doses of medicinal iron. J. Pediatr. **79:** 569.
25. HARRIS, E. R., L. A. BOXER & R. L. BAEHNER. 1980. Consequences of vitamin E deficiency on the phagocytic and oxidative functions of the rat polymorphonuclear leukocyte. Blood **55:** 338.

DISCUSSION

H. J. KAYDEN (*New York University School of Medicine, New York, N.Y.*): I have two questions. First, I wonder if you would tell us whether the phospholipid and cholesterol abnormalities of the thalassemic patients were altered with vitamin E. Second, were there any abnormalities in the red cells of the patients with Gaucher's disease? Did they have evidence of increased hemolysis or shortened life span?

E. A. RACHMILEWITZ: Regarding your first question, I'm afraid we didn't do the study.

F. A. OSKI (*State University of New York, Syracuse, N.Y.*): You said that the clinical results with vitamin E were disappointing but in a very narrow sense, from the hematologic standpoint. Did you look to see if the patients were better in any other way as a consequence of it?

E. A. RACHMILEWITZ: No. Now as to Dr. Kayden's second question, Gaucher patients have anemia, but how much of this is related to vitamin E deficiency is unknown.

L. J. MACHLIN (*Hoffmann-La Roche, Inc., Nutley, N.J.*): I'd like to comment about this question of why the E is low in both the hemolytic anemia and Gaucher's disease. I don't think we have a very good explanation. As far as malabsorption goes, you mentioned that in some of your patients malabsorption is not a problem. I believe that in Dr. Natta's group too there was no evidence for malabsorption. As far as the concept that the presence of hemoglobin or iron circulating may catalyze the destruction of E, there's really no clear evidence. We've done a very preliminary experiment where we've simply incubated blood at 37° in the air. Over a three-day period, there was absolutely no destruction of vitamin E. In the literature one of the mysteries of E is generally that it simply doesn't disappear. There's very little evidence for its destruction in tissues where you might expect its destruction, such as after carbon tetrachloride. Perhaps tocopherols or tocopheryl esters are to some extent picked up by the reticular endothelial system.

S. B. SHOHET (*University of California, San Francisco, Calif.*): It occurred to me that vitamin E is indeed necessary but not sufficient to prevent the damage. As Dr. Pryor pointed out and other questioners have suggested, there are two or maybe more phases, but certainly a lipid phase and a protein phase. Vitamin E seems to have cleaned up the lipid phase, at least as measured by MDA levels. Wouldn't it be a nice idea now to add some of those water-soluble antioxidants like vitamin C or maybe uric acid to see if by giving them a double treatment you can get rid of this problem?

E. A. RACHMILEWITZ: Vitamin C is definitely a complicated story in thalassemia.

F. A. OSKI: And those patients have an awful lot of their own uric acid.

E. A. RACHMILEWITZ: That's right.

L. A. BOXER (*Indiana University, Indianapolis, Ind.*): A comment and then a question. Not too long ago I happened to study an Israeli child with Von Gierke's disease and marked hepatosplenomegaly who turned out to have neutropenia. We weren't able to find out the mechanism, and as I look in the literature it's not an uncommon problem to see severe neutropenia. I would be interested to know if you studied any white cell functions in these patients. And, as a control, have you looked at vitamin E levels in patients with hypersplenism?

E. A. RACHMILEWITZ: Yes, we have looked at other patients with hypersplenism, and the E levels are not different from normal. We looked at two patients with Niemann-Pick disease, which is another lipid storage disease, and their E levels are also very low. It is possible that the lipids in Gaucher's disease may activate the macrophage and use up vitamin E.

F. A. OSKI: Actually there's another circumstance where you see Gaucher cells, although the patient doesn't have Gaucher's disease, and that's diserythropoiesis type II. These patients have very low vitamin E levels as well.

G. J. HANDELMAN (*University of California, Santa Cruz, Calif.*): Why did your patients have rather low serum vitamin E, on the order of 2 to 3 μg/ml plasma, but normal red cell vitamin E?

E. A. RACHMILEWITZ: That's a very good point. But you have to understand that our main concern was to see whether the E that we give to the patients could be found in the cells and membranes. And the answer to that is positive.

H. J. MEVWISSEN (*Albany Medical College, Albany, N.Y.*): Have you checked the dietary intake of vitamin E?

E. A. RACHMILEWITZ: Yes. In the normal Israeli diet, we don't seem to have a big problem with vitamin E deficiency.

CHRONIC HEMOLYTIC ANEMIA DUE TO GLUCOSE-6-PHOSPHATE DEHYDROGENASE DEFICIENCY OR GLUTATHIONE SYNTHETASE DEFICIENCY: THE ROLE OF VITAMIN E IN ITS TREATMENT*

Laurence M. Corash,† Michael Sheetz,‡ John G. Bieri,§
Christos Bartsocas,¶ Shimon Moses,‖ Nava Bashan,‖
and Joseph D. Schulman**

National Institutes of Health
Bethesda, Maryland 20205

INTRODUCTION

Rose and György observed 30 years ago that vitamin E can act *in vitro* to protect red blood cells (RBCs) from oxidant-induced lysis.[1] It is now well recognized that vitamin E deficiency in both man and animals is associated with increased red cell susceptibility to oxidant-induced damage and shortened red cell survival.[2-5] Repletion with vitamin E improves red cell survival and restores cellular resistance to oxidant stress. In light of these observations, we felt that supplementation with oral vitamin E could be of benefit to individuals with genetic disorders of red cell metabolism that are associated with increased cellular susceptibility to oxidant stress. Red cells deficient in either glucose-6-phosphate dehydrogenase (G6PD, EC 1.1.1.49) or glutathione synthetase (GS, EC 6.3.2.3) activity share a common defect of increased sensitivity to oxidant stress.[6,7]

G6PD deficiency, a sex-linked trait, has been reported worldwide and exhibits extensive genotypic and phenotypic polymorphism.[8] G6PD-deficient red cells generate abnormally small quantities of reduced nucleotides in response to oxidant stress, which results in an increased sensitivity to oxidants.[6] The most prevalent forms of G6PD deficiency are the African (Gd^{A-}) and the Mediterranean (Gd^{B-}) variants.[8] Individuals with these genotypes are generally well but may develop severe, acute hemolysis after an oxidative stress. Routine hematologic examination of these subjects at first glance appears normal in the absence of acute hemolysis, although closer scrutiny demonstrates that baseline autologous red cell survival may be slightly decreased in the Gd^{A-} form and is significantly reduced in the Gd^{B-} variant.[9,10] Careful comparison of the hematologic status of a Gd^{B-} population versus a normal population (Gd^{B+}) reveals that a

*Portions of this work were supported by Hoffmann-La Roche, Inc.
†Present affiliation: Hematology Service, Department of Laboratory Medicine, University of California, San Francisco, Calif. 94143.
‡Department of Physiology, University of Connecticut, Fairfield, Conn. 06032.
§Nutritional Biochemistry Section, National Institute of Arthritis, Metabolism and Digestive Diseases.
¶Department of Pediatrics, University of Athens, Athens, Greece 138.
‖Department of Pediatrics, Ben Gurion School of Medicine, Beersheva, Israel.
**National Institutes of Child Health and Human Development.

348

small, but statistically significant, degree of chronic hemolysis is present among the Gd^{B-} subjects even under nonstress conditions.[11]

Rare forms of G6PD deficiency associated with moderate to severe constant chronic hemolytic anemia have also been described.[12] In addition to constant chronic hemolysis, these patients undergo an exacerbation of hemolysis with exposure to oxidant stress. Many of these variants have undergone partial biochemical characterization, and recently a secondary defect in membrane protein structure has been identified in some chronic hemolysis variants.[13]

Red cell GS deficiency is a less common cause of chronic hemolytic anemia and may occur with or without oxoprolinuria depending upon the specific nature of the enzyme deficiency.[14] Individuals with this disorder have a significant reduction in red cell survival and moderately severe anemia.[7] GS-deficient red cells synthesize inadequate levels of glutathione to protect cellular components against oxidants. During periods of increased oxidative stress, there is further acceleration of the hemolytic process as in G6PD-deficient subjects.

The present report reviews our experience over the past four years in evaluating the effect of oral supplementation with vitamin E on the hemolysis in subjects with GS deficiency, chronic hemolytic G6PD deficiency, and the common Gd^{B-} variant of G6PD deficiency.

METHODS

Hemoglobin concentration, hematocrit, red blood cell count, reticulocyte count, haptoglobin concentration, and radiochromium red cell survival were performed as previously described.[15] Enzymatic assays for GS and G6PD were measured on platelet- and leukocyte-free red cells as before.[14,15] Serum vitamin E as total tocopherols was measured colorimetrically.[15] Serum and red cell α- and γ-tocopherol concentrations were measured by high-pressure liquid chromatography as reported by Bieri *et al.*[16] Statistical analysis of red cell survival was performed as previously reported.[15]

RESULTS

Glutathione Synthetase Deficiency

We have studied two brothers (AR and JR), both under six years of age, who had an established diagnosis of GS deficiency with oxoprolinuria,[14] and a third adult male without oxoprolinuria (RC) previously reported by Mohler *et al.*[7] The pediatric patients received 30 IU of vitamin E (*all-rac-α*-tocopheryl acetate, Hoffmann-La Roche, Nutley, N.J.) per kg per day, and the adult 1,000 IU/day as a total oral dose.

Two subjects (AR and RC) who were available for study before treatment demonstrated shortening of red cell survival and moderate anemia (TABLE 1). JR was placed on vitamin E shortly after birth and could not be studied before initiating this medication. After vitamin E supplementation, AR and RC had a significant improvement in red cell survival. AR demonstrated a statistically significant, but small, reduction in his reticulocyte count with little improvement in hematocrit. However, on several occasions when free of other medical problems, both AR and JR had improved hemoglobin concentrations (TABLE 1). JR had a normal red cell half-life while receiving vitamin E supplementation. The

TABLE 1

GLUTATHIONE SYNTHETASE DEFICIENCY: HEMATOLOGIC VALUES AND RED CELL SURVIVAL
BEFORE AND AFTER VITAMIN E SUPPLEMENTATION

Subject	Hemoglobin (g/dl)	Reticulocyte (%)	RBC Half-Life (days)
Baseline Values			
AR*	10.0 ± 0.6 (20)†	2.0 ± 0.2 (20)	14.2
JR*	NA‡	NA	NA
RC	13.5 ± 0.2 (2)	7.9 ± 0.2 (3)	8.5
After Vitamin E			
AR§	11.1	0.6	19.8, 18.3¶
JR§	11.2	1.1	24.6‖
RC	14.3 ± 0.1 (5)	4.4 ± 0.3 (7)	13.3¶

*Siblings with oxoprolinuria, below six years of age at time of study.

†Number of observations given in brackets when available, means ± SEM.

‡NA, data not available as subject treated from birth, data after vitamin E obtained at two to three years of age.

§Posttreatment values represent single observations obtained during periods when subjects were free of other medical complications.

¶Different from baseline p < 0.005 by comparison of slopes of the regression analysis by t-test.

‖Not statistically different from normal value.

third subject, RC, was never severely anemic and due to unavailability could only be followed sporadically. He did demonstrate a significant increase in red cell half-life and hemoglobin concentration and a reduction in reticulocyte count after treatment with vitamin E.

Chronic Hemolytic G6PD Deficiency

We initially studied a single G6PD-deficient subject, age 7½ years (TABLE 2), with severe chronic hemolysis.[17] He was treated with 800 IU of vitamin E per day and had an increase in red cell half-life as well as a small increase in hematocrit and a significantly reduced reticulocyte count. Although hemolysis was somewhat improved, vitamin E clearly failed to abolish the hemolytic process. Subsequently, we studied three additional G6PD-deficient kindreds with chronic

TABLE 2

G6PD DEFICIENCY WITH CHRONIC HEMOLYSIS: EFFECT OF VITAMIN E
SUPPLEMENTATION ON HEMATOLOGIC STATUS

Subject	Hematocrit (%)	Reticulocyte (%)	Mean RBC Life Span (days)
Baseline			
AW	29 ± 0.7 (7)*	15 ± 2 (7)	6.6
After Vitamin E			
AW	31 ± 0.5 (7)	8 ± 2 (7)†	10.4‡

*Numbers in parentheses indicate number of observations, means ± SEM.

†Different from baseline p < 0.005 by Student's t-test.

‡Different from baseline p < 0.005 by comparison of slopes for the regression analysis by t-test.

TABLE 3

G6PD Deficiency with Chronic Hemolysis: Hematologic Values
before and after Vitamin E Supplementation*

	Subject	Baseline Values†			Post-Vitamin E†		
		Hemoglobin (g/dl)	Reticulocyte (%)	RBC Half-Life (days)	Hemoglobin (g/dl)	Reticulocyte (%)	RBC Half-Life (days)
A	KS	13.3	15.7	7.1	13.4	6.3	7.5
	RS	13.5	15.7	6.9	13.0	15.6	5.7
	MP	11.2	18.5	4.5	11.5	15.4	5.7
	KF	12.0	11.0	6.2	13.1	6.0	6.1
	LP‡	14.3	4.4	24.2	13.5	3.7	25.7
B	MH	13.0	10.1	9.4	12.9	9.7	7.4, 9.8§
	CF	12.7	9.1	7.1	11.5	10.6	7.6
C	BB‡	12.0	11.2	13.8	11.8	12.6	11.4
	JB	12.4	14.3	4.4	11.9	11.2	5.9

*A, B, and C represent the three separate kindreds.
†Values are mean of three determinations.
‡Heterozygote.
§Two separate survivals while on vitamin E were performed.

hemolysis designated A, B, and C consisting of seven hemizygous males and two heterozygous females. As would be expected, the males were severely affected. One of the females (BB) was also severely affected, while the other (LP) had moderate hemolysis. These subjects were treated with 1,000 IU of all-rac-α-tocopheryl acetate per day in divided doses for six months before repeat routine hematology testing and red cell survivals were performed. Unlike the first G6PD-deficient subject, no patient in this larger group showed any consistent improvement in either the degree of anemia or the rate of red cell destruction (TABLE 3). We were able to measure serum and red cell vitamin E concentrations before and after treatment (TABLE 4). In all subjects, the vitamin E content of both

TABLE 4

G6PD Deficiency with Chronic Hemolysis: Plasma and Red Cell α-Tocopherol
Levels before and after Vitamin E Supplementation

	Subject	Pretherapy		Posttherapy	
		Plasma*	Red Cell	Plasma	Red Cell
A	KS	1214	271	1485	616
	RS	1002	255	1482	400
	MP	522	305	1094	493
	KF	860	340	NA†	NA
	LP	684	279	1464	564
B	MH	NA	NA	4103	1018
	CF	NA	NA	1650	NA
C	BB	1078	312	3057	660
	JB	756	367	1740	662

*Vitamin E expressed as μg/100 ml plasma and μg/100 ml of packed red blood cells.
†NA, not available.

serum and red cells was within normal limits prior to vitamin E supplementation and rose appropriately when the vitamin was administered. No adverse effects of vitamin E supplementation were observed, and continued administration for an additional six months showed no further improvement in any hematologic parameter. Two subjects were also treated with 1,200 IU/day of oral vitamin E in the alcohol form for several months but still showed no improvement.

Mediterranean (Gd^{B-})-Type G6PD Deficiency

A group of G6PD-deficient subjects were recruited from the Athens metropolitan area and from Patras, a smaller city in western Greece.[15] These subjects were referred with a documented clinical diagnosis of G6PD deficiency of the Mediterranean phenotype. This diagnosis was reconfirmed at the time of study by a quantitative assay on red cells free of leukocytes and platelets. Twenty-three patients were initially recruited into the study, 20 males and 3 homozygous females. They ranged in age from 4 to 43 years of age, with an average age of 15 years. Nineteen patients had an antecedent history of severe hemolysis, and 13

TABLE 5

MEDITERRANEAN G6PD DEFICIENCY: EFFECT OF THREE MONTHS OF VITAMIN E SUPPLEMENTATION ON HEMATOLOGIC STATUS OF GREEK SUBJECTS (n = 23)

Parameter	Before Therapy	After Therapy	Mean Difference of Paired Values	n	p*
Hemoglobin (g/dl)	13.3 ± 0.2	13.8 ± 0.2	+0.5 ± 0.1	23	<0.001
Reticulocyte count (%)	2.8 ± 0.2	2.2 ± 0.1	−0.6 ± 0.1	23	<0.001
RBC half-life (days)	22.9 ± 0.7	25.1 ± 6	+4.2 ± 1.0	20	<0.025
Serum vitamin E (mg/dl)	0.53 ± 0.04	1.6 ± 0.6	+1.1 ± 0.17	18	<0.001

*Single-tailed paired t-test analysis.

had a history of at least one hemolytic episode requiring transfusion. Routine hematologic tests and radioisotopic red cell survivals were measured initially, three months after vitamin E supplementation with 800 IU per day, and nine months later after continuous vitamin E supplementation at the same dosage for one year.

Initial evaluation (TABLE 5) demonstrated the presence of low-grade chronic hemolysis similar to the observations of Piomelli and Siniscalco on Sardinian Gd Mediterranean subjects.[11] The mean reticulocyte count of 2.8% and the mean red cell half-life of 22.9 days were significantly different from the control values. Of specific note was the observation that the mean serum α-tocopherol concentration was significantly less than that of a group of G6PD-normal controls drawn from the same households (0.53 mg/dl versus 0.80 mg/dl).

After three months of vitamin E supplementation, there was a small, but statistically significant, rise in hemoglobin and red cell half-life with a corresponding decline in the reticulocyte count for G6PD-deficient subjects (TABLE 5).

Due to the brief treatment time and in consideration of possible seasonal variation in the hemolytic rate, we elected to restudy this patient population after one year of vitamin E supplementation (TABLE 6). Thirteen patients from the

TABLE 6

MEDITERRANEAN G6PD DEFICIENCY: EFFECT OF VITAMIN E SUPPLEMENTATION ON HEMATOLOGIC STATUS OF GREEK SUBJECTS AFTER THREE MONTHS AND ONE YEAR OF THERAPY*

Hematologic Parameter	Before Therapy	Three Months after Therapy	One Year after Therapy	Mean Difference of Paired Values†	p‡
Hemoglobin (g/dl)	13.2 ± 0.3	13.7 ± 0.3	14.5 ± 0.3	+1.3 ± 0.3	<0.001
Packed cell volume (%)	39.1 ± 0.7	40.1 ± 0.9	42.0 ± 0.7	+2.9 ± 0.7	<0.001
Reticulocyte count (%)	2.7 ± 0.3	2.1 ± 0.2	1.5 ± 0.1	−1.2 ± 0.3	<0.001
Serum vitamin E (mg/dl)	0.55 ± 0.07	1.59 ± 0.14	1.49 ± 0.20	+0.94 ± 0.23	<0.001

*Values stated as the mean ± SEM; $n = 3$.

†Comparison based on values before therapy and after one year.

‡One-tailed t-test for paired samples.

initial study were available for evaluation after one year of treatment and were shown to be representative of the entire initial study population. After one year of vitamin E administration, there was continued improvement in all hematologic values with achievement of a normal mean hemoglobin concentration and normal mean reticulocyte count.

Because of reported variation in the frequency and severity of hemolysis among the Mediterranean populations with G6PD deficiency, we decided to study a second Gd^{B-} population of different ethnic origin from the Greek patients, a group of Kurdish-Iraqi G6PD-deficient subjects living near Beersheva, Israel. The original intent of the study was to duplicate the design of the Greek study, but due to problems of patient compliance it was not possible to perform red cell survivals or a paired study before and after vitamin E administration.

The Israeli study population consisted of 34 hemizygous G6PD-deficient males, 12 heterozygous G6PD-deficient females, and 16 G6PD normal controls composed of 7 females and 9 males who were drawn from the same households as the G6PD-deficient subjects. Examination of routine hematologic values demon-

TABLE 7

MEDITERRANEAN G6PD DEFICIENCY: BASELINE HEMATOLOGIC STATUS OF
KURDISH-IRAQI PATIENTS*

	Homozygotes	Heterozygotes	Male Controls†	Controls
n	34	12	9	16
Hemoglobin (g/dl)	13.3 ± 0.3	12.7 ± 0.2	14.9 ± 0.3	14.4 ± 0.3
Packed cell volume (%)	39.7 ± 0.7	38.8 ± 0.9	44.3 ± 0.9	42.6 ± 0.8
Reticulocyte count (%)	3.0 ± 0.3	2.9 ± 0.3	1.6 ± 0.3	1.8 ± 0.3
Haptoglobin (mg/dl)	59.3 ± 6.6	79.8 ± 11.6	80.7 ± 14.6	96.6 ± 13.0

*Values represent mean ± SEM.
†Two-tailed t-test comparing G6PD-deficient males to male controls demonstrates the following differences: hemoglobin, p < 0.02; hematocrit, p < 0.001; reticulocyte count, p < 0.05.

strated the presence of low-grade chronic hemolysis among this population (TABLE 7) similar to our prior observation among the Greek subjects.

Because of our earlier observation of lower than normal total serum tocopherol concentrations among Greek G6PD deficients, we measured both serum α- and γ-tocopherol concentrations of the Israeli subjects (TABLE 8).

Serum α-tocopherol levels were significantly lower among male G6PD-deficient subjects compared to male G6PD-normal controls. Heterozygous G6PD-deficient females demonstrated intermediate α-tocopherol levels compared to the mixed-sex control group. A mixed-sex control group was used since no sex-related differences in serum tocopherol have been described. There was no difference in mean serum γ-tocopherol concentrations between any of the study subgroups. The control subjects were recruited from the patients' households to eliminate dietary differences. The ratio of γ- to α-tocopherol was significantly higher for the G6PD deficients than for the Israeli controls. For additional comparison, the $\gamma:\alpha$ ratio among American controls is 0.21 ± 0.02 (standard error of the mean, SEM) in our laboratory.

TABLE 8

MEDITERRANEAN G6PD DEFICIENCY: SERUM α- AND γ-TOCOPHEROL CONCENTRATIONS AMONG KURDISH-IRAQI
G6PD-DEFICIENT SUBJECTS AND G6PD-NORMAL CONTROLS*

	Homozygotes	Heterozygotes	Controls	Male Controls	p†
n	34	12	16	9	
Plasma lipids (mg/dl)	822 ± 35	807 ± 70	949 ± 71	1,000 ± 111	NS
α-Tocopherol [μg/dl]	637 ± 29	761 ± 45	836 ± 35	884 ± 77	<0.001
γ-Tocopherol [μg/dl]	224 ± 13	225 ± 23	229 ± 21	249 ± 28	<0.80
γ- to α-tocopherol ratio	0.37 ± 0.02	0.31 ± 0.04	0.27 ± 0.02	0.28 ± 0.02	<0.005

*All values mean ± SEM.
†Two-tailed t-test comparing homozygous male G6PD-deficient to male G6PD-normal controls.

DISCUSSION

Vitamin E functions as a biological antioxidant when red cells are subjected to *in vitro* oxidant stresses. Moreover, red cells from vitamin E–deficient subjects have an increased susceptibility to oxidant stress both *in vitro* and *in vivo*, and supplementation with the vitamin corrects this defect.[3] It is attractive to speculate that in genetic disorders where cellular defenses against oxidation are compromised, vitamin E could have a therapeutic role as a protective agent. Three hereditary disorders of red cell metabolism are discussed in the present paper, and although of variable severity and of differing causes, they serve as a model to evaluate the efficacy of vitamin E as a protective antioxidant for red cells with compromised oxidant resistance.

The three subjects with GS deficiency have moderate chronic hemolytic disease with clinical evidence of acute exacerbation during periods of stress. Earlier work showed that the biochemical basis of the enzyme deficiency is different for the two phenotypes,[14] but vitamin E supplementation improved red cell survival in both types.

Of additional interest are the observations made on the granulocytes of the two GS-deficient children. One of the subjects (AR) had had severe recurrent neutropenia during infections.[18] Supplementation with vitamin E prevented neutropenia and protected the patient's granulocytes both *in vitro* and *in vivo* against oxidant damage,[19] and it was subsequently shown that a defect in microtubule assembly was corrected.[20] Thus, vitamin E preserved or improved cellular function in two different cell lines from patients with this disorder.

All eight male subjects with chronic hemolytic G6PD deficiency had marked hemolytic disease, while one female subject was mildly affected and the other was moderately severe. In only one case did vitamin E improve red cell survival and provide minimal hematologic improvement. Pretreatment plasma and red cell tocopherol levels are normal and rose appropriately with therapy. We had previously identified high-molecular-weight protein aggregates in the membranes of these subjects' red cells,[21] similar to the observations of Johnson et al.[13] Vitamin E treatment did not change the membrane protein pattern in our patients. Recently Johnson et al. reported two additional patients with chronic hemolytic G6PD deficiency who also failed to improve their red cell half-life with vitamin E supplementation.[22]

The results of vitamin E supplementation for Mediterranean variants indicate that in less severe disease, vitamin E improves red cell survival. It is important to note that the degree of anemia due to chronic hemolysis is minimal and continuous vitamin E supplementation has not yet been shown to be efficacious in ameliorating the acute hemolytic episodes. Stockman and coworkers reported that vitamin E did prolong survival of nonstressed Gd Mediterranean red cells after cross transfusion into normal subjects but it was not protective during primaquine exposure.[23]

Our second study of the Mediterranean variant carried out in a different ethnic subgroup reconfirmed the presence of mild chronic hemolysis. As for the Greek subjects, the G6PD-deficient Israeli males had lower serum vitamin E levels than did the control group, and fractionation of total tocopherols into α- and γ-fractions revealed that this decrease was selective for the α-isomer. The γ-tocopherol concentrations were virtually identical among all groups tested. Thus, in two separate populations of G6PD-deficient Mediterranean variants, we have observed decreased serum tocopherol concentrations.

The significance of decreased serum α-tocopherol levels in Gd Mediterranean is unclear at present. We speculate that it may be due to increased utilization at the red cell membrane with a secondary reduction of serum levels. Reduced serum tocopherol would be expected to be associated with reduced red cell tocopherol, perhaps with increased oxidant damage to these cells. Recent reports by other laboratories have demonstrated reduced serum tocopherol concentrations in sickle-cell anemia and thalassemia as well.[24,25] In both instances, evidence of increased lipid peroxidation was also observed.

These findings of reduced serum tocopherol levels for the Gd Mediterranean variant are in sharp contrast with the normal levels observed in the more severely affected chronic hemolytic G6PD-deficient variants. This apparent paradox could be explained by the possibility that in the chronic hemolytic type, the molecular lesion is different, as evidenced by the membrane protein aggregates, and is so severe that increased utilization of vitamin E by the red cell membrane plays no role in the subsequent pathologic process.

The role for vitamin E in the treatment of these disorders remains largely theoretical. The strongest case can be made for treatment of GS deficiency, because both red cell life span and polymorphonuclear cell function seem greatly improved. In spite of the failure to improve chronic hemolytic G6PD patients, the role of vitamin E as a potential antioxidant in this disorder requires further study, as only a small number of kindreds have been studied and the response could vary with the specific molecular lesion. The magnitude of hematologic improvement due to vitamin E in Gd^{B-} is small, and the ability of tocopherol to protect these cells against severe oxidant stress remains unproven. Thus, its routine use in these patients is unwarranted at this time.

Neonatal hyperbilirubinemia in G6PD-deficient subjects is reportedly increased, and we are currently evaluating the efficacy of vitamin E to reduce the degree of hemolysis and hyperbilirubinemia in this patient group.

ACKNOWLEDGMENTS

The authors thank Mrs. Lynda Ray and Ms. Laurie Tuchman for assistance in preparation of the manuscript and Ms. Brenda Shafer for technical assistance. We are especially grateful for the cooperation of Drs. Myron Brin and Dietrich Hornig.

REFERENCES

1. ROSE, C. S. & P. GYÖRGY. 1950. Hemolysis with alloxan and alloxan-like compounds, and the protective action of tocopherol. Blood **5:** 1062–1074.
2. BROWNLEE, N. R., J. J. HUTTNER, R. V. PANGANAMALA & D. G. CORNWELL. 1977. Role of vitamin E in glutathione-induced oxidant stress: methemoglobin, lipid peroxidation and hemolysis. J. Lipid Res. **18:** 635–644.
3. DALLMAN, P. R. 1974. The nutritional anemias. *In* Hematology of Infancy and Childhood. D. G. Nathan & F. A. Oski, Eds.: 97–105. W. B. Saunders Co. Philadelphia, Pa.
4. FARRELL, P. M., J. G. BIERI, J. F. FRATANTONI, R. E. WOOD & P. A. DI SANT'AGNESE. 1977. The occurrence and effects of human vitamin E deficiency: a study in patients with cystic fibrosis. J. Clin. Invest. **60:** 233–241.
5. LEONARD, P. J. & M. S. LOSOWSKY. 1971. Effect of alpha-tocopherol administration on red cell survival in vitamin E deficient human subjects. Am. J. Clin. Nutr. **24:** 388–393.

6. LUZZATO, L. & U. TESTA. 1978. Human erythrocyte glucose-6-phosphate dehydrogenase: structure and function in normal and mutant subjects. In Current Topics in Hematology. S. Piomelli & S. Yachnin, Eds. 1: 1–70. Alan R. Liss. New York, N.Y.

7. MOHLER, D. N., P. W. MAJERUS, V. MINNICK, C. E. HESS & M. D. GARRICK. 1970. Glutathione synthetase deficiency as a cause of hereditary hemolytic disease. N. Engl. J. Med. 283: 1253–1257.

8. BEUTLER, E. 1978. Hemolytic Anemias in Disorders of Red Cell Metabolism. Plenum Medical Book Co. New York, N.Y.

9. PIOMELLI, S. 1974. G6PD deficiency and related disorders of the pentose pathway. In Hematology of Infancy and Childhood. D. G. Nathan & F. A. Oski, Eds.: 363. W. B. Saunders Co. Philadelphia, Pa.

10. BERNINI, L., B. LATTE & M. SINISCALCO. 1964. Survival of ^{51}Cr labelled red cells in subjects with thalassemia trait or G6PD deficiency or both abnormalities. Br. J. Haematol. 10: 171–180.

11. PIOMELLI, S. & M. SINISCALCO. 1969. The hematologic effects of glucose-6-phosphate dehydrogenase deficiency and thalassemia trait: interaction between two genes at the phenotype level. Br. J. Haematol. 16: 537–549.

12. PIOMELLI, S. 1974. G6PD deficiency and related disorders of the pentose pathway. In Hematology of Infancy and Childhood. D. G. Nathan & F. A. Oski, Eds.: 359–361. W. B. Saunders Co. Philadelphia, Pa.

13. JOHNSON, G. J., D. W. ALLEN, S. CADMAN, V. F. FAIRBANKS, J. G. WHITE, B. C. LAMPKIN & M. E. KAPLAN. 1979. Red cell membrane polypeptide aggregates in glucose-6-phosphate dehydrogenase mutants with chronic hemolytic disease. N. Engl. J. Med. 301: 552.

14. SPIELBERG, S. P., M. D. GARRICK, L. M. CORASH, J. D. BUTLER, F. TIETZE, L. V. ROGERS & J. D. SCHULMAN. 1978. Biochemical heterogeneity in gluthathione synthetase deficiency. J. Clin. Invest. 61: 1417–1420.

15. CORASH, L., S. SPIELBERG, C. BARTSOCAS, L. BOXER, R. STEINBERG, M. SHEETZ, M. EGAN, J. SCHLESSLEMAN & J. D. SCHULMAN. 1980. Reduced chronic hemolysis during high dose vitamin E administration in Mediterranean type glucose-6-phosphate dehydrogenase deficiency. N. Engl. J. Med. 303: 416–420.

16. BIERI, J. R., T. T. TOLLIVER & G. L. CATIGNANI. 1979. Simultaneous determination of α-tocopherol and retinol in plasma or red cells by high pressure liquid chromatography. Am. J. Clin. Nutr. 32: 2143–2149.

17. SPIELBERG, S. P., L. A. BOXER, L. M. CORASH & J. D. SCHULMAN. 1979. Improved erythrocyte survival with high dose vitamin E in chronic hemolyzing G6PD and glutathione synthetase deficiencies. Ann. Intern. Med. 90: 53–54.

18. SPIELBERG, S. P., L. A. BOXER, J. M. OLIVER, J. M. ALLEN & J. D. SCHULMAN. 1979. Oxidative damage to neutrophiles in glutathione synthetase deficiency. Br. J. Haematol. 42: 215–223.

19. BOXER, L. A., J. M. OLIVER, S. P. SPIELBERG, J. M. ALLEN & J. D. SCHULMAN. 1979. Protection of granulocytes by vitamin E in glutathione synthetase deficiency. N. Engl. J. Med. 301: 901–905.

20. OLIVER, J. M., S. P. SPIELBERG, C. B. PEARSON & J. D. SCHULMAN. 1978. Microtubule assembly and function in normal and glutathione synthetase deficient human polymorphonuclear leukocytes. J. Immunol. 120: 1181–1186.

21. SHEETZ, M. 1980. Glucose-6-phosphate dehydrogenase deficiency. Ann. Intern. Med. 93: 341–343. (Section of a review entitled Genetic disorders of glutathione and sulfur amino acid metabolism: new biochemical insights and therapeutic approaches. J. D. Schulman, moderator.)

22. JOHNSON, G. J., B. FINKEL, G. VATASSERY, J. G. WHITE & D. W. ALLEN. 1981. Shortened erythrocyte survival in chronic hemolytic disease due to glucose-6-phosphate dehydrogenase deficiency is not corrected by high dose vitamin E therapy. Blood 58(Suppl. 29a).

23. STOCKMAN, J. A., III, S. LANDAU & F. A. OSKI. 1979. Primaquine induced hemolysis in glucose-6-phosphate dehydrogenase (G6PD) deficiency, effect of vitamin E. (abst.). Pediatr. Res. 13: 442.

24. NATTA, C. L. & L. J. MACHLIN. 1979. Plasma levels of tocopherol in sickle cell anemia subjects. Am. J. Clin. Nutr. **32:** 1359–1362.
25. CHIU, D. & B. LUBIN. 1979. Abnormal vitamin E and glutathione peroxidase levels in sickle cell anemia: evidence for increased susceptibility to lipid peroxidation in vivo. J. Lab. Clin. Med. **94:** 542–545.

———————————◆———————————

DISCUSSION

E. A. RACHMILEWITZ (*Hadassah University Hospital, Jerusalem, Israel*): I understand that you do not recommend constant vitamin E treatment to the so-called mild hemolyzer?

L. M. CORASH: That's right.

E. A. RACHMILEWITZ: Okay, but I must say I'm very puzzled by the fact that you didn't find any changes in the severe hemolyzer. The vitamin E levels in these patients were normal.

L. M. CORASH: That's right, in the group that we studied, they were normal.

E. A. RACHMILEWITZ: Did you study some other parameters in the chronic hemolyzers in red cells, like lipids or proteins?

L. M. CORASH: We did look at some of our patients, and we found high-molecular-weight protein aggregates on polyacrylamide gel.

I agree with you that I'm perplexed as to why the vitamin E levels are not lower. Maybe we are looking at a defect so severe that vitamin E utilization may play no role in this; maybe that's not part of the mechanism of the hemolysis; maybe peroxidation itself may not have anything to do with the rapid elimination of these cells. I don't know. We certainly don't see very severe lowering of vitamin E in other chronic hemolytic disorders; in patients with spherocytosis, for example, vitamin E is not dramatically lowered. So I think it's a puzzle, and I don't understand why.

I. D. DESAI (*University of British Columbia, Vancouver, B.C., Canada*): Your observations regarding α- and γ-tocopherol are quite interesting. I'm just wondering as to how you explain the differences between the subjects and the controls, in one case α being reduced quite significantly but not γ. What is the significance of this?

L. M. CORASH: First of all, of course, α-tocopherol is the more predominant form and is also the more predominant form in the red cell, so this may just reflect the relative ratio. There is greater utilization of α because more of it is around. Or perhaps, as one of the speakers in an earlier session suggested, the receptors on the red cell membrane may have greater affinity for α. Perhaps that's why you may have selective utilization of α-tocopherol.

L. A. BOXER (*Indiana University, Indianapolis, Ind.*): I have a brief comment. When your paper dealing with mild G6PD deficiency was published in the *New England Journal of Medicine*, Dr. Oski wrote a very lovely editorial called "A Radical Defense." I would maintain that in the patient with glutathione synthetase deficiency, we were able to show very clearly that vitamin E protected the integrity of the granulocyte membrane as well as some of its cytoplasmic constituents from peroxide damage. Originally, Drs. Schulman and Spielberg observed that when this infant, over the first couple of years of life, had mild infections, unexplained neutropenia developed. We observed that the granulocyte from patients whose glutathione levels were only about 20% normal released 50% more peroxide, when stimulated, to the extracellular milieu. In turn, Dr. Oliver from the University of Connecticut observed that the peroxide destroyed and affected the assembly of sulfhydryl-bearing microtubules. When this child was placed on vitamin E, not only were we able to normalize the red cell survival, but we observed that vitamin E in this situation was able to subserve the role of intracellular gluthathione and protect microtubule assembly in the granulocytes as well as normalize other aspects of granulocyte function. Concomitantly, Dr. Baehner and I along with John McAllister developed a selenium-deficient model in rats that leads to glutathione peroxidase deficiency, and replicated the same findings we saw in the human patient.

F. A. OSKI (*State University of New York, Syracuse, N.Y.*): Dr. Corash, have you had an opportunity to get the newborn study under way, and is there any preliminary information that you could share with us?

L. M. CORASH: We have just gotten the first batch of slides and data, and nothing has been analyzed yet, so I think it's a little too premature to say. About 60 patients have been recruited into that study so far.

L. BOWIE (*Evanston Hospital, Evanston, Ill.*): I would like to support your findings with regard to G6PD deficiency. We were interested a couple of years ago in looking at whether or not vitamin E might be effective at the membrane level. As a result, we studied whether or not vitamin E given externally could affect gluthathione stability within the cell, that is to say, whether or not it might have some protective effect in the cytoplasm as opposed to just at the level of the membrane. In general, we did not find the counterprotection. At the same time, we did study one particular patient with G6PD deficiency and observed 15% reticulocytosis, chronic hemolysis; in that same patient, vitamin E given at 400 units per day over a period of three months was not effective.

So the suggestion is that perhaps in those patients where E is not effective, it may be due to the lack of an effect at the cytoplasmic level as opposed to the lack of an effect at the membrane level.

F. A. OSKI: Stimulated and encouraged by Dr. Corash and Dr. Schulman, Dr. Stockman at our institute took the blood from a patient with a severe form of G6PD deficiency of the chronic hemolyzing type and did a slightly different study. We took this patient's blood, transfused it into five recipients, and measured the red cell life span in those individuals. Then we put those individuals on 800 units of vitamin E for about a month and then retransfused the cells into the recipients. We found that the original subject's red cells now survived significantly longer in the recipients who had been taking large quantities of vitamin E. When each of the subjects, however, took primaquine, the cells were rapidly destroyed, so they certainly could not withstand a primaquine challenge although they seemed to fare better in the recipients.

THE EFFECT OF VITAMIN E ON WARFARIN-INDUCED VITAMIN K DEFICIENCY*

James J. Corrigan, Jr.

Department of Pediatrics
Section of Pediatric Hematology-Oncology
University of Arizona Health Sciences Center
Tucson, Arizona 85724

INTRODUCTION

Vitamin E has no measurable adverse effect on the coagulation mechanism of normal animals and humans.[1-6] However, the administration of vitamin E to vitamin K–deficient rats, dogs, chicks, and humans enhances the coagulation defect.[7-12] The effect is the same whether the vitamin K–deficient state is induced by drug or by diet. In addition, this coagulopathy can be corrected with exogenous sources of vitamin K.

The mechanism by which vitamin E causes a further reduction in the vitamin K–dependent functional proteins is not known. In this study on warfarin-treated rats, dogs, and humans, the data suggest that vitamin E may interfere somehow with the vitamin K–carboxylase reaction and not with the synthesis of the precursor proteins.

METHODS AND MATERIALS

In the animal studies, whole blood was obtained from the vena cava of the rat and hind limb vein of the dog and anticoagulated using one part 3.8% sodium citrate to nine parts of whole blood. In the humans, blood was obtained by sterile venipuncture and anticoagulated using one part of a sodium citrate–citric acid anticoagulant and nine parts whole blood. Platelet-poor plasma was obtained by centrifugation of the anticoagulated blood in plastic tubes at 8,000 rpm, 4°C, for 20 minutes. The platelet-poor plasma was used for the determination of the prothrombin time,[13] prothrombin and proconvertin (P&P) test,[14] factor II coagulant assay using thromboplastin and *Echis* venom,[14,15] and factor II antigen by electroimmunoassay.[15] The results are expressed as percent of pooled normal rat, dog, or human time, which is expressed as seconds [mean ± standard error of the mean (SEM)].

The warfarin employed was the oral and parenteral preparation supplied by Endo Laboratories, Inc., Garden City, N.Y. (Coumadin). Vitamin E (*all-rac-*α-tocopherol) in sesame oil for injection was obtained from Rugby Laboratories, Inc., Rockville Center, N.Y., and vitamin E capsules from Whiteworth, Inc., Gardena, Calif.

In the animal studies, 250-gram Sprague-Dawley male rats fed a standard rat chow and mongrel dogs weighing 25–30 kilograms also fed a standard diet were used.

*Supported by research grants from the National Institutes of Health (HL 21431) and from the American Heart Association (Arizona Affiliate), Phoenix, Arizona.

361

Humans studied were 12 cardiology patients who had been receiving warfarin on a long-term basis and who had mild to moderate prolongation of their prothrombin times (range, 16.0–21.5 seconds). None of these patients had known liver disease, nor were they self-administering vitamin E. In addition, 19 patients with cystic fibrosis were investigated. During the investigation, no human developed a clinical bleeding state. For the human studies, 50 adult patients without known liver disease or vitamin K deficiency were used as controls. The data were statistically analyzed using the "t"-test for nonpaired experiments; a "p" value of less than 0.05 was considered a significant change.

RESULTS

Dog Experiments

Dogs were given warfarin either intravenously or orally at a dose that would maintain the prothrombin time at 1½ to 2 times their baseline values.[11] The normal

TABLE 1

EFFECT OF VITAMIN E IN THREE DOGS*

	1		2		3	
Warfarin (mg/day)	0	0	15	15	7.5	7.5
Vitamin E (IU/day)	0	800	0	800	0	800
Prothrombin time (seconds)	7.0	6.8	14.1	25.5	11.0	13.3
Assays (%):†						
P&P	100	110	3	<1	9	3
Factor II	100	110	21	6	27	10
Factor VII	100	80	4	3	10	2
Factor V	100	150	150	140	130	160

*Warfarin and vitamin E were administered orally. For each dog, the first column represents the mean coagulation values for two to three weeks prior to the addition of vitamin E. The second column represents mean coagulation values after one week of vitamin E.

†Percent of normal dog plasma.

prothrombin time for the dogs was 7.0 ± 0.5 seconds [mean ± standard deviation (SD)]; and for the P&P assay, 50–150%. The coagulation data on dogs given warfarin orally at two different dosages for two to three weeks and then the addition of vitamin E are shown in TABLE 1. In dog no. 1, which did not receive warfarin, the vitamin E imparted no significant change in the vitamin K–dependent coagulation factors. Dog no. 2 received 15 mg/day of warfarin and showed a significant increase in the prothrombin time and a further reduction in the vitamin K coagulation factors; most pronounced was the reduction in factor II. Dog no. 3, which received 7.5 mg/day of warfarin, showed similar changes, however not as marked as dog no. 2. Factor V, being a non–vitamin K–dependent factor, did not change significantly in any of these animals. The effect of a single intravenous dose of warfarin in dogs with and without vitamin E is shown in TABLE 2. In this experiment, the dogs were given an injection of 25 mg of warfarin with or without 400 or 800 IU of vitamin E. As can be seen, the prothrombin time

TABLE 2

EFFECT OF VITAMIN E IN DOGS GIVEN ONE INTRAVENOUS DOSE OF WARFARIN (W)

	Prothrombin Time (seconds)			P&P (%)*		
Day	W	W + vit E (400 IU)	W + vit E (800 IU)	W	W + vit E (400 IU)	W + vit E (800 IU)
1	7.1	7.2	7.1	105	100	100
2	9.2	10.9	10.2	30	23	24
3	9.1	15.7	16.7	32	9	10
4	8.1	8.2	7.7	70	46	64
5	7.7	7.1	7.7	82	73	60

*Percent of normal dog plasma.

increased and the P&P assay decreased in those animals receiving vitamin E as compared to those dogs who received only warfarin. The changes were most marked by day 3. There did not appear to be a difference between the two doses of vitamin E. Normal dogs given 800 IU of vitamin E orally showed a significant increase in the plasma levels of vitamin E [before the vitamin, 2.42 ± 0.41 mg/dl; with the vitamin, 3.95 ± 0.74 (mean ± SD); p < 0.01].

Rat Experiments

Rats were given vitamin E (100 units/100 g body weight per day) for seven days intramuscularly.[12] Control animals were given either saline or sesame oil intramuscularly. The animals were fasted for 24 hours on the sixth day and given warfarin (0.01 mg/100 g body weight) intraperitoneally, and the blood collected 24 hours later. The results of this experiment are shown in TABLE 3. Those animals receiving warfarin and vitamin E demonstrated a more severe reduction in factor II coagulant activity as measured with thromboplastin than did those given warfarin without the vitamin. Factor II levels measured by using Echis venom,

TABLE 3

WARFARIN-TREATED RATS: EFFECT OF VITAMIN E ON
FACTOR II COAGULANT ACTIVITY (CA)

Number of Rats	Warfarin*	Vitamin E†	Factor II CA (%)‡	
			Thromboplastin	Echis Venom
20	0	0	130 ± 5	125 ± 4
10	0	0 (oil × 7 days)§	105 ± 5	190 ± 5
10	0	+ (7 days)	180 ± 8	130 ± 4
20	+	0	74 ± 3	110 ± 4
5	+	0 (oil × 7 days)	70 ± 4	200 ± 8
10	+	+ (7 days)	9 ± 3	150 ± 5

*Warfarin, 0.01 mg/100 g intraperitoneally.
†Vitamin E, 100 IU/100 g intramuscularly.
‡Percent of pooled normal rat plasma (mean ± SEM).
§Sesame oil without vitamin E.

however, were not reduced. There was no significant difference for functional factor II coagulant activity between the control rats given warfarin and those given sesame oil. In addition, those animals given vitamin E alone did not have *Echis* factor II levels below the untreated controls.

Human Studies

Factor II coagulant activity in the cardiology patients was 52% ± 10; and factor II antigen, 84 ± 6.8%.[12] These data, when compared to normal humans, revealed a significant reduction in factor II coagulant levels but normal antigen. TABLE 4 shows the results on the factor II coagulant activity, antigen levels, and ratios of coagulant activity to antigen in the patients given vitamin E. Factor II antigen did not change throughout the testing period, and these levels were no different from controls. Factor II coagulant activity measured with thromboplastin declined by the first week and remained at this level for the remainder of the four-week testing period. As can be seen from the table, there was no significant difference between the two doses of vitamin E employed in this experiment. The initial coagulation studies performed on the warfarin-treated cardiology patients prior to vitamin E showed the prothrombin time to be 19 ± 0.8 seconds compared to 12.0 ± 0.2 for controls. The standard prothrombin times changed slightly during this period of time, the pretreatment value being 19 seconds, increasing to 21 seconds in the 400-IU group and 22 seconds in the 100-IU group. None of the patients experienced a bleeding diathesis, and in no case was the warfarin dose discontinued or reduced.

Nineteen patients with cystic fibrosis were evaluated.[16] These particular patients were found to fall into three major groups: those not receiving supplemental vitamin E or K; those receiving vitamin E alone (100–200 IU/day perorally); and those receiving both vitamin E and K (5 mg twice a week perorally). Analysis of the factor II levels in these patients can be seen in TABLE 5. As is noted, those patients without supplementation had a 56% frequency of vitamin K deficiency as defined by a factor II coagulant activity to antigen ratio of less than 0.75. Those receiving both vitamin K and vitamin E had a similar frequency; however, the patients receiving vitamin E alone without vitamin K supplementation showed a much higher frequency of vitamin K deficiency. It is interesting to note that the factor II antigen levels in the three groups of patients were not

TABLE 4

WARFARIN-TREATED PATIENTS: EFFECT OF VITAMIN E ON FACTOR II
COAGULANT ACTIVITY (CA) TO ANTIGEN RATIO

| Vitamin E (IU/day) | Factor II (%)* | | | p |
	CA	Antigen	Ratio (CA:Antigen)	
None (baseline) (12)†	52 ± 10‡	84 ± 6‡	0.63 ± 0.07	—
400 (6)	33 ± 4	83 ± 4	0.40 ± 0.04	<0.02
100 (6)	37 ± 5	83 ± 3	0.45 ± 0.04	<0.05

*Percent of normal plasma.
†Number of patients given in parentheses.
‡Mean ± SEM.

TABLE 5

FACTOR II DATA: CYSTIC FIBROSIS PATIENTS WITHOUT LIVER DISEASE

| Group | Vitamin | | Factor II (%)* | | | Vitamin K Deficiency† |
	K	E	CA	Antigen	Ratio (CA:Antigen)	
I	0	0 (9)‡	68§	87	0.78	56%
			45–90¶	70–105	0.54–1.00	
II	0	+ (5)	65	98	0.65	80%
			46–86	70–125	0.45–0.84	
III	+	+ (5)	80	102	0.78	60%
			45–100	68–140	0.66–1.11	
Controls	0	0 (50)	83	91	0.91	—
			60–150	60–150	0.77–1.00	

*Percent of pooled normal plasma.
†CA:antigen ratio <0.75.
‡Number of patients is given in parentheses.
§Mean.
¶Range.

significantly different and that the severity of the functional coagulation abnormalities appeared to be the same between group I and group II patients.

DISCUSSION

Studies in numerous animal models made vitamin K deficient have shown that the administration of vitamin E will enhance the vitamin K–deficient state and the animal can subsequently die a hemorrhagic death. Other studies have shown that excess vitamin E in normal humans, rats, and dogs does not affect the prothrombin time, however. In the studies reported here in dogs, rats, and humans, the vitamin K–deficiency state was induced by warfarin or fat malabsorption, and the addition of vitamin E did allow for a further reduction of the vitamin K–dependent coagulation factors. In the rat and human studies, a detailed analysis of prothrombin levels demonstrated that the biologically active functional factor II was decreased but that immunoreactive protein and the assays of the factor employing *Echis carinatus* venom were normal. This suggests that the site of action of vitamin E is at the vitamin K–carboxylase step (FIGURE 1) and is not interfering with the production of the precursor protein by the liver. In addition, it seems unlikely that vitamin E was interfering with vitamin K intestinal absorption, since the hypoprothrombinemic effect can be produced by oral or intramuscular administration of vitamin E. It is known that the vitamin K reaction requires a carboxylase enzyme, oxygen, and a source of carbon dioxide.[17] Vitamin K exists in two forms—a reduced and an epoxide form. The reduced form appears to be metabolically active, and the energy to drive the carboxylation reaction may come from the oxidation of the reduced vitamin K to the epoxide in the system. It is known from animal studies that warfarin appears to inhibit the reductase reaction. Thus, during anticoagulation therapy, there is a high ratio of K-oxide to vitamin K in the liver. Vitamin E could interact in this system by interfering with the oxidation of the reduced vitamin K. It is also possible, however, that vitamin E may exert its effect at the microsomal level by interfering with the reaction that needs to take place on a phospholipid bilayer surface. It should be noted that the vitamin E effect can be overcome by either stopping vitamin E or by administering vitamin K. Although doses of vitamin E of 400 IU or less per day in the humans did not induce a clinical bleeding state in moderate vitamin K deficiency, the data suggest that large doses of vitamin E should be used with caution in such patients.

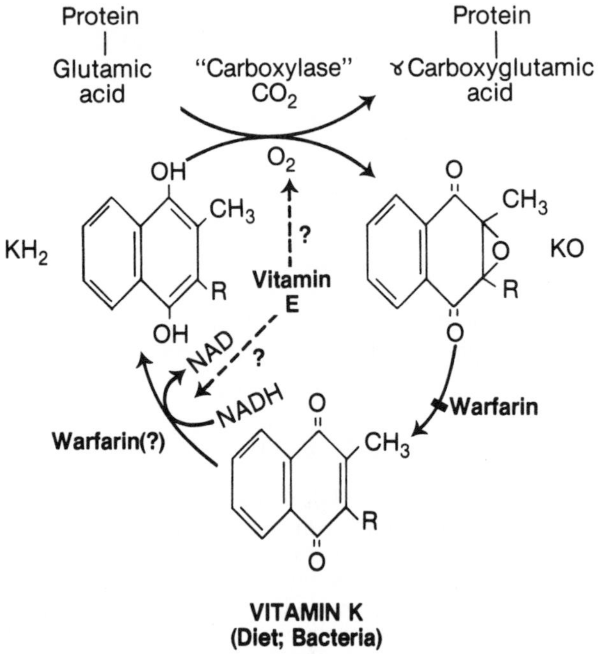

FIGURE 1. Vitamin K cycle and the vitamin K-carboxylase reaction. Possible site(s) of action of vitamin E.

SUMMARY

Vitamin K-deficient animals and humans developed a more severe coagulopathy when treated with vitamin E, which was due to further reduction in the vitamin K-dependent coagulation factors (II, VII, IX, and X). This phenomenon was not seen in normal vitamin K-sufficient animals or human subjects. The mechanism by which vitamin E causes this effect is not known. These coagulation factors are produced by the liver in precursor forms and are converted to functional proteins by a vitamin K-dependent reaction. Analysis of one of these coagulation factors, prothrombin (factor II), in plasma of vitamin K-deficient animals and humans treated with vitamin E was done in this study. The precursor of factor II is antigenically similar to biologically active factor II and can be activated to form thrombin by *Echis carinatus* venom. The data showed that functional factor II coagulant activity was reduced below base in warfarin-treated humans and animals given vitamin E. Factor II antigen as determined by electroimmunoassay in humans and factor II coagulant activity as measured using *Echis* venom in animals were unchanged and no different from untreated controls. The data suggest that vitamin E acts at the vitamin K–carboxylase step of carboxylation of precursor prothrombin and not in the synthesis of the precursor protein.

REFERENCES

1. HILLMAN, R. W. 1957. Tocopherol excess in man: creatinuria associated with prolonged ingestion. Am. J. Clin. Nutr. **5:** 597–600.
2. AYERS, S. & R. MIHAN. 1969. Pseudoxanthoma elasticuns and epidermolysis bullosa: response to vitamin E (tocopherol). Cutis **5:** 287–294.
3. GOODMAN, L. S. & A. GILMAN, Eds. 1970. The Pharmacological Basis of Therapeutics. 4th edit.: 1694–1697. Macmillan Publishing Co., Inc. New York, N.Y.
4. ANDERSON, T. W. 1974. Vitamin E in angina pectoris. Can. Med. Assoc. J. **110:** 401–408.
5. 1975. Vitamin E. Med. Lett. **17:** 69–70.
6. TSAI, A. C., J. J. KELLY, B. PENG & N. COOK. 1978. Study on the effect of mega–vitamin E supplementation in man. Am. J. Clin. Nutr. **31:** 831–837.
7. MILLETTE, S. J. & L. A. LEONE. 1960. Influence of age, sex, strain of rat and fat-soluble vitamins on hemorrhagic syndromes in rats fed irradiated beef. Fed. Proc. **19:** 1045–1049.
8. DOISY, E. A., JR. 1961 Nutritional hypoprothrombinemia and metabolism of vitamin K. Fed. Proc. **20:** 989–994.
9. MARCH, B. E., E. WONG, L. SEIER, et al. 1973. Hypervitaminosis E in the chick. J. Nutr. **103:** 371–377.
10. CORRIGAN, J. J., JR. & F. I. MARCUS. 1974. Coagulopathy associated with vitamin E ingestion. J. Am. Med. Assoc. **230:** 1300–1301.
11. CORRIGAN, J. J., JR. 1979 Coagulation problems relating to vitamin E. Am. J. Pediatr. Hematol. Oncol. **1:** 169–173.
12. CORRIGAN, J. J., JR. & L. L. ULFERS. 1981. Effect of vitamin E on prothrombin levels in warfarin-induced vitamin K deficiency. Am. J. Clin. Nutr. **34:** 1701–1704.
13. QUICK, A. J. 1957. Hemorrhagic Diseases: 379–387. Lea & Febiger. Philadelphia, Pa.
14. OWREN, P. A. & K. AAS. 1951. Control of dicumarol therapy and quantitative determination of prothrombin and proconvertin. Scand. J. Clin. Lab. Invest. **3:** 201–208.
15. CORRIGAN, J. J., JR. & D. L. EARNEST. 1980. Factor II antigen in liver disease and warfarin-induced vitamin K deficiency: correlation with coagulant activity using *Echis* venom. Am. J. Hematol. **8:** 249–255.
16. CORRIGAN, J. J., JR., L. M. TAUSSIG, R. BECKERMAN & J. S. WAGENER. 1981. Factor II (prothrombin) coagulant activity and immunoreactive protein: detection of vitamin K deficiency in patients with cystic fibrosis. J. Pediatr. **99:** 254–256.
17. SUTTIE, J. W., Ed. 1980. Vitamin K Metabolism and Vitamin K–Dependent Proteins. University Park Press. Baltimore, Md.

———◆———

DISCUSSION

R. E. OLSON (*St. Louis University School of Medicine, St. Louis, Mo.*): I'd like to make one comment about the *Echis* thromboplastin assays, because the extent to which precursor is secreted varies according to species. The key to the posttranslational modification of prothrombin was really illuminated by the immunoassays of patients taking dicumarol in Sweden. Stenflo took this idea and compared prothrombin from cows given warfarin with prothrombin from cows that were not given warfarin.

In man, in the cow, in the dog, and in most strains of rodents, the precursor protein accumulates in the reticulum and makes the reticulum a very good source for the study of the enzyme. In your studies, it appears that in warfarinized rats, the Echis activity remained high as thromboplastic activity went low; that's very atypical for rats. In our case, the rat is a species in which the two activities parallel the vitamin K deficiency. It may well be, however, that very large doses of vitamin E could alter the reticulum enough to permit the precursor to be secreted.

J. J. CORRIGAN: I appreciate the views you have on the rats, and this was a concern for us when we were trying to find the right model. However, in our model it seems to be working.

V. S. HUBBARD (National Institutes of Health, Bethesda, Md.): In regard to the data that you presented on the cystic fibrosis patients, do you have the absolute α-tocopherol levels in these patients? Were they receiving vitamin E supplementation or antibiotics that may interfere with vitamin K levels?

J. J. CORRIGAN: We presented these data at the cystic fibrosis meeting last year, and they've also been published. We found no correlation between the clinical staging or antibiotics at the time these studies were performed. When these patients were on vitamin E at 200 IU, serum E levels were normal. Those who were not on E had low levels but not less than 0.5 mg/dl.

B. LUBIN (Children's Hospital Medical Center, Oakland, Calif.): What about the premature infant? We're considering high doses of vitamin E to prevent intraventricular hemorrhage. This seems to be exactly the opposite of your recommendations.

J. J. CORRIGAN: I am saying this as a caution—that vitamin K-deficient humans if given vitamin E can develop a bleeding disorder or at least an enhancement of the vitamin K-deficient state. However, it can be overcome with exogenous vitamin K. As you know all babies, at least most of them in the United States, are given vitamin K at the time of birth. I would think that unless you had extenuating circumstances, that would be sufficient.

V. S. HUBBARD: I have to emphasize the point again, because I think not all hospitals and not all states practice the administration of phylloquinone to infants at birth. But certainly the question Dr. Lubin raises is very important—that these children who are given high doses of vitamin E when they are at risk for vitamin K deficiency in the neonatal period must be given vitamin K.

J. J. CORRIGAN: We would hope that there would be no infants at risk for vitamin K deficiency if physicians follow the recommendations of the American Academy of Pediatrics Committee on Nutrition.

A. R. BRASH (Vanderbilt University, Nashville, Tenn.): The activity of warfarin is strictly related to the free fraction of the drug in plasma. It's very highly bound in plasma. Do you know if vitamin E affects the binding of warfarin?

J. J. CORRIGAN: I'm sorry, I didn't study that.

A. R. BRASH: So it could be that vitamin E changes the free fraction of warfarin in plasma.

J. J. CORRIGAN: I guess it's possible.

R. E. OLSON: The point of my remarks was to show that this effect can be gotten independently of warfarin. It is likely that the effect is mediated at the K-dependent carboxylation step by some competition with a vitamin E metabolite. At least that's a working hypothesis. On the other hand, it could be that vitamin E has some effect on warfarin binding, but that would be independent of the main competition.

LONG-TERM STUDY OF α-TOCOPHEROL IN INTERMITTENT CLAUDICATION

Knut Haeger

Slottsstaden Clinic
S-21748 Malmö, Sweden

In 1949, Boyd published his first results on the use of α-tocopherol (vitamin E) in patients with intermittent claudication (review by Boyd and Marks).[1,2] During the following years, a large number of reports confirmed the favorable impression of the efficacy of the drug on that indication. For example, we were able to prove that patients on α-tocopherol had a significantly longer walking distance than did patients given either vasodilator agents or anticoagulant therapy, or a placebolike regimen of multivitamin tablets excluding vitamin E.[3] Larsson and Haeger demonstrated a lower content of α-tocopherol in the soleus muscle of elderly men with peripheral arterial flow and also found that the increase of α-tocopherol in the soleus muscle was related to the clinical improvement,[4] creating a foundation for a dose-response relationship. In 1978, Haeger demonstrated a significant difference in the effects on arterial flow between one group of patients treated with α-tocopherol and a control group.[5] In this series, 17% of the controls and 88% of the treated patients demonstrated an improved arterial flow in the lower leg.

In a survey of the vitamin E complex, Bieri and Farrell summarized, "It is clear that although these studies favor the use of large doses of vitamin E in intermittent claudication, further clinical studies are needed."[6]

The aim of this report is to follow up our earlier studies, giving the results of continuous α-tocopherol treatment for up to 16 years.

MATERIALS AND METHODS

Some of the patients reported here were reported earlier.[3,5,7] The present cumulative series consists of 158 patients (130 males, 28 females) with a presenting complaint of intermittent dysbasia. In all cases, diagnosis was confirmed by one or more of the following examinations: arteriography, measurement of lower leg arterial flow, measurement of peripheral arterial blood pressure at the ankle and big toe levels, and a check of the walking distance under standardized conditions. Patients with severe rest pain or manifest gangrene were excluded from the study and referred to surgery.

All patients were instructed to perform active muscular exercise, including walks at least twice daily and home gymnastics, and were forbidden to smoke. One hundred twenty-two patients were given vitamin E in the form of RRR-α-tocopheryl acetate (Ido E®, Ferrosan) 100 mg three times a day. No other vasoactive drug or any drug possibly interfering with the peripheral vascular state was given. However, in approximately 40% of the cases, minor analgesics (acetyl salicylate, sodium salicylate, paracetamol, or diflunisal) were given for at least part of the treatment period. Thirty-six patients did not receive α-tocopherol. Some of these patients received vasoactive drugs ordered by doctors beyond our control.

After the initiation of treatment, physiological parameters were checked once

369

0077-8923/82/0393-0369 $01.75/0 © 1982, NYAS

a year except for the first year, in which an additional control was made after six months. In patients with subjective deterioration of symptoms, further checks were made according to clinical demands.

Arterial flow was measured by lower leg plethysmography in exercise and rest. Walking distance was measured according to standardized conditions, with step velocity monitored by metronome. Peripheral blood pressure was measured according to the method of Gundersen.[8]

Observation time ranged from 1 to 16 years. The geometric mean observation period was 4 years. The distribution of observation periods is demonstrated in FIGURE 1. During this lengthy period of study, some patients died. Since the cause

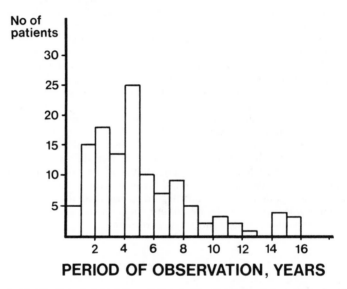

PERIOD OF OBSERVATION, YEARS

FIGURE 1. Distribution of observation periods in 94 patients receiving α-tocopherol and 26 control patients.

of death was not known in the majority of cases, no conclusions could be drawn as to the role of atherosclerotic disease.

RESULTS

The effect of the treatment on *standardized walking distance* is presented in TABLE 1. From the table, it is evident that the overall results were markedly better in the α-tocopherol group than in the control group. Thus, there were significantly less patients on α-tocopherol classified as becoming worse and, inversely, considerably more patients in the treated group developing a walking distance improved by more than 30%. The results of *arterial flow* measurements are given in TABLES 2 and 3. Even after 12 months of medication, there was no significant difference in flow between the treated group and the control group, whereas a

TABLE 1

WALKING DISTANCE

	Controls	Vitamin E
Worse	6 (16%)	6 (5%)
≤10% Better	20 (55%)	17 (13%)
10–30% Better	7 (19%)	40 (32%)
≥30% Better	4 (11%)	62 (50%)
	36	122

TABLE 2

ARTERIAL FLOW*

	Control	Vitamin E
Number of patients	26	94
Initial flow	7.2 ± 2.4	7.4 ± 2.6
After 12 months	6.9 ± 2.3	7.2 ± 2.4
After 18 months	6.4 ± 3.0	10.8 ± 3.9
After 36 months†	6.6 ± 2.8	9.2 ± 3.0

*Milliliters per 100 g per minute.
†Twenty controls; 71 treated.

highly significant difference appeared after 18 months of treatment. The small number of patients controlled by plethysmography after this period does not permit a calculation of means and statistical significance, but it is our clinical impression that patients on α-tocopherol also get along better in the long run. A graphic representation of the development of lower leg flow over the first three years of treatment is given in FIGURE 2.

In a series of patients with severe dysbasia, it is inescapable that some will develop symptoms and signs indicating surgery. Criteria for operation were intractable rest pain and manifest gangrene. Nine patients were submitted to surgical measures, including three cases of amputation of the lower leg. In TABLE 4 the rates of surgical interventions are listed, again demonstrating better results in the group treated with α-tocopherol than in the control group.

TABLE 3

ARTERIAL FLOW*

	Controls	Vitamin E
Improved	5	69
No change	4	11
Diminished	17	14
	26	94
% Improved	19.2	73.4

p < 0.01

*Milliliters per 100 g per minute.

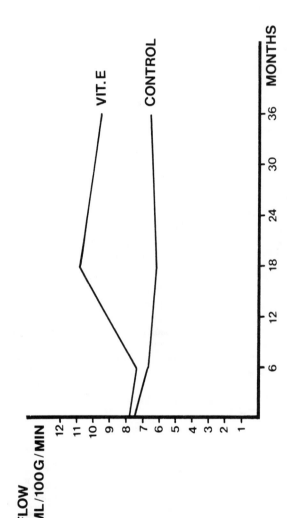

FIGURE 2. Average lower leg arterial flow in patients treated with vitamin E and in control patients respectively. The upper curve is based on the plethysmographic evaluation of 71 patients, the lower curve based on 20 control patients.

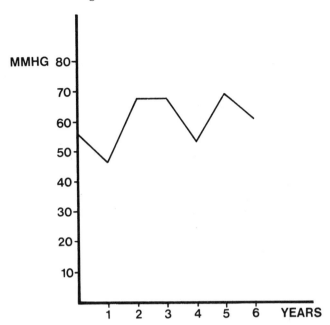

FIGURE 3. Systolic blood pressure in the big toe of the worst leg in six patients receiving α-tocopherol. (Also see text.)

The technique using peripheral blood pressure as an index of therapy results was introduced fairly recently in our laboratory. Only six patients so far have been followed for six years. In FIGURE 3, a graphic representation is given of the development of the mean of their pressures in the big toe of the worst leg. The general impression based on this parameter is that peripheral blood pressure after an initial depression during the first year rises to a fairly acceptable level for the following years. The dip of the curve at four years is due to one patient, who developed a pressure of less than 20 mm Hg and was referred for amputation.

No serious *side effects* were observed even in patients who received α-tocopherol three times daily during 16 years. In three cases, patients complained of transient slight nausea, but in no case did this symptom cause a discontinuation of medication.

TABLE 4

SURGICAL RECONSTRUCTION OR AMPUTATION

	Control	Vitamin E
Surgical Reconstruction	4 (11%)	2 (1.6%)
Amputation	2 (6%)	1 (0.8%)

difference significant

DISCUSSION

There is no doubt in our mind that α-tocopherol is a valuable addition to the treatment of peripheral arterial occlusive disease causing intermittent dysbasia. This series, as well as our previous reports,[3,5,7] speaks in favor of this conclusion. Our results agree with those reported by Livingstone and Jones, who performed a double-blind study of 34 patients over 40 weeks,[9] and by Williams et al., who demonstrated clinical improvement in 19 out of 30 patients on α-tocopherol and in 2 out of 15 on placebo.[10]

On the other hand, Hamilton et al. were not able to demonstrate a benefit from α-tocopherol treatment in intermittent dysbasia.[11] Their observation period, however, was restricted to 3 months. As shown in this series, we were not able to prove any increase of lower leg flow until after 18 months of medication; consequently, a 3-month study is not long enough to permit conclusions on the long-term results of the treatment. A more valid conflicting report is that by Hutchison and Williams, who studied calf blood flow and ankle blood pressure every 6 months over a five-year period and did not find any statistically significant change after a regime including α-tocopherol.[12] These authors discussed the possible reasons for the discrepancy of their results and our previously reported findings.[5,12] They thought it might be due to the fact that their subjects were not on an active exercise regimen. We tend to agree with this explanation and will use this opportunity to stress the importance of active exercise, evident from this series in which 55% of the control patients improved their walking distance without vitamin E. Hutchison and Williams did not measure their subjects' walking distance.

CONCLUSION

Our results indicate that the administration of α-tocopherol 100 mg three times daily in connection with active muscular training improves the state of patients with peripheral occlusive arterial disease presenting the symptom of intermittent claudication.

REFERENCES

1. BOYD, A. M. 1949. (As cited in Reference 2.)
2. BOYD, A. M. & G. MARKS. 1963. Angiology **14**: 198.
3. HAEGER, K. 1968. Vasc. Dis. **5**: 199.
4. LARSSON, H. & K. HAEGER. 1968. Pharmacol. Clin. **1**: 72.
5. HAEGER, K. 1974. Am. J. Clin. Nutr. **27**: 1179.
6. BIERI, J. G. & P. M. FARRELL. 1978. Vitam. Horm. **34**: 31.
7. HAEGER, K. 1978. In Tocopherol, Oxygen and Biomembranes. C. de Duve & O. Hayaishi, Eds.: 329–339. Elsevier/North Holland Biomedical Press. Amsterdam, the Netherlands.
8. GUNDERSEN, J. 1972. Acta Chir. Scand. Suppl. 426.
9. LIVINGSTONE, P. D. & C. JONES. 1958. Lancet **2**: 602.
10. WILLIAMS, H. T., D. FENNA & R. A. MACBETH. 1971. Surg. Gynecol. Obstet. **132**: 662.
11. HAMILTON, M., G. M. WILSON, P. ARMITAGE & J. T. BOYD. 1953. Lancet **1**: 367.
12. HUTCHISON, K. J. & H. T. G. WILLIAMS. 1978. Angiology **29**: 719.

DISCUSSION

F. A. OSKI (*State University of New York, Syracuse, N.Y.*): During the period of observation, in the controls as opposed to the vitamin E-treated group, was there any other advance of an arterial obstructive nature? Did the patients who were on vitamin E have any myocardial infarcts? Did the controls have any infarcts during this period of time?

K. HAEGER: Yes there were some during this long period of observation, and of course there were some patients who died in both groups. The rates in the two groups were equal. However, all these patients are outpatients and we don't know the exact cause of death in all of them, so I have no specific data to answer your question with.

F. A. OSKI: How much vitamin E were the patients taking each day?

K. HAEGER: One hundred milligrams three times daily.

P. B. McCAY (*Oklahoma Medical Research Foundation, Oklahoma City, Okla.*): Do you know what the mechanism of improvement in circulation is? Is it related to the collateral circulation? And what about exercise?

K. HAEGER: I don't know, and I have not made any experiments to clarify this in my mind. But vitamin E is not a vasodilator, so that could not explain it. There is a very small vasodilating effect, but that cannot in any way explain the results. I believe that this treatment in connection with muscular exercise opens up the collaterals. We have some scattered evidence from arteriograms that show, after a long time, better vascularization of the calf muscles.

G. A. FITZGERALD (*Vanderbilt University, Nashville, Tenn.*): Were any of your observations randomized in double blind or was it an entirely open study? How did you control for patients in either group taking other medications or being exposed to other factors besides their exercise regimen at home that might have altered or improved their blood flow in their lower limbs?

K. HAEGER: In a way, our study is single blind because the evaluator of the walking distance and the arterial flow has not known what treatment the patient is on. In both groups, we permitted the patients to take minor analgesics, such as aspirin, paracetamol, etc., but that was only done for short periods in small doses, and I don't think it had any influence.

In our control group, we know that some patients were taking vasoactive drugs, because they went to their own doctors. I'm fairly sure that at least the patients who had been in my office for 10 years or more have not taken any vasoactive drugs or drugs that could possibly interfere with these results.

G. A. FITZGERALD: If the treatment groups weren't randomized, how did you decide which patients would be the control patients?

K. HAEGER: By chance. The initial flows and the initial walking distances in the control group and the treatment group were very similar, and there was certainly no statistical difference between them.

THE EFFECTS OF VITAMIN E ON ARACHIDONIC ACID METABOLISM*

Rao V. Panganamala and David G. Cornwell

Department of Physiological Chemistry
The Ohio State University
Columbus, Ohio 43210

INTRODUCTION

A number of enzyme reactions are involved in the biosynthesis of prostanoids and hydroxy fatty acids from arachidonic acid (5,8,11,14–20:4). These reactions are outlined in FIGURE 1. Arachidonic acid is released from phospholipids and glycerides by a variety of lipases.[1-6] Prostanoids are then synthesized from the free fatty acid by a series of enzymatic reactions beginning with the formation of endoperoxides.[7,8] The enzyme cyclooxygenase catalyzes oxygen insertion and rapid cyclization of arachidonic acid into the hydroperoxy derivative prostaglandin G_2 (PGG_2). This short-lived hydroperoxy endoperoxide is transformed by a peroxidase into the hydroxy endoperoxide PGH_2. Prostacyclin (PGI_2), thromboxane A_2 (TxA_2), and prostaglandins E and F (PGE_2 and $PGF_{2\alpha}$) are synthesized from PGH_2 by a number of enzymes that are relatively tissue specific. Hydroperoxy fatty acids are synthesized from the free fatty acid by several lipoxygenases.[9-11] These enzymes, which are also relatively tissue specific, synthesize several isomers of the hydroperoxy fatty acid. Hydroperoxy fatty acids are converted to hydroxy fatty acids by a peroxidase. The 5-hydroperoxy fatty acid can also be incorporated into a leukotriene.[12]

Vitamin E and other lipid antioxidants modulate the biosynthetic pathways in arachidonic acid metabolism at a number of different points (FIGURE 1). Vitamin E has no effect on arachidonic acid incorporation into different lipid classes. Vitamin E inhibits both fatty acid release and lipoxygenase activity. Vitamin E does not inhibit cyclooxygenase. Indeed, low concentrations of some antioxidants enhance endoperoxide biosynthesis by prolonging cyclooxygenase activity. Finally, vitamin E and other antioxidants elevate PGI_2 by blocking the inhibitory effects of lipid peroxides on prostacyclin synthetase. These physiologic effects of vitamin E are related to its properties as an antioxidant. Vitamin E is a surfactant,[13-17] and high concentrations of vitamin E *in vitro* may function as a detergent. Antioxidant and detergent properties must be separated in a discussion of the effects of vitamin E on arachidonic acid metabolism. Data from our laboratory and data from other investigators supporting these observations are summarized in this review.

FATTY ACID INCORPORATION AND RELEASE

Vitamin E had no effect on the uptake and distribution of arachidonic acid in the major cellular lipid fractions of medial cells in tissue culture (TABLE 1). The

*These studies were supported in part by Grants HL-23439 and HL-11897 from the National Institutes of Health.

376

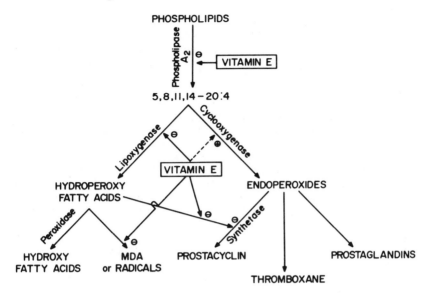

FIGURE 1. A model for the effects of vitamin E on the biosynthesis of prostanoids and hydroxy fatty acids from arachidonic acid.

absence of a vitamin E effect was found when cells were incubated with either 120 μM fatty acid or 0.6 μM fatty acid.[19] Even the total polar lipid fraction, presumably a fraction containing various oxidation products of the fatty acid, was unchanged in the presence or absence of vitamin E. Arachidonic acid is incorporated initially into choline phosphoglycerides rather than ethanolamine phosphoglycerides.[19] The ratio of arachidonic acid in phospholipid fractions decreases from 25 to 2 during a 24-hour incubation period. Vitamin E has no effect on this ratio. These data show that vitamin E does not alter the uptake and distribution of arachidonic acid. Vitamin E has profound effects on arachidonic acid metabolism, but these effects are exerted on biosynthetic pathways involving lipid fractions containing small amounts of specific fatty acid derivatives.

The release of arachidonic acid from phospholipids (FIGURE 1) is a rate-

TABLE 1

UPTAKE AND DISTRIBUTION OF 5,8,11,14–20:4 IN LIPIDS
OF MEDIAL CELLS IN TISSUE CULTURE*

Fraction	Without Vitamin E	With 10 μM Vitamin E
Total lipid (uptake in %)	81.4 ± 12.2	80.7 ± 9.3
Cholesteryl esters	0.3 ± 0.1	0.3 ± 0.1
Triglyceride	81.2 ± 3.5	81.1 ± 1.6
Free fatty acids	0.3 ± 0.1	0.2 ± 0.1
Polar lipids	0.9 ± 0.2	0.9 ± 0.2
Phospholipids	17.3 ± 3.7	17.5 ± 1.6

*Confluent cultures were incubated with 120 μM fatty acid for 24 hours. Figures are means ± standard deviations (SD). (Data from Reference 18.)

limiting step in the biosynthesis of prostanoids and hydroxy fatty acids. Considerable evidence has accumulated that a phospholipase A_2 is activated for arachidonic acid release from choline phosphoglycerides.[20] The release of arachidonic acid from inositol phosphoglycerides requires the sequential action of phospholipase C and a diglyceride lipase.[21,22] Diglyceride lipase activity may be inhibited by arachidonic acid metabolites.

A vitamin E deficiency in the rat resulted both in increased serum PGE_2 and $PGF_{2\alpha}$ levels[23] and in enhanced platelet aggregation in response to collagen.[24] Vitamin E-deficient children also demonstrated hyperaggregability to collagen, and this condition was corrected by supplementation with vitamin E.[25] Several early studies had suggested that very large amounts of vitamin E inhibited cyclooxygenase.[26,27] Nevertheless, it had not been established with certainty whether a vitamin E deficiency raised serum prostaglandin levels through enhanced phospholipase A_2 activity or enhanced cyclooxygenase activity.

We have measured the biosynthesis of TxA_2 in platelets from vitamin

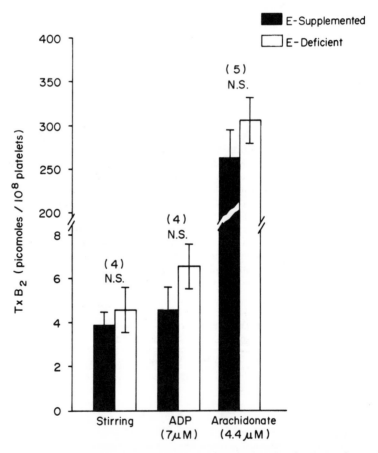

FIGURE 2. Generation of TxB_2 from washed platelets incubated with stirring alone, ADP, or arachidonic acid. (Reproduced from Reference 28 with permission from the publisher.)

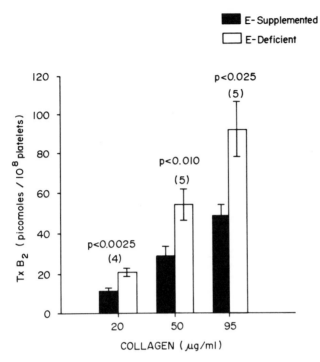

FIGURE 3. Generation of TxB_2 from washed platelets incubated with different concentrations of collagen. (Reproduced from Reference 28 with permission from the publisher.)

E-deficient and vitamin E-supplemented rats.[28] The same amounts of TxA_2, measured as TxB_2, were formed in platelets from E-deficient and E-supplemented rats when the platelets were supplied with unesterified arachidonic acid (FIGURE 2). However, platelets from E-deficient rats generated significantly more TxA_2 than did platelets from E-supplemented rats when the platelets were challenged with collagen (FIGURE 3). These data strongly suggest that phospholipase A_2 activity is enhanced in vitamin E deficiency.

The mechanism by which vitamin E diminishes arachidonic acid release from phospholipid has not been established. The oxidizing agent diazenedicarboxylic acid (bis) dimethylamide increases sulfhydryl cross-linking and enhances arachidonic acid release in platelet membranes.[5] Lipid peroxides enhance fatty acid release from mitochondria.[29] Vitamin E inhibits lipid peroxidation, and this inhibitory effect of vitamin E may decrease the sulfhydryl group cross-linking that enhances deacylase activity. The diglyceride lipase pathway does not explain enhanced release in a vitamin E deficiency since diglyceride lipase is apparently inhibited by lipid peroxides.[3]

Alternatively, vitamin E may also function indirectly by affecting cyclic nucleotide levels since phospholipase activity varies inversely with adenosine 3',5'-cyclic monophosphate (cAMP).[20] Vitamin E in high concentrations potentiates fatty acid release in platelets.[30] However, vitamin E in this concentration range probably functions as a surfactant rather than as a physiologic antioxidant.[31,32]

CYCLOOXYGENASE

The role of vitamin E in cyclooxygenase reactions has been disputed for some time. Early investigators reported that high concentrations of vitamin E inhibited oxygen uptake and prostaglandin biosynthesis in microsomal systems.[26,27] Several later investigators have reported that added vitamin E *in vitro* inhibited platelet aggregation.[33-39] We have found high concentrations of vitamin E are required to inhibit platelet aggregation, and vitamin E in this high concentration range is equally effective in the inhibition of either arachidonic acid–induced or adenosine diphosphate (ADP)-induced platelet aggregation (FIGURE 4). The fluidity of the platelet membrane is altered when platelets are incubated with vitamin E in this concentration range.[40] Some antioxidants, such as α-naphthol, propyl gallate, and butylated hydroxy anisole, inhibit prostaglandin biosynthesis, and these antioxidants discriminate between arachidonic acid–induced and ADP-induced platelet aggregation.[37,39] These data further support the concept that vitamin E in high concentrations functions as a surfactant that alters the platelet membrane

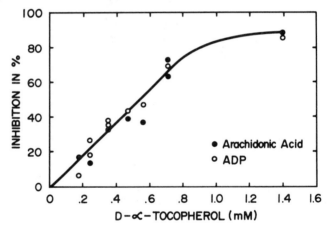

FIGURE 4. *RRR*-α-Tocopherol inhibition of arachidonic acid–induced and ADP-induced platelet aggregation. (Reproduced from Reference 37 with permission from the publisher.)

rather than as a physiologic antioxidant that inhibits prostaglandin biosynthesis in the platelet.

A number of investigators have measured the effects of added vitamin E and other antioxidants on prostaglandin biosynthesis from exogenous arachidonic acid in microsomes, tissue homogenates, and platelets. These studies are summarized in TABLE 2. Vitamin E, even in high concentrations, has very little effect on prostaglandin biosynthesis. Antioxidants such as α-naphthol are highly effective inhibitors of microsomal cyclooxygenase. Other antioxidants such as propyl gallate either stimulate or inhibit prostaglandin biosynthesis, depending on the source of tissue and the antioxidant concentration.

The studies with vitamin E added to tissue (TABLE 2) were confirmed and extended in studies where cells were grown in tissue cultures with and without added vitamin E or other antioxidants (TABLE 3). The inhibitory antioxidant α-naphthol stimulated cell growth and inhibited prostaglandin formation. Vita-

TABLE 2

EFFECT OF ANTIOXIDANTS ON PROSTAGLANDIN BIOSYNTHESIS

Antioxidant*	Molarity	Inhibiton $(-)$ or Stimulation $(+)$ (in %)
BVG microsomes[37]		
α-Naphthol	4×10^{-5}	-96
Propyl gallate	4×10^{-4}	-94
Vitamin E	4×10^{-3}	0
Rat testis microsomes[41]		
Propyl gallate	5×10^{-5}	$+79$
Vitamin E	1×10^{-4}	-3
SVG microsomes[42]		
Vitamin E	2.3×10^{-3}	-12
Rat renal medullary homogenate[43]		
Vitamin E	5×10^{-3}	$+21$
Washed platelets[30]		
Vitamin E	1.1×10^{-3}	-5
Washed platelets[39]		
Butylated hydroxy anisole	1.4×10^{-5}	-50
Vitamin E	1×10^{-3}	-15

*BVG is bovine vesicular gland; SVG is sheep vesicular gland.

min E stimulated cell growth without inhibiting prostaglandin formation. Prostaglandin–cell colony ratios were very similar in the presence and absence of vitamin E. Finally, several studies have shown that microsomes isolated from vitamin E–supplemented animals synthesize greater amounts of prostaglandins from added arachidonic acid than do microsomes from vitamin E–deficient animals.[41,45]

Antioxidants may inhibit, have no effect on, or stimulate cyclooxygenase. The more water-soluble antioxidants, such as α-naphthol or propyl gallate, both inhibit and stimulate prostaglandin biosynthesis (TABLES 2 and 3). A number of water-soluble antioxidants inhibit prostaglandin biosynthesis when present in high concentrations and enhance prostaglandin biosynthesis at low concentrations.[46–48] High concentrations of these antioxidants may lower the concentrations of the oxygen-centered radicals necessary for cyclooxygenase activity,[46,47,49–52] while low concentrations of these antioxidants may protect cyclooxygenase from

TABLE 3

EFFECT OF ANTIOXIDANTS ON PROSTAGLANDIN BIOSYNTHESIS AND CELL PROLIFERATION WITH MEDIAL CELLS IN TISSUE CULTURE*

Treatment	PGE (pg/ml)	Number of Colonies (mean ± SD)	PGE/Colonies
Medial	2700	420 ± 25	6.4
+10 μM α-naphthol	590	920 ± 76	0.6
+10 μM vitamin E	4400	1120 ± 109	3.9
Medial cells + 5,8,11,14–20:4	2500	470 ± 31	5.3
+50 μM α-naphthol	725	720 ± 37	1.0
+10 μM vitamin E	5750	970 ± 63	5.9

*Data from Reference 44.

TABLE 4

EFFECT OF ANTIOXIDANTS ON THE INHIBITION OF LIPOXYGENASE

Treatment	Molarity	Inhibition (%)
Soybean lipoxidase[37]		
+ Vitamin E	7×10^{-6}	61
+ α-Naphthol	9×10^{-5}	94
+ Propyl gallate	3×10^{-4}	78
Platelet lipoxygenase[31]		
+ Vitamin E	2×10^{-3}	77
+ Vitamin E acetate	2×10^{-3}	79
Neutrophile lipoxygenase[57]		
+ Vitamin E	3×10^{-5}	elevated
+ Vitamin E	1×10^{-3}	inhibited
Platelet lipoxygenase[31]		
Vitamin E	dietary supplement	53

inactivation resulting from autoxidation.[53-55] Vitamin E is a highly lipid-soluble surfactant that apparently protects cyclooxygenase from autoxidation without diminishing the concentrations of oxygen-centered radicals in the aqueous phase. Thus, depending on the system, vitamin E either has no effect on or enhances prostaglandin biosynthesis from arachidonic acid (FIGURE 1).

LIPOXYGENASE

Early experiments with vitamin E showed it to be a highly effective inhibitor of partially purified soybean lipoxidase.[56] This observation has been confirmed in studies from our laboratory, which showed vitamin E is more effective than either α-naphthol or propyl gallate as an inhibitor of diene conjugation produced by soybean lipoxidase (TABLE 4).

Studies with vitamin E and mammalian lipoxygenase are more difficult to interpret. Vitamin E added at a high concentration inhibits platelet lipoxygenase, but vitamin E and vitamin E acetate are equally effective as inhibitors at this concentration (TABLE 4). The surfactant Tween 20 also inhibits platelet lipoxygenase.[31] Vitamin E in the same millimolar concentration range inhibits neutrophile lipoxygenase, while lower concentrations of vitamin E actually enhance neutrophile lipoxygenase (TABLE 4). These data suggest that vitamin E added in high concentrations functions *in vitro* as a nonphysiologic surfactant. These data do not prove that vitamin E functions *in vivo* as a lipoxygenase inhibitor.

We have found that less hydroxy eicosatetraenoic acid (HETE) is formed when arachidonic acid is added to platelets from vitamin E-supplemented animals than when arachidonic acid is added to platelets from vitamin E-deficient animals (TABLE 4). Platelet lipoxygenase is an active enzyme, and a significant vitamin E effect was seen in experiments only with low concentrations of platelet protein. These data and other indirect experiments, such as the formation of the lipid peroxide breakdown product malondialdehyde (MDA), suggest that vitamin E inhibits mammalian lipoxygenase (FIGURE 1). However, there are problems with the use of MDA data in estimating the inhibition of mammalian lipoxygenase with vitamin E.

MALONDIALDEHYDE

The thiobarbituric acid test for the detection of MDA is used extensively to measure lipid peroxidation in polyunsaturated fatty acids.[58-62] Agents that diminish the MDA yield are generally considered to be agents that inhibit both enzymatic and nonenzymatic lipid peroxidation reactions. Vitamin E and other antioxidants have been shown to block the formation of MDA in many biological systems.[58-62] It is not clear whether these antioxidants block enzymatic lipid peroxidation or the breakdown of lipid peroxides to MDA (FIGURE 1). This problem is illustrated by studies with cells in tissue culture.

Confluent medial cells generate large amounts of MDA when incubated with a polyunsaturated fatty acid for 24 hours (TABLE 5). MDA formation is blocked when cells are preincubated with the antioxidants vitamin E or vitamin E quinone. These data suggest that the antioxidant has blocked lipid peroxidation. However, medial cells preincubated with a polyunsaturated fatty acid form less MDA from lipid peroxides when the incubation is continued in the presence of added antioxidant (TABLE 5). The effect is most dramatic with butylated hydroxytoluene (BHT). This antioxidant does not interfere with the thiobarbituric acid assay of MDA generated from 1,1,3,3-tetramethoxypropane, yet added BHT immediately blocks MDA formation from preformed lipid peroxides in cells (TABLE 5).

Acyclic hydroperoxides are formed during the enzymatic oxidation of polyunsaturated fatty acids by lipoxygenase. Acyclic hydroperoxides undergo a series of radical rearrangement reactions to form bicyclic endoperoxides that decompose to MDA.[63,64] MDA, like ethylene,[65] is formed from the breakdown of lipid peroxides during assay. Antioxidants may prevent radical formation from lipid peroxides[66,67] and the radical rearrangement reactions that ultimately generate MDA.[62] We suggest that antioxidants such as vitamin E or BHT, which block MDA formation without blocking cyclooxygenase, prevent peroxide decomposition without necessarily inhibiting lipoxygenase activity.[62]

TABLE 5

MDA FORMATION IN CONFLUENT MEDIAL CELLS TREATED WITH ANTIOXIDANTS*

	Incubation Time	
Treatment	0 Hours	24 Hours
a. Preincubate cells 24 hours with/without antioxidant then incubate with 120 μM 8,11,14-20:3		
no antioxidant	0.7 ± 0.5	9.2 ± 0.8
10 μM vitamin E	0.6 ± 0.3	0.3 ± 0.3†
10μM vitamin E quinone	0.2 ± 0.4	0.3 ± 0.1†
b. Preincubate cells 24 hours with 120 μM 8,11,14-20:3 then incubate with/without antioxidant		
no antioxidant	10.5 ± 0.8	9.9 ± 1.8
10 μM vitamin E	11.3 ± 1.5	7.5 ± 0.8‡
10 μM vitamin E quinone	10.8 ± 0.5	1.1 ± 0.4†
10 μM BHT	1.9 ± 0.2	1.5 ± 0.5†

*Figures are nmoles MDA/culture, means $\pm$ SD. (Data from Reference 62.)
†$p < 0.005$.
‡$p < 0.01$.

PROSTACYCLIN SYNTHETASE

Several studies in the recent literature show that PGI_2 levels are diminished in tissues from vitamin E-deficient animals. Antiaggregatory activity is lowered and MDA is elevated in tissue from vitamin E-deficient rats.[68] We find that PGI_2 levels, measured as 6-keto-$PGF_{1\alpha}$, are diminished when aorta from vitamin E-deficient rats is incubated either with or without added unesterified arachidonic acid (FIGURES 5 and 6). The experiments with unesterified arachidonic acid prove that inhibition occurs at the cyclooxygenase–prostacyclin synthetase steps rather than at the fatty acid release step in arachidonic acid metabolism. Vitamin E restores the aorta PGI_2 level without altering the PGE_2 level.[28] Thus, prostacyclin synthetase activity is highly sensitive to the vitamin E status of the experimental animal. Prostacyclin synthetase activity is diminished only in a long-term nutritional deficiency. We have found in preliminary experiments that rabbits cannot be maintained on a vitamin E-deficient diet for sufficient time to establish the effect of vitamin E on prostacyclin synthetase.

Prostacyclin synthetase (FIGURE 1) is sensitive to inactivation by hydroperoxy fatty acids[69,70] and to inactivation by hydroperoxy endoperoxides.[71] Inhibition is mediated through formation of oxygen-centered radicals from these hydroperoxy derivatives.[72]

Vitamin E acts either to inhibit hydroperoxide formation or to inhibit hydroperoxide decomposition in preventing the long-term inhibition of prostacyclin

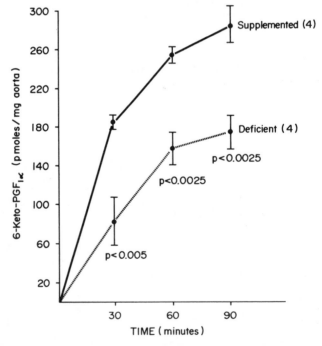

FIGURE 5. Generation of 6-keto-$PGF_{1\alpha}$ from aorta incubated with 17.2 μM 1-^{14}C-arachidonic acid for 30, 60, and 90 minutes. (Reproduced from Reference 28 with permission from the publisher.)

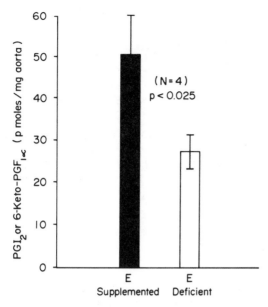

FIGURE 6. Generation of 6-keto-PGF$_{1\alpha}$ from aorta incubated without added arachidonic acid. (Reproduced from Reference 28 with permission from the publisher.)

synthetase (FIGURE 1). Water-soluble antioxidants such as propyl gallate have immediate effects on both cyclooxygenase and prostaglandin synthetase in microsomes.[41] Lipid-soluble antioxidants such as BHT have an immediate effect only on the decomposition of lipid peroxides to MDA.[62] We suggest that the long-term effect of a vitamin E deficiency on prostacyclin synthetase activity[28,68] is correlated with the ability of this antioxidant to prevent the decomposition of lipid hydroperoxides.

PHYSIOLOGIC CONSEQUENCES

Vitamin E has two clear and significant effects on arachidonic acid metabolism. Arachidonic acid release from phospholipid is diminished and, consequently, platelet TxA$_2$ biosynthesis is lowered by vitamin E. Arachidonic acid peroxidation and/or radical formation from hydroperoxy arachidonic acid would be diminished, resulting in elevated PGI$_2$ biosynthesis in the presence of vitamin E. It is apparent that vitamin E may have profound effects in physiologic states that are associated with platelet aggregation.

Diabetes mellitus is characterized both by the hyperaggregability of washed platelets[73,74] and by diminished tissue PGI$_2$ biosynthesis.[75,76] We have found in preliminary experiments that the critical balance between TxA$_2$ and PGI$_2$ is altered to favor platelet aggregation in experimental diabetes. We also found platelets from diabetic rats to be deficient in vitamin E. Finally, the balance between TxA$_2$ and PGI$_2$ was restored when diabetic rats received vitamin E as a dietary supplement. These studies will be reported elsewhere.

The progression of the atherosclerotic lesion is a complex network of biologic

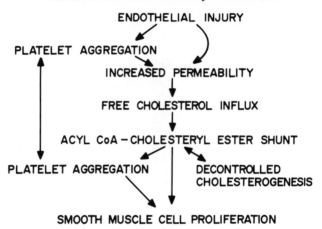

FIGURE 7. A model for the development of the atherosclerotic lesion. (Reproduced from Reference 77 with permission from the publisher.)

events. No single model or scheme explains the process. There is increasing evidence that the progression of the lesion begins with injury to the endothelium and platelet aggregation (FIGURE 7). The progression of the lesion ends with the proliferation of smooth muscle cells (FIGURE 7). Vitamin E may diminish platelet aggregation and the subsequent release of the platelet-derived growth factor that stimulates the proliferation of smooth muscle cells.[78] However, vitamin E is itself

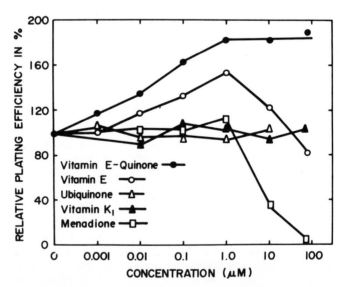

FIGURE 8. Extent of cell proliferation (relative plating efficiency) in medial cells treated with increasing concentrations of α-tocopherol or specified quinones. (Reproduced from Reference 62 with permission from the publisher.)

a growth factor that stimulates the proliferation of medial cells.[18,44,62] The stimulation of cell proliferation with two antioxidants, vitamin E and vitamin E quinone, is demonstrated in FIGURE 8. Vitamin E may suppress initiating events and enhance the terminal event in the development of the atherosclerotic lesion (FIGURE 7). The positive and negative effects of vitamin E are characteristic of the "antioxidant paradox."

REFERENCES

1. BILLAH, M. M., E. G. LAPETINA & P. CUATRECASAS. 1979. Phosphatidylinositol-specific phospholipase-C of platelets: association with 1,2-diacylglycerol-kinase and inhibition by cyclic AMP. Biochem. Biophys. Res. Commun. **90:** 92–98.
2. BELL, R. L., D. A. KENNERLY, N. STANFORD & P. W. MAJERUS. 1979. Diglyceride lipase: a pathway for arachidonic release from human platelets. Proc. Nat. Acad. Sci. USA **76:** 3238–3241.
3. RITTENHOUSE-SIMMONS, S. 1980. Indomethacin-induced accumulation of diglyceride in activated human platelets. J. Biol. Chem. **255:** 2259–2262.
4. BILLAH, M., E. G. LAPETINA & P. CUATRECASAS. 1980. Phospholipase A_2 and phospholipase C activities of platelets. Differential substrate specificity, Ca^{++} requirement, pH dependence, and cellular localization. J. Biol. Chem. **255:** 10227–10231.
5. SILK, S. T., K. T. H. WONG & A. J. MARCUS. 1981. Arachidonic acid releasing activity in platelet membranes: effects of sulfydryl-modifying reagents. Biochemistry **20:** 391–397.
6. BILLAH, M. M., E. G. LAPETINA & P. CUATRECASAS. 1981. Phospholipase A_2 activity specific for phosphatidic acid. A possible mechanism for the production of arachidonic acid in platelets. J. Biol. Chem. **256:** 5339–5403.
7. SAMUELSSON, B., M. GOLDYNE, E. GRANSTROM, M. HAMBERG, S. HAMMARSTROM & C. MALMSTEN. 1978. Prostaglandins and thromboxanes. Annu. Rev. Biochem. **47:** 997–1029.
8. LANDS, W. E. M. 1979. The biosynthesis and metabolism of prostaglandins. Annu. Rev. Physiol. **41:** 633–652.
9. HAMBERG, M. & B. SAMUELSSON. 1974. Prostaglandin endoperoxides. Novel transformation of arachidonic acid in human platelets. Proc. Nat. Acad. Sci. USA **71:** 3400–3404.
10. BORGEAT, P., M. HAMBERG & B. SAMUELSSON. 1976. Transformation of arachidonic acid and homo-γ-linolenic acid by rabbit polymorphonuclear leukocytes. Monohydroxy acids from novel lipoxygenase. J. Biol. Chem. **251:** 7816–7820.
11. GARDNER, H. W. 1980. Lipid enzymes: lipases, lipoxygenases, and "hydroperoxidases." In Autoxidation in Food and Biological Systems. M. G. Simic & M. Karel, Eds.: 447–504. Plenum Press. New York, N.Y.
12. SAMUELSSON, B., P. BORGEAT, S. HAMMARSTRON & R. C. MURPHY. 1980. Leukotrienes: a new group of biological active compounds. Adv. Prostglandin Thromboxane Res. **6:** 1–18.
13. PATIL, G. S. & D. G. CORNWELL. 1978. Interfacial oxidation of α-tocopherol and the surface properties of its oxidation products. J. Lipid Res. **19:** 416–422.
14. MAGGIO, B., A. T. DIPLOCK & J. A. LUCY. 1977. Interactions of tocopherols and ubiquinones with monolayers of phospholipids. Biochem. J. **161:** 111–121.
15. FUKUZAWA, K., K. HAYASHI & A. SUZUKI. 1977. Effects of α-tocopherol analogs on lysosome membranes and fatty acid monolayers. Chem. Phys. Lipids **18:** 39–48.
16. FUKUZAWA, K., H. IKENO, A. TOKUMURA & H. TSUKATANI. 1979. Effect of α-tocopherol incorporation on glucose permeability and phase transition of lecithin liposomes. Chem. Phys. Lipids **23:** 13–22.
17. FUKUZAWA, K., H. CHIDA & A. SUZUKI. 1980. Fluorescence depolarization studies of phase transition and fluidity in lecithin liposomes containing α-tocopherol. J. Nutr. Sci. Vitaminol. **26:** 427–434.
18. MILLER, J. S., V. C. GAVINO, G. A. ACKERMAN, H. M. SHARMA, G. E. MILO, J. C. GEER &

D. G. CORNWELL. 1980. Triglycerides, lipid droplets, and lysosomes in aorta smooth muscle cells during the control of cell proliferation with polyunsaturated fatty acids and vitamin E. Lab. Invest. **42:** 495-506.

19. GAVINO, V. C. 1981. Polyunsaturated fatty acids, lipid accumulation, and oxidant stress in cells in culture. Ph.D. Dissertation. Ohio State University. Columbus, Ohio.

20. LAPETINA, E. G., C. J. SCHMITGES, K. CHANDRABOSE & P. CUATRECASAS. 1978. Regulation of phospholipase activity in platelets. Adv. Prostaglandin Thromboxane Res. **3:** 127-135.

21. BELL, R. L. & P. W. MAJERUS. 1980. Thrombin-induced hydrolysis of phosphoinositol in human platelets. J. Biol. Chem. **255:** 1490-1792.

22. LAPETINA, E. G., M. M. BILLAH & P. CUATRECASAS. 1981. The initial action of thrombin on platelets. Conversion of phosphatidylinositol to phosphatidic acid preceding the production of arachidonic acid. J. Biol. Chem. **256:** 5037-5040.

23. HOPE, W. C., C. DALTON, L. J. MACHLIN, R. J. FILIPSKI & F. M. VANE. 1975. Influence of dietary vitamin E on prostaglandin biosynthesis in rat blood. Prostaglandins **10:** 557-571.

24. MACHLIN, L. J., R. FILIPSKI, A. L. WILLIS, D. C. KUHN & M. BRIN. 1975. Influence of vitamin E on platelet aggregation and thrombocythemia in the rat. Proc. Soc. Exp. Biol. Med. **149:** 275-277.

25. LAKE, A. M., M. J. STUART & F. A. OSKI. 1977. Vitamin E deficiency and enhanced platelet function: reversal following E supplementation. J. Pediatr. **90:** 722-725.

26. NUGTEREN, D. H., R. K. BEERTHUIS & D. A. VAN DORP. 1966. The enzymatic conversion of all-cis 8,11,14-eicosatrienoic acid into prostaglandin E_1. Recl. Trav. Chim. Pays-Bas **85:** 405-419.

27. LANDS, W. E. M., P. R. LETELLIER, L. H. ROME & J. Y. VANDERHOEK. 1972. Inhibition of prostaglandin biosynthesis. Adv. Biosci. **9:** 15-28.

28. KARPEN, C. W., A. J. MEROLA, R. W. TREWYN, D. G. CORNWELL & R. V. PANGANAMALA. 1981. Modulation of platelet thromboxane A_2 and arterial prostacyclin by dietary vitamin E. Prostaglandins **22:** 651-661.

29. YASUDA, M. & T. FUJITA. 1977. Effect of lipid peroxidation on phospholipase A_2 activity of rat liver mitochondria. Jpn. J. Pharmacol. **27:** 429-435.

30. BUTLER, A. M., J. M. GERRARD, J. PELLER, S. F. STODDARD, G. H. R. RAO & J. G. WHITE. 1979. Vitamin E inhibits the release of calcium from a platelet membrane fraction in vitro. Prostaglandins Med. **2:** 203-216.

31. GWEBU, E. T., R. W. TREWYN, D. G. CORNWELL & R. V. PANGANAMALA. 1980. Vitamin E and the inhibition of platelet lipoxygenase. Res. Commun. Chem. Pathol. Pharmacol. **28:** 361-376.

32. GUTTERIDGE, J. M. C. 1978. The membrane effects of vitamin E, cholesterol and their acetates on peroxidative susceptibility. Res. Commun. Chem. Pathol. Pharmacol. **22:** 563-572.

33. HIGASHI, O. & Y. KIKUCHI. 1974. Effects of vitamin E on the aggregation and the lipid peroxidation of platelets exposed to hydrogen peroxide. Tohoku J. Exp. Med. **112:** 271-278.

34. FONG, J. S. C. 1976. Alpha-tocopherol: its inhibition on human platelet aggregation. Experientia **15:** 639-641.

35. STEINER, M. & J. ANASTASI. 1976. Vitamin E—an inhibitor of the platelet release reaction. J. Clin. Invest. **57:** 732-737.

36. HIGASHI, O. & Y. KIKUCHI. 1977. A comparative study of the effect of vitamin E-nicotinate and the combination of vitamin E and nicotinic acid on the hydrogen peroxide-induced platelet aggregation. Tohoku J. Exp. Med. **121:** 81-84.

37. PANGANAMALA, R. V., J. S. MILLER, E. T. GWEBU, H. M. SHARMA & D. G. CORNWELL. 1977. Differential inhibitory effects of vitamin E and other antioxidants on prostaglandin synthetase, platelet aggregation and lipoxidase. Prostaglandins **14:** 261-271.

38. STEINER, M. 1978. Inhibition of platelet aggregation by alpha-tocopherol. In Tocopherol, Oxygen and Biomembranes. C. de Duve & O. Hayaishi, Eds.: 143-163. Elsevier/North-Holland Biomedical Press. Amsterdam, the Netherlands.

39. AGRADI, E., A PETRONI, A. SOCINI & C. GALLI. 1981. In vitro effects of synthetic antioxidants and vitamin E on arachidonic acid metabolism and thromboxane formation in human platelets and platelet aggregation. Prostaglandins **22:** 255-266.

40. STEINER, M. 1981. Vitamin E changes the membrane fluidity of human platelets. Biochim. Biophys. Acta **640:** 100–105.
41. CARPENTER, M. P. 1981. Antioxidant effects on the prostaglandin endoperoxide synthetase product profile. Fed. Proc. **40:** 189–194.
42. RAO, G. H. R., S. M. BURRIS, J. M. GERRARD & J. G. WHITE. 1979. Inhibition of prostaglandin (PG) synthesis in sheep vesicular gland microsomes (SVGM) by nitroblue tetrazolium (NBT) and vitamin E (VE). Prostaglandins Med. **2:** 111–121.
43. ZENSER, T. V. & B. B. DAVIS. 1978. Antioxidant inhibition of prostaglandin production by rat renal medulla. Metabolism **27:** 227–233.
44. CORNWELL, D. G., J. J. HUTTNER, G. E. MILO, R. V. PANGANAMALA, H. M. SHARMA & J. C. GEER. 1979. Polyunsaturated fatty acids, vitamin E, and the proliferation of aortic smooth muscle cells. Lipids. **14:** 194–207.
45. CHAN, A. C., C. E. ALLEN & P. V. J. HEGARTY. 1980. The effects of vitamin E depletion and repletion on prostaglandin synthesis in semitendinosus muscle of young rabbits. J. Nutr. **110:** 66–73.
46. PANGANAMALA, R. V., H. J. SHARMA, R. E. HEIKKILA, J. C. GEER & D. G. CORNWELL. 1976. Role of hydroxyl radical scavengers dimethyl sulfoxide, alcohols and methional in the inhibition of prostaglandin biosynthesis. Prostaglandins **11:** 599–607.
47. PANGANAMALA, R. V., V. C. GAVINO & D. G. CORNWELL. 1979. Effect of low and high methional concentrations on prostaglandin biosynthesis in microsomes from bovine and sheep vesicular glands. Prostaglandins **17:** 155–162.
48. DEBY, C. & C. DEBY-DUPONT. 1980. Oxygen species in prostaglandin biosynthesis in vitro and in vivo. Dev. Biochem. **11B:** 84–97.
49. PANGANAMALA, R. V., N. R. BROWNLEE, H. SPRECHER & D. G. CORNWELL. 1974. Evaluation of superoxide anion and singlet oxygen in the biosynthesis of prostaglandins from eicosa-8,11,14-trienoic acid. Prostaglandins **7:** 21–28.
50. PANGANAMALA, R. V., H. M. SHARMA, H. SPRECHER, J. C. GEER & D. G. CORNWELL. 1974. A suggested role for hydrogen peroxide in the biosynthesis of prostaglandins. Prostaglandins **8:** 3–11.
51. COOK, H. W. & W. E. M. LANDS. 1976. Mechanism for suppression of cellular biosynthesis of prostaglandins. Nature **260:** 630–632.
52. HEMLER, M. E., G. GRAFF & W. E. M. LANDS. 1978. Accelerative autoactivation of prostaglandin biosynthesis by PGG$_2$. Biochem. Biophys. Res. Commun. **85:** 1325–1331.
53. EGAN, R. W., P. H. GALE & F. A. KUEHL, JR. 1979. Reduction of hydroperoxides in the prostaglandin biosynthetic pathway of a microsomal peroxidase. J. Biol. Chem. **254:** 3295–3302.
54. EGAN, R. W., P. H. GALE, G. C. BEVERIDGE, L. J. MARNETT & F. A. KUEHL, JR. 1980. Direct and indirect involvement of radical scavengers during prostaglandin biosynthesis. Adv. Prostaglandin Thromboxane Res. **6:** 153–155.
55. LAPETINA, E. G. & P. CUATRECASAS. 1979. Rapid inactivation of cyclooxygenase activity after stimulation of intact platelets. Proc. Nat. Acad. Sci. USA **76:** 121–125.
56. TAPPEL, A. L., W. O. LUNDBERG & P. D. BOYER. 1953. Effect of temperature and antioxidants upon the lipoxidase-catalyzed oxidation of sodium linoleate. Arch. Biochem. Biophys. **42:** 293–297.
57. GOETZL, E. J. 1980. Vitamin E modulates the lipoxygenation of arachidonic acid in leukocytes. Nature **288:** 183–185.
58. BERNHEIM, F. 1963. Biochemical implications of prooxidants and antioxidants. Radiat. Res. Suppl. **3:** 17–32.
59. MEAD, J. F. 1976. Free radical mechanism of lipid damage and consequences for cellular membranes. In Free Radicals in Biology. W. A. Pryor, Ed. **1:** 51–68. Academic Press, Inc. New York, N.Y.
60. McCAY, P. B. & M. M. KING. 1980. Vitamin E: its role as a biologic free radical scavenger and its relationship to the microsomal mixed-function oxidase system. In Vitamin E, A Comprehensive Treatise. L. J. Machlin, Ed. **1:** 289–317. Marcel Dekker, Inc. New York, N.Y.
61. WALTON, J. R. & L. PACKER. 1980. Free radical damage and protection: relationship to

cellular aging and cancer. *In* Vitamin E, A Comprehensive Treatise. L. J. Machlin, Ed. **1:** 495–517. Marcel Dekker, Inc. New York, N.Y.

62. GAVINO, V. C., J. S. MILLER, S. O. IKHAREBHA, G. E. MILO & D. G. CORNWELL. 1980. Effect of polyunsaturated fatty acids and antioxidants on lipid peroxidation in tissue cultures. J. Lipid Res. **22:** 763–769.

63. PRYOR, W. S., J. P. STANLEY & E. BLAIR. 1976. Autoxidation of polyunsaturated fatty acids. II. A suggested mechanism for the formation of TBA-reactive materials from prostaglandin-like endoperoxides. Lipids **11:** 370–379.

64. PORTER, N. A. 1980. Prostaglandin endoperoxides. *In* Free Radicals in Biology. W. A. Pryor, Ed. **4:** 261–294. Academic Press, Inc. New York, N.Y.

65. DUMELIN, E. E. & A. L. TAPPEL. 1977. Hydrocarbon gases produced during *in vitro* peroxidation of polyunsaturated fatty acid and decomposition of preformed hydroperoxides. Lipids **12:** 894–900.

66. SVINGEN, B. A., J. A. BUEGE, F. O. O'NEAL & S. D. AUST. 1979. The mechanism of NADPH-dependent lipid peroxidation. J. Biol. Chem. **254:** 5892–5899.

67. NAKAMURA, T. 1980. Formation and inhibition of lipid peroxides *in vivo*. Oil Chem. Jpn **29:** 309–315.

68. OKUMA, M., H. TAKAYAMA & H. UCHINO. 1980. Generation of prostacyclin like substance and lipid peroxidation in vitamin E–deficient rats. Prostaglandins **19:** 527–536.

69. MONCADA, S., R. J. GRYGLEWSKI, S. BUNTING & J. R. VANE. 1976. A lipid peroxide inhibits the enzyme in blood vessel microsomes that generates from prostaglandin endoperoxides the substance (prostaglandin X) which prevents platelet aggregation. Prostaglandins **12:** 715–733.

70. SALMON, J. A., D. R. SMITH, R. J. FLOWER, S. MONCADA & J. R. VANE. 1978. Further studies on the enzymatic conversion of prostaglandin endoperoxide into prostacyclin by porcine aorta microsomes. Biochim. Biophys. Acta **523:** 250–262.

71. HAM, E. A., R. W. EGAN, D. D. SODERMAN, P. H. GALE & F. A. KUEHL, JR. 1979. Peroxidase-dependent deactivation of prostacyclin synthetase. J. Biol. Chem. **254:** 2191–2194.

72. WEISS, S. J., J. TURK & P. NEEDLEMAN. 1979. A mechanism for the hydroperoxide-mediated inactivation of prostacyclin synthetase. Blood **53:** 1191–1196.

73. COLWELL, J. A., P. V. HALUSHKA, K. SARJI, J. LEVINE, J. SAGEL & R. M. G. NAIR. 1976. Altered platelet function in diabetes mellitus. Diabetes 25(Suppl.): 826–831.

74. ELDOR, A., S. MERIN & H. BAR-ON. 1978. The effects of streptozotocin diabetes on platelet function in rats. Thromb. Res. **13:** 703–714.

75. CARRERAS, L. O., D. A. F. CHAMONE, P. KLERCK & J. VERMYLEN. 1980. Decreased vascular prostacyclin (PGI_2) in diabetic rats. Stimulation of PGI_2 release in normal and diabetic rats by the antithrombotic compound Bay 6575. Thromb. Res. **19:** 663–670.

76. HARRISON, H. E., A. H. REECE & M. JOHNSON. 1978. Decreased vascular prostacyclin in experimental diabetes. Life Sci. **23:** 351–356.

77. CORNWELL, D. G. & R. V. PANGANAMALA. 1981. Atherosclerosis: an intracellular deficiency in essential fatty acids. Prog. Lipid Res. (In press.)

78. ROSS, R. & B. KARIYA. 1980. Morphogenesis of vascular smooth muscle in atherosclerosis and cell culture. *In* Handbook of Physiology. The Cardiovascular System. D. F. Bohr, A. P. Somlyo & H. V. Sparks, Jr., Eds. (Section 2): 69–91. American Physiological Society. Bethesda, Md.

DISCUSSION

C. C. REDDY *(Pennsylvania State University, University Park, Pa.)*: You mentioned something about the hydroxyl radicals being modulators of cyclooxygenase and prostacyclin synthetase and lipoxygenase. I don't think there is any direct evidence that hydroxy radicals are responsible for that. In fact, all the evidence suggests that the lipid radicals or fatty acid radicals are responsible, at low concentrations, for inactivation of the cyclooxygenase and, at higher concentrations, for the inhibition of cyclooxygenase.

When you see the effect of vitamin E deficiency in a given tissue on a given pathway, I think it is more tissue specific and it's not general. In some tissues, the prostaglandin biosynthesis seems to be increased; in other tissues, it seems to be decreased.

R. V. PANGANAMALA: We have shown that hydroxyl radicals are indeed involved in the metabolism of arachidonic acid. We used specific radical scavengers. The level of hydroxyl radicals is crucial.

C. C. REDDY: You mentioned that in vitamin E deficiency, prostacyclin synthetase is affected whereas cyclooxygenase is not affected.

R. V. PANGANAMALA: The prostacyclin synthetase is the one that is sensitive to the peroxides. The high levels of peroxides or hydroxyl radicals inhibit the prostacyclin synthetase, which is a sulfhydryl enzyme. Cyclooxygenase is not as sensitive to peroxides.

D. H. HWANG (*Louisiana State University, Baton Rouge, La.*): Could you explain why the formation of 12-HETE in vitamin E deficiency decreases only when platelet protein concentration is low.

R. V. PANGANAMALA: We think it is the saturation of the substrate. You can increase the substrate concentration or you can lower the protein.

D. H. HWANG: We measured endogenous formation of 12-HETE in vitamin E-deficient rats and found that there is no difference between the control group and the vitamin E-deficient group, although endogenous formation of the thromboxane B_2 and PGF_1 increased in the vitamin E-deficient group.

R. V. PANGANAMALA: If you used rats, then there is some problem with the lipoxygenase. We see the difference in the rabbit where we do not see the differences in the rat.

D. H. HWANG: And I think we have to be careful in interpreting the data if we use exogenous arachidonic acid as compared to endogenous formation, because the substrate pool might be different.

R. V. PANGANAMALA: I agree with you.

J. DUPONT (*Iowa State University, Ames, Iowa*): I'd like to caution about extrapolating your results with the diabetic rat model to the human population. With Dr. Peter Chase at Colorado, I've just completed a study with children's diabetes. Supplementation with vitamin E, 400 IU per day for six months, does not correct the excess thromboxane synthesis and it causes increased hyperlipidemia.

M. STEINER (*The Memorial Hospital, Pawtucket, R.I.*): Did you find that the platelet aggregation of these animals that you put on vitamin E was increased or decreased?

R. V. PANGANAMALA: We found that the platelets obtained from the vitamin E-deficient animals have enhanced aggregation.

M. STEINER: How does that fit in with the theory that the cyclooxygenase pathway and the products of this pathway are stimulatory for aggregation?

R. V. PANGANAMALA: Aggregation is one of the most confusing things because when you talk about aggregation, you're not talking only about thromboxane. You have other reactions that you have to take into consideration and that are affected by the levels of vitamin E. For example, as Fong has shown, ADP and 5-HT [5-hydroxytryptamine] are indeed affected by vitamin E. So you have to take into consideration that these reactions from the granules as well as other reactions are going on. Therefore, platelet aggregation is not always directly related to the cyclooxygenase effect.

EXPERIMENTAL AND CLINICAL RESULTS IN SHOCK LUNG TREATMENT WITH VITAMIN E

Hellmut R. D. Wolf* and H. Werner Seeger†

*Department of Internal Medicine
†Department of Clinical Chemistry
Justus-Liebig University
D-6300 Giessen, Federal Republic of Germany

The so-called shock lung syndrome, or respiratory distress syndrome of the adult (ARDS), has become the main cause of death in the course of severe shock states since the management of acute circulatory failure and anuria was improved.[1,2] A very uniform pattern of pulmonary lesions consisting of progressive deterioration of gas exchange and lung compliance, increased pulmonary vascular resistance, and severe interstitial edema develops after hours or days in the course of different shock forms, e.g., traumatic, hypovolemic, and septic shock, as well as in severe intoxications with various drugs and poisons. Furthermore this pattern is seen as the main complication in premature newborns.[3] At least in the adult respiratory distress syndrome, pulmonary microembolism in combination with disseminated intravascular coagulation is the outstanding pathogenetic event, with subsequent increase of pulmonary vascular resistance and permeability.[4,5]

Oxidizing agents such as ozone (O_3), nitrogen dioxide (NO_2), and hyperbaric oxygen as well as enteral poisoning with chlorate or paraquat (1,1'-dimethyl-4,4'-bipyridylium dichloride) cause quite similar pulmonary lesions.[6-8] Thomas et al. demonstrated in rats that high enteric doses of α-tocopheryl acetate protected pulmonary lipids from peroxidation evoked by NO_2 inhalation.[9] If pulmonary lipid peroxidation has any significance for the pathogenesis of the described pulmonary lesions, high doses of tocopherol should also be able to prevent them in the absence of oxidizing agents. In a microembolization model with rabbits, we have investigated this question.[10-13]

FIRST EXPERIMENT

Model

Awake rabbits of either sex, weighing 2.13 ± 0.34 kg and breathing ambient room air, were intermittently microembolized with particles of aggregated human albumin—such as those, charged with ^{99}Tc, that are used for pulmonary perfusion scintigrams in minute doses (Tecepart®, gift from Behringwerke, Marburg, Federal Republic of Germany)—via an auricular vein catheter placed in the right atrium. Most (86%) of the particles had diameters between 10 and 40 μm. During the first 3 hours, 13.5 mg/kg body weight were administered, suspended in Ringer's solution. From hours 6 to 8, 12 to 14, and 18 to 20, 4 mg/kg were added. Thus about 80% of pulmonary microvessels were occluded throughout the experiment. Surviving animals were sacrificed after 24 hours. Blood gas parameters, cardiac output (thermodilution method), and shunt volume of cardiac output were measured hourly. Pressure-volume (PV) diagrams were drawn from the

392

immediately postmortem isolated lung as classical PV diagrams (FIGURE 1) and as pneumoloop diagrams (FIGURE 2) under nearly static pressure conditions with maximum air flow of 0.5 ml/second at 25°C. PV parameters referred to are (1) V_{max}/k (ml/kg) = inflated air volume per kg body weight in classical PV diagrams at a constant maximum pressure of 35 cm H_2O; (2) P_K (cm H_2O) = pressure at the bending point of the deflation curve—the bisector of the angle formed by the tangents in the flattest and steepest parts of the deflation curve intersects this curve in the bending point; (3) $C_{Q/pv}$ = compliance quotient of the classical PV diagrams, i.e., the compliance of the steepest part (T_0) divided by the compliance of the flattest part (T_{max}) of the deflation curve; and (4) $C_{Q/pl}$ = compliance quotient of the pneumoloops, i.e., the quotient of the compliances of corresponding loops

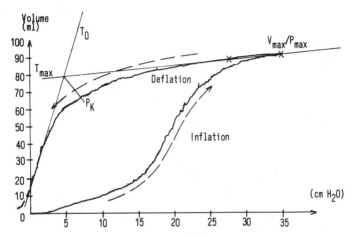

FIGURE 1. Classical pressure-volume (PV) diagrams of a normal rabbit lung, inflated to a constant maximum pressure of 35 cm H_2O (V_{max}) and subsequently deflated (25°C; maximum air flow, 0.5 ml/second). The tangent at the flattest part of the deflation curve (between 35 and 27.5 cm H_2O) = T_{max}; the tangent at the steepest part = T_0. The compliance quotient $C_{Q/pv}$ is calculated as T_0/T_{max}. The bisector of the angle between T_0 and T_{max} hits the deflation curve in P_K (cm H_2O). $C_{Q/pv}$ is diminished by deterioration of the surfactant system. P_K allows the discrimination between functional impairment of the system and lack of surfactant material.

in the deflation ($C_{Defl/K}$) and inflation ($C_{Infl/K}$) parts at one-third maximum volume.

Animal Groups

Group A (n = 9) consisted of control animals without microembolization but with equal amounts of Ringer's solution. Group B (n = 19) consisted of reference animals microembolized in the above-mentioned manner. Group C (n = 8) consisted of microembolized animals that received all-rac-α-tocopheryl acetate (Merck, Darmstadt, Federal Republic of Germany) by gastric tube in a dosage of 50 mg/kg body weight dissolved in 5 ml vegetable oil at 18 hours and again at 1 hour prior to the beginning of the microembolization. Group D (n = 9) consisted of microembolized reference animals that received only vegetable oil in the same manner without tocopherol.

Statistics

One- and two-way analyses of variance were calculated with a Tektronix 4051 processor.

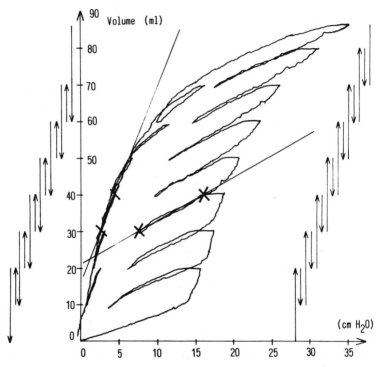

FIGURE 2. Pneumoloop diagram of a normal rabbit lung, inflated and deflated stepwise according to the arrows (maximum pressure, 35 cm H_2O; 25°C; maximum air flow, 0.5 ml/second). The quotient of the compliances of a deflation loop ($C_{Defl/K}$) and an inflation loop ($C_{Infl/K}$) at one-third maximum volume $C_{Q/pl}$ reflects hysteresis of the pulmonary surfactant system.

Results

There were highly significant deteriorations of surface-tension and gas-exchange parameters in the microembolized reference groups as well as cardiac output reduction (FIGURES 3–5) compared to the control group. Microembolized animals that received vegetable oil only (D) did not show any difference from the reference animals (B), whereas the tocopherol group (C) differed significantly from both reference groups (B and D). In the pneumoloop diagrams (FIGURE 3), the compliance quotient, $C_{Q/pl}$, as well as the compliance of the deflation part, $C_{Defl/K}$, showed significantly ($p < 10^{-5}$) higher levels in the tocopherol-treated animals.

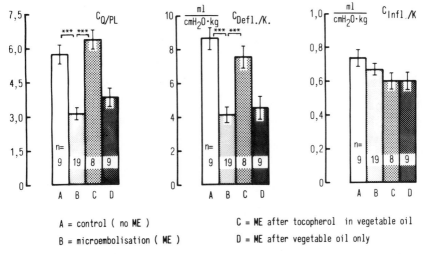

A = control (no ME)   C = ME after tocopherol in vegetable oil

B = microembolisation (ME)   D = ME after vegetable oil only

FIGURE 3. Compliances ($C_{Defl/K}$; $C_{Infl/K}$) and compliance quotient ($C_{Q/pl}$) of pneumoloops obtained from the different animal groups with (B–D) and without microembolization (A). Tocopherol pretreated animals (C) show highly significant ($p < 10^{-5}$) higher $C_{Q/pl}$ due to higher $C_{Defl/K}$, indicating much better hysteresis of their surfactant systems. [Means $\pm$ standard errors of the mean (SEM).] (Reproduced from Reference 11 with permission from the publisher.)

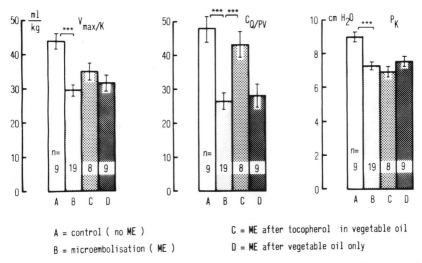

A = control (no ME)   C = ME after tocopherol in vegetable oil

B = microembolisation (ME)   D = ME after vegetable oil only

FIGURE 4. V_{max}/k, $C_{Q/pv}$, and P_K of classical PV diagrams from the animal groups with (B–D) and without microembolization (A). Tocopherol pretreated animals (C) show a highly significant ($p < 10^{-5}$) higher $C_{Q/pv}$. V_{max} being only partly improved and P_K being even lower, this implies the conclusion that tocopherol prevented the predominant functional impairment of the surfactant system, but did not influence the slight depletion of surface active material. (Means $\pm$ SEM.) (Reproduced from Reference 11 with permission from the publisher.)

On the other hand, the compliance of the inflation part, $C_{Infl/K}$, did not differ significantly; thus, hysteresis was significantly improved in the tocopherol group. In the classical PV diagrams (FIGURE 4), the compliance quotient, $C_{Q/pv}$, of the tocopherol group exceeded the values of both reference groups significantly $(p < 10^{-5})$, reaching those of the nonmicroembolized control animals. Taking into consideration the even lower pressure at the bending point, P_K, and the only partially improved maximum volume, V_{max}/k, these findings imply that tocopherol prevented the predominant functional impairment of the surfactant system, but did not influence the slight depletion of surfactant material in the microembolization model.

Gas exchange was significantly better in the tocopherol group $(p < 0.01)$, as is indicated by the higher values of arterial oxygen partial pressure (P_{aO_2}) and the less increased alveolar-arterial O_2 difference $(A\text{-}a_{D_{O_2}})$ of the tocopherol group (FIGURE 5). This corresponds to less interstitial edema and less thrombocyte and leukocyte aggregates in the histological specimens of the tocopherol animals' lungs. Cardiac output and the shunt volume of cardiac output were not altered by tocopherol (FIGURE 6).

Conclusions

Significant protective effects of tocopherol could be demonstrated in the microembolization model concerning various parameters. An explanation for the

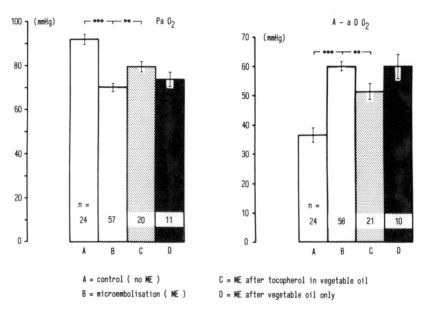

A = control (no ME)   C = ME after tocopherol in vegetable oil
B = microembolisation (ME)   D = ME after vegetable oil only

FIGURE 5. Arterial O_2 pressure (P_{aO_2}) and alveolar-arterial O_2 difference $(A\text{-}a_{D_{O_2}})$ of the animal groups with (B–D) and without microembolization (A) during the experiment. Tocopherol pretreated animals (C) have significantly higher P_{aO_2} and $A\text{-}a_{D_{O_2}}$ (both $p < 0.01$), indicating better O_2 diffusion. (Means ± SEM.)

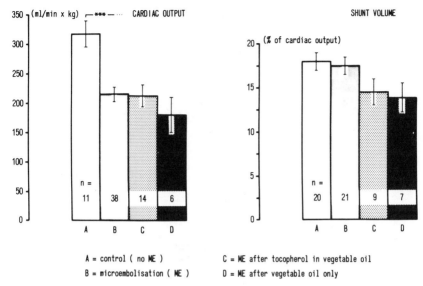

A = control (no ME)   C = ME after tocopherol in vegetable oil
B = microembolisation (ME)   D = ME after vegetable oil only

FIGURE 6. Cardiac output (CO) and shunt volume of CO of the animal groups with (B–D) and without microembolization (A) during the experiment. CO is significantly (p < 0.001) reduced by microembolization, but not altered by tocopherol pretreatment. (Means ± SEM.)

pathophysiological role of tocopherol, however, was still lacking. Discussion of the possible sites of tocopherol influence in the ARDS extended over several pathophysiological mechanisms:

1. Prevention of peroxidation of unsaturated fatty acid components of the surfactant film.[11,14]

2. Prevention of damage to vascular endothelial and alveolar epithelial cell membranes.[15]

3. Stabilization of such circulating components as thrombocytes or leukocytes; inhibition of their aggregation and neutralization of released oxygen radicals.[16,11]

SECOND EXPERIMENT

Free radical chain reactions and peroxidation of unsaturated fatty acids might damage lung tissue and surfactant at various sites. In the meantime, we have carried out further experiments on peroxidation effects in isolated surfactant films and have tested the influence of free unsaturated fatty acids on the pulmonary vasculature and surface tension conditions.[17–23] The most convincing effects were seen in consequence of arachidonic acid (AA) oxygenation in isolated, perfused rabbit lungs.

It is known that different oxygenation pathways of free AA yield very different, partly adversely acting bioactive products of high efficacy, as there are prostaglandins, thromboxanes, leukotrienes, and other lipoxygenase products (FIGURE 7). Release of AA from membrane phospholipids has turned out to be an unspecific response to a variety of stimulating conditions at membrane surfaces.

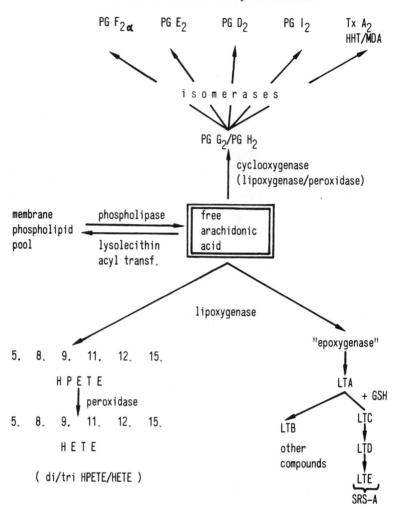

FIGURE 7. Schematic pathways of arachidonic acid (AA) liberation and AA metabolism. PG, prostaglandin; Tx, thromboxane; LT, leukotriene; HPETE, hydroperoxy-eicosatetraenoic acid; HETE, hydroxy-eicosatetraenoic acid; HHT, hydroxy-heptadecatrienoic acid; MDA, malondialdehyde; GSH, glutathione; SRS-A, slow-reacting substance of anaphylaxis.

We investigated the biological effects in consequence of increased availability of free AA in the pulmonary vasculature.[17,18,21,22]

In a model of isolated, ventilated rabbit lungs, perfused with Krebs-Henseleit-albumin buffer (KHAB) (4% bovine albumin; free fatty acid content, 2.5–5 μg/g) with a pulsatile flow of 200 ml/minute in a recirculating system (FIGURE 8), the addition of AA to the perfusion fluid or its release by the calcium-ionophore A 23187, for example, causes a biphasic increase in vascular resistance (pulmonary arterial pressure reaction, PaPR) and an increase in vascular permeability (gain of organ weight) (FIGURE 9). The PaPR could be ascribed to cyclooxygenase products, and the vascular leakage to lipoxygenase products, of AA.[21] For example by addition of indomethacin, which selectively inhibits cyclooxygenase, the PaPR is completely suppressed, whereas pulmonary weight gain is considerably enhanced. We have evidence that this phenomenon is due to an AA shift from the inhibited cyclooxygenase to the noninhibited lipoxygenase pathways.

The first steps of all AA metabolic pathways are oxygenation reactions with intermediate formation of arachidonate radicals and possibly oxygen radicals.[24-26] These steps may be influenced by antioxidants and oxygen radical scavengers. In our isolated lung model, we investigated the influence of α-tocopherol, α-tocopheryl quinone, the chromane compound of α-tocopherol (6-hydroxy-2,5,7,8-tetramethyl-chroman-2-carboxylic acid, Trolox®, gift from Hoffmann-La Roche, Basel, Switzerland), phytol (3,7,11,15-tetramethyl-2-hexadecen-1-ol), vitamin K_1 (2-methyl-3-phytyl-1,4-naphthoquinone), vitamin K_3 (2-methyl-1,4-naphthoqui-

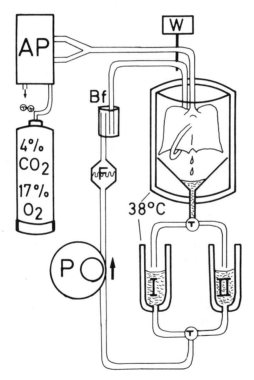

FIGURE 8. Model of isolated rabbit lung. The lung is freely hanging down from an electronic force transducer (W), continuously perfused by pump (P) (pulsatile flow of 200 ml/minute) with Krebs-Henseleit-albumin (4%) buffer through a 40-mm filter (F) and a bubble trap (Bf), ventilated by a Starling pump (AP) (tidal volume, 30 ml; frequency, 45/minute) with a special gas mixture allowing maintenance of physiological acid-base conditions. Two different fluid containers allow multiple consecutive perfusion phases with fresh fluid, with or without stimulus and additional inhibitor. (Reproduced from Reference 21 with permission from the publisher.)

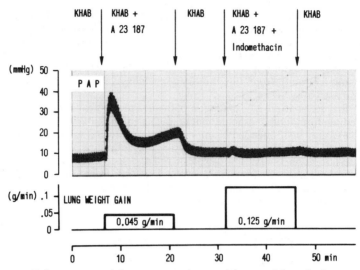

FIGURE 9. Pulmonary arterial pressure and rate of lung weight gain in response to calcium-ionophore A 23187 (2 μM). Cyclooxygenase inhibition by indomethacin (44 μM) inhibits the pressure reaction (PaPR) completely, whereas the rate of lung weight gain is increased.

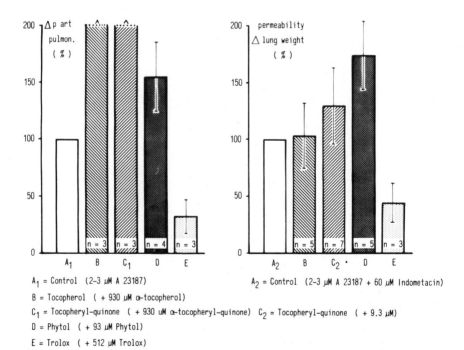

A_1 = Control (2–3 μM A 23187) A_2 = Control (2–3 μM A 23187 + 60 μM Indometacin)

B = Tocopherol (+ 930 μM α-tocopherol)

C_1 = Tocopheryl-quinone (+ 930 uM α-tocopheryl-quinone) C_2 = Tocopheryl-quinone (+ 9.3 μM)

D = Phytol (+ 93 μM Phytol)

E = Trolox (+ 512 μM Trolox)

FIGURE 10. Relative increase/decrease of PaPR (left) and the rate of lung weight gain (right) after stimulation with A 23187 in the presence of α-tocopherol, α-tocopheryl quinone, phytol, and Trolox. (Means ± SEM.)

none), and superoxide dismutase (SOD, Orgotein®, gift from Grünenthal, Aachen, Federal Republic of Germany) on the increase of pulmonary vascular resistance and permeability due to increased availability of free AA.

Results

Pulmonary Arterial Pressure Reaction

The addition of α-tocopherol in a concentration of 9.3 μM (related to the perfusion fluid, = 4 μg/ml) had no definite influence on the PaPR. A hundredfold higher dose (930 μM) brought about unexpected results: PaPR was increased to more than 200%, both after addition of free AA and after stimulation with A 23187. An even augmentation of PaPR was seen after the addition of α-tocopheryl quinone (930 μM). So we suspected that, not the antioxidative function of the molecule, but rather the phytyl chain was responsible for that effect. Pure phytol (93 μM) indeed augmented PaPR to more than 150% (FIGURE 10, left). In contrast, Trolox reduced both parts of the biphasic PaPR dose dependently (FIGURE 11). In accordance with these results, PaPR was augmented by phytyl-methylnaphtho-quinone (vitamin K_1), whereas PaPR was diminished by methylnaphthoquinone (vitamin K_3). Furthermore, SOD (48 U/ml) reduced PaPR after both stimuli, AA and A 23187, to less than 50%.[20,22]

Pulmonary Vascular Permeability

Concentrations between 9.3 μM and 930 μM of α-tocopherol had no influence on the increased vascular permeability after AA or A 23187 in the presence of indomethacin (60 μM). α-Tocopheryl quinone in low concentrations (9.3 μM), however, markedly increased vascular leakage. According to the PaPR effects, phytol increased, and Trolox in contrast decreased, the rate of weight gain after A 23187 stimulation (FIGURE 10, right, and FIGURE 12). Comparison between vitamins K_1 and K_3 again confirmed that in the presence of a phytyl side chain, the rate of weight gain was increased after A 23187 stimulation. Again, SOD (48 U/ml) reduced vascular permeability to about 65% of its initial value.

There were no effects of all the test substances without A 23187 stimulation on PaPR or weight gain up to the highest concentrations used.

Discussion

These results clearly demonstrated that the two components of the tocopherol molecule exert opposite effects on PaPR as well as on vascular permeability after added or released AA in the isolated rabbit lung: the chromane compound reduced both parameters, whereas phytol augmented them. The Trolox effect is in accordance with investigations showing an inhibition of cyclooxygenase activity and lipoxygenase activity by antioxidants in general, and especially by tocopherol.[24-28] The site of interference may be the formation of an adduct of the chromane compound with an initial arachidonate radical in these oxygenation pathways.[29] The mode of phytol action is open for speculation. Its known penetration into the membrane lipids[30,31] and the postulated physicochemical interaction preferably with AA might result in an increased availability of

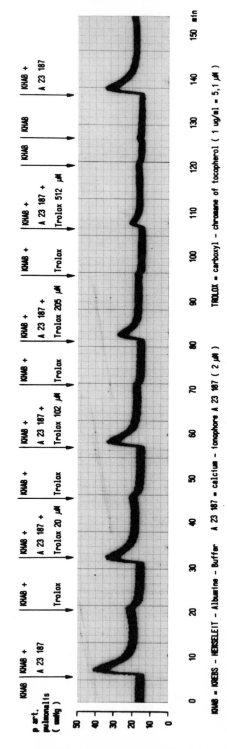

FIGURE 11. PaPR inhibition by different concentrations of Trolox. After rinsing, the initial PaPR is nearly reobtained. (Reproduced from Reference 18 with permission from the publisher.)

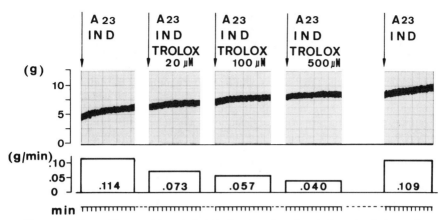

FIGURE 12. Rate of lung weight gain (original registration above) after stimulation with A 23187 in the presence of indomethacin (IND; 44 μM) and different concentrations of Trolox. After rinsing, the initial reaction is nearly reobtained. (Reproduced from Reference 22 with permission from the publisher.)

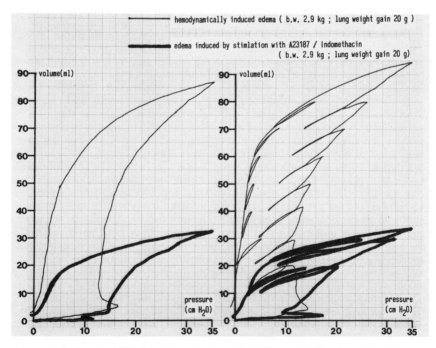

FIGURE 13. Classical PV diagrams and pneumoloop diagrams of two lungs (each from an animal of 2.9 kg) after the same amount of total weight gain (20 g), the one by throttling pulmonary venous outflow (= hemodyamically induced edema), the other by repeated stimulation with A 23187 in the presence of indomethacin without any rise in pulmonary arterial pressure (= increased vascular permeability). It is obvious that increased permeability is followed by severe deterioration of surface tension conditions.

phospholipid-bound arachidonate to phospholipase attack and/or an increased motility of free AA to the sites of cyclooxygenase or lipoxygenase metabolism. In our model of isolated lungs, the two components of α-tocopherol appear to "neutralize" each other. This is a surprising finding, in view of the remarkably beneficial effect of α-tocopherol in the microembolization model. It must be considered, however, that in the whole organism, not only the cell membranes of the inner vascular surface but also lung tissue itself as well as corpuscular and other circulating components offer multiple sites for the antioxidative and oxygen radical-scavenging properties of tocopherol. The total of the different tocopherol effects, after all, has turned out beneficial in the described pathophysiological conditions.

In any case, it is remarkable that the antioxidative chromane compound as well as SOD significantly diminished vascular leakage in the isolated rabbit lung, which can be ascribed to lipoxygenase products of AA, among which the leukotrienes C_4, D_4, and E_4 appeared to be of major importance.[20] For it is edema formation following increased vascular permeability that causes massive deterioration of the surfactant function in contrast to pure hemodynamically induced edema (FIGURE 13). Such protein-rich edema must be regarded as an initial, crucial step in ARDS development. The efficacy of SOD, an enzyme with a high molecular weight (32,000 daltons), suggests accessibility of this initial step from the luminal surface of the vascular membranes.

CLINICAL STUDIES

Since 1977, we have administered all-rac-α-tocopheryl acetate (6–8 × 300–500 mg/day) by gastric tube together with the diet to patients with manifest or threatening ARDS in addition to the individually required complex therapy. FIGURE 14 shows the time each patient was subjected to artificial ventilation and the final outcome of all our patients who were ventilated for at least four days. Diagnoses have been manifold, including mainly posttraumatic and postoperative states with renal failure; septic, hypovolemic, and cardiogeneic shock; severe intoxications with different drugs and poisons; but also malignant hyperthermia, massive hemolysis, intracerebral hemorrhage, etc. By 1977, we had the strong impression of being more successful with the additional tocopherol therapy. We have about 30–40 long-term ventilated patients a year who are very inhomogeneous as to diagnosis and age. So a clinical trial with well-matched collectives was decided to be impossible with our patients. Since tocopherol was assumed to be helpful, at least not harmful, in these patients, it was administered predominantly to those who were considered to have a dubious prognosis. It must be emphasized that therapeutic techniques and means have been improved during the last five years, especially hemofiltration and hemodialysis techniques. What we can present here should be looked upon as casuistic, to be followed up with well-prepared clinical trials. Out of 176 patients between 16 and 82 years of age (mean, 53 ± 18) in the past five years, 87 received tocopherol therapy and 89 did not. Distribution of age, sex, duration of artificial ventilation, maximum oxygen fraction of inspired gas ($F_{I_{O_2}}$), and maximum positive end-expiratory ventilation pressure (PEEP) is shown in TABLE 1. Surviving tocopherol patients are the youngest in mean, but the group also contains the oldest survivors (2 patients 78 years old, ventilated for 8 and 11 days). Mean $F_{I_{O_2}}$ and PEEP values confirm the assumption that tocopherol patients were more severely ill in the beginning than were the nontocopherol patients. We were struck by the observation that we were

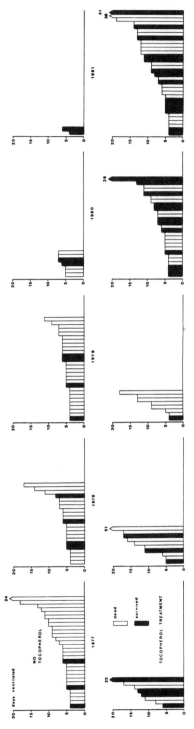

FIGURE 14. Duration of artificial ventilation and final outcome of all patients treated in the Internal Intensive Care Unit, Giessen, who had been ventilated for at least four days (1977–1981). The upper row shows patients without tocopherol therapy, the lower row with additional tocopherol therapy (6–8×300–500 mg/day all-rac-α-tocopheryl acetate by gastric tube).

TABLE 1
PATIENTS VENTILATED AT LEAST FOUR DAYS (1977–1981)

With Tocopherol	Without Tocopherol
$n = 87$	$n = 89$
$F_{I_{O_2}}$ ($n = 86$): 0.77 ± 0.21	$F_{I_{O_2}}$ ($n = 80$): 0.61 ± 0.21
PEEP ($n = 79$): 8.2 ± 2.9	PEEP ($n = 50$): 6.8 ± 3.1
Survivors: $34 = 39\%$	**Survivors**: $15 = 17\%$
Female: 9	Female: 6
Male: 25	Male: 9
Age: 42 ± 21	Age: 57 ± 15
Ventilation days: 10.0 ± 7.7	Ventilation days: 5.5 ± 1.1
$F_{I_{O_2}}$: 0.72 ± 0.20	$F_{I_{O_2}}$: 0.54 ± 0.17
PEEP: 7.8 ± 2.6	PEEP: 4.6 ± 2.1
Dead: $53 = 61\%$	**Dead**: $74 = 83\%$
Female: 19	Female: 22
Male: 34	Male: 52
Age: 50 ± 18	Age: 61 ± 13
Ventilation days: 10.3 ± 7.9	Ventilation days: 6.8 ± 3.6
$F_{I_{O_2}}$: 0.80 ± 0.20	$F_{I_{O_2}}$: 0.63 ± 0.22
PEEP: 8.7 ± 2.9	PEEP: 7.2 ± 3.0

able to ventilate tocopherol-treated critically ill patients for very long periods of time with rather high $F_{I_{O_2}}$ and saw pulmonary improvement instead of the expected progressive pulmonary failure. There were tocopherol patients surviving 25, 28, and even 41 days of artificial ventilation, whereas not one of the nontocopherol patients survived after more than 8 days of ventilation.

Only recently are we able to measure serum tocopherol levels by gas chromatography. Our ventilated patients do absorb tocopherol, but not as rapidly as is known from healthy controls (FIGURE 15).[32]‡ We are convinced that further investigations on tocopherol and, in general, on antioxidant therapy of ARDS patients would be very reasonable. Moreover, it should be considered that antioxidant therapy might be useful in other exudative diseases.

SUMMARY

The adult respiratory distress syndrome (ARDS) is not confined only to late shock states but is a typical finding in intoxications with such oxidizing agents as O_3, NO_2, chlorate, or paraquat. Under experimental conditions, α-tocopherol in a high enteric dosage (2×50 mg/kg) was able to prevent alterations of pulmonary surface tension parameters ($p < 10^{-5}$) induced by microembolization of pulmonary vessels in awake rabbits. Parameters of gas exchange ($P_{a_{O_2}}$, A-a$_{D_{O_2}}$) were

‡These results will be part of a thesis to be presented by Achim Ziegler, Justus-Liebig University.

significantly less impaired ($p < 0.01$) in the tocopherol group. Since there was no additional oxidative stress, the protective effect of tocopherol suggests an involvement of pathophysiologically occurring peroxidation mechanisms. Arachidonic acid (AA) metabolism is known to be a physiological oxygenation process yielding products with utmost biological efficacy. In a model of isolated, ventilated, and continuously perfused rabbit lungs, release or addition of AA resulted in an increase of pulmonary vascular resistance and permeability. The former could be ascribed to cyclooxygenase products, the latter to lipoxygenase products, of AA. The α-tocopherol effect in this model was a complex one: the antioxidative chromane structure (Trolox) as well as superoxide dismutase (SOD) decreased both pulmonary vascular resistance and permeability induced by AA metabolism dose dependently to a large degree, whereas the phytyl side chain augmented both effects. Pharmacological efficacy of high-dose α-tocopherol is not yet completely understood. Since 1977, we have applied all-rac-α-tocopheryl acetate (6–8 × 300–500 mg/day by gastric tube) to patients with manifest or threatening ARDS in addition to the required conventional complex therapy. Out of 176 patients being artificially ventilated for at least four days in the Internal Intensive Care Unit, Giessen University, 87 received tocopherol and 89 did not. There was no statistically valid stratification or randomization of the patients. In general, the tocopherol-treated patients were considered to have the worse prognosis, as is confirmed by higher maximum $F_{I_{O_2}}$ and PEEP values. Thirty-four tocopherol patients (39%) and 15 nontocopherol patients (17%) survived. Surviving tocopherol patients were ventilated for a mean of 10.0 ± 7.7 days (with maxima of 25, 28, and 41 days), whereas surviving nontocopherol patients were ventilated only for 5.5 ± 1.1 days (none of these for more than 8 days). Absorption of α-tocopherol by these severely ill patients was shown by gas chromatography. A well-prepared clinical trial for tocopherol therapy of ARDS is suggested.

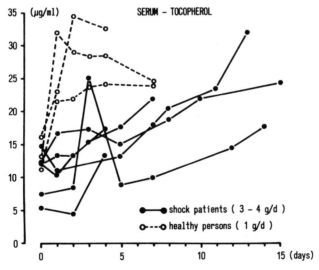

FIGURE 15. Serum tocopherol levels of six shock patients and three healthy controls before (day 0) and during oral tocopherol application (days 1–15).

REFERENCES

1. BREDENBERG, C. E., P. M. JAMES, J. COLLINS, R. W. ANDERSON, A. M. MARTIN & R. M. HARDAWAY. 1969. Respiratory failure in shock. Ann. Surg. 169(3): 392.
2. BLAISDELL, F. W. & R. M. SCHLOBOHM. 1973. The respiratory distress syndrome: a review. Surgery 74(2): 251-262.
3. EDWARDS, D. K., W. M. DYER & W. H. NORTHWAY, JR. 1977. Twelve years' experience with bronchopulmonary dysplasia. Pediatrics 59:839-846.
4. SALDEEN, T. 1979. The microembolism syndrome: a review. In The Microembolism Syndrome. T. Saldeen Ed.: 7-44. Almqvist & Wiksell International. Stockholm, Sweden.
5. WOLF, H. & H. NEUHOF. 1977. The role of microembolism on the genesis of shock lung. Curr. Top. Crit. Care Med. 3: 2-8.
6. DOWELL, A. R., K. H. KILBURN & P. C. PRATT. 1971. Short-term exposure to nitrogen dioxide. Arch. Intern. Med. 128: 74.
7. WILLIAMS, R. A., R. A. RHOADES & W. S. ADAMS. 1971. The response of lung tissue and surfactant to nitrogen dioxide exposure. Arch. Intern. Med. 128: 101.
8. WITSCHI, H.-P., K.-I. HIRAI & M. G. COTE. 1977. Primary events in lung following exposure to toxic chemicals. In Biochemical Mechanisms of Paraquat Toxicity. A. P. Autor, Ed.: 1-20. Academic Press. New York, San Francisco & London.
9. THOMAS, H. V., P. K. MÜLLER & R. L. LYMAN. 1968. Lipoperoxidation of lung lipids in rats exposed to nitrogen dioxide. Science 159: 532.
10. WOLF, H., N. SUTTORP, W. SEEGER & H. NEUHOF. 1977. Effects of methylprednisolone, bromhexin metabolite VIII, and α-tocopherol on surfactant activity and hemodynamic parameters in a standardised shock lung model in rabbits. Intensive Care Med. 3(3): 115.
11. WOLF, H., W. SEEGER, N. SUTTORP & H. NEUHOF. 1981. Experimental results in the prevention of RDS with α-tocopherol. Prog. Respir. Res. 15: 308-316.
12. SUTTORP, N. 1980. Veränderungen der Hämodynamik und des Gasaustausches am tierexperimentellen Modell der Schocklunge und Möglichkeiten zur therapeutischen Beeinflussung. Doctoral Thesis. Justus-Liebig University. Giessen, Federal Republic of Germany.
13. SEEGER, W. 1980. Veränderungen der alveolären Oberflächenspannung und Möglichkeiten ihrer therapeutischen Beeinflussung am tierexperimentellen Modell der Schocklunge. Doctoral Thesis. Justus-Liebig University. Giessen, Federal Republic of Germany.
14. SEEGER, W., U. MOSER & L. ROKA. Measurement of organic hydroperoxides in animal tissue by glutathione peroxidase and glutathione reductase. (Submitted for publication.)
15. CHOW, C. K., K. REDDY & A. TAPPEL. 1973. Effect of dietary vitamin E on the activities of the glutathione peroxidase system in rat tissues. J. Nutr. 103: 618.
16. STEINER, M. & J. ANASTASI. 1976. Vitamin E: an inhibitor of the platelet release reaction. J. Clin. Invest. 57: 732-737.
17. SEEGER, W., H. WOLF, G. STÄHLER, H. NEUHOF & L. ROKA. 1981. Zunahme des Strömungswiderstandes und der Gefässpermeabilität in der pulmonalen Strombahn als Folge des Metabolismus freier Arachidonsäure. Klin. Wochenschr. 59: 459-461.
18. WOLF, H., W. SEEGER, G. STÄHLER, H. NEUHOF & L. ROKA. 1981. Protektiver Effekt der antioxidativ wirksamen Chromanstruktur des Tocopherols auf die Folgen stimulierter Arachidonsäre-Freisetzung in der pulmonalen Strombahn. Klin. Wochenschr. 59: 463-465.
19. SEEGER, W., H. WOLF, G. STÄHLER, H. NEUHOF & L. ROKA. 1981. Pulmonary vascular leakage induced by lipoxygenase metabolism of free arachidonic acid. Abstract no. 86, International Symposium on Leukotrienes and Other Lipoxygenase Products, Florence, Italy, June 10-12.
20. WOLF, H., W. SEEGER, G. STÄHLER, H. NEUHOF & L. ROKA. 1981. Chromane compound and SOD decrease lung vascular leakage caused by lipoxygenase metabolism of

arachidonic acid. Abstract no. 101, International Symposium on Leukotrienes and Other Lipoxygenase Products, Florence, Italy, June 10–12.

21. SEEGER, W., H. WOLF, G. STÄHLER, H. NEUHOF & L. ROKA. 1982. Increased pulmonary vascular resistance and permeability due to arachidonate metabolism in isolated rabbit lungs. Prostaglandins **23:** 157–173.

22. SEEGER, W., H. WOLF, G. STÄHLER, H. NEUHOF & L. ROKA. 1982. Influence of tocopherol, its chromane compound, phytyl chains and superoxide dismutase on increased vascular resistance and permeability due to arachidonate metabolism in isolated rabbit lungs. Prostaglandins **23:** 175–184.

23. SEEGER W., H. WOLF, G. STÄHLER, H. NEUHOF & L. ROKA. Alteration of pressure-volume characteristics due to different modes of edema development in isolated lungs. (Submitted for publication.)

24. MACLOUF, J., H. SORS & M. RIGAUD. 1977. Recent aspects of prostaglandin biosynthesis: a review. Biomedicine **26:** 362.

25. HEMLER, M. E. & W. E. M. LANDS. 1980. Evidence for a peroxide initiated free radical mechanism of prostaglandin biosynthesis. J. Biol. Chem. **255:** 6253.

26. PORTER, N. A. 1980. Prostaglandin endoperoxides. In Free Radicals in Biology. W. A. Pryor, Ed. **4:** 261–295. Academic Press, Inc. New York, N.Y.

27. VANDERHOEK, J. Y. & W. E. M. LANDS. 1978. The inhibition of fatty acid oxygenase of sheep vesicular gland by antioxidants. Biochim. Biophys. Acta **296:** 382.

28. EGAN, R. W., P. H. GALE, C. G. BEVERIDGE, L. J. MARNETT & F. A. KUEHL, JR. 1980. Direct and indirect involvement of radical scavengers during prostaglandin biosynthesis. Adv. Prostaglandin Thromboxane Res. **6:** 153.

29. LOSCHEN, G. 1981. α-Tocopherol traps an intermediate of the enzymatic peroxidation of arachidonic acid. Abstract no. 67, International Symposium on Leukotrienes and Other Lipoxygenase Products, Florence, Italy, June 10–12.

30. LUCY, A. T. 1978. Structural interactions between vitamin E and polyunsaturated lipids. In Tocopherol, Oxygen and Biomembranes. C. de Duve & O. Hayaishi, Eds.: 109–120. Elsevier/North-Holland Biomedical Press. Amsterdam, the Netherlands.

31. FUKUZAWA, K. & K. HAIASHI. 1977. Effects of α-tocopherol analogues on lysosome membranes and fatty acid monolayers. Chem. Phys. Lipids **18:** 39.

32. GALLO-TORRES, H. E. 1980. Absorption of vitamin E. In Vitamin E, A Comprehensive Treatise. L. J. Machlin. Ed.: 170. Marcel Dekker, Inc. New York, N.Y.

DISCUSSION

A. E. KITABCHI (*University of Tennessee, Memphis, Tenn.*): How did you decide which patients to put on tocopherol?

H. R. D. WOLF: It was up to the doctor on duty in the intensive-care unit to decide whether he would give tocopherol. Once they had tocopherol, they had it all the time.

C. C. TANGNEY (*Rush University, Chicago, Ill.*): How many of your patients were on hyperalimentation?

H. R. D. WOLF: Some of them were, especially those with septic shock. A few of the patients had hyperalimentation of up to 8,000 to 9,000 calories a day.

C. C. TANGNEY: Were you using intravenous fat emulsions at the same time?

H. R. D. WOLF: In the last 1½ years, we have, but from 1977 through 1980, we did not.

F. VOGEL (*BASF Wyandotte, Parsippany, N.J.*): You had some differences in age between the groups of untreated and treated people. How much of the increased survival rate would you attribute to age?

H. R. D. WOLF: This is very difficult to calculate. We had among surviving tocopherol patients, two patients 78 years of age who survived 8 days and even 11 days of artificial ventilation. This was not common in the non-tocopherol-treated patients.

CLINICAL AND PHARMACOLOGIC INVESTIGATION OF THE EFFECTS OF α-TOCOPHEROL ON ADRIAMYCIN CARDIOTOXICITY*

Sewa S. Legha, Yeu-Ming Wang,† Bruce Mackay,‡
Michael Ewer, Gabriel N. Hortobagyi,
Robert S. Benjamin, and Mohammed K. Ali

*Division of Medical Services
The University of Texas System Cancer Center
M. D. Anderson Hospital and Tumor Institute
Houston, Texas 77030*

Adriamycin (doxorubicin) is one of the most effective antitumor drugs presently in clinical use. The major limitation of its clinical usefulness is a dose-related cardiomyopathy, which prevents its use beyond a total cumulative dose of 500–550 mg/m². The incidence of cardiomyopathy is between 1 and 2% at this dose level but rises steeply to, for instance, 20–40% at 600 mg/m² or higher.[1] This has led to the common practice of discontinuing adriamycin at or before a maximum total dose of 550 mg/m².

The mechanism of adriamycin-induced cardiac injury is poorly understood. The histological changes are most obvious with the electron microscope and consist of loss of myofilaments, cytoplasmic vacuolization, and ultimately cellular necrosis and disappearance of myocytes. This lesion is strikingly similar to the muscle pathology produced by α-tocopherol deficiency in both rabbit and mouse.[2,3] In α-tocopherol deficiency, the lesions seen in skeletal as well as cardiac muscle are in part the result of unrestrained free radical reactions that lead to peroxidation of membrane lipids.[4] A similar process of free radical–mediated lipid peroxidation characterizes the tissue damage elicited by a number of drugs containing quinone and hydroxyquinone groups.[5] Since adriamycin contains both quinone and hydroxyquinone groups on adjacent aromatic rings, Myers *et al.* investigated the possibility of lipid peroxidation in mice and proved the formation of lipid peroxides in the myocardium of adriamycin-treated animals.[6] The similarity in the mechanism of action as well as pathological changes of adriamycin-induced cardiac injury to those seen in vitamin E deficiency in animals led Myers *et al.* to try α-tocopherol as a measure to prevent adriamycin-induced cardiac toxicity.[6,7] By using intraperitoneal injection of α-tocopherol 24 hours prior to adriamycin, they were able to prevent the formation of malondialdehyde in the myocardium. Further, they showed that α-tocopherol administration significantly reduced the incidence and severity of histological changes observed in adriamycin cardiotoxicity. Although effective in preventing the cardiac toxicity of adriamycin, α-tocopherol did not interfere with the inhibition of DNA

*This research was supported in part by Grant CA 05831 from the National Institutes of Health and by a grant from Hoffmann-La Roche, Inc., Nutley, N.J.
†Department of Experimental Pediatrics.
‡Department of Pathology.

0077-8923/82/0393-0411 $01.75/0 © 1982, NYAS

synthesis of P388 leukemia cells by adriamycin, and accordingly its antitumor effect was not compromised.[6] Similar effects of α-tocopherol in amelioration of adriamycin cardiac toxicity without interfering with its antitumor effects have been reported in a rat model bearing acute myeloid leukemia.[8] We have demonstrated the effectiveness of α-tocopherol in reducing the cardiac toxicity of adriamycin in a rabbit model.[9] We have also demonstrated that the generation of superoxide radicals from adriamycin therapy reduced glutathione (GSH) levels in red cells and other cells and that α-tocopherol effectively blocked the drop in GSH levels in α-tocopherol-treated cells in vitro and in vivo.[9,10] Furthermore, we have shown that a fourfold increase in serum α-tocopherol level was effective in decreasing the acute cardiac toxicity of adriamycin in the rabbit model.[9]

Although the cardiotoxicity of adriamycin is dose related, it does not affect all patients receiving the drug, there being considerable individual variation in the dose that may be cardiotoxic. A number of invasive and noninvasive means have been used to measure the left ventricular function in order to detect early damage to the myocardium. Unfortunately, there is no one method that has uniformly and reproducibly detected subclinical cardiac damage from adriamycin. This has led to utilization of endomyocardial biopsy from the right ventricle, and the results of this procedure have indicated a dose-related damage to the myocardial cells, which can be detected with the electron microscope at adriamycin doses as low as 180 to 240 mg/m^2.[11,12] We feel that endomyocardial biopsy is at present the most sensitive way of detecting early myocardial toxicity of adriamycin. Other complementary procedures that appear to add to the predictive value of endomyocardial biopsy are echocardiographic determination of left ventricular contractility and radioisotopic cardiac scanning to determine the left ventricular ejection fraction.[13] Abnormality in any one of these tests, if supported by one or both of the other tests, is currently the best guide to safe administration of adriamycin.

In this study we wanted to determine whether α-tocopherol offered significant protection against adriamycin-induced cardiotoxicity in humans. Furthermore, we wished to determine whether the oral ingestion of α-tocopherol concurrently with an adriamycin-containing chemotherapy regimen interfered with its antitumor activity.

MATERIALS AND METHODS

Patients

This study was conducted in 21 patients with histological diagnosis of metastatic breast cancer who were treated with a triple drug combination of 5-fluorouracil, adriamycin, and cyclophosphamide.[14] All patients entered in this study had had no prior therapy with adriamycin. They were ambulatory and had a performance score close to normal. Patients with brain metastases or with impaired cardiac reserve secondary to organic heart disease (such as coronary insufficiency, hypertension, or valvular heart disease) were excluded. Informed consent indicating the investigational nature of the study, including endomyocardial biopsies, was obtained from each participant. The majority of our patients were in good general physical condition and had the usual sites of metastases that characterize patients with metastatic breast cancer. The characteristics of these patients are summarized in TABLE 1.

Treatment Regimen

α-Tocopherol was provided by Hoffmann-La Roche, Inc., Nutley, N.J. It was given orally at a dose of 2 g/m² daily, starting seven days prior to adriamycin therapy. The vitamin therapy was started as soon as the diagnosis of metastatic breast cancer was confirmed. This was to ensure that the serum α-tocopherol level rose to at least four times the baseline level before the patient was exposed to adriamycin. This was based on our experience in the animal study.[9] α-Tocopherol therapy was continued as long as each patient received adriamycin, which was continued as long as the tumor responded to chemotherapy. All patients had blood counts, SMA-12, and repeat staging studies to determine the response to therapy as stipulated in standard chemotherapy protocols. Cardiac function studies including electrocardiogram, echocardiogram, and cardiac scan were repeated at cumulative adriamycin doses of 250 mg/m² and 450 mg/m² and at other times whenever there was a need for endomyocardial biopsy or if there was suggestion of cardiac impairment. Patients whose tumor failed to respond to therapy after a minimum of two or more courses of therapy were taken off the protocol. Patients whose tumor was responsive to therapy continued on adriamy-

TABLE 1

PATIENT CHARACTERISTICS

Number of patients	21
Age	50 (37–73)
Performance status	
0–2	15 (71%)
3–4	6 (29%)
Dominant site of metastasis	
Visceral	9 (43%)
Osseous	8 (38%)
Soft tissue	4 (19%)

cin as long as the cardiac biopsy revealed no significant damage (< grade 2 changes) and the left ventricular function was normal by other parameters.

Assessment of Cardiac Biopsies

The histopathological grading system used to define the severity of cardiac lesions induced by adriamycin was a modification of Billingham's method.[11,14] It is a semiquantitative assessment of the distribution of the three characteristic electron-microscopic findings, which include distension of the sarcoplasmic reticulum leading to vacuolization, myofibrillar dropout, and necrosis of the myocardial cells. All biopsies were given a pathologic score of cardiac toxicity ranging from 0 to 3, using a half-point scale (TABLE 2). The average number of fibers per block, showing each type of change, was determined, and grade was assessed according to criteria shown in this table. When more than one type of pathologic change reached the defined magnitude, the next higher grade was assigned. At least six blocks of tissue each containing approximately 400 myocar-

TABLE 2

MORPHOLOGIC GRADING OF ENDOMYOCARDIAL BIOPSY SPECIMENS

	Muscle Fibers Showing Changes*		
Grade	Vacuoles	Myofibrillar Dropout	Necrosis
0.5	<4	0	0
1	4–10	<3	0
1.5	>10	3–5	<2
2		6–8	2–5
3		>8	>5

*Reflects average number of abnormal muscle fibers per grid, based on an examination of a minimum of six grids obtained from six blocks.

dial muscle fibers were selected from each biopsy, so that the total number of fibers evaluated ultrastructurally was close to 2,000. Since the average biopsy grade at the usual dose that could be safely utilized with a low incidence of heart failure was about 2, we decided to treat our patients with adriamycin up to cumulative doses that resulted in a biopsy grade of 2, rather than to a fixed cumulative dose.

Quantitation of a-Tocopherol

Serum tocopherol level was determined by the methods of colorimetry[15] and high-performance liquid chromatography.[16]

RESULTS AND DISCUSSION

The response to treatment was assessed using the standard criteria proposed by the International Union Against Cancer. Fifteen of 21 patients achieved an objective response, for a response rate of 71%. This response rate was similar to that achieved with this chemotherapeutic regimen in our previous experience. The spectrum of toxicity observed with this treatment program is shown in TABLE 3. No obvious side effects were observed that could be related to the vitamin E therapy. The incidence of nausea, vomiting, and stomatitis was quite similar to that usually observed with this chemotherapeutic regimen, indicating that vita-

TABLE 3

TOXICITIES OF THE 5-FLUOROURACIL, ADRIAMYCIN, CYCLOPHOSPHAMIDE, AND α-TOCOPHEROL COMBINATION REGIMEN

Symptom	Percent of Patients
Nausea/vomiting	95
Stomatitis	14
Alopecia	100
Myelosuppression	
Median lowest granulocyte count $\times$ $10^3/mm^3$	0.8 (0.1–1.5)
Median lowest platelet count $\times$ $10^3/mm^3$	168 (36–460)

TABLE 4

CARDIAC TOXICITY OF 5-FLUOROURACIL, ADRIAMYCIN, CYCLOPHOSPHAMIDE,
AND α-TOCOPHEROL COMBINATION

Adriamycin Dose (mg/m^2)	Number of Patients	Heart Failure
100–380	7	0
450–550	8	2
560–660	5	0
820	1	1
Total	21	3 (14%)

min E offered no protection from the gastrointestinal toxicity of chemotherapy. Similarly, the incidence of alopecia and the degree of myelosuppression were not influenced by the concomitant administration of vitamin E.

The clinical cardiac toxicity of adriamycin at various dose levels is illustrated in TABLE 4. Three of 21 patients developed congestive heart failure, the first patient at an adriamycin dose level of 470 mg/m^2, the second after 550 mg/m^2, and the third at 820 mg/m^2. The heart failure occurred prior to a scheduled cardiac biopsy in the first patient and three months after the last adriamycin dose in the second and third patients. Two of these patients had previously received mediastinal irradiation, and the third was receiving chest wall irradiation for a local tumor recurrence when congestive heart failure developed. Although six patients exceeded the traditional adriamycin dose limit of 550 mg/m^2, four of these showed significant pathologic changes in the biopsy.

The cardiac biopsy findings among 12 patients who had a total of 19 cardiac biopsies are summarized in TABLE 5. We observed pathologic changes of grade 1.5 or 2 in approximately half of the biopsies carried out at adriamycin dose levels in the range of 450 to 660 mg/m^2, with a median dose of 550 mg/m^2. These results are similar to our current experience with the conventional use of adriamycin, where approximately 50% of patients develop changes of grade 1.5 to 2 at a cumulative adriamycin dose of 450 mg/m^2.[14] Therefore, vitamin E therapy may have at best allowed administration of an additional 100 mg/m^2 of adriamycin.

Serum α-tocopherol levels before and during chemotherapy are shown in TABLE 6. There was generally a six- to eightfold increase in blood levels within 5–6 days of starting α-tocopherol therapy, and the levels were sustained with maintenance therapy. Therefore, despite the achievement of the targeted increase in serum α-tocopherol levels, our study failed to show significant protection of the myocardium from adriamycin toxicity. This study was designed based on experimental evidence in rabbit of protective effects of α-tocopherol

TABLE 5

CARDIAC BIOPSY FINDINGS FOLLOWING THERAPY WITH 5-FLUOROURACIL, ADRIAMYCIN,
CYCLOPHOSPHAMIDE, AND α-TOCOPHEROL COMBINATION REGIMEN

Adriamycin Dose (mg/m^2)	Number of Biopsies	Percent with Biopsy Grade			
		<1	1	1.5	≥ 2
450–550	14	29	29	42	0
560–660	5	20	20	0	60

against acute adriamycin cardiac toxicity. More recent studies by Breed et al. using the rabbit model, however, have shown that α-tocopherol fails to protect against the cardiac toxicity due to the chronic administration of adriamycin.[17] Furthermore, one preliminary report has provided evidence that overdosage of α-tocopherol diminishes its protective effects against adriamycin-induced cardiac toxicity.[18]

In conclusion, our data revealed that use of vitamin E prophylaxis against adriamycin cardiac toxicity is not a clinically useful undertaking. A similar conclusion was reached in another clinical study recently reported by Weitzman and associates.[19]

TABLE 6

SERUM VITAMIN E LEVELS DURING TREATMENT

	Number of Patients	Vitamin E Levels (mg/100 ml)	
		Median	Range
Baseline	8	1.1	0.4–1.9
Prechemotherapy (days 5–6)	7	6.0	1.0–7.0
Maintenance	7	8.5	1.6–15.8

SUMMARY

Our data indicate that α-tocopherol used in an oral dose of 2 g/m^2 daily results in a six- to eightfold increase of the vitamin E levels in serum. The occurrence of congestive heart failure in three patients and the observation of significant pathologic changes in endomyocardial biopsies in approximately half of the patients treated with a median cumulative adriamycin dose level of 550 mg/m^2 indicate that α-tocopherol does not offer substantial protection against adriamycin-induced cardiac toxicity. The antitumor activity of the drug, however, is not compromised by the concomitant administration of the vitamin.

REFERENCES

1. LENAZ, L. & J. A. PAGE. 1976. Cancer Treatment Rev. 3: 111–120.
2. VAN VLEET, J. F., B. V. HALL & J. SIMON. 1968. Am. J. Pathol. 52: 1067–1079.
3. HOWES, E. L., H. H. PRICE & J. M. BLUMBERG. 1964. Am. J. Pathol. 45: 599–631.
4. WITTING, L. A. 1975. Am. J. Clin. Nutr. 27: 952–959.
5. JACOB, H. S., S. H. INGBAR & J. H. JANDL. 1965. J. Clin. Invest. 44: 1187–1199.
6. MYERS, C. E., W. P. MCGUIRE, R. H. LISS et al. 1977. Science 197: 165–167.
7. MYERS, C. E., W. MCGUIRE & R. YOUNG. 1976. Cancer Treatment Rep. 60: 961–962.
8. SONNEVALD, P. 1978. Cancer Treatment Rep. 62: 1033–1035.
9. WANG, Y. M., F. F. MADANAT, J. C. KIMBALL, C. A. ORTEISE, M. K. ALI, M. W. KAUFMAN & J. VAN EYS. 1980. Cancer Res. 40: 1022–1027.
10. KIMBALL, J. C., E. LANTIN & Y. M. WANG. 1979. (abst.). Proc. Am. Assoc. Cancer Res. 20: 188.
11. BRISTOW, M. R., J. W. MASON, M. E. BILLINGHAM & J. R. DANIELS. 1978. Ann. Intern. Med. 88: 168–175.

12. FRIEDMAN, M. A., M. J. BOZDECH, M. E. BILLINGHAM & A. K. RIDER. 1978. J. Am. Med. Assoc. **240:** 1603–1606.
13. GOTTDIENER, J. S. 1978. Cancer Treatment Rep. **62:** 949–953.
14. LEGHA, S. S., R. S. BENJAMIN, B. MACKAY, M. EWER, S. WALLACE, M. VALDIVIESO, S. L. RASMUSSEN, G. R. BLUMENSCHIEN & E. J. FREIREICH. 1982. Ann. Intern. Med. **96:** 133–139.
15. O'BRIEN, D., F. A. IBBOTT & D. O. RODGERSON. 1968. Laboratory Manual of Pediatric Microbiochemical Techniques. 4th edit.: 358–360. Harper and Row. New York, N.Y.
16. HOWELL, S. K. & Y. M. WANG. 1982. J. Chromatogr. **227:** 174–180.
17. BREED, J. C. S., A. N. E. ZIMMERMANN, J. A. M. A. DORMANS & H. M. PINEDO. 1980. Cancer Res. **40:** 2033–2038.
18. MCGUINESS, J. E., R. S. BENJAMIN & Y. M. WANG. 1980. (abst.). Proc. Am. Assoc. Cancer Res. **21:** 288.
19. WEITZMAN, S. A., B. LORELL, R. W. CAREY, S. KAUFMAN & T. P. STOSSEL. 1980. Curr. Ther. Res. **28:** 682–686.

———————◆———————

DISCUSSION

C. E. MYERS (*National Cancer Institute, Bethesda, Md.*): Since our initial description in 1977 of the activity of vitamin E in protecting the mouse against adriamycin toxicity, there have been a number of studies that have or have not duplicated that report. The people who have duplicated our observation of protection have all worked in acute animal models, and the negative studies have been in chronic animal models which are more akin to the chronic cardiomyopathy we're all worried about. I'm rather convinced at this point that there are complications that arise when one goes from an acute adriamycin cardiac toxicity to the chronic setting. At least one thing that develops is a progressive depletion of myocardial glutathione peroxidase. A progressive decrease in cardiac glutathione peroxidase with time in the chronic rabbit model has been described by Oak Ridge workers. How effective vitamin E is in the absence of glutathione peroxidase I think is an interesting question.

Y. M. WANG: The Oak Ridge study showed depletion of selenium, is that right?

C. E. MYERS: Yes. They showed that selenium became unavailable.

F. L. KRETZER (*Baylor College of Medicine, Houston, Tex.*): Over the last two years, with John McGinnis of your institute, we've been studying retinal toxicity of adriamycin in the albino rat, and it seems to be very age dependent and hormonally modulated. In the prepubescent rat, there's no photoreceptor toxicity, while in the sexually mature older rat that's nine months, 450 grams, there's a severe retinal toxicity where there is photoreceptor atrophy within six days after a single intraperitoneal injection. Apparently you can modulate this with daily injections of estradiol benzoate in the prepubescent rat and then modulate that rat to the same sensitivity as found in the sexually mature.

I think with regard to some of your data, it would be very interesting to know if the severe cardiac myopathies were in your older patients who were postmenopausal or in your young ones who were still sexually immature.

Y. M. WANG: I cannot answer that. Only 21 patients entered this study on a first-come, first-served basis.

S. B. SHOHET (*University of California, San Francisco, Calif.*): In your review, did you say that as the dose of vitamin E was increased, the protective effect was reduced as you got too high a level of vitamin E?

Y. M. WANG: That's correct.

S. B. SHOHET: Given that unusual paradox, I'd like to know if either you or Dr. Myers could suggest a possible mechanism with regard to the suppression.

C. E. MYERS: I'm very skeptical of the idea that vitamin E is going to have a very simple linear dose-response curve because I don't think it acts by itself. I think it's a component of a very complex system, and it is the integration of that whole system that is responsible for successful action. For example, glutathione peroxidase is obviously very important in vitamin E's protective effect; it can't act alone.

S. B. SHOHET: I would just like to make a gentle plea. It would be a good idea with vitamin E to be concerned about the minimal effective dose as opposed to the maximum tolerated dose.

EFFECT OF TOCOPHEROL AND SELENIUM ON DEFENSES AGAINST REACTIVE OXYGEN SPECIES AND THEIR EFFECT ON RADIATION SENSITIVITY

Charles E. Myers,* Aspandiar Katki,* and Elizabeth Travis†

*Clinical Pharmacology Branch
†Radiation Biology Branch
Clinical Oncology Program
Division of Cancer Treatment
National Cancer Institute
National Institutes of Health
Bethesda, Maryland 20205

INTRODUCTION

It is clear from the papers presented in this symposium that a large portion of the interest in vitamin E arises from the fact that radical species appear to be involved in a wide range of normal and pathologic biologic processes. The tocopherols, as naturally occurring radical quenchers, are often proposed as antagonists of these radical processes. As a specific example, our interest in tocopherols arose out of work in our laboratory on the cardiac toxicity of the anthracycline anticancer agents, daunorubicin and doxorubicin (adriamycin). In 1976 and 1977, we documented that doxorubicin administration led to the formation of malondialdehyde in cardiac muscle and that pretreatment with a preparation of mixed tocopherols suppressed both malondialdehyde formation and pathologic evidence of subacute cardiac injury.[1,2] Subsequent to that publication, both malondialdehyde formation and the protective effects of tocopherol in acute and subacute models of doxorubicin-mediated cardiac injury have been confirmed by others.[3-5] In addition, other antioxidants such as N-acetyl-cysteine[6,7] and ascorbic acid[8] have also been shown to lessen the cardiac toxicity of the anthracyclines. Considerable progress has been made on the biochemical basis for this anthracycline-induced cardiac lipid peroxidation. Handa and Sato, Bachur et al., and Goodman and Hochstein have shown that cytochrome P_{450} reductase will catalyze the reduced nicotinamide-adenine dinucleotide phosphate (NADPH)-dependent reduction of doxorubicin to a semiquinone radical that can, in turn, reduce oxygen to superoxide.[9-11] Doroshow and Reeves have shown that this reaction is also catalyzed by cardiac mitochondria and cardiac sarcoplasmic reticulum.[12]

In spite of all of this supportive evidence, there were a number of odd observations about the cardiac toxicity that were unexplained. First, why is the drug such a unique cardiac toxin? Other tissues such as liver have higher P_{450} reductase levels than does cardiac tissue, yet liver toxicity does not occur with these drugs. Second, cardiac doxorubicin levels peak 3 hours after drug administration and fall to negligible levels by 24 hours, yet lipid peroxidation is barely detectable until day 2 and peaks on day 4 (FIGURE 1). In order to explain these observations, we sought to reexamine how oxygen radicals interact with cardiac, as opposed to hepatic, tissue. In the process, we have uncovered some interesting aspects of these tissues' oxygen radical defenses.

0077-8923/82/0393-0419 $01.75/0 © 1982, NYAS

HEPATIC VERSUS CARDIAC DETOXIFICATION OF REACTIVE OXYGEN SPECIES

The results of this comparison are summarized, from previous publications by our group, in TABLE 1.[13,14] Superoxide dismutase (SOD) activity in cardiac cytosol was approximately half that of liver cytosol. In contrast, cytosol glutathione peroxidase (GSH-PX) activity was equivalent in the two tissues. On the other

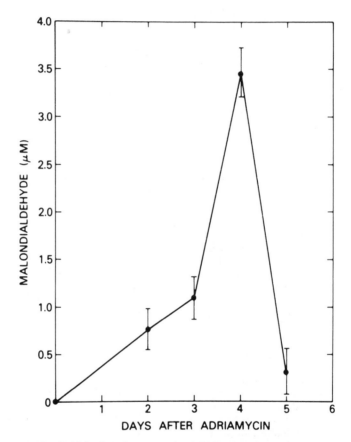

FIGURE 1. Malondialdehyde in heart muscle of CDF₁ mice after an intravenous adriamycin dose of 15 mg/kg. Malondialdehyde was measured by the 2-thiobarbituric acid technique as previously described.[2] The values reported represent the mean ± standard error of the mean.

hand, catalase activity was nearly absent from cardiac tissue, whereas it is abundant in liver. At this point we were struck by the fact that cardiac tissue, because it lacked catalase, appeared to be heavily dependent upon glutathione peroxidase for the detoxification of hydrogen peroxide.

Doxorubicin also binds to DNA and alters DNA, RNA, and protein synthesis rates. We reasoned that if glutathione peroxidase were either a rapidly turning

TABLE 1

OXYGEN RADICAL DEFENSES OF LIVER AS COMPARED TO HEART

	Liver	Heart
1. Cytosol		
SOD	100%	43%
GSH-PX	100%	86%
2. Mitochondria		
(a) Matrix		
SOD	present	present
GSH-PX	present	absent
(b) Membrane		
GSH-PX	present	present
3. Catalase	100%	0.6%
4. Effect of adriamycin on GSH-PX	none	decrease

over enzyme or were sensitive to one of the radical species generated by doxorubicin, the drug could well result in a drop in glutathione peroxidase activity. The consequence of this would be to leave cardiac tissue with no mechanism of peroxide removal at a time when drug-induced peroxide generation was occurring. For this reason, we measured cytosol glutathione peroxidase activity after doxorubicin. As is apparent from TABLE 2, a drop in glutathione peroxidase activity did occur after doxorubicin. It is interesting to note that the rise in FIGURE 1 correlates temporally with the fall in cytosol glutathione peroxidase shown in TABLE 2.

Because of these results, we next examined the subcellular distribution of glutathione peroxidase in cardiac muscle. Because this enzyme was also known to be selenium dependent, the subcellular distribution was studied in selenium deficiency as well as in normal mice. The results, presented in TABLE 3, show the expected drop in cytosol glutathione peroxidase with selenium deficiency. The surprising observation was that activity was found in mitochondria and pellet that increased slightly, rather than declined, with selenium deficiency. Because one of the coauthors had had extensive experience with isolation and fractionation of

TABLE 2

EFFECT OF DOXORUBICIN ON GLUTATHIONE PEROXIDASE*

Organ	Doxorubicin Dose (mg/kg ip)	Hours after Doxorubicin Treatment				
		4	24	48	72	96
Heart	5		93 ± 9 (NS)			
	10		63 ± 6 (p < 0.02)			
	15	104 ± 13 (NS)	43.9 ± 4.4 (p < 0.01)	77 ± 2 (p < 0.05)	53 ± 7 (p < 0.05)	84 ± 8 (NS)

*Glutathione peroxidase activity in doxorubicin-treated animals compared to simultaneous controls receiving physiologic saline, percent control ± 1 standard error; p, values of Student's t-test.

mitochondria (A.K.), the decision was made to study the nature of the selenium-independent enzyme activity in mitochondria first. Glutathione peroxidase activity in liver mitochondria had been extensively studied and found to exist in the mitochondrial matrix. This enzyme has been isolated and been shown to be a selenoprotein similar to the cytosol enzyme.[15] In fact, we were able to confirm that liver mitochondrial matrix had a selenium-dependent glutathione peroxidase. This matrix enzyme was absent from cardiac mitochondria. In the latter, the entire activity resided in the mitochondrial membrane. A similar membrane-bound selenium-independent enzyme activity was apparent in liver mitochondria isolated from selenium-deficient mice. In normal liver mitochondria, this

TABLE 3

SUBCELLULAR DISTRIBUTION OF GLUTATHIONE PEROXIDASE ACTIVITY IN HEART MUSCLE
WITH DIFFERENT SUBSTRATES IN CONTROL AND SELENIUM-DEFICIENT CDF$_1$ MICE*

Cell Fraction	Control		Selenium Deficient	
	Hydrogen Peroxide as Substrate†	Cumene Hydroperoxide as Substrate†	Hydrogen Peroxide as Substrate†	Cumene Hydroperoxide as Substrate†
Pellet	5.31	6.96	7.51	8.38
Mitochondria	10.30	9.48	11.25	10.80
Microsome	0	0	1.22	1.86
Soluble	4.33	5.11	1.28	2.85

*Subcellular fractionation was done by preparing 10% heart homogenate in 250 mM sucrose, 1 mM tris, 10 mM EDTA, pH 7.2, in a Brinkmann model PCU-2-110 Polytron 3 times for 5 seconds at 5.5 settings with cooling in between cycles. After sedimentation of the nuclear fraction (700 × g for 10 minutes), the supernatant was centrifuged at 10,000 × g for 15 minutes to sediment mitochondria. The postmitochondrial supernatant was centrifuged at 105,000 × g for 60 minutes to sediment microsomes. Nuclear, mitochondrial, and microsomal pellets were resuspended in the initial buffer. Glutathione peroxidase activity was determined by the decrease in absorbance at 340 nm by incubating enzyme in 100 mM tris, 3 mM EDTA, pH 7.0, 1.2 units glutathione reductase, 0.25 mM GSH, 3.0 mM NaN$_3$, 0.25 mM NADPH, and 0.04 mM H$_2$O$_2$ or 0.75 mM cumene hydroperoxide in 1 ml final volume. Blank reactions with the enzyme source replaced by distilled water were subtracted from each assay. The activity is expressed as nmoles NADPH oxidized/minute per mg protein using the extinction coefficient for NADPH of 6.22 × 10^3 mol^{-1} cm^{-1}. Succinate-cytochrome c reductase and rotenone-insensitive NADH-cytochrome c reductase activities were determined as mitochondrial and microsomal marker enzymes, respectively.
†Nanomoles per minute per milligram protein.

activity was quantitatively minor compared to the selenium-dependent activity, and for this reason had probably escaped detection.

The technique of digitonin fractionation of mitochondria has been extensively used to determine whether enzymes are located on the inner membrane, outer membrane, or in the space between the membranes. When such techniques are applied to the mitochondrial membrane, the selenium-independent enzyme activity is found to reside predominantly in the intermembrane space. There are relatively few proteins in this intermembrane space, and partial purification of the enzyme has been relatively easy. The partially purified enzyme has been subjected to study for selenium content by neutron activation and found to be selenium free and iron free. This indicates that this is a new class of peroxidase that differs from the selenium-dependent glutathione peroxidase and from the heme-centered peroxidases. We are now trying to purify this enzyme to homogeneity so that its properties may be studied in detail.

These studies have revealed multiple differences between cardiac tissue and liver in terms of defenses against oxygen radical detoxification. These are tabulated in TABLE 3. In summary, cytosol superoxide dismutase in heart was 50% of that in liver. Catalase was absent in heart muscle and abundant in liver. Mitochondrial matrix glutathione peroxidase was abundant in liver but absent in heart. These results all indicate that cardiac muscle is relatively speaking much more heavily dependent upon cytosol selenium-dependent glutathione peroxidase for protection against oxygen radical–induced damage. In addition to providing a basis for the selective cardiac toxicity of doxorubicin, these results may explain why cardiac damage is a common manifestation of selenium deficiency.

ROLE OF SELENIUM AND VITAMIN E IN THE RADIATION RESPONSE

Because of the above results and our previously published observation on the ability of tocopherol to protect against doxorubicin cardiac toxicity, we were interested in examining the relative contributions of tocopherol and selenium to tissue defenses against oxygen radical attack. For this purpose, doxorubicin has undesirable characteristics. It is a very complex drug in terms of its biochemistry and can engage in a variety of nonradical reactions capable of causing tissue damage.[16] Acute radiation injury, on the other hand, represents a well-defined universally accepted model for radical-induced tissue damage. As a result of our work with doxorubicin, we had developed detailed information on selenium and tocopherol deficiency in the CDF_1 mouse strain. For the studies on selenium deficiency or tocopherol deficiency, the torula yeast and lard-based diet previously described by us was used.[17] This diet is both selenium and tocopherol free. For dietary controls, some mice were also placed on Ralston Purina NIH rat and mouse ration no. 5108. This diet contained 0.33 ppm of selenium and 80 U/kg of α-tocopherol and used soybean and fish oil as major sources of fat. When newly weaned CDF_1 mice were placed on the selenium-deficient diet in the presence or absence of tocopherol, cardiac glutathione peroxidase reached a nadir of 10–20% of initial enzyme activity by 6 weeks. Thereafter, enzyme activity remained stable at this level for as long as 4 months. Over the same 6 weeks, cardiac and liver tocopherol concentration dropped from 1.2×10^{-5} M to 1.1×10^{-6} M. The animals on this diet remained in apparent good health, but exhibited impaired growth for 6–8 months, after which their health declined. Most animals were dead by the end of the 12 months. The cardiac glutathione peroxidase activity in these animals responded rapidly to selenium supplementation: 40 μg of sodium selenite intraperitoneally per day for 3 days followed by a 2-day wait resulted in restoration of normal enzyme activity. In a similar fashion, cardiac tocopherol concentration returned to normal 1 week after 85 units of RRR-α-tocopherol was administered intraperitoneally. With this animal model, we have examined the effect of selenium and tocopherol on radiation sensitivity. Animals deficient in both selenium and tocopherol exhibited an LD_{50} of 3.5 gray as compared to 6 gray for repleted mice. These results show dose modification factors of 1.8 for mice with combined deficiency and 1.4 for selenium-repleted tocopherol-deficient mice. Tocopherol-repleted, selenium-deficient mice showed the same enhanced radiation sensitivity as did the mice with combined deficiency. Thus, in the absence of selenium, tocopherol had no measurable effect on bone marrow radiation sensitivity. In the presence of selenium, however, tocopherol exhibited measurable protection. Studies are in progress on gut and skin toxicity. Tocopherol is clearly only a part of a rather complex system that defends cells against free radical damage. The results presented here suggest that the state of one of the other components of the system, the selenium-dependent glutathione peroxidase, can markedly alter the effect of tocopherol. These results suggest that it may be an error to study the role of tocopherol out of the full biochemical context in which it operates.

REFERENCES

1. MYERS, C. E., W. McGUIRE & R. C. YOUNG. 1976. Cancer Treatment Rep. **60:** 961.
2. MYERS, C. E., R. H. LISS, J. IFRIM, K. GROTZINGER & R. C. YOUNG. 1977. Science **197:** 165.
3. WANG, Y. M., F. F. MADANAT, J. G. KIMBALL, C. A. GLEISER, M. W. KAUFMAN & J. V. VANEYS. 1980. Cancer Res. **40:** 1022.
4. POGGI, A., F. DELAINI & M. D. DONATI. 1980. In Internal Medicine (Part 1): 386. Excerpta Medica. Amsterdam, the Netherlands.
5. SONNEVELD, P. 1978. Cancer Treatment Rep. **62:** 1033.
6. OLSON, R. D., J. S. MacDONALD, R. D. HARBISON, J. C. VONBOXTEL, R. C. BOERTH, A. E. SLONIM & J. A. OATES. 1977. Fed. Proc. **36:** 303.
7. DOROSHOW, J. H., G. Y. LOCKER, J. IFRIM & C. E. MYERS. 1981. J. Clin. Invest. **64:** 1053.
8. FUJITA, K., K. SHINPO, K. YAMADA, T. SATO, H. NIIMI, M. SHAMOTO, T. NAGATAU, T. TAKEUCHI & H. UMEZAWA. 1982. Cancer Res. **42:** 309.
9. HANDA, K. & S. SATO. 1975. Gann **66:** 43.
10. BACHUR, N. A., S. L. GORDON, M. V. GEL & H. KON. 1979. Proc. Nat. Acad. Sci. **76:** 954.
11. GOODMAN, J. & P. HOCHSTEIN. 1977. Biochem. Biophys. Res. Commun. **77:** 797.
12. DOROSHOW, J. H. & J. REEVES. 1980. Proc. Am. Assoc. Cancer Res. **21:** 1067.
13. DOROSHOW, J. H., G. Y. LOCKER & C. E. MYERS. 1980. J. Clin. Invest. **65:** 128.
14. KATKI, A. G. & C. E. MYERS. 1980. Biochem. Biophys. Res. Commun. **96:** 85.
15. ZAKOWSKI, J. J. & A. L. TAPPEL. 1978. Biochim. Biophys. Acta **197:** 31.
16. YOUNG, R. C., R. F. OZOLS & C. E. MYERS. 1981. N. Engl. J. Med. **305:** 139.
17. LOCKER, G. Y., J. H. DOROSHOW, J. C. BALDINGER & C. E. MYERS. 1979. Nutr. Rep. Int. **19:** 671.

DISCUSSION

B. D. GOLDSTEIN (*College of Medicine and Dentistry of New Jersey, Piscataway, N.J.*): Do you have a metal requirement for this? Is there any metal at all associated with it?

C. E. MYERS: By neutron activation analysis, there was no selenium and no iron, the two things we expected to find in there. There was a lot of cobalt, but that needs to be confirmed by other techniques.

V. SRINIVASAN (*National Naval Medical Center, Bethesda, Md.*): The point that you made about the gut microcolonies not showing an effect was perhaps because of the doses that you measured. Radiation doses that you've used are in the range of 700 rads, which would bring about changes in the hematological parameters as you have shown. Probably if you had taken a higher radiation dose, you might have observed some changes with the gut microcolonies.

C. E. MYERS: The major purpose of this first set of experiments was to find out what the lesion was that was killing the animals that were deficient. It wasn't to answer the question, Does selenium deficiency affect the radiation response with every tissue?

There was at least a possibility that the gut might have been so increased in sensitivity that it now became the most sensitive tissue. And I think we've excluded that, but I think that in this system one would need to examine in a formal way the radiation dose response of each tissue.

R. L. BAEHNER (*Indiana University, Indianapolis, Ind.*): I wanted to compliment you on your animal model and acquaint the audience with some of the differences in species between the catalase and glutathione peroxidase systems. Your model may not be directly applicable to the human situation. In 1979, Colleen Higgins in our laboratory noted that there was a reciprocal relationship between the catalase and glutathione peroxidase activities in polymorphonuclear leukocytes. She found that in the human as well as in the guinea pig, there were close parallelisms between catalase and glutathione peroxidase and that in those two species, there was much more catalase activity relative to the glutathione peroxidase.

However, in the rat and mouse models, there was much more glutathione peroxidase activity and virtually no catalase activity. It would be of interest to develop an animal model in a guinea pig as well, to see if we can then make some conclusions that might also be applicable to human situations.

C. E. MYERS: Yes, I think that the catalase–glutathione peroxidase story we've put together has been shown in rats and rabbits. Each species is a study in and of itself. But I think that the big need is for information on the concentration of these various enzymes in a variety of human tissues. The blood elements have been fairly well studied, but we don't have any data on the human heart and the various zones of the kidney, for example. The liver has been studied; but those are the three tissues that we particularly would like to know something about.

R. L. BAEHNER: You mentioned that cardiac muscle was deficient in catalase. I'm assuming that was in your mouse model?

C. E. MYERS: Yes, that's true in mouse, rat, and rabbit, but no one has studied the human heart.

R. BRYANT (*George Washington University Medical School, Washington, D.C.*): Have you measured a K_m for the non-selenium-dependent enzyme for glutathione?

C. E. MYERS: No we have not measured a K_m at the present time. We're a little reluctant to begin that. If you notice, I only showed you an SDS [sodium dedecyl sulfate] gel of the purified protein, and that's because the "purified" protein exists as such in multiple states of aggregation. The one Michaelis curve that we did was very curvilinear and difficult to interpret.

C. C. REDDY (*Pennsylvania State University, University Park, Pa.*): This makes it more complicated. I don't known how many glutathione peroxidases exist in the cell. Did you measure the transferase activity of this purified protein?

C. E. MYERS: No, we haven't done that yet. I think that would be very interesting.

C. C. REDDY: Is there a selenium-dependent protein in mitochondria?

C. E. MYERS: In cardiac mitochondria, we can detect no evidence of a selenium-dependent glutathione peroxidase. People have reported in heart mitochondria the incorporation of radioactive selenium into the electron transport schema, then speculated on its involvement in the iron sulfur protein steps. But we haven't looked at that.

DIETARY VITAMIN E AND CELLULAR
SUSCEPTIBILITY TO CIGARETTE SMOKING*

Ching K. Chow

Department of Nutrition and Food Science
University of Kentucky
Lexington, Kentucky 40506

INTRODUCTION

Cigarette smoke comprises a large variety of chemical substances, and approximately 3,000 compounds have been identified.[1] It has been implicated to contribute to the causation and exacerbation of various chronic respiratory diseases and to affect the blood vessels, heart, and various disorders in man. However, relatively little is known concerning the biological consequences of cigarette smoking.

As cigarette smoke contains a large variety of compounds, it is not surprising that many of them are oxidants or prooxidants capable of initiating or enhancing free radical lipid peroxidation. For example, Pryor has identified alkoxy, aroyoxy, and nitrogen dioxide free radicals in the gaseous phase of cigarette smoke.[2] Nitrogen dioxide, one of the major oxidant air pollutants present in photochemical smog, is found in smoke at the level of up to 250 parts per million. Animal experiments indicate that nitrogen dioxide can have irreversible effects on the respiratory system at a concentration as low as 1 ppm.[3]

As nutrients are essential for all fundamental cellular processes, their role in modulating the action and metabolism of chemicals, drugs, and environmental pollutants has gained considerable recent research interest. For example, administration of vitamin E to experimental animals has been shown to lessen the toxicity of a variety of compounds such as ozone,[4,5] oxygen,[6] lead,[7] paraquat,[8] adriamycin,[9] nitrofurantoin,[10] nitrosamine,[11] methyl mercury,[12] and cadmium.[13] While the precise mechanism of such effects is not yet clear, vitamin E may protect cellular components from the adverse effects of those compounds either via a free radical–scavenging mechanism or as a component of cell membrane.[14] In both animals and humans, vitamin E deficiency has been shown to be associated with platelet hyperaggregability and to increase the synthesis of platelet endoperoxide and prostaglandins *in vivo*.[15] Thus vitamin E may exert its protective effect against smoke-induced myocardial infarction via the suppression of prostaglandin synthesis and prevention of platelet hyperaggregability. Similarly, the cigarette-smoking-induced aggregate formation has been shown to be preventable by aspirin administration.[16]

The studies reported herein deal primarily with the influence of dietary vitamin E on cellular susceptibility of rats to cigarette smoking. Efforts were also made to examine the possible role of lipid peroxidation in the toxicity of cigarette smoking.

*Supported by the University of Kentucky Agricultural Experiment Station and by Hoffmann-La Roche, Inc.

0077-8923/82/0393-0426 $01.75/0 © 1982, NYAS

Male Sprague-Dawley rats were used as experimental animals. Weanling rats received from the supplier (Harlan Industries, Inc., Indianapolis, Ind.) were initially maintained on Purina rat chow for 5–10 days. They were then randomly divided into two groups and fed a basal vitamin E–deficient diet[17] supplemented with either nothing or 100 ppm vitamin E (as all-rac-α-tocopheryl acetate) for four to eight weeks prior to smoking treatment. As determined spectrophotofluorometrically,[18] the selenium content of the basal diet averaged 0.02 ppm. The nutritional status of vitamin E was monitored by measuring the degree of erythrocyte hemolysis[19] and activity of plasma pyruvate kinase.[20]

Animals were exposed to either sham smoke, gaseous phase of smoke, or whole smoke at 10–120 puffs/exposure (one exposure per day) for up to seven days using either a single-port reverse-phase smoking machine[21] or a peristaltic pump smoking machine designed by Dr. Robert Griffith of the College of Pharmacy, University of Kentucky. Additional animals were also maintained to serve as room controls. The single-port reverse-phase smoking machine generates a retilinear puff of 2 seconds duration and 35 ml volume once per minute. The puff is diluted to 10% concentration with fresh air in the inhalation chamber and is held there for 15 seconds. The smoke-air mixture is then removed from the chamber, and fresh air is introduced for the remaining 45 seconds. The nonfiltered University of Kentucky reference cigarette A1, which contains low nicotine, was employed for this type of exposure. The peristaltic pump smoking machine also generates a 35-ml puff volume per minute. The initial puff at the concentration of up to 50% is delivered to the exposure system and remains there for 2 seconds. In the next 2 seconds, smoke in the recycle loop is diluted by air from the pump head, and one-half concentration of the initial smoke is delivered to the exposure system. The concentration of smoke is continuously decreased by half every 2 seconds until the next puff is generated. The gaseous phase of smoke is generated and total particulate matter of smoke is monitored by using a Cambridge filter. The University of Kentucky reference cigarette 2R1 was used for this type of smoking exposure.

Sixteen hours following each exposure period, animals from each group were killed following ethereal anesthetization and withdrawal of blood. Tissues (lung, kidney, heart, liver, spleen, and testis) were examined for abnormal changes and were removed, blotted, and weighed. Lungs and in some cases kidneys were homogenized with isotonic phosphate buffer, pH 7.4. The tissue homogenates and 9,000 × g supernatant fraction as well as blood plasma and/or serum were then pipetted for the measurement of various biochemical parameters. The significance of difference between sample means was determined using Student's t-test at a 95% confidence interval.

RESULTS

Animal Mortality, Body Weight, and Tissue Weight

When one-month-old male rats maintained on a vitamin E–deficient diet for five weeks were exposed to 10% cigarette smoke at 120 puffs/exposure using a single-port reverse-phase smoking machine, 5 out of 16 animals died within 24 hours following the single exposure, as compared with 1 out of 13 from the

TABLE 1

EFFECT OF DIETARY VITAMIN E AND CIGARETTE SMOKE ON RATS*

Exposure Period (days)	Parameter	Without Vitamin E		With Vitamin E (100 ppm)	
		Smoke	Sham	Smoke	Sham
3	Animal mortality	5/16	0/10	1/13	0/10
	Body weight (g)	175 ± 19†	187 ± 14	186 ± 16	183 ± 12
	Lung weight (g)	0.89 ± 0.07	0.87 ± 0.09	0.86 ± 0.11	0.87 ± 0.07
	Lung protein (mg/lung cyt.)‡	63 ± 4	62 ± 6	63 ± 4	64 ± 4
7	Animal mortality	0/5	0/5	0/6	0/6
	Body weight (g)	168 ± 19	183 ± 12	194 ± 13	210 ± 12
	Lung weight (g)	0.99 ± 0.10	0.91 ± 0.10	0.92 ± 0.05	0.94 ± 0.09
	Lung protein (mg/lung cyt.)	68 ± 4	64 ± 6	65 ± 5	67 ± 5

*One-month-old male rats maintained on the respective diets for five weeks were exposed to 120 puffs of cigarette smoke or sham for the first day and 50 puffs/day from day 2.

†Mean ± standard deviation.

‡Cyt. is cytosol.

vitamin E-supplemented group (TABLE 1). No animal mortality occurred when animals were exposed to 60 puffs/exposure or less for up to seven days by either type of smoking machine. None of the sham exposed animals from both dietary groups died during the experimental periods.

The body weight, tissue weight (lung, liver, kidney, spleen, testis, and heart), and protein contents in the lungs and kidneys of both dietary groups of animals were not significantly altered by smoking exposure under the experimental conditions.

Blood Cell Concentrations

The lung with airway and alveolar surface exposed directly to the external environment is vulnerable to injury from a variety of agents, including cigarette smoke. However, the blood cells may become exposed to cigarette smoke at the lung parenchymal gas-exchange surface. Increased carboxyhemoglobin levels in blood with secondary tissue hypoxia have been suggested to be associated with increased hematocrit values in smokers.[22] In patients who stopped smoking, hematocrit values were found to decrease from a mean of 56% down to 46%.[23] Smoking has also been linked to an increase in white blood cell count and red cell mean corpuscular volume.[24] As expected, animals exposed to either whole smoke or gaseous phase of smoke exhibited a marked increase in the blood levels of carboxyhemoglobin when measured immediately after each exposure. The levels of carboxyhemoglobin were proportionate to the concentration of smoke inhaled, and were not affected by the nutritional status of vitamin E. Smoke-exposed animals were found to have higher red cell counts, mean cell volume, and hematocrit and hemoglobin levels, while white blood cell counts were either unchanged or depressed. The magnitude of the alterations was more profound in the blood of animals fed the vitamin E–deficient diet than in the supplemented group.

Plasma/Serum Enzymes and Lipids

To determine if biochemical alterations in the easily accessible blood plasma/serum can be employed as sensitive parameters for monitoring the cellular effect of cigarette smoking, the activities of plasma/serum enzymes known to be increased by the deprivation of vitamin E were determined. While the activities of pyruvate kinase, lactate dehydrogenase, glutamic oxaloacetic transaminase, alkaline phosphatase, and creatine phosphokinase were found to increase significantly in the plasma/serum of vitamin E-deficient rats, the activities of these enzymes and levels of serum cholesterol and triglyceride were not significantly affected by cigarette smoking under the experimental conditions.

Ascorbic Acid and Vitamin E

Studies have shown lower blood vitamin C levels[25] and decreased urinary excretion of vitamin C[26] among human smokers. Although the mechanism of the decreases is not yet known, it appears to be a reduced bioavailability of vitamin C in cigarette smokers. As in the human studies, the plasma levels of L-ascorbic acid in rats were found to decrease following smoking exposure (TABLES 2 and 3). The degree of the decline was of a greater magnitude in animals fed the vitamin E-deficient diet than in the supplemented group. On the other hand, the levels of ascorbic acid in the lungs of vitamin E-deficient rats, but not the supplemented animals, were found to increase significantly following smoking exposure. It appears that an increased amount of ascorbic acid may be synthesized in the lungs of smoke-exposed rats to meet their increased need. A marked stimulation of hepatic ascorbic acid biosynthesis in rats and mice has been reported upon exposure to various noxious compounds.[27,28]

The functional interrelationship between ascorbic acid and vitamin E has been known for many years.[29] While our results indicate that cigarette smoking

TABLE 2

EFFECT OF CIGARETTE SMOKE AND DIETARY VITAMIN E ON PLASMA
LEVELS OF ASCORBIC ACID AND VITAMIN E*

| | | Three Days | | Seven Days | |
| | | Dietary Vitamin E (ppm) | | Dietary Vitamin E (ppm) | |
	Exposure	0	100	0	100
Ascorbic	sham	847 ± 29 (6)†	1,156 ± 28 (6)	813 ± 18 (5)	1,250 ± 34 (7)
acid	smoke	665 ± 47 (6)	1,095 ± 40 (6)	708 ± 62 (7)	1,064 ± 51 (7)
	p‡	<0.005	NS§	<0.05	<0.005
Vitamin E	sham	151 ± 24 (6)	640 ± 25 (6)	172 ± 11 (5)	679 ± 23 (7)
	smoke	146 ± 23 (6)	679 ± 54 (6)	144 ± 11 (7)	718 ± 22 (7)
	p	NS	NS	NS	NS

*One-month-old male rats were fed the respective diets for 5 weeks and were exposed to cigarette smoke or sham for three or seven days.

†Mean ± standard error; number in parentheses represents number of animals per group. The data are expressed as μg/100 ml.

‡Student's t-test.

§Not significant (p > 0.05).

TABLE 3

DIETARY VITAMIN E AND LEVELS OF ASCORBIC ACID IN THE PLASMA, LUNG,
AND KIDNEY OF CIGARETTE-SMOKE-EXPOSED RATS*

Dietary Vitamin E (ppm)	Treatment	Plasma (mg/100 ml)	Lung (mg/g)	Kidney (mg/ml)
0	smoke	1.29 ± 0.12 (8)†	147.0 ± 9.3	82.3 ± 5.3
	sham	1.53 ± 0.14 (6)	115.8 ± 9.3	80.5 ± 7.8
		$p < 0.01$‡	$p < 0.001$	NS§
100	smoke	1.37 ± 0.11 (8)	119.5 ± 8.5	74.3 ± 6.8
	sham	1.56 ± 0.10 (4)	130.3 ± 11.0	72.5 ± 4.5
		$p < 0.02$	NS	NS

*One-month-old male rats maintained on the respective diets for eight weeks were exposed to either sham or cigarette smoke for seven days.

†Mean ± standard deviation; number in parentheses represents number of animals in each group.

‡Student's t-test.

§Not significant ($p > 0.05$).

did not significantly affect the plasma levels of vitamin E (TABLE 2), vitamin E supplementation appears to aid in maintaining plasma ascorbic acid of smoke-exposed animals at a higher level.

Lipid Peroxidation Products and the Glutathione Peroxidase System

Cigarette smoke contains a large variety of compounds including oxidants and free radicals.[1,2] The aqueous phase of the cigarette smoke has been shown to be capable of initiating autoxidation of unsaturated lipids of alveolar macrophages in vitro.[30] The activities of the potentially protective enzymes, glutathione (GSH) peroxidase and its metabolically related enzymes, have been reported to increase in the lungs of cigarette-smoke-exposed rats.[31] The reduction of the elastase-inhibiting capability of α_1-antitrypsin in the lung lavage fluid of cigarette-smoke-exposed rats has been shown to be preventable by reducing agents.[32] These findings suggest that an oxidative damage mechanism may be involved in the adverse effects of cigarette smoking.

TABLE 4

DIETARY VITAMIN E AND THIOBARBITURIC ACID REACTANTS
IN THE LUNGS OF CIGARETTE-SMOKE-EXPOSED RATS*

Exposure Period (days)	Without Vitamin E		With Vitamin E (100 ppm)	
	Smoke	Sham	Smoke	Sham
3	7.1 ± 0.8†	8.9 ± 0.8‡	6.2 ± 0.9†	7.1 ± 0.8†
7	6.4 ± 0.8†	8.7 ± 1.1‡	5.8 ± 0.4	6.5 ± 0.7†

*One-month-old male rats maintained on the respective diets for five weeks were exposed to 120 puffs of cigarette smoke or sham on day 1 and 50 puffs/day from day 2. The data are expressed as μmoles/lung; mean ± standard deviation. Figures with different symbols (†, ‡) are significantly different ($p < 0.05$).

In our attempt to determine the possible role of free radical lipid peroxidation in smoke-induced toxicity, we measured the levels of lipid peroxidation products—thiobarbituric acid reactants—in the lung homogenate with or without prior incubation at 37°C for one hour. Contrary to our expectation, the levels of thiobarbituric acid reactants were found to be decreased, rather than increased, in the lungs of cigarette-smoke-exposed rats as compared with those of the sham-smoke-exposed animals (TABLE 4). Such a depression effect, however, was observed only when animals were exposed to whole smoke, and not to the gaseous phase of smoke.

Similar to the report of York et al.,[31] the levels of GSH and the activities of GSH peroxidase, GSH reductase, and glucose 6-phosphate dehydrogenase in the lungs were variably increased following cigarette-smoking exposure (TABLE 5).

TABLE 5

DIETARY VITAMIN E AND THE GSH PEROXIDASE SYSTEM IN THE LUNGS
OF CIGARETTE-SMOKE-EXPOSED RATS*

Dietary Vitamin E (ppm)	Biochemical Parameter	Sham Smoke	Gaseous Phase	Whole Smoke
0	GSH (μmoles/lung)	0.99 ± 0.08†	1.29 ± 0.24‡	1.40 ± 0.33‡
	GSH peroxidase (μmoles/minute per lung)	1.44 ± 0.20†	1.54 ± 0.28†	1.56 ± 0.20†
	GSH reductase (μmoles/minute per lung)	1.53 ± 0.23†	1.45 ± 0.12†	1.53 ± 0.19†
	G-6-P dehydrogenase (μmoles/minute per lung)	1.64 ± 0.14†	1.74 ± 0.18†	2.00 ± 0.19‡
100	GSH (μmoles/lung)	1.09 ± 0.16†	1.10 ± 0.12†	1.29 ± 0.14‡
	GSH peroxidase (μmoles/minute per lung)	1.46 ± 0.32†	1.62 ± 0.24†	1.50 ± 0.16†
	GSH reductase (μmoles/minute per lung)	1.53 ± 0.20†	1.58 ± 0.20†	1.58 ± 0.15†
	G-6-P dehydrogenase (μmoles/minute per lung)	1.83 ± 0.21†	1.79 ± 0.19†	1.95 ± 0.23†

*One-month-old male rats maintained on the respective diets for four weeks were exposed to 10 puffs/day for four days. Figures are mean ± standard deviation; eight animals in each group. Figures with different symbols (†, ‡) differ significantly ($p < 0.05$).

However, the magnitude of the changes was, in general, dose dependent and was greater in the lungs of animals fed the vitamin E–deficient diet than in those of the supplemented groups.

Aryl Hydrocarbon Hydroxylase and GSH-S-transferase

Aryl hydrocarbon hydroxylase is the most thoroughly studied microsomal monooxygenase, and is considered to be a good indicator of cytochrome P_{450}-mediated metabolism. Induction of this mixed-function oxidase has been shown to be a biochemical change that occurs in the lung and other tissues as a direct response to cigarette smoking in humans and animals.[33,34] As expected, the activity of aryl hydrocarbon hydroxylase was found to be significantly increased in the lungs of cigarette-smoke-exposed rats fed either the vitamin E-deficient or the supplemented diet. The activity of this enzyme was also found to be significantly increased in the kidney of smoke-exposed rats maintained on the vitamin E-deficient diet, but not those on the supplemented diet.

GSH-S-transferases are important enzymes that catalyze the metabolism of diverse foreign compounds, including carcinogens.[35] They are also known to bind certain drugs nonenzymatically both reversibly and covalently and thereby decrease the drugs' potential toxicity.[36] The activity of GSH-S-transferase was found to increase significantly in the lungs of cigarette-smoke-exposed rats maintained on the vitamin E-deficient diet, but not in the supplemented group (TABLE 6). The enzyme activity in the kidneys was not significantly altered by cigarette-smoke exposure in either dietary group of animals.

TABLE 6

EFFECT OF DIETARY VITAMIN E AND CIGARETTE SMOKE
ON GSH S-TRANSFERASE ACTIVITY*

Tissue	Dietary Vitamin E (ppm)	Enzyme Activity (nmoles/minute per g tissue)		
		Sham	Smoke	p‡
Lung	0	729 ± 116 (6)†	1,016 ± 91 (8)	<0.001
	100	724 ± 50 (4)	795 ± 116 (8)	NS§
Kidney	0	1,489 ± 60 (6)	1,444 ± 121 (8)	NS
	100	1,796 ± 111 (4)	1,675 ± 1.1 (8)	NS

*One-month-old rats maintained on the respective diets for eight weeks were exposed to sham or cigarette smoke for seven days.

†Mean ± standard deviation; number in parentheses represents number of animals in each group.

‡Student's t-test.

§Not significant (p > 0.05).

DISCUSSION

Increasing evidence indicates that diet plays an important role in modulating the action and metabolism of a number of chemicals, drugs, and environmental agents. While the metabolic machinery of the affected subject is able to reverse or prevent most of the adverse effects due to noxious agents under normal conditions, irreversible damage may occur when the cellular defense capability is weakened due to nutritional deficiency or inadequacy. On the other hand, optimal nutrient intake may enhance the defense systems and thus minimize the cellular effects or tissue damage. Thus it is possible that dietary inadequacy of such nutrients as vitamin E may enhance cellular susceptibility to cigarette smoking and lead to the development of respiratory disease, and that dietary vitamin E may afford protection against the adverse effects of cigarette smoking.

Coupled with the higher animal mortality rate, greater increases in the levels of GSH, GSH reductase, GSH-S-transferase, and ascorbic acid in the lungs of vitamin E-deficient rats following smoke exposure suggest that deprivation of dietary vitamin E renders rats more susceptible to the effect of cigarette smoke. Although the mechanism of such an effect is not clear in view of the proposed antioxidant function of vitamin E, it is possible that vitamin E deprivation may alter cellular stability and permeability of pulmonary tissue and thus alter the cellular effect of cigarette smoking. Vitamin E has been shown to alter the toxicity of a large variety of compounds.[4-13]

While the available information suggests that an oxidative damage mechanism may be involved in the toxicity of cigarette smoking, the results obtained, however, showed that the levels of thiobarbituric acid reactants were decreased, rather than increased, in the lungs of cigarette-smoke-exposed rats. Our results also showed that only whole smoke, and not the gaseous phase of smoke, caused a decrease in the levels of thiobarbituric acid reactants in the lungs. The findings suggest an overall reducing nature of cigarette smoke, and that the reducing compounds present in the particulate fraction may be mainly responsible for the observed decline of thiobarbituric acid reactants. Thus, despite the presence of a number of free radicals and oxidants in smoke, lipid peroxidation does not appear to be a major factor contributing to the adverse effects of smoke exposure.

While the gaseous phase of smoke was found to be as effective as whole smoke in raising the levels of blood carboxyhemoglobin, the biochemical changes resulting from smoke exposure were more severe in the lungs of rats exposed to whole smoke than in those exposed to the gaseous phase of smoke. These results indicate that the Cambridge filter employed was effective in removing portions of the reactive or harmful substances from the whole smoke, and that the smoke particulate matter may be mainly responsible for the pulmonary effect of cigarette smoking.

The mechanism of the biochemical changes observed is yet to be elucidated. It is possible that the increased activities of enzymes in the lungs of smoke-exposed rats may be an adaptive response to counteract further damage. However, it is also possible that the biochemical changes may simply result from nonspecific injury-response processes of pulmonary cells, as in the case of insults resulting from a variety of irritants.[37-40] Further morphometric and histochemical studies are needed to provide a better understanding as to the role of alveolar macrophages, type 2 cells, and other types of cells in the biochemical responses to cigarette smoking and the biological significance of the biochemical changes.

ACKNOWLEDGMENTS

The author is grateful for the collaboration and assistance of Dr. R. Griffith, Dr. L. Chen, Dr. C. Gairola, Dr. M. Reese, and Mr. R. Thacker and for the technical assistance provided by the University of Kentucky Tobacco and Health Research Institute.

REFERENCES

1. PETTERSSON, B., M. CURVALL & C. R. ENZELL. 1980. Effects of tobacco smoke compounds on the noradrenaline induced oxidative metabolism in isolated brown fat cells. Toxicology 18: 1–15.
2. PRYOR, W. A. 1978. Bio-organic chemistry of ozone, nitrogen dioxide and tobacco smoke. In Directory of Ongoing Research in Smoking and Health: 242–243. U.S. Department of Health, Education and Welfare, Public Health Service. Rockville, Md.

3. PARKINSON, D. R. & R. J. STEPHENS. 1973. Morphological surface changes in the terminal bronchial regions of NO_2-exposed rat lung. Environ. Res. **6**: 37-51.
4. GOLDSTEIN, B. D., R. D. BUCKLEY, R. CARDENAS & O. J. BALCHUM. 1970. Ozone and vitamin E. Science **169**: 605-606.
5. MENZEL, D. B., J. N. ROEHM & S. D. LEE. 1972. Vitamin E: the biological and environmental antioxidant. J. Agric. Food Chem. **20**: 481-486.
6. MINO, M. 1973. Oxygen poisoning and vitamin E deficiency. J. Nutr. Sci. Vitaminol. **19**: 95-104.
7. LEVANDER, O. A., V. C. MORRIS & R. J. FERRETTI. 1977. Comparative effects of selenium and vitamin E in lead-poisoned rats. J. Nutr. **107**: 378-382.
8. BLOCK, E. R. 1979. Potentiation of acute paraquat toxicity by vitamin E deficiency. Lung **156**: 195-203.
9. DOROSHOW, J. H., G. Y. LOCKER & C. E. MYERS. 1979. Experimental animal models of adriamycin cardiotoxicity. Cancer Treatment Rep. **63**: 855-860.
10. BOYD, M. R., G. L. CATIGNANI, H. A. SASAME, J. R. MITCHELL & A. W. STIKO. 1979. Acute pulmonary injury in rats by nitrofurantoin and modification by vitamin E, dietary fat and oxygen. Am. Rev. Respir. Dis. **120**: 93-99.
11. DASHMAN, T. & J. J. KAMM. 1979. Effects of high doses of vitamin E on dimethylnitrosamine hepatotoxicity and drug metabolism in the rat. Biochem. Pharmacol. **28**: 1485-1490.
12. WELSH, S. O. 1979. The protective effect of vitamin E and N,N'-diphenyl-p-phenylenediamine (DPPD) against methyl mercury toxicity in the rat. J. Nutr. **109**: 1673-1681.
13. KORKEALA, H. 1980. The effect of vitamin E on the toxicity of cadmium in cadmium-sensitive Staphylococcus aureus. Acta Vet. Scand. **21**: 224-228.
14. LUCY, J. A. 1972. Functional and structural aspects of biological membranes: a suggested structural role for vitamin E in the control of membrane permeability and stability. Ann. N.Y. Acad. Sci. **203**: 4-11.
15. STUART, M. J. & F. A. OSKI. 1979. Vitamin E and platelet function. Am. J. Pediatr. Hematol. Oncol. **1**: 77-82.
16. DAVIS, J. W. & R. F. DAVIS. 1981. Prevention of cigarette smoking-induced platelet aggregate formation by aspirin. Arch. Intern. Med. **141**: 206-207.
17. SCHWARZ, K. & A. FREDGA. 1969. Biological potency of organic selenium compounds. J. Biol. Chem. **244**: 2103-2110.
18. SPALLHOLZ, J. E., G. F. COLLINS & K. SCHWARZ. 1978. A single-test-tube method for the fluorometric microdetermination of selenium. Bioinorg. Chem. **9**: 453-459.
19. DRAPER, H. H. & A. S. CSALLANY. 1969. A simplified hemolysis study for vitamin E deficiency. J. Nutr. **98**: 390-394.
20. CHOW, C. K. 1975. Increased activity of pyruvate kinase in plasma of vitamin E-deficient rats. J. Nutr. **105**: 1221-1224.
21. GRIFFITH, R. B., J. F. BENNER, S. S. OWENS & R. L. HANCOCK. 1972. The design and construction of machines for the controlled generation of smoke. Proc. Univ. Kentucky Tobacco Health Res. Inst. Conf. Rep. **3**: 71-84.
22. SMITH, J. R. & S. A. LANDAW. 1978. Smokers' polycythemia. N. Engl. J. Med. **298**: 6-10.
23. MCALOON, E. J., R. R. STREIFF & C. S. KITCHENS. 1980. Erythrocytosis associated with carboxyhemoglobinemia in smokers. South. Med. J. **73**: 137-139.
24. HELMAN, N. & L. S. RUBENSTEIN. 1975. The effect of age, sex and smoking on erythrocytes and leukocytes. Am. J. Clin. Pathol. **63**: 35-44.
25. PELLETIER, O. 1970. Vitamin C status of cigarette smokers and nonsmokers. Am. J. Clin. Nutr. **23**: 520-528.
26. PELLETIER, O. 1969. Smoking and vitamin C levels in humans. Am. J. Clin. Nutr. **21**: 1259-1267.
27. BOYLAND, E. & P. L. GROVE. 1961. Stimulation of ascorbic acid synthesis and excretion by carcinogenic and other foreign compounds. Biochem. J. **81**: 163-168.
28. CONNEY, A. H. & J. J. BURNS. 1959. Stimulatory effects of foreign compounds on ascorbic acid biosynthesis and on drug-metabolizing enzymes. Nature **184**: 363-364.
29. CHOW, C. K. 1979. Nutritional influence on cellular antioxidant defense systems. Am. J. Clin. Nutr. **32**: 1066-1081.

30. LENTZ, P. E. & N. R. DI LUZIO. 1974. Peroxidation of lipids in alveolar macrophages. Production by aqueous extracts of cigarette smoke. Arch. Environ. Health **28:** 279–282.

31. YORK, G. K., T. H. PEIRCE, L. W. SCHWARTZ & C. E. CROSS. 1976. Stimulation by cigarette smoke of glutathione peroxidase system enzyme activities in rat lung. Arch. Environ. Health **31:** 286–290.

32. JANOFF, A., H. CARP & D. K. LEE. 1979. Cigarette smoke inhalation decreases α_1-antitrypsin activity in rat lung. Science **206:** 1313–1314.

33. AKIN, F. J. & J. F. BENNER. 1976. Induction of aryl hydrocarbon hydroxylase in rodent lung by cigarette smoke: a potential short-term bioassay. Toxicol. Appl. Pharmacol. **36:** 331–337.

34. CONTRELL, E. T., G. A. WARR, D. L. BUSBEE & R. R. MARTIN. 1973. Induction of aryl hydrocarbon hydroxylase in human alveolar macrophages by cigarette smoking. J. Clin. Invest. **52:** 1881–1884.

35. SMITH, G. J., V. S. OHL & G. LITWACK. 1977. Ligandin, the glutathione S-transferases, and chemically induced hepatocarcinogenesis: a review. Cancer Res. **37:** 8–14.

36. CHASSEAUL, L. F. 1976. Conjugation with glutathione and mercapturic acid excretion. In Glutathione: Metabolism and Function. I. M. Arias & B. B. Jacob, Eds.: 77–114. Raven Press. New York, N.Y.

37. EVANS, M. J., R. B. BILS & C. G. LOOSLI. 1971. Effects of ozone on cell renewal in pulmonary alveoli of aging mice. Arch. Environ. Health **22:** 450–453.

38. BUS, J. A., A. VINEGAR & S. M. BROOKS. 1978. Biochemical and physiologic changes in lungs of rats exposed to a cadmium chloride aerosol. Am. Rev. Respir. Dis. **118:** 573–580.

39. WITSCHI, H. & W. SAHEB. 1974. Stimulation of DNA synthesis in mouse lung following intraperitoneal injection of butylated hydrotoluene. Proc. Soc. Exp. Biol. Med. **147:** 690–693.

40. BOWDEN, D. H. & I. Y. R. ADAMSON. 1974. Endothelial regeneration as a marker of the differential vascular responses in oxygen-induced pulmonary edema. Lab. Invest. **30:** 350–357.

DISCUSSION

B. D. GOLDSTEIN (*College of Medicine and Dentistry of New Jersey, Piscataway, N.J.*): Why did your animals die that were exposed to cigarette smoke? They didn't have any more lung edema, so they didn't die in pulmonary edema, and there didn't seem to be any more carboxyhemoglobin. What is it about vitamin E deficiency that makes them more susceptible?

C. K. CHOW: We don't know the cause of the deaths.

B. D. GOLDSTEIN: Do you think that vitamin E deficiency makes one more prone to carboxyhemoglobinemia?

C. K. CHOW: No, smoke-exposed animals in both dietary groups had similar carboxyhemoglobin levels.

V. SRINIVASAN (*National Naval Medical Center, Bethesda, Md.*): Do you wash the lungs before doing the thiobarbituric acid measurement?

C. K. CHOW: No.

V. SRINIVASAN: I have a comment. The thiobarbituric acid test is not really sensitive by itself. But if you apply a stress, such as using NADPH plus ferrous or ascorbate plus ferrous, it will be much more sensitive.

W. A. PRYOR (*Louisiana State University, Baton Rouge, La.*): You said that particulate matter was primarily responsible. Why did you conclude that?

C. K. CHOW: Only whole smoke, but not the gaseous phase, suppresses the thiobarbituric acid reactants.

W. A. PRYOR: The gaseous phase is what comes through a Cambridge filter?

C. K. CHOW: Right. It does have the same effect on carboxyhemoglobin content as whole smoke does, but it doesn't suppress thiobarbituric acid reactants in the lung.

W. A. PRYOR: One thing I didn't mention in my presentation is that when you try to measure the free radical content of gas-phase smoke, you find that the radicals in gas-phase smoke react very rapidly with a tar component, and the only way you can get an estimate of the free radical content of gas-phase smoke is by filtering out particulate matter. That doesn't mean that in whole smoke the gas-phase free radicals aren't there. The detection method we use requires that you first dissolve the material in a liquid. In that liquid phase, the gas-phase radicals and the particulate matter react together, and in fact we studied that reaction and it's very fast. So I think some caution is necessary in interpreting these results that you're quoting.

C. K. CHOW: I agree, particularly when you are dealing with the thousands of compounds here.

VITAMIN E AND IMMUNE REGULATION*

Laurence M. Corwin and Richard K. Gordon

Department of Microbiology
Boston University School of Medicine
Boston, Massachusetts 02118

Introduction

An assessment of the minimal daily requirement (MDR) of a nutrient involves a determination of the least amount of the nutrient that will prevent clinical symptoms of a deficiency or support a well-defined physiological or biochemical response. The requirement for vitamin E of human adults set forth by the National Research Council is 15 IU/day or about 30 IU/kg of diet. In humans and animals, measurements of erythrocyte hemolysis[1] and peroxidation[2] in hepatic microsomes have been used to determine the MDR. Such values are similar and are dependent upon the intake of polyunsaturated fats (PUFA). We will show that in mice fed a semipurified diet containing 50 IU vitamin E/kg, the diet is not optimal for several parameters of the immune response, although the animal is healthy in all other respects. It has been demonstrated by Tengerdy et al. that addition of vitamin E to normal laboratory chow will enhance the antibody response to several antigens.[3,4] We have shown that cell-mediated responses are similarly enhanced by levels of vitamin E much higher than the MDR when added to semipurified rations that contain fats either rich or low in PUFA.[5]

Although vitamin E has been shown to enhance both humoral and cell-mediated immunity (CMI), this paper will be limited to studies of only the latter. Specifically, a demonstration of the effect and experiments to show the mechanisms of action of the vitamin will be presented.

Methods and Materials

Mice and Diets

Male CBA/J mice were obtained from Jackson Laboratories at 5–7 weeks of age and immediately placed on the appropriate diet. Semipurified diets contained 4 or 8% fat and 20% casein according to the formula of Csallany and Ayaz.[6] Fat was supplied either as hydrogenated coconut oil (HCO), corn oil (CO), or lard that had been stripped of tocopherol. Vitamin E, when included, was added at a level of 0.5 g all-rac-α-tocopheryl acetate/kg diet, except as described in the Results section. After four weeks on diet, experiments were performed.

Mitogenic Assay

These assays have been described previously.[5] Details concerning specific labeling conditions and time of harvesting are given in the figures and tables.

*Supported by a grant from the National Institutes of Health, No. AM 21618.

437

Mixed Lymphocyte Reaction

CBA/J spleen cells were used as the responder population at 0.5×10^6 cells per 0.2 ml. The BALB/c stimulator cells were treated with mitomycin C (25 μg/ml) for 1 hour at 37°C in the absence of fetal calf serum (FCS). The cells were washed twice with 5% FCS in MEM and added in different ratios to the CBA/J cells. After 96 hours at 37°C, the cells were pulsed with 0.5 μCi/0.2 ml ^{3}H-thymidine (^{3}H-TdR) for 18 hours.

Ultrafiltration

The splenic supernatant fraction was separated into fractions less than 10,000 daltons (eluant) and greater than 10,000 daltons (retentate) by ultrafiltration with a PM 10 membrane (Amicon Corp., Lexington, Mass.).

Time Course Addition of Vitamin E

Spleen cell suspensions at 2×10^7 cells/ml were plated at 4 ml/dish in 60-mm^2 dishes in the presence or absence of concanavalin A (Con A) for 18 hours. After incubation, the cells were removed from the dishes and washed three times with 25 mM α-methyl-mannoside and once with medium. The cells were added at 10^6/well, and α-tocopherol was added at different times at a final concentration of 1 mg/ml.

Treatment with Anti-Ia^k Serum + C'

A.Th anti.TL antiserum (anti-Ia^k, courtesy of the National Institutes of Health, Bethesda, Md.) and "low-tox" rabbit complement (C'; 1/15 final dilution) were used to deplete spleen populations of Ia$^+$ cells. (Ia is a surface antigen of some cells. See Results: Cell Fractionation Experiments.) Appropriate dilutions of antiserum were added to the spleen cell suspension for one hour at 4°C, and the cells washed and incubated for one hour at 37°C with C' in FCS-free media. Control populations were treated identically except for the absence of antiserum.

RESULTS

Effect of Vitamin E on Mitogenesis

CBA/J mice were fed diets containing 20% casein, 4% lard, and either 0, 5, or 50 mg all-rac-α-tocopheryl acetate/100 g diet for four weeks. Spleen cells from these mice were tested for their response to suboptimal (0.125 μg/0.2 ml) or optimal (0.5 μg/0.2 ml) Con A to phytohemagglutinin (PHA) and to lipopolysaccharide (LPS). Con A and PHA are T cell mitogens, and LPS is a B cell mitogen. It was found (FIGURE 1) that 5 mg/100 g diet, which is a moderate dose found in most chow diets, increased the response about 2.5-fold, but high levels (50 mg/100 g diet) increased the response by more than eightfold. In vitro addition of α-tocopherol (1 μM) to spleen cells from mice fed no vitamin E or moderate levels

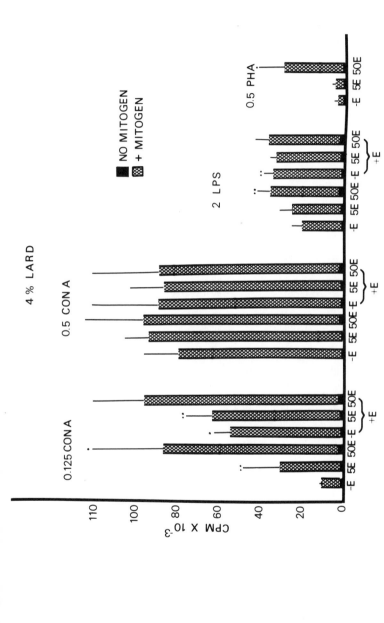

FIGURE 1. Effect of dietary and *in vitro* addition of vitamin E on the mitogenic response of spleen cells from CBA/J mice fed diets containing 4% lard. The results are the means of six mice per group ± standard error of the mean (SEM). With each mitogen, the first three bars represent the results of different dietary levels of *all-rac-α*-tocopheryl acetate: −E = 0; 5E = 5 mg/100 g diet; and 50E = 50 mg/100 g diet. The second group of three bars indicates the effect of the addition of 1 μM *RRR-α*-tocopherol *in vitro* to the spleen cells from −E, 5E, and 50E mice. Significance determined by Student's *t*-test is indicated (two dots, p ≤ 0.05 and one dot, p ≤ 0.01) over the SEM lines. The comparisons in the first three bars are with the −E; those in the second three bars test the effect of *in vitro* addition of the vitamin with the results of diet alone. Mitogen addition given in μg/0.2 ml. [Reproduced from Reference 5 with permission from the publisher; © *Journal of Nutrition*, American Institute of Nutrition.]

increased the suboptimal Con A response, but was ineffective when the diet contained high levels of the vitamin. A similar, but less dramatic, effect of vitamin E was seen when LPS was used as the mitogen. The response to PHA was low when the diet contained either no vitamin or moderate levels of vitamin E. At high levels of the vitamin, there was a significant increase in the response to PHA. Of interest is the fact that these experiments have been repeated using spleen cells from mice fed diets containing 8% lard, corn oil, or hydrogenated coconut oil, diets that have a wide range of polyunsaturated fatty acids. Vitamin E was found to be effective in stimulating mitogenesis in all of these diets.[5] This raised the question of whether vitamin E might be acting in ways other than as an antioxidant.

TABLE 1

EFFECT OF ANTIOXIDANTS ON MITOGENESIS IN SPLEEN CELLS
OF MICE FED CORN OIL DIETS*

Mitogen		^{3}H-TdR Incorporation (cpm $\times$ 10^{-3})	
(μg/0.2 ml)	Antioxidant†	$-$E Diet‡	$+$E Diet‡
2 LPS	—	5.1 ± 1.5^{ab}	13.4 ± 0.2^a
	DPPD	13.6 ± 2.8^b	17.3 ± 2.1
	BHT	6.1 ± 0.5^c	11.4 ± 0.3^c
0.125 Con A	—	7.5 ± 0.4^{ab}	35.0 ± 10.1^a
	DPPD	37.1 ± 13.0^b	54.0 ± 16.9
	BHT	15.9 ± 6.8	28.4 ± 8.8
0.5 Con A	—	82.8 ± 23.7	84.0 ± 0.8^a
	DPPD	90.0 ± 21.4	112.6 ± 7.9^a
	BHT	63.9 ± 2.1	93.5 ± 3.4
0.5 PHA	—	2.6 ± 0.1^{ab}	6.9 ± 0.7^{ab}
	DPPD	10.8 ± 1.3^{bd}	20.8 ± 1.6^{cd}
	BHT	5.1 ± 1.4	10.6 ± 2.6

*Results are the mean of three mice per group ± standard error of the mean (SEM). In each group, numbers with the same letter superscript differ significantly, as determined by Student's t-test, p < 0.05. All results have been subtracted for controls without mitogen. (Table reproduced from Reference 7 with permission from the publisher. © *Journal of Nutrition*, American Institute of Nutrition.)

†DPPD was added at 0.1 μg/0.2 ml; BHT at 0.5 μg/0.2 ml.

‡CBA/J mice were fed diets containing 8% corn oil ± 0.5 g/kg diet *all-rac-α*-tocopheryl acetate.

Does Stimulation of Mitogenesis Involve Antioxidant Function?

By comparing the activity of tocopherol with other antioxidants and tocopherol analogs on mitogenesis of murine spleen cells, an attempt was made to understand the mechanism of tocopherol stimulation.[7] N,N'-Diphenyl-p-phenylenediamine (DPPD) was very active in this system, whereas butylated hydroxytoluene (BHT), another antioxidant, was much less active (TABLE 1). Trolox C, an analog of α-tocopherol with a carboxyl group instead of the isoprene side chain, was totally inactive (FIGURE 2). Tocopheryl quinone, an oxidized form of tocopherol, was almost as active as tocopherol. Menadione (vitamin K$_3$), a quinone without a side chain, was also active. It is suggested that although in tocopherol-like compounds the side chain seems important, the activities of DPPD and

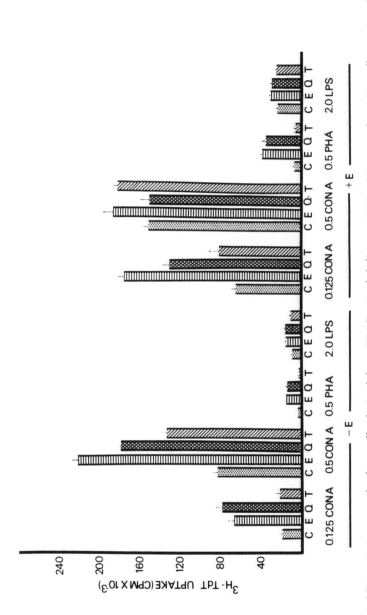

FIGURE 2. Mitogenic response of spleen cells obtained from CBA/J mice fed diets containing 8% corn oil ± 0.05 g *all-rac-α-tocopheryl* acetate/kg diet. The effects *in vitro* of adding 1 µg/ml *RRR-α-tocopherol* (E), tocopheryl quinone (Q), or Trolox C (T) were studied [C is control]. The − E and + E below the mitogen additions represent whether vitamin E is included in the diet. The vertical lines above the bars indicate the SEM. [Reproduced from Reference 7 with permission from the publisher; © *Journal of Nutrition*; American Institute of Nutrition.]

TABLE 2

EFFECTS OF VITAMIN E AND INDOMETHACIN ON MITOGENIC RESPONSE*

Mitogen (μg/0.2 ml)	^{3}H-TdR Incorporation (cpm × 10^{-3})			
	5% FCS†	+E†	+I†	+E+I†
Control	1.9 ± 0.5	10.6 ± 1.0	2.0 ± 0.3	9.5 ± 1.7
0.1 Con A	19.4 ± 6.0	53.6 ± 7.0‡	20.8 ± 7.5	53.4 ± 8.2‡
0.5 Con A	107.8 ± 9.0	152.7 ± 5.5	132.7 ± 5.7	98.6 ± 25.7
0.6 PHA	5.9 ± 0.8	25.2 ± 1.2§	5.9 ± 0.6	27.1 ± 1.1‡

*Mitogenic response of spleen cells from CBA/J mice fed an 8% lard diet without vitamin E for four weeks. Results expressed as means ± SEM. (Table reproduced from Reference 7 with permission from the publisher. © *Journal of Nutrition*, American Institute of Nutrition.)

†Additions: E = RRR-α-tocopherol at a concentration of 2 μM; I = indomethacin at 5 μM.

‡Significantly different from FCS control as determined by Student's t-test, p < 0.03.

§Significantly different from FCS control, p < 0.01.

menadione clearly do not require it. On the other hand, the stimulation by tocopheryl quinone and menadione, the lack of stimulation by BHT, and the effectiveness of tocopherol whether dietary fat was unsaturated or saturated appear to rule out a requirement for antioxidant function in mitogenic stimulation. A comparison of the stimulation by tocopherol with the lack of effect of indomethacin on mitogenesis ruled out regulation of the peroxidation step leading to prostaglandin synthesis as the mechanism for the tocopherol effect (TABLE 2).

Cell Fractionation Experiments

Vitamin E stimulates the response to Con A and PHA of murine spleen cells. Removal of plastic adherent cells did not prevent the stimulation by the vitamin.[5] The response to low levels of Con A is under genetic control and is absent from C_3H/HeJ mice, which are LPS nonresponders. Normal C_3H/Tif mice lose responsiveness to low levels of Con A when treated with anti-Ia serum.[8] We therefore investigated whether the stimulation of the response to low levels of Con A by vitamin E requires Ia^+ cells either as direct targets of the vitamin or as accessory cells.

Using graded dilutions of anti-Ia^k serum, it was found that the response to suboptimal Con A was almost maximally inhibited at the highest dilution used (1/200): about 75% (FIGURE 3). The response to optimal Con A was only inhibited by 11%. Vitamin E stimulated the response to low level Con A by threefold when 1/200 anti-Ia^k was used. At higher concentrations of antiserum, stimulation by the vitamin was about the same as without antiserum. Removal of plastic adherent cells prior to treatment with anti-Ia serum did not prevent the response of the resulting Ia^--nonadherent cells to stimulation by vitamin E (FIGURE 4).

Effect of Washing Spleen Cells

It should be noted that in the previous experiment, the effect of vitamin E on the response of control spleen cells treated with complement without anti-Ia serum to suboptimal Con A was not very marked. This is to be contrasted with previous results, when the stimulation was quite marked. The major difference is that the spleen cells in the antiserum experiments were subjected to washing procedures involved in the removal of antiserum and complement. To confirm that washing was responsible for the difference, the effect of vitamin E on unwashed spleen cells (SCs) and washed spleen cells (WSCs) in their response to Con A and PHA was measured (TABLE 3). SCs were strongly stimulated by vitamin E when the mitogen was suboptimal Con A or PHA. Washing enhanced these mitogenic responses, but vitamin E could not further stimulate these responses. Restoration of the vitamin E effect could be partially achieved by adding back the medium in which the spleen cells were originally suspended prior to washing. It was found that this supernatant fraction was stable to boiling for 10 minutes and contained an active factor that went through an Amicon PM 10 filter with a cutoff of 10,000 daltons.

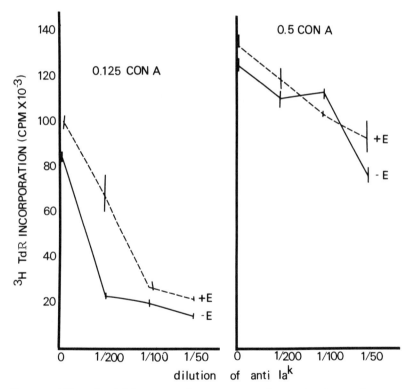

FIGURE 3. Effect of anti-Ia^k serum on the response to suboptimal and optimal concentration of Con A (0.125 and 0.5 µg/0.2 ml respectively) and on the stimulation by vitamin E. CBA/J spleen cells (2 × 10^7/ml) were treated with the indicated dilutions of A.Th anti A.TL serum plus low-tox rabbit complement. The ability of treated and untreated cells to respond to indicated Con A concentrations was measured in a 72-hour period. ^{3}H-TdR was added during the last 18 hours of incubation. Results are means of triplicate samples ± SEM. Mice were fed a diet containing 8% HCO without added vitamin E. Vitamin E added *in vitro* was at 1 µg/ml. (Reproduced from Reference 25 with permission from the publisher.)

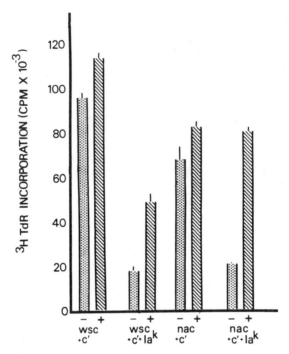

FIGURE 4. Effect of anti-Ia^k serum on the ability of vitamin E to stimulate response of CBA/J spleen cells (wsc) and plastic dish nonadherent cells (nac) to a suboptimal concentration (0.125 μg/0.2 ml) of Con A. Mice were fed 8% CO diets deficient in vitamin E. Vitamin E was added (+) or not added (−) in vitro at a concentration of 1 μg/ml. Anti-Ia^k serum was used at a dilution of 1:150. (Reproduced from Reference 25 with permission from the publisher.)

TABLE 3

EFFECT OF WASHING ON MITOGENESIS AND VITAMIN E STIMULATION*

| | | | ^{3}H-TdR Incorporation (cpm × 10^{-3}) | |
Spleen Cell Washing	Added Splenic Factor	Vitamin E†	0.125 Con A‡	1 PHA‡
−	−	−	30.3	1.0
−	−	+	67.4	14.1
+	−	−	88.4	50.4
+	−	+	87.2	51.4
+	+	−	56.9	8.6
+	+	+	71.8	27.9

*Results are the means of 10 experiments. (Table modified from Reference 25.)
†Vitamin E added at 1 μg/ml to spleen cells from −E CBA/J mice.
‡Mitogen addition given as μg/well (0.2 ml).

Spermine as the Splenic Suppressor Factor

High-voltage electrophoresis of the <10,000-dalton filtrate revealed a number of compounds, including amino acids and the polyamines spermine and spermidine. High-performance liquid chromatographic (HPLC) separations also revealed several nucleotides. In brief, only spermine fulfilled all the criteria of the splenic inhibitory factor: it produced an inhibition of the response of washed spleen cells, which was mostly reversible by vitamin E (TABLE 4). The concentration of spermine in the splenic supernatant was 0.65 ± 0.09 μg/0.2 ml. Over a very narrow range around this concentration, spermine was found to be inhibitory. A dose-response curve was found to be sigmoid in nature.

Our studies of mitogenesis were performed in media containing 5% FCS. In the absence of FCS or when FCS was heated to 70°C for one hour, spermine was no longer effective (TABLE 4). FCS contains a polyamine oxidase that has been shown to be heat inactivated.[9] Sera that do not contain the enzyme, such as horse, mouse, or human sera, do not permit spermine to be effective. Furthermore, the

TABLE 4

EFFECT OF FETAL CALF SERUM ON INHIBITION BY SPERMINE*

Spleen Cell Washing	Spermine	E	^{3}H-TdR Incorporation (cpm $\times$ 10^{-3} $\pm$ SEM)†			
			−FCS		+FCS	
			Con A	PHA	Con A	PHA
−	−	−	28.2 ± 0.2	2.2 ± 0.4	17.0 ± 1.2	0.6 ± 0.1
−	−	+	19.8 ± 5.0	7.4 ± 0.8	47.2 ± 3.0	10.5 ± 2.7
+	−	−	60.0 ± 6.3	14.6 ± 0.6	55.5 ± 4.4	54.7 ± 6.2
+	−	+	57.5 ± 9.9	12.5 ± 1.0	57.3 ± 2.5	60.3 ± 5.4
+	+	−	72.6 ± 9.0	14.4 ± 0.2	43.9 ± 2.4	7.3 ± 1.5
+	+	+	67.4 ± 3.6	13.0 ± 0.6	53.8 ± 1.5	50.8 ± 7.6

*Spermine added at 0.52 μg/0.2 ml, vitamin E at 1 μg/ml, Con A at 0.06 μg/0.2 ml, and PHA at 0.5 μg/0.2 ml.

†Incubation was for 72 hours with 10^6 cells/0.2 ml and ^{3}H-TdR added during the last 18 hours.

splenic factor itself was less effective in sera other than FCS. It did produce some suppression of the PHA response, which was reversible by vitamin E, but did not suppress the suboptimal Con A response. The residual activity may be due to preformed oxidized products of spermine produced by polyamine oxidase in organs such as the liver.[10] We have shown that when spermine or splenic factor was added with commercial porcine kidney amine oxidase to heat-inactivated FCS, it produced an inhibition of the mitogenic response reversible by vitamin E. From these experiments, then, it would appear that the splenic factor is spermine, but it must be oxidized to an active form. The factor is not species specific, since a rat splenic factor is equally effective under these conditions.

Kinetics of Splenic Factor Inhibition and Vitamin E Protection

Vitamin E is known to affect membranes, and it is possible that some of the enhancing effects of the vitamin could be explained by altering the membrane to

TABLE 5

EFFECT OF TIME OF VITAMIN E ADDITION ON MITOGENESIS AFTER
PRECOMMITMENT TO MITOGEN FOR 18 HOURS*

Time of Vitamin E Addition (hours)	^{3}H-TdR Incorporation (cpm $\times$ 10^{-3} $\pm$ SEM)		
	0.125 Con A†	0.5 Con A†	1.0 PHA†
Not added	3.4 ± 0.1	47.9 ± 4.9	0.8 ± 0.2
18	12.4 ± 0.7	42.0 ± 1.5	3.3 ± 0.2
24	12.1 ± 1.2	46.0 ± 1.5	3.2 ± 0.5
42	9.4 ± 1.2	40.7 ± 3.3	0.1 ± 0.6
49	7.3 ± 0.5	46.8 ± 1.5	0.3 ± 0.2

*Cells were incubated with indicated mitogen for 18 hours, washed with αMM, and plated in microtiter dishes in triplicate in the absence of mitogen. Vitamin E was added (1 μg/ml) at indicated times. (Table reproduced from Reference 25 with permission from the publisher.)
†Mitogen (μg/0.2 ml).

enhance binding of the mitogen. To test this hypothesis, the ability of vitamin E to effect a response after washing the cells free of mitogen at 18 hours was measured (TABLE 5). Washing was performed with α-methyl-mannoside to remove residual Con A. PHA was effectively removed just by the washing procedure. The results indicate that vitamin E can stimulate the committed response to low-level Con A and to PHA after they have been removed. Vitamin E enhanced mitogenesis by low Con A as late as 49 hours, although the optimum was at the 18- to 24-hour period. PHA mitogenesis could be enhanced at 18–24 hours, but not beyond that point.

TABLE 6

TIMING OF SPERMINE AND SPLENIC FACTOR (SF) ADDITION TO MITOGENIC ASSAYS*

Cells	^{3}H-TdR Incorporation (cpm $\times$ 10^{-3} $\pm$ SEM)		
	0†	24†	48†
0.0625 μg Con A/0.2 ml			
W	63.2 ± 2.9	70.2 ± 2.0	73.8 ± 7.8
W + E	52.6 ± 6.1	ND	ND
W + SF	2.8 ± 0.6	6.0 ± 0.4	31.2 ± 0.7
W + E + SF	13.3 ± 0.3	14.2 ± 1.5	35.5 ± 1.2
W + spermine	3.3 ± 0.3	7.5 ± 0.8	18.6 ± 2.8
W + spermine + E	17.9 ± 1.9	22.3 ± 1.2	36.4 ± 2.8
0.5 μg PHA/0.2 ml			
W	10.6 ± 1.7	ND	ND
W + E	14.3 ± 2.2	ND	ND
W + SF	0.0 ± 0.1	0.0 ± 0.1	1.3 ± 1.1
W + E + SF	2.3 ± 0.3	2.5 ± 0.1	4.3 ± 0.0
W + spermine	0.0 ± 0.1	0.0 ± 0.1	0.8 ± 0.6
W + spermine + E	3.3 ± 0.5	1.4 ± 0.6	2.0 ± 0.1

*Conditions identical to TABLE 5. Spermine added at 0.6 μg/0.2 ml. W = washed spleen cells.
†Time of factor addition (hours).

Of interest is the fact that washing at 18 hours still allowed vitamin E stimulation although the splenic factor would have been removed as well. This indicates that the effects of the factor cannot be abrogated by washing at 18 hours. The possibility existed that spermine oxidation products acted early to produce their inhibitory effects. A kinetic experiment in which the factor was added to washed cells at different times during the mitogenic cycle was performed (TABLE 6). It indicated that, like vitamin E, spermine oxidation products can act late in the cycle.

Mixed Lymphocyte Response

The mixed lymphocyte response (MLR) is considered to be an *in vitro* system for recognition of potential allograft rejection. The responder cell in this reaction

TABLE 7

EFFECT OF VITAMIN E ON THE MIXED LYMPHOCYTE RESPONSE OF WASHED CELLS

BALB/c Stimulators*	^{3}H-TdR Incorporation (cpm $\times$ 10^{-3} $\pm$ SEM)			
	WSC†		NAC†	
	−E	+E‡	−E	+E
WSC (1.25×10^5)	2.3 ± 0.2	5.3 ± 0.1	14.7 ± 2.2	29.7 ± 0.8
WSC (2.5×10^5)	3.4 ± 0.1	10.7 ± 0.7	26.7 ± 0.1	44.6 ± 0.3
NAC (1.25×10^5)	3.0 ± 0.4	5.6 ± 0.4	4.1 ± 0.9	15.2 ± 0.6
NAC (2.5×10^5)	3.3 ± 0.3	13.8 ± 3.5	8.1 ± 0.6	25.0 ± 2.0
No stimulators	0.3 ± 0.0	1.1 ± 0.1	0.6 ± 0.1	1.8 ± 0.0

*BALB/c stimulator cells were treated with mitomycin C and mixed with CBA/J spleen cells at the indicated cell concentrations for 96 hours including an 8-hour pulse of ^{3}H-TdR. Both stimulator and responder cells were washed.

†CBA/J responders (5×10^5); WSC = whole spleen cells; NAC = cells nonadherent to plastic dishes.

‡Vitamin E as RRR-α-tocopherol was added at 1 μg/ml to spleen cells obtained from mice fed diets deficient in vitamin E.

is known to be an Ia$^-$ cell, whereas the stimulator cells are Ia$^+$. Since we have shown that vitamin E stimulates the mitogenic response of Ia$^-$ cells even in the absence of the splenic factor, we chose the MLR as a functional assay to test the vitamin's effect on Ia$^-$ cells. Accordingly, both stimulator and responder cells were washed free of splenic factor prior to mixing. In addition, the effect of removal of plastic adherent cells (macrophages) was also studied since they are known to be effective stimulator Ia$^+$ cells in the MLR. In these experiments, responder-stimulator ratios of 2:1 and 4:1 were used (TABLE 7). The general result was that vitamin E stimulated the MLR response under all conditions. When adherent cells were removed from both stimulator and responder cells, the stimulation by tocopherol was three- to fourfold. Removal of adherent cells from only the responder cells greatly enhanced the MLR, but the vitamin E stimulation was still maintained.

The main features of these experiments are (1) that vitamin E, in higher than normal amounts, enhances mitogenesis and the mixed lymphocyte response of murine spleen cells; (2) that it enhances mitogenesis of spleen cells by overcoming the effects of splenic factors, probably spermine oxidation products; and (3) that these effects of stimulation by vitamin E and inhibition by the splenic factor may occur late during the mitogenic cycle. In addition, cell fractionation experiments revealed that there is an Ia⁻-spleen cell population that responds to vitamin E even in the absence of the splenic factor.

In these experiments, using two models of cell-mediated immunity, vitamin E enhanced the response whether added *in vivo* or *in vitro*. Optimal effects were not observed unless dietary levels were in excess of the vitamin content of ordinary laboratory chow diets. In this respect, our results were similar to the results obtained by Campbell *et al.* in studies of the humoral response.[4] They showed that addition of vitamin E to normal laboratory chow increased the antibody response to certain antigens.[4] The implication from these experiments, therefore, is that as far as the immune response is concerned, normal dietary levels may not be sufficient to maintain an optimal host defense against disease. In fact, Nockels has demonstrated the effectiveness of increased dietary vitamin E in stimulating the host protection against several infectious agents.[11]

The mechanisms by which vitamin E enhances the immune system are not clearly defined. The immune system is normally regulated by several systems of checks and balances. Two such mechanisms include the formation of specific suppressor cells and the presence of soluble inhibitory factors. Some of the known inhibitory factors are substances known as chalones.[12,13] Chalones by definition must be tissue specific, but not species specific. They should not be cytotoxic, and the effects should be reversible by washing. The best-characterized lymphocyte chalone has been described by Lenfant.[14-16] It was prepared from bovine spleen extracts and has a molecular weight less than 2,000 daltons. It suppresses mouse humoral and cell-mediated responses, even when injected *in vivo*. We have shown that washing spleen cells increases the mitogenic response to a level that cannot be enhanced further by vitamin E. The inhibitory factor that is removed by washing appears to have many of the properties of spermine. Addition of spermine, in the concentration found in the splenic wash, to washed spleen cells inhibits the mitogenic response, and this inhibition is prevented by vitamin E. In addition, both splenic factor and spermine are effective in FCS, but the inhibition is much less pronounced in the absence of FCS or in heat-inactivated FCS. Spermine, however, is not a chalone in that it is not cell specific.[17,12] Furthermore, Lenfant has shown that spermine is not as potent an inhibitor *in vivo* as the bovine spleen chalone.[18]

Thus, mitogenesis can be stimulated by vitamin E in the presence of spermine. However, spermine, to be inhibitory, must be converted into oxidation products by a polyamine oxidase. Fortuitously, our *in vitro* measurements took place in fetal calf serum, which contains the enzyme. In the absence of FCS, spermine is ineffective and the splenic factor loses effectiveness in the inhibition of mitogenesis.

Preformed spermine oxidation products could be produced in other organs such as the liver, where spermine oxidase exists mainly in the peroxisomal fraction.[10] Once formed, the spermine oxidation products(s) such as 3-aminopropionaldehyde may interact with proteins to form Schiff bases,[19,20] which may be the active product. Several mechanisms of inhibition by spermine products have

been proposed including interference with the cross-linking of membrane components necessary for the mitogenic response and interference with Ca^{++}
binding, which is required for early events in mitogenesis.[21]

We have discovered that an Ia^- population of T cells exists that is responsive
to vitamin E even after washing. This has been demonstrated both with spleen
cells treated with anti-Ia serum and with nylon-wool-filtered cells, which are
mostly Ia^- cells. In addition, we have demonstrated that the Ia^- responder cell in
the mixed lymphocyte reaction is also stimulated by vitamin E after washing.
Whether these Ia^- populations respond to vitamin E in a different manner than
other T cells do or whether they somehow fix the inhibitory splenic factor such
that it is resistant to washing has not been determined. In our *in vitro* studies, it
has been determined that incubation of the splenic factor with spleen cells for 18
hours prevents removal of inhibitory effects by washing.

It has been discovered that addition of vitamin E after precommitment to and
removal of Con A still allows for stimulation of the mitogenic response. In other
words, the vitamin can act late in the mitogenic response. However, it is not clear
what acting "late" means. Con A can be removed with α-methyl-mannoside
(αMM). Adding αMM at 6 hours to spleen cells results in lower levels of DNA
synthesis than when added at 24 hours. This has been interpreted to mean that
fewer cells have been committed to entering S phase at 6 hours than at 24 hours.[22]
Addition of vitamin E after removal of Con A at 18 hours with αMM produced
higher levels of DNA synthesis. This could mean that vitamin E increases the
number of cells entering S phase. This effect would be produced by affecting
some stage late in the G1 phase of the mitogenic cycle required for preparing the
cell for DNA synthesis. Such a proposal assumes a direct effect on a single cell
population. Since our experiments have not dealt with purified preparations,
alternative proposals that include interactions between cells must be considered.
For example, it is known that T cell mitogens do enhance B cell proliferation and
plasmablast differentiation, a process requiring T cells.[23] In addition, these
mitogens stimulate the production of soluble growth factors, such as IL2, as well
as receptors for these factors.[24] Where vitamin E acts in this maze of sequelae after
exposure to mitogens will be the subject of future studies in our laboratory.

The puzzling result that vitamin E stimulates an Ia^- cell population without
the need for the inhibitory splenic factor but can only stimulate a whole spleen
cell population when the factor is present has led us to the following hypothesis.
An Ia^- population can be stimulated by Ia^+ accessory cells or by vitamin E. When
Ia^+ cells are removed by anti-Ia antiserum or by nylon wool, the Ia^- cells can be
stimulated by vitamin E. In addition, we postulate that the Ia^+-cell accessory
activity is inhibited by the splenic factor, thereby permitting vitamin E stimulation.

SUMMARY AND CONCLUSIONS

Dietary vitamin E, in higher than normal doses, can stimulate the response to
T cell mitogens as well as the mixed lymphocyte response to murine spleen cells.
It was discovered that the vitamin E stimulation of the mitogenic responses is
dependent on the presence of splenic inhibitory factors, probably oxidation
products of spermine. In addition, it was found that vitamin E can also stimulate
the responses of selected T cell populations, including the MLR responding cells,
which lack the Ia antigen. This stimulation occurs even when the splenic factor
was absent. It is suggested that this Ia^- population can be stimulated either by Ia^+

accessory cells or vitamin E. When Ia$^+$ accessory cells are missing or inhibited by splenic factor, then vitamin E stimulation is enhanced.

REFERENCES

1. HORWITT, M. K. 1962. Vitam. Horm. **20:** 541–558.
2. COMBS, G. F., JR. & M. L. SCOTT. 1974. J. Nutr. **104:** 1292–1296.
3. TENGERDY, R. P., R. H. HEINZERLING, G. L. BROWN & M. M. MATHIAS. 1973. Int. Arch. Allergy **44:** 221–232.
4. CAMPBELL, P. A., H. R. COOPER, R. A. HEINZERLING & R. P. TENGERDY. 1974. Proc. Soc. Exp. Biol. Med. **146:** 465–469.
5. CORWIN, L. M. & J. SHLOSS. 1980. J. Nutr. **110:** 916–923.
6. CSALLANY, A. A. & K. L. AYAZ. 1977. J. Nutr. **107:** 1792–1799.
7. CORWIN, L. M. & J. SHLOSS. 1980. J. Nutr. **110:** 2497–2505.
8. BICK, P. H., U. PERSSON, E. SMITH, E. MOLLER & L. HAMMERSTROM. 1977. J. Exp. Med. **146:** 1146–1151.
9. TABOR, C. W., H. TABOR & S. M. ROSENTHAL. 1953. J. Biol. Chem. **208:** 645–661.
10. HOLTTA, E. 1977. Biochemistry **16:** 91–110.
11. NOCKELS, C. F. 1979. Fed. Proc. **38:** 2134–2138.
12. PATT, L. M. & J. C. HOUCK. 1980. FEBS Lett. **120:** 163–170.
13. BULLOCK, W. W. & E. MOLLER. 1972. Eur. J. Immunol. **2:** 514–517.
14. LENFANT, M., E. GARCIA-GIRALT, L. DI GIUSTO & M. THOMAS. 1980. Mol. Immunol. **17:** 119–126.
15. MILLERIOUX, L., M. LENFANT, D. OLESON & E. MAYADOUX. 1981. Int. Arch. Allergy Appl. Immunol. **64:** 128–137.
16. MILLERIOUX, L., N. DUCHANGE, A. MASSON & M. LENFANT. 1981. Cell Immunol. **58:** 209–215.
17. ALLEN, J. C., C. J. SMITH, J. I. HUSSAIN, J. M. THOMAS & J. M. GAUGAS. 1979. Eur. J. Biochem. **102:** 153–158.
18. LENFANT, M., L. DI GIUSTO, D. L. OLESON, E. GARCIA-GIRALT, E. MAYADOUX, V. VILLANUEVA & R. C. ADLAKHA. 1979. Biomedicine **31:** 110–113.
19. LABIB, R. S. & T. B. TOMASI, JR. 1981. Eur. J. Immunol. **11:** 266–269.
20. DWYER, D. S. 1979. Med. Hypoth. **5:** 1169–1181.
21. THEOHARIDES, T. C. 1980. Life Sci. **27:** 703–713.
22. McCLAIN, D. A. & G. M. EDELMAN. 1976. J. Exp. Med. **144:** 1494–1508.
23. PIGUET, P. F., H. K. DEWEY & P. VASSALLI. 1976. J. Immunol. **117:** 1817–1823.
24. LARSSON, E. L. & A. COUTINHO. 1979. Nature **280:** 239–241.
25. CORWIN, L. M., R. K. GORDON & J. SCHLOSS. 1981. Scand. J. Immunol. **14:** 565–571.

DISCUSSION

A. E. KITABCHI (*University of Tennessee, Memphis, Tenn.*): Have you tried to see if some of the lymphocyte effects could occur in humans? You have done these mainly in spleen cells, right?

L. M. CORWIN: Yes. Just recently we have begun some human studies, and we have only some preliminary results.

A. E. KITABCHI: The cells in the spleen are apparently responsive to vitamin E. Do they develop receptors to vitamin E?

L. M. CORWIN: We know that in the liver, there is a great deal of spermine oxidase, and we think it's possible that preformed spermine oxidation products have come to the spleen from other sources. We can't find the spermine oxidase in the spleen. But your hypothesis is also valid.

S. S. SHAPIRO (*Hoffmann-La Roche, Inc., Nutley, N.J.*): Do these lectins induce ornithine decarboxylase activity in the spleen cell?

L. M. CORWIN: Yes.

S. S. SHAPIRO: What does vitamin E do to ornithine decarboxylase activity?

L. M. CORWIN: We haven't measured the effect of vitamin E, but we think that anything that stimulates cell growth will stimulate ornithine decarboxylase.

EFFECT OF VITAMIN E ON THE DEVELOPMENT OF OXYGEN-INDUCED LUNG INJURY IN NEONATES*

Richard A. Ehrenkranz,† Ronald C. Ablow,‡
and Joseph B. Warshaw

Division of Perinatal Medicine
Departments of Pediatrics and Obstetrics and Gynecology
Yale University School of Medicine and
Yale–New Haven Hospital
New Haven, Connecticut 06510

Bronchopulmonary dysplasia (BPD) is a form of chronic pulmonary insufficiency in infants. Since its description by Northway *et al.* in 1967,[1] the development of BPD has been attributed primarily to the duration and intensity of oxygen exposure and to positive-pressure mechanical ventilation. In addition, other factors including endotracheal intubation, barotrauma such as pneumothoraces or pulmonary interstitial emphysema, fluid overload, and a patent ductus arteriosus with congestive heart failure have been considered. The role of these factors has recently been reviewed.[2,3] In 1978 we reported that vitamin E administration during the acute phase of therapy for respiratory distress syndrome (RDS) appeared to ameliorate the development of BPD, and suggested that vitamin E decreased the extent of oxygen-induced pulmonary damage.[4]

The hypothesis tested in that investigation was based upon several lines of reasoning.[2,4,5] First, vitamin E is thought to function as an antioxidant, protecting lipid membranes from peroxidation by scavenging free radicals[6,7] or by becoming incorporated into biological membranes in proportion to the content of polyunsaturated fatty acids and rendering them more resistant to oxygen-induced injury.[8] Second, vitamin E–deficient animals had more oxygen-induced damage to the lungs, red blood cells, and central nervous system than did animals receiving a control diet,[9–12] and vitamin E treatment of vitamin E–deficient rats decreased that damage.[10] Third, the chemical vitamin E deficiency common in many premature infants[5] would predispose them to oxygen-induced pulmonary injury if they had RDS and required treatment with high inspiratory oxygen concentrations ($F_{I_{O_2}}$). Therefore, we had suggested that early vitamin E administration might limit oxygen-induced damage and minimize the risk of BPD by increasing endogenous antioxidant protection.

In an effort to verify our preliminary findings,[4] a randomized, double-blind study was initiated.[13] This paper describes the results of that study.

MATERIALS AND METHODS

One hundred neonates with the diagnosis of RDS as defined by standard clinical, radiographic, and laboratory criteria[14] were admitted to the study and

*Supported in part by a grant (RR-00125 NIH) from the Children's Clinical Research Center and by a grant (HD 10949) from the United States Public Health Service.
†Address correspondence to the Department of Pediatrics.
‡Department of Diagnostic Radiology.

were treated within the first 24 hours of life with either vitamin E or the vitamin E placebo (Vitamin E Injectable and the vehicle for Vitamin E Injectable, Hoffmann-La Roche, Inc., Nutley, N.J., respectively) in a randomized, double-blind manner. Doses of 20 mg/kg (0.4 ml/kg) were administered intramuscularly upon admission to the study and then 24, 48, and 168 hours later. Additional doses were then given twice weekly as long as the infant remained in an oxygen-enriched environment and could not tolerate feedings and vitamin supplements. Permission to include each infant in the study was obtained by informed consent of the parents. This protocol was approved by the Human Investigation Committee, Yale University School of Medicine. Although any infant with the diagnosis of RDS was a candidate for this study, parental consent was sought primarily for those infants with moderate to severe RDS requiring early treatment with high $F_{I_{O_2}}$ and ventilatory assistance.

Except for the investigational drug, all the infants received similar care and were managed in accordance with presently accepted methods for the treatment of RDS. The $F_{I_{O_2}}$ and the extent of ventilatory assistance were adjusted to maintain an arterial P_{O_2} ($P_{a_{O_2}}$) between 50 and 75 mm Hg and an arterial P_{CO_2} ($P_{a_{CO_2}}$) between 30 and 45 mm Hg. An initial application of continuous distending airway pressure (CDAP) by nasal prongs was considered if an $F_{I_{O_2}}$ greater than 0.45 was required to maintain a $P_{a_{O_2}}$ greater than 50 mm Hg and if the infant did not have apnea. An initial application of CDAP by an endotracheal tube was considered if an $F_{I_{O_2}}$ greater than 0.70 was required to maintain a $P_{a_{O_2}}$ greater than 50 mm Hg and if the infant did not have apnea. Positive-pressure mechanical ventilation with CDAP was initiated if an $F_{I_{O_2}} = 1.00$ was required to maintain a $P_{a_{O_2}}$ greater than 50 mm Hg and/or if the infant had apnea, a persistent acidosis (pH < 7.2), or a $P_{a_{CO_2}}$ greater than or equal to 60 mm Hg or that was rising. Ventilatory assistance was provided primarily by a time-cycled ventilator (Bourns Infant Pressure Ventilator, Model BP200, Bourns, Inc., Life Systems, Riverside, Calif.) and occasionally by a volume-cycled ventilator (Bourns Infant Ventilator, Model LS 104-150), both of which were pressure limited and operated in an intermittent mandatory ventilation mode. Other ventilator settings—including the respiratory frequency, the inspiratory-expiratory ratio, the peak proximal airway pressure, and the end-expiratory pressure or CDAP—were adjusted as per the recommendations of Taghizadeh and Reynolds.[15,16] In addition, while requiring supplemental oxygen, each infant's hematocrit was maintained over 40% with packed red blood cell transfusions.

Furthermore, all of the infants were exposed to nutritional sources of vitamin E. During the acute phase of therapy for RDS, they received an intravenous protein alimentation solution that contained 2.5 IU vitamin E/liter. A lipid emulsion was administered if the infants continued to require intravenous nutrition following the acute stages of RDS, provided that they were not hyperbilirubinemic or did not require an $F_{I_{O_2}} > 0.30$. Enteral feedings with a proprietary formula designed for the premature infant (16 IU vitamin E/liter) or human milk (approxmately 3 IU vitamin E/liter) were initiated and advanced as tolerated. In addition, a daily supplement of an oral multivitamin preparation and an oral vitamin E preparation (Aquasol E®, USV Pharmaceutical Corp., Tuckahoe, N.Y.) was begun once the infants regularly tolerated feedings. The daily dose of the oral vitamin E preparation provided 50 IU vitamin E to infants weighing less than 1,000 g and 25 IU to infants weighing over 1,000 g.[5]

Clinical data relating to the entire study population are shown in TABLE 1. The vitamin E-treated and placebo-treated groups were compared on a variety of covariant factors. No statistically significant differences in race, gestational age,

TABLE 1

PATIENT PROFILE

Variable	Study Population		Patients Surviving >10 Days	
	Vitamin E	Placebo	Vitamin E	Placebo
Number	47	53	38 (80)*	43 (81)
Males:females	27:20	21:32	21:17	16:27
White:nonwhite	44:3	45:8	35:3	35:8
Gestational age (weeks)	30.3 ± 0.4†	30.5 ± 0.4	30.8 ± 0.4	30.6 ± 0.4
Birth weight (g)	1427 ± 63	1425 ± 69	1492 ± 72	1483 ± 79
Apgar score:				
1 minute	4.4 ± 0.3	3.9 ± 0.3	4.7 ± 0.4	4.0 ± 0.4
5 minute	6.3 ± 0.3	5.9 ± 0.3	6.8 ± 0.3	5.8 ± 0.3
Inborn:transport	26:21	36:17	22:16	31:12
Air leaks	18 (38)	27 (50)	12 (32)	19 (44)
Patent ductus arteriosus	29 (62)	33 (62)	27 (71)	32 (74)
Number requiring Rx‡	12 (41)	25 (76)	11 (41)	25 (78)
Intraventricular hemorrhage	16/27§ (59)	21/39 (54)	7/18 (39)	14/29 (48)
Age (hours) at treatment	14.3 ± 0.9	13.8 ± 0.9	14.1 ± 1.0	13.5 ± 0.9
Number of doses	6.3 ± 0.9	4.8 ± 0.4	7.3 ± 1.0	5.5 ± 0.4

*Figures in parentheses denote %.

†Mean ± SEM.

‡Number of infants in whom the patent ductus arteriosus was closed with indomethacin and/or ductal ligation.

§Denominator denotes number of infants evaluated by computer tomography scan and/or ultrasound.

birth weight, one- and five-minute Apgar scores, the occurrence of a patent ductus arteriosus (PDA) and intraventricular hemorrhage, age at treatment, and number of doses were found. However, differences in the male-female ratio, the number of infants born at Yale–New Haven Hospital vs. those transferred to the Newborn Special Care Unit, the incidence of air leaks (pneumothorax and/or pneumomediastinum), and the number of infants with a PDA that was closed with indomethacin treatment and/or ductal ligation were noted between the groups. None of these differences were significant, except for the number of infants with a PDA that required treatment with indomethacin and/or surgery ($\chi^2 = 7.58$, df = 1, p = 0.006).

TABLE 1 also provides descriptive data about those patients in each group who lived for more than 10 days and whose hospital courses were analyzed for this report. As previously described,[4] patients living for less than 10 days were excluded from analysis of the hospital course because of the difficulty in differentiating the radiologic changes seen in severe RDS from BPD during that time period. Of the 100 study patients, 19 died at less than 10 days of age; 9 vitamin E-treated and 7 placebo-treated infants as a result of intraventricular hemorrhages. Three other placebo-treated infants died: 1 with sepsis, 1 with a tension pneumopericardium and cardiac tamponade, and 1 with a pulmonary hemorrhage. The similarities and differences noted between the treatment groups in the total study population tended to remain between the patients in each group living for longer than 10 days.

Serum vitamin E levels were determined by the micromethod of Fabianek et al.[17] on blood samples obtained prior to treatment and during the treatment period. As shown in TABLE 1, vitamin E-treated and placebo-treated patients received the first dose at mean ages of 14.3 and 13.8 hours respectively, and received an average of six and five doses respectively.

The hospital course of each of the 38 vitamin E-treated and 43 placebo-treated patients living for more than 10 days was analyzed for the duration in hours of supplemental oxygen, positive-pressure mechanical ventilation, and endotracheal CDAP. Chest radiographs of each of the patients obtained during the first two months of the hospital course were interpreted independently by a pediatric radiologist (R.C.A.), who did not know which infants were treated with vitamin E. As previously described,[4] persistent or chronic findings noted during that time period were used to place each infant into one of the categories of radiologic abnormalities defined in TABLE 2. Transient abnormalities were not used to classify patients. The moderate and severe categories are consistent with the radiologic description of BPD, stage IV, as reported by Northway *et al.*[1] The mild and normal categories are not consistent with BPD even though such a possibility cannot be completely eliminated without histologic evaluation.

Student's t-test for unpaired data, chi-square analysis, and the Fisher's exact test were used to test the significance of the study results. When data were not normally distributed, appropriate transformations were applied before statistical analysis. Data analyses were performed with the CLINFO data management and analysis system.

RESULTS

The effect of vitamin E administration on serum vitamin E levels is shown in TABLE 3. Upon admission to the study, the overall mean pretreated serum vitamin E level was 0.44 ± 0.03 mg/100 ml [mean $\pm$ standard error of the mean (SEM)]; 0.45 ± 0.04 mg/100 ml and 0.43 ± 0.03 mg/100 ml in the vitamin E-treated and placebo-treated infants, respectively. The mean level in the placebo-treated infants was 0.78 ± 0.08 mg/100 ml 168 hours after the first dose and 1.11 ± 0.17 mg/100 ml on the fourteenth day. However, in the vitamin E-treated patients, the mean value rose to 2.18 ± 0.16 mg/100 ml ($p < 0.001$) 24 hours after one dose, and to 5.48 ± 0.60 mg/100 ml ($p < 0.001$) 24 hours after the third dose. Serum vitamin E levels remained elevated with a mean of 3.89 ± 0.24 mg/100 ml ($p < 0.001$) prior to

TABLE 2

RADIOGRAPHIC LUNG ABNORMALITIES

Categories	Definitions
Severe	Irregular strands of increased density with an overall large increase in thoracic volume. May have more diffuse areas of opacification.
Moderate	Thinner strands of increased density, less diffuse in distribution, with unequal aeration of localized areas. May have a small increase in thoracic volume.
Mild	A few small residual parenchymal densities, of varying configurations. May have a small region of decreased volume. No overall increase in thoracic volume.
None	Normal lung fields.

TABLE 3

SERUM VITAMIN E LEVELS

Treatment	Serum Vitamin E (mg/100 ml)			
	Pretreatment	+ 24 Hours*	+ 72 Hours	+ 168 Hours
Vitamin E	0.45 ± 0.04†	2.18 ± 0.16	5.48 ± 0.60	3.89 ± 0.24
	(37)	(31)	(14)	(30)
Placebo	0.43 ± 0.03	0.60 ± 0.05	0.60 ± 0.06	0.78 ± 0.08
	(46)	(33)	(18)	(21)

*Hours after the first dose.
†Mean ± SEM of the number of determinations shown in parentheses.

the fourth dose of vitamin E at 168 hours after the first dose. Infants who received four doses of vitamin E had mean serum levels of 2.23 ± 0.20 mg/100 ml on the fourteenth day after the first dose, whereas infants who received five doses had mean levels of 2.84 ± 0.34 mg/100 ml on the fourteenth day.

The duration of exposure to oxygen and of ventilatory assistance was not significantly different in the first five days of the hospital course and in the total hospital course between the vitamin E-treated and placebo-treated groups (TABLES 4 and 5 respectively). There was also no significant difference between the peak $F_{I_{O_2}}$, peak proximal inspiratory pressures, and peak CDAP to which the

TABLE 4

DURATION OF OXYGEN EXPOSURE AND VENTILATORY ASSISTANCE
IN THE FIRST FIVE DAYS OF THE HOSPITAL COURSE

Variable	Vitamin E Treated (37)*	Placebo Treated (43)
$F_{I_{O_2}}$		
0.21–0.39	52.8 ± 4.4†	50.8 ± 3.9
0.40–0.69	41.0 ± 4.2	46.7 ± 3.3
≥0.70	8.8 ± 2.2	9.0 ± 2.8
Total >0.21‡	102.1 ± 3.3	106.6 ± 1.4
Positive-pressure mechanical ventilation (cm H₂O)		
<20	20.2 ± 4.9	15.3 ± 3.6
20–24.9	31.2 ± 4.8	41.5 ± 4.5
≥25	25.5 ± 5.4	26.5 ± 4.6
Total	76.9 ± 5.7	83.3 ± 3.9
Endotracheal CDAP (cm H₂O)		
<5	29.5 ± 5.6	25.8 ± 4.4
5–7.9	49.8 ± 6.3	57.7 ± 5.0
≥8	2.3 ± 1.0	2.2 ± 1.2
Total	81.5 ± 5.3	85.7 ± 3.6

*Number of patients surviving more than 10 days.
†Mean ± SEM (hours) of inspired oxygen, positive-pressure mechanical ventilation, or endotracheal CDAP.
‡Total exposure to each treatment modality.

groups were exposed: 0.79 ± 0.03 vs. 0.80 ± 0.03; 23.7 ± 1.7 vs. 24.5 ± 0.9 cm H_2O; and 5.6 ± 0.4 vs. 6.2 ± 0.2 cm H_2O, respectively, in the vitamin E-treated and placebo-treated groups. Complete data for the duration of oxygen exposure and of ventilatory assistance were not available for 1 vitamin E-treated patient because parts of the medical record had been lost. Therefore, these analyses for the vitamin E-treated group are based upon 37 instead of 38 patients.

Most infants required supplemental oxygen in excess of their need for ventilatory assistance. This finding can be inferred from TABLE 5 and is demonstrated in TABLES 6 and 7. While approximately 20% of the vitamin E-treated and placebo-treated patients required ventilatory assistance for more than 250 hours, about 50% of the infants in each treatment group required supplemental oxygen for more than 250 hours. Furthermore, about 20% of the infants in each group

TABLE 5

DURATION OF OXYGEN EXPOSURE AND VENTILATORY
ASSISTANCE IN THE TOTAL HOSPITAL COURSE

Variable	Vitamin E Treated (37)*	Placebo Treated (43)
$F_{I_{O_2}}$		
0.21–0.39	409.8 ± 94.5†	290.8 ± 43.5
0.40–0.69	154.5 ± 86.9	75.3 ± 11.7
≥0.70	18.8 ± 10.6	16.0 ± 7.3
Total >0.21‡	582.7 ± 140.6	382.1 ± 50.5
Positive-pressure mechanical ventilation (cm H_2O)		
<20	83.8 ± 25.5	80.6 ± 21.9
20–24.9	59.6 ± 12.9	57.4 ± 6.6
≥25	74.1 ± 42.0	32.8 ± 8.0
Total	217.5 ± 59.0	170.8 ± 24.8
Endotracheal CDAP (cm H_2O)		
<5	139.9 ± 38.0	103.9 ± 25.3
5–7.9	85.4 ± 27.7	70.8 ± 8.9
≥8	2.3 ± 1.0	2.2 ± 1.2
Total	227.6 ± 58.7	176.9 ± 25.3

*Number of patients surviving more than 10 days.
†Mean ± SEM (hours) of inspired oxygen, positive-pressure mechanical ventilation, or endotracheal CDAP.
‡Total exposure to each treatment modality.

required supplemental oxygen for longer than 30 days (720 hours). Chi-square analyses of these data did not demonstrate any significant differences in the frequency distributions between each treatment group ($\chi^2 = 0.65$, df = 2, p = 0.726 and $\chi^2 = 1.76$, df = 2, p = 0.582 for TABLES 6 and 7 respectively).

Since none of the infants who were exposed to less than 250 hours of supplemental oxygen developed the clinical picture of BPD with moderate or severe radiologic abnormalities, TABLE 8 summarizes the radiologic findings in the remaining vitamin E-treated and placebo-treated infants according to TABLE 2. Of the 21 vitamin E-treated patients, moderate x-ray changes developed in 1

TABLE 6

TOTAL EXPOSURE TO OXYGEN IN VITAMIN E-TREATED AND
PLACEBO-TREATED PATIENTS DURING THE HOSPITAL COURSE

Treatment	≤250 Hours*	>250–720 Hours	>720 Hours	Total
Vitamin E	17 (45)†	12 (32)	9 (24)	38
Placebo	23 (53)	12 (28)	8 (19)	43

*Mean (hours) of inspired oxygen.
†Number (percent) of patients.

infant and severe x-ray changes in 1 infant. Both of these infants required supplemental oxygen for longer than 30 days. One of the 21 patients expired; that infant had severe radiologic abnormalities and BPD on postmortem examination.

Of the 20 placebo-treated patients who were exposed to supplemental oxygen for more than 250 hours, chest x-rays from 19 infants could be classified as being normal or only mildly abnormal. However, the remaining infant died with an indeterminate radiologic picture after requiring 100% oxygen and high inspiratory pressures throughout the 13 days of her life. Although a postmortem examination revealed pathological evidence of BPD in multiple areas of the lungs, she was excluded from TABLE 8 because only persistent radiologic abnormalities were used to classify patients. Two other placebo-treated infants who required supplemental oxygen for more than 250 hours expired. Both infants died from necrotizing enterocolitis, one at 4 weeks of age and the other at 6 weeks. At that time, each still required supplemental oxygen and had been classified as having mild radiologic findings; unfortunately autopsies were not obtained. Since the moderate and severe radiologic findings are characteristic of BPD, while the mild and normal findings are not, the data in TABLE 8 were collapsed into a 2 × 2 matrix for statistical analysis. No significant difference was found between the distribution of x-ray findings (p = 0.488, Fisher's exact test).

TABLE 9 summarizes the incidence of BPD with respect to the duration of exposure to supplemental oxygen and the occurrence of radiologic and/or pathologic findings characteristic of BPD. We have defined clinical BPD as the need for supplemental oxygen for longer than 30 days without evidence of a patent ductus arteriosus, fluid overload, the development of moderate or severe radiologic abnormalities, or a finding of pathologic evidence of BPD on postmortem examination. Seven of 21 vitamin E-treated and 8 of 20 placebo-treated infants requiring supplemental oxygen for longer than 250 hours had only clinical BPD. Three other patients, 2 vitamin E treated and 1 placebo treated, demon-

TABLE 7

TOTAL EXPOSURE TO POSITIVE-PRESSURE MECHANICAL VENTILATION IN VITAMIN E-
TREATED AND PLACEBO-TREATED PATIENTS DURING THE HOSPITAL COURSE

Treatment	≤250 Hours*	>250–720 Hours	>720 Hours	Total
Vitamin E	31 (82)†	4 (11)	3 (8)	38
Placebo	35 (81)	7 (16)	1 (2)	43

*Mean (hours) of positive-pressure mechanical ventilation.
†Number (percent) of patients.

TABLE 8

RADIOLOGIC FINDINGS* IN VITAMIN E-TREATED AND PLACEBO-TREATED
PATIENTS EXPOSED TO SUPPLEMENTAL OXYGEN >250 HOURS

Treatment	None	Mild	Moderate	Severe	Total
Vitamin E	5†	14	1	1	21
Placebo	9	10	0	0	19

*Classified according to TABLE 2.
†Number of patients.

strated radiologic and/or pathologic findings characteristic of BPD. Thus, no significant difference in the occurrence of BPD was noted between the treatment groups ($\chi^2 = 0.42$, df = 2, p = 0.813).

DISCUSSION

Oxygen-induced lung injury results from excessive exposure to oxygen. The pathologic findings associated with this injury have been well established and have been the subject of a number of reviews.[18-20] Factors contributing to its development include the concentration (or partial pressure) of the inspired oxygen, the duration of exposure to oxygen, and an individual's susceptibility to oxygen damage, which is related to such factors as the metabolic rate, endocrine and nutritional status, and the level of endogenous antioxidant protection.[2,18-22] Endogenous antioxidant defenses include the various physiological barriers confronting oxygen as it travels from the inspired air in the alveolar air space to the cells, the activity of protective enzyme systems, and tissue levels of antioxidant compounds.[2,18-24]

Experiments with perfused rat lung[25] and intact rats[26,27] indicate that adaptation or tolerance to hyperoxia requires an increase in the activity of such protective antioxidant enzymes as superoxide dismutase, catalase, glutathione peroxidase, glutathione reductase, and glucose-6-phosphate dehydrogenase. This enzymatic response varies with the animal species and is age dependent.[27-29] Neither neonatal nor adult guinea pigs respond to hyperoxia by increasing the activity of these enzymes. However, neonatal mice, rabbits, and rats react with significant increases in their activity as compared to the adults of those species. Although Bucher and Roberts recently reported that histological evidence of oxygen-induced lung injury in the newborn rat could be described as dose

TABLE 9

INCIDENCE OF BRONCHOPULMONARY DYSPLASIA IN VITAMIN E-TREATED AND PLACEBO-
TREATED PATIENTS EXPOSED TO SUPPLEMENTAL OXYGEN >250 HOURS

Treatment	No Evidence of BPD	Only Clinical Evidence of BPD*	Radiologic and/or Pathologic Evidence of BPD	Total
Vitamin E	12 (57)†	7 (33)	2 (10)	21
Placebo	11 (55)	8 (40)	1 (5)	20

*As defined in the text.
†Number (percent) of patients.

dependent, they noted that changes in antioxidant enzyme activities and lung compliance were not consistent with a dose-response relationship.[29]

Optimum tissue levels of antioxidant compounds, such as vitamin E, selenium, sulfur amino acids, and vitamin C, should help to maximize protection against oxygen-induced injury.[6,7,22-24] Vitamin E-deficient animals have been shown to have more oxygen-induced damage to the lungs, red blood cells, and central nervous system than do animals receiving a control diet.[9-12] In addition, vitamin E treatment of vitamin E-deficient rats significantly decreased the lung damage and prevented red cell hemolysis and central nervous system effects.[10] Although the precise mode of action of vitamin E has not been elucidated, it is thought to function as an antioxidant, protecting lipid membranes from peroxidation by scavenging free radicals[6,7] or by becoming incorporated into biological membranes in proportion to the content of polyunsaturated fatty acids and thereby making them more resistant to oxygen-induced injury.[8] The mechanism of action of vitamin E has recently been reviewed.[5]

Wender and his coworkers from our laboratory examined the effect of vitamin E treatment on the biochemical and morphologic response to hyperoxia in lungs from newborn rabbits fed an artificial diet.[30] A dose of 20 mg/kg per day given intramuscularly significantly increased serum and lung tissue vitamin E levels and was found to inhibit in vitro lipid peroxidation as assessed by malondialdehyde production and to blunt the hyperoxia-induced antioxidant enzyme response in animals exposed to 100% oxygen for 72 hours. But, when the lungs of these rabbits were compared morphologically to nontreated animals after the 72-hour exposure to 100% oxygen, there was no evidence of protection from oxygen-induced injury. With a vitamin E dose of 60 mg/kg per day, however, lung specimens were indistinguishable after the 72-hour oxygen exposure from the lungs of animals maintained in room air. These findings suggested that the pulmonary antioxidant protection provided by vitamin E involved the inactivation or scavenging of free radicals, the likely stimuli for antioxidant enzyme induction. This would account for the blunted biochemical response to hyperoxia. Furthermore, since morphologic oxygen-induced injury occurred with the lower dose of vitamin E and not with the higher dose, a certain minimal tissue concentration of vitamin E might be necessary to achieve maximal antioxidant protection and to prevent morphologic injury.

In view of the factors noted above, and since vitamin E deficiency is common in many premature neonates,[5] we thought that a premature infant with RDS who required high inspired-oxygen concentrations would be predisposed to the development of such oxygen-related disorders as BPD and retinopathy of prematurity (or retrolental fibroplasia). And furthermore, that early vitamin E administration might be expected to increase endogenous antioxidant protection and to reduce the incidence and/or severity of these complications of oxygen use in the neonates by altering the effect of acute hyperoxia. Findings from our preliminary investigation suggested that parenteral vitamin E administration during the acute phase of therapy for RDS ameliorated the development of BPD.[4] This report describes the findings of a randomized, double-blind study that was initiated to further evaluate that suggestion.

As shown in TABLE 3, the first dose of vitamin E increased serum vitamin E levels significantly when measured 24 hours later. The other three doses, administered according to our treatment schedule 24, 48, and 168 hours afterward, maintained serum vitamin E levels over 2 mg/100 ml throughout the first 14 days of life in the vitamin E-treated patients. The serum vitamin E level in the placebo-treated patients reached the normal adult mean of 1.05 mg/100 ml [the 2 standard deviations (SD) range is 0.5 to 1.6 mg/100 ml][31] during the second week of life, apparently in response to the nutritional sources of vitamin E that all the infants received. Thus, during the initial period of exposure to increased $F_{I_{O_2}}$, the vitamin E–treated infants had serum vitamin E levels that were significantly higher than the levels in the placebo-treated infants. However, many placebo-treated infants did not have chemical vitamin E deficiency during that time interval. Furthermore, since daily oral vitamin E supplements maintain serum vitamin E levels within the normal adult range,[5,32] vitamin E adequacy would be anticipated in all patients once feedings and vitamin supplements were tolerated.

The similarity between the vitamin E–treated and placebo-treated groups with respect to the duration of oxygen exposure, positive-pressure mechanical ventilation, and endotracheal CDAP in the first five days of the hospital course (TABLE 4) demonstrates that both groups had RDS of comparable severity. This is further supported by a similar occurrence of air leaks and PDAs in each treatment group. Although significantly more placebo-treated patients required treatment with indomethacin and/or surgery for a problematic PDA, all infants were managed in the same manner.

Persistent radiologic abnormalities characteristic of BPD were noted only in two vitamin E–treated infants (TABLE 8). However, as shown in TABLE 9, the incidence of BPD was similar in each treatment group. Since the chest x-ray tends to underestimate the pathological extent of BPD,[33] and since lung injury would seem to be indicated by the prolonged supplemental oxygen requirement associated with clinical BPD, the possibility that pathologic evidence of BPD might exist in lungs that would be classified by radiologic appearance as normal or mildly abnormal (TABLE 2) cannot be completely eliminated without histologic evaluation. Therefore, in contrast to our preliminary findings,[4] administration of vitamin E as described in this study did not prevent the development of BPD. A similar finding has also been reported recently by several other investigators.[34-38]

However, several differences between our preliminary and current investigations may account for the contrasting results. The effect of a change in the management of inspiratory pressure during mechanical ventilation in which an effort has been made to keep the proximal inspiratory peak pressure less than 35 cm H_2O has been discussed previously.[2,13] Futhermore, a marked difference in the vitamin E status of the infants is apparent. In our preliminary study,[4] the mean serum vitamin E level was 0.28 mg/100 ml prior to treatment and remained less than 0.36 mg/100 ml during the first 14 days of the study in the nontreated patients. In comparison, mean serum vitamin E levels in the placebo-treated infants rose from 0.43 mg/100 ml pretreatment to 0.78 mg/100 ml 168 hours later and to 1.11 mg/100 ml on the 14th day of the current study. Therefore, the nontreated infants in the first study had markedly lower serum vitamin E levels initially and remained chemically vitamin E deficient for at least the first 2 weeks of life, while many of the placebo-treated infants in the second study were chemically vitamin E deficient for only a short period of time. The higher pretreatment serum vitamin E level in the second study may represent changes in the maternal diet, for example, consumption of foods that contain increased amounts of polyunsaturated fatty acids with the associated increased content of total tocopherols,[39] and the use of prenatal vitamins that have been supplemented with vitamin E. In addition, serum vitamin E levels within the normal adult range may also reflect improvements in nutritional management, which have resulted in such changes as the earlier initiation of a vitamin E–supplemented intravenous protein alimentation solution to infants with RDS.

In an attempt to further understand the differences between our two studies, data from 16 vitamin E–treated and 20 placebo-treated infants from the current investigation with pretreatment serum vitamin E levels ≤ 0.4 mg/100 ml were analyzed. The mean pretreatment serum vitamin E level was similar to the pretreatment level in the preliminary study.[4] As seen in TABLE 10, little difference was noted between these subgroups, and also between each subgroup and its respective larger treatment group (TABLE 1). In addition, no significant difference was noted with respect to the incidence of radiologic abnormalities characteristic of BPD (p = 0.444, Fisher's exact test), with only 1 infant, a vitamin E–treated infant, developing persistent moderate findings. Furthermore, although 6 of the

TABLE 10

COMPARISON OF INFANTS WITH PRETREATMENT
SERUM VITAMIN E LEVELS ≤0.4 MG/DL

Variable	Vitamin E Treated	Placebo Treated
Number	16	20
Pretreatment serum vitamin E level	0.24 ± 0.03*	0.28 ± 0.02
Males:females	7:9	9:11
Gestational age (weeks)	31.1 ± 0.7	29.6 ± 0.6
Birth weight (g)	1509 ± 113	1389 ± 130
Apgar score:		
1 minute	4.7 ± 0.6	3.7 ± 0.6
5 minute	6.6 ± 0.5	5.0 ± 0.5
Air leaks	4 (25)†	11 (55)
Patent ductus arteriosus	11 (69)	18 (90)
Number requiring Rx‡	2 (18)	15 (83)
Intraventricular hemorrhage	5/10§ (50)	7/13 (54)
Age (hours) at treatment	12.1 ± 1.2	10.8 ± 1.1
Number of doses	6.6 ± 1.4	6.8 ± 0.8
Total O_2 ≥0.21 (hours)	516 ± 235	538 ± 88
Total positive-pressure mechanical ventilation (hours)	201 ± 74	222 ± 42
Total endotracheal CDAP (hours)	207 ± 74	232 ± 43

*Mean ± SEM.
†Figures in parentheses denote %.
‡Number of infants in whom the patent ductus arteriosus was closed with indomethacin and/or ductal ligation.
§Denominator denotes number of infants evaluated by computer tomography scan and/or ultrasound.

placebo-treated infants required supplemental oxygen for longer than 720 hours compared to only 2 of the vitamin E–treated infants (1 of whom had the persistent x-ray changes), this difference was not significant (p = 0.257, Fisher's exact test). However, since the mean serum vitamin E levels in these placebo-treated infants had risen to 0.72 mg/100 ml 168 hours after the first placebo dose, this subgroup cannot be considered equivalent to the control group in our first study, which remained chemically vitamin E deficient during that time period.

Thus, these data might imply that the administration of vitamin E to infants who have serum levels within the normal adult range does not provide additional protection against the development of oxygen-induced lung injury. This possibility is supported by Yam and Roberts, who have reported that supplemental doses of vitamin E (20 and 50 mg/kg intramuscularly every 12 hours) to adult rats maintained on a normal diet did not protect against the development of oxygen-induced lung injury.[40] Furthermore, Bucher and Roberts have noted that the content of vitamin E in neonatal rat lung reflected the dietary concentration of vitamin E plus the dose of any supplemental vitamin E administered.[41] Starving newborn rats by denying them access to dams prevented the normal increase in lung vitamin E content and significantly increased mortality. Although administration of pharmacologic doses of vitamin E to newborn rats significantly increased lung vitamin E content, these levels were not directly related to the cumulative dose. In addition, lung vitamin E content in the vitamin E-treated and nontreated animals did not change during exposure to hyperoxia. Data concerning the lungs of infants were consistent with newborn rat findings; lung vitamin E content correlated with dietary and pharmacologic vitamin E exposure and was not influenced by hyperoxia.[41] Additional studies by Bucher and Roberts found that administration of vitamin E (100 mg/kg subcutaneously on days 0, 2, and 4) to newborn rats allowed free access to dams did not prevent the development of oxygen-induced morphologic abnormalities, but did prevent the development of some functional abnormalities, such as alterations in lung compliance.[42]

Although these findings differ from those of Wender *et al.*,[30] the explanation is probably related to the nutritional and vitamin E status of the animals. The newborn rabbits described by Wender *et al.* received an artificial diet that did not support growth well,[30] while the newborn rats studied by Bucher and Roberts were allowed free access to dams.[42] Thus, the newborn rabbits were vitamin E deficient, poorly nourished, and highly sensitive to oxygen-induced lung injury, which was diminished by vitamin E treatment. In comparison, since the newborn rats had normal levels of vitamin E and were well nourished, supplemental vitamin E treatment did not provide additional protection against the development of oxygen-induced lung injury. A similar analogy can be constructed concerning the nutritional and vitamin E status of the infants participating in our preliminary study and in the current one, and might be related to the different findings.

In conclusion, although this study did not demonstrate that supplemental vitamin E administration during the acute phase of therapy for RDS modified the development of BPD, the incidence of BPD in the placebo-treated infants was only 2.5% (1/43), markedly lower than the 30% incidence in the nontreated infants in our preliminary study, and similar to the 5% (2/38) incidence in the current vitamin E-treated group. Therefore, taken together with our preliminary findings,[4] these data emphasize the multifactorial basis for BPD and the need to optimize nutritional support for sick premature infants. They also appear to support a role for vitamin E in the defense against the development of oxygen-induced lung injury.

ACKNOWLEDGMENTS

We are grateful to Hoffmann-La Roche, Inc., for supplying the vitamin E and the vitamin E placebo and to Debra Camputaro for preparation of the manuscript.

REFERENCES

1. NORTHWAY, W. H., JR., R. C. ROSAN & D. Y. PORTER. 1967. Pulmonary disease following respirator therapy of hyaline membrane disease: bronchopulmonary dysplasia. N. Engl. J. Med. **276:** 357–368.
2. EHRENKRANZ, R. A., R. C. ABLOW & J. B. WARSHAW. 1978. Oxygen toxicity: the complication of oxygen use in the newborn infant. Clin. Perinatol. **5:** 437–450.
3. EHRENKRANZ, R. A. & J. B. WARSHAW. Chronic lung disease in the newborn. In The Diagnosis and Management of Respiratory Disorders in the Newborn. L. Stern, Ed. Addison-Wesley Publishing Company. Menlo Park, Calif. (In press.)
4. EHRENKRANZ, R. A., B. W. BONTA, R. C. ABLOW & J. B. WARSHAW. 1978. Amelioration of bronchopulmonary dysplasia after vitamin E administration. A preliminary report. N. Engl. J. Med. **299:** 564–569.
5. EHRENKRANZ, R. A. 1980. Vitamin E and the neonate. Am. J. Dis. Child. **134:** 1157–1166.
6. TAPPEL, A. L. 1962. Vitamin E as the biological lipid antioxidant. Vitam. Horm. **20:** 493–510.
7. TAPPEL, A. L. 1973. Lipid peroxidation damage to cell components. Fed. Proc. **32:** 1870–1874.
8. LUCY, J. A. 1972. Functional and structural aspects of biological membranes: a suggested structural role for vitamin E in the control of membrane permeability and stability. Ann N.Y. Acad. Sci. **203:** 4–11.
9. TAYLOR, D. W. 1953. Effects of vitamin E deficiency on oxygen toxicity in the rat. J. Physiol. **121:** 47p–48p.
10. TAYLOR, D. W. 1956. The effects of vitamin E and methylene blue on the manifestations of oxygen poisoning in the rat. J. Physiol. **131:** 200–206.
11. KANN, H. E., JR., C. E. MENGEL, W. SMITH & B. HORTON. 1964. Oxygen toxicity and vitamin E. Aerosp. Med. **35:** 840–844.
12. POLAND, R. L., R. O. BOLLINGER, M. E. BOZYNSKI, P. KARNA & E. V. D. PERRIN. 1977. Effect of vitamin E deficiency on pulmonary oxygen toxicity. Pediatr. Res. **11:** 577.
13. EHRENKRANZ, R. A., R. C. ABLOW & J. B. WARSHAW. 1979. Prevention of bronchopulmonary dysplasia with vitamin E administration during the acute stages of respiratory distress syndrome. J. Pediatr. **95:** 873–878.
14. FARRELL, P. M. & M. E. AVERY. 1975. Hyaline membrane disease. Am. Rev. Respir. Dis. **111:** 657–688.
15. TAGHIZADEH, A. & E. O. R. REYNOLDS. 1976. Pathogenesis of bronchopulmonary dysplasia following hyaline membrane disease. Am. J. Pathol. **82:** 241–264.
16. REYNOLDS, E. O. R. 1974. Pressure waveform and ventilator settings for mechanical ventilation of severe hyaline membrane disease. Int. Anesthesiol. Clin. **12:** 259–280.
17. FABIANEK, J., J. DEFILIPPI, T. RICKARDS & A. HERP. 1968. Micromethod for tocopherol determination in blood serum. Clin. Chem. **14:** 456–462.
18. CLARK, J. M. & C. J. LAMBERTSEN. 1971. Pulmonary oxygen toxicity: a review. Pharmacol. Rev. **23:** 37–133.
19. WINTERS, P. M. & G. SMITH. 1972. The toxicity of oxygen. Anesthesiology **37:** 210–241.
20. WOLFE, W. G. & W. C. DEVRIES. 1975. Oxygen toxicity. Annu. Rev. Med. **26:** 203–217.
21. BEAN, J. W. 1965. Factors influencing clinical oxygen toxicity. Ann. N.Y. Acad. Sci. **117:** 745–755.
22. DENEKE, S. M. & B. L. FANBURG. 1980. Normobaric oxygen toxicity of the lung. N. Engl. J. Med. **303:** 76–86.
23. GILBERT, D. L. 1963. The role of pro-oxidants and antioxidants in oxygen toxicity. Radiat. Res. 3 (Suppl.): 44–53.
24. GILBERT, D. L. 1972. Introduction: oxygen and life. Anesthesiology **37:** 100–111.
25. NISHIKI, K., D. JAMIESON, N. OSHINO & B. CHANCE. 1976. Oxygen toxicity in the perfused rat liver and lung under hyperbaric conditions. Biochem. J. **160:** 343–355.
26. KIMBALL, R. E., K. REDDY, T. H. PEIRCE, L. W. SCHWARTZ, M. G. MUSTAFA & C. E. CROSS. 1976. Oxygen toxicity. Augmentation of antioxidant defense in rat lung. Am. J. Physiol. **230:** 1425–1431.

27. YAM, J., L. FRANK & R. J. ROBERTS. 1978. Oxygen toxicity: comparison of lung biochemical responses in neonatal and adult rats. Pediatr. Res. **12:** 115–119.
28. FRANK, L., J. R. BUCHER & R. J. ROBERTS. 1978. Oxygen toxicity in neonatal and adult animals of various species. J. Appl. Physiol. **45:** 699–704.
29. BUCHER, J. R. & R. J. ROBERTS. 1981. The development of the newborn rat lung in hyperoxia: a dose-response study of lung growth, maturation, and changes in antioxidant enzyme activities. Pediatr. Res. **15:** 999–1008.
30. WENDER, D. F., G. E. THULIN, G. J. W. SMITH & J. B. WARSHAW. 1981. Vitamin E affects lung biochemical and morphological response to hyperoxia in the newborn rabbit. Pediatr. Res. **15:** 262–268.
31. BIERI, J. G. & P. M. FARRELL. 1976. Vitamin E. Vitam. Horm. **34:** 31–75.
32. BELL, E. F., E. J. BROWN, R. MILNER, J. C. SINCLAIR & A. ZIPURSKY. 1979. Vitamin E absorption in small premature infants. Pediatrics **63:** 830–832.
33. EDWARDS, D. K., T. V. COLBY & W. H. NORTHWAY, JR. 1979. Radiographic-pathologic correlations in bronchopulmonary dysplasia. J. Pediatr. **85:** 834–836.
34. MCCLUNG, H. J., C. BACKES, A. LAVIN & B. KERZNER. 1980. Prospective evaluation of vitamin E therapy in premature infants with hyaline membrane disease (HMD). Pediatr. Res. **14:** 604.
35. ABBASI, S., L. JOHNSON & T. BOGGS. 1980. Effect of vit. E by infusion in sick small premature infants at risk for BPD. Pediatr. Res. **14:** 638.
36. SALDANHA, R. L., E. E. CEPEDA & R. L. POLAND. 1980. Effect of prophylactic vitamin E on the development of bronchopulmonary dysplasia in high-risk neonates. Pediatr. Res. **14:** 650.
37. FINER, N. N., K. L. PETERS, R. F. SCHINDLER & G. D. GRANT. 1981. Vitamin E, retrolental fibroplasia (RLF) and bronchopulmonary dysplasia (BPD). Pediatr. Res. **15:** 660.
38. WATTS, J. L., B. A. PAES, R. A. MILNER, A. ZIPURSKY, G. J. GILL & B. D. FLETCHER. 1981. Randomized controlled trial of vit. E and bronchopulmonary dysplasia (BPD). Pediatr. Res. **15:** 686.
39. WITTING, L. A. 1972. Recommended dietary allowance for vitamin E. Am. J. Clin. Nutr. **25:** 257–261.
40. YAM, J. & R. J. ROBERTS. 1979. Pharmacological alteration of oxygen-induced lung toxicity. Toxicol. Appl. Pharmacol. **47:** 367–375.
41. BUCHER, J. R. & R. J. ROBERTS. 1981. α-Tocopherol (vitamin E) content of lung, liver, and blood in the newborn rat and human infant: influence of hyperoxia. J. Pediatr. **98:** 806–811.
42. BUCHER, J. R. & R. J. ROBERTS. 1981. The influence of vitamin E on oxygen-induced lung injury and dysfunction in the neonatal rat. Pediatr. Res. **15:** 653.

DISCUSSION

B. LUBIN (*Children's Hospital Medical Center, Oakland, Calif.*): I agree with your conclusions on oxygen toxicity. Do you think that vitamin E therapy in premature infants might enhance spontaneous closure of a patent ductus?

R. A. EHRENKRANZ: I don't have enough numbers to comment on this. Nathan Rudolph at Downstate Medical Center tested the hypothesis and was not able to demonstrate a significant benefit by E therapy. I'm very intrigued by the data, and I'm going to try to follow up on them, but I just think the numbers are too small at this point for me to draw a conclusion.

L. A. BARNESS (*University of South Florida, Tampa, Fla.*): Did you notice any difference in the infection rate in your treated or your placebo groups?

R. A. EHRENKRANZ: I can't really comment on that because almost every infant in our intensive-care nursery with respiratory distress syndrome is placed on antibiotics very early. In the whole group, there were one or two bacterial infections, not enough to draw conclusions.

M. A. GUGGENHEIM: (University of Colorado Medical Center, Denver, Colo.): I'm curious how you arrived at your dose. Did you obtain any data regarding volume of distribution or serum half-life?

R. A. EHRENKRANZ: I picked this dose based upon a study by Nitowsky, Hsu, and Gordon [1962. Vitam. Horm. **20:** 559–571], in which they injected into the umbilical vein the polyethylene glycol succinate ester of tocopherol. The dose they used was 20 mg/kg, and it gave them adequate E levels. There are some pharmacokinetic data that I obtained with this dose on well infants at 1,500 ± 100 g birth weight by giving one intramuscular dose within the first several days of life and then following the E level for one week. A dose of 20 mg/kg resulted in a half-life of elimination that ranged from 60–160 hours, a volume of distribution (V_β) of 0.2 to 0.6 l/kg, and a serum clearance of about 0.1 ml/kg per minute. Therefore, a loading dose of 20 mg/kg followed by an additional 10 mg/kg 48 to 72 hours later should maintain E levels in the 3 to 4 mg/dl range.

H. J. MEVWISSEN (Albany Medical College, Albany, N.Y.): I'd like to ask about the acute respiratory distress syndrome you observed. Did you have any conclusions about the cause and the possible improvement?

R. A. EHRENKRANZ: There did not appear to be any effect of vitamin E on the acute course of respiratory distress syndrome. That's based on observations in the present study and in our preliminary report. There are many variables during acute respiratory distress syndrome, and you can alter the course very easily depending upon your therapeutic approach independent of E status.

H. R. D. WOLF (Justus-Liebig University, Giessen, Federal Republic of Germany): Did you have hematomas due to the intramuscular injection of vitamin E? We wouldn't dare to give intramuscular injections to our patients since they are heparinized.

R. A. EHRENKRANZ: Each of these infants received 1 milligram of vitamin K intramuscularly very early on in life. The dose of E is administered as a split dose, half into each thigh. There is occasionally some erythema around the injection site, but there is no significant adverse effect. I did not do clotting studies on these babies. Sick infants with respiratory syndrome often have some abnormalities in clotting tests. Clinically, there were no bleeding phenomena.

If I could make one additional comment to the last questioner. One of the major problems with the study is that we're really looking at a very late effect. We're looking at the development of a chronic condition. We have very little information available to us with which to measure acute changes. I think one of the intriguing things would be to use the type of system that Dr. Cohen and Dr. Lawrence demonstrated in their poster session of trying to look for ethane or pentane in the expired air of these infants. I have tried that, but I have not been very successful to date. I think that a way of looking for some acute evidence of either lipid peroxidation or oxygen injury would give us a much better handle on whether vitamin E therapy is beneficial.

THE EFFECT OF VITAMIN E ON LIPOPROTEIN CHOLESTEROL DISTRIBUTION

William J. Hermann, Jr.

Department of Pathology
Memorial City General Hospital
Houston, Texas 77024

The concept of a lower risk of coronary heart disease among persons with a relatively higher portion of their cholesterol present in the high-density lipoprotein (HDL) fraction, as opposed to the low-density lipoprotein (LDL) and very low-density lipoprotein (VLDL) fractions, has been well established.[1] It has, therefore, been a goal to identify agents that affect the lipoprotein cholesterol distribution, especially those that cause a relative increase in the HDL-cholesterol content. Some of these factors include jogging, moderate alcohol intake, and carbohydrate restriction.[2] My studies to date indicate that vitamin E in the form of synthetic all-rac-α-tocopheryl acetate is also a significant agent in increasing the HDL-cholesterol content. My hope is to recruit additional interest in the further investigation and explanation of the apparent beneficial effect.

In August 1978, I completed method-development research on the electrophoretic determination of lipoprotein cholesterol concentration. Using my own serum as testing material, I found my HDL-cholesterol content to be consistently between 9 and 11%. I then began taking an over-the-counter preparation of all-rac-α-tocopheryl acetate in a single daily dose of 600 IU for completely unrelated reasons. Approximately 30 days later, I again used my serum as a control in the method and found that my HDL-cholesterol had increased to 40%. For 2 days, I seriously questioned the validity of the method until I realized that there was a significantly different factor between the two sampling periods. That factor was the vitamin E. I purchased more of the same vitamin E preparation and began a similar experiment on an associate. He had a type IV hyperlipoproteinemia and a low HDL-cholesterol of 6%. On retesting after only 10 days, a marked improvement was observed to 22%, with a final level of 29% achieved in 49 days. In addition to the dramatic improvement in the HDL-cholesterol content, we both experienced reduced pre-β lipoproteins and triglycerides with little change in total cholesterol. After this first 10-day evaluation, realizing the effect was consistent and, therefore, possibly valid, I placed numerous other colleagues on a similar regimen with their initial values acting as their own controls. The results were published in July 1979.[3]

The resulting data made it immediately apparent that persons with initially low HDL-cholesterol (<15%) responded more predictably and to a greater degree to vitamin E. Therefore, two groups were formed on this basis and the first modifying variable was defined. A second modifying variable also became evident by the time the galley proof was reviewed. The one overweight person with initially low HDL-cholesterol had a somewhat delayed response, which extended over six months, indicating body weight to be a modifier concerning the rapidity of the full response (TABLE 1).

A second study utilizing placebos was organized with a group of cardiologists.

467

0077-8923/82/0393-0467 $01.75/0 © 1982, NYAS

TABLE 1

CHANGES IN LIPID PARAMETERS (PERCENT OF INITIAL VALUES)

	n	ΔHDL-Cholesterol	Δ HDL	Δ VLDL	Δ Triglycerides	Δ Cholesterol
Group 1—normal parameters, average risk	5	167%	107%	109%	111%	103%
Group 2—low HDL-cholesterol (<15%), high risk	5	321%	121%	69%	82%	105%

TABLE 2

SECOND STUDY: CHANGES IN LIPID PARAMETERS (PERCENT OF INITIAL VALUES)

	n	ΔHDL-Cholesterol	Δ HDL	Δ VLDL	Δ Triglycerides	Δ Cholesterol
Placebo group	10	103%	114%	99%	99%	97%
Treated group (all)	14	110%	110%	101%	98%	95%
average HDL-cholesterol	7	94%	109%	95%	103%	93%
low HDL-cholesterol	7	127%	112%	108%	94%	96%

TABLE 3

THIRD STUDY: CHANGES IN LIPID PARAMETERS (PERCENT OF INITIAL VALUES)

	n	ΔHDL-Cholesterol	Δ HDL	Δ VLDL	Δ Triglycerides	Δ Cholesterol
Placebo group	3	82%	99%	94%	88%	95%
Treated group (all)	7	121%	104%	109%	91%	90%
average HDL-cholesterol	5	110%	95%	122%	105%	86%
low HDL-cholesterol	2	148%	127%	75%	56%	99%

TABLE 4

ANALYSIS OF TREATED GROUP FOR AGE VARIABLE

	Second Study ($\overline{X}$ = 53 years)		Third Study ($\overline{X}$ = 26 years)	
	Average Risk	High Risk	Average Risk	High Risk
ΔHDL-cholesterol	94%	127%	110%	148%
ΔVLDL	95%	108%	122%	75%
ΔTriglycerides	103%	94%	105%	56%

After discovering that the first 24 responses were of a much lower magnitude than the original observation, the code was broken and the data analyzed. The only significant difference found between the original group and the second group was age. The average age in this second study was 49 years with only 2 persons under 35 years, as compared to 34 years for the original study with only 3 of 10 over 35 years (TABLE 2).[4]

Before completely accepting age as a modifying variable, a third, double-blind, controlled study was performed specifically on a younger age group (average, 26 years old). After the code was broken and the data analyzed, the degree of change was much greater than in the older population of the second study. Therefore, age became an important modifying variable (TABLES 3 and 4).[5]

TABLE 5 represents the modifying variables that are thought to play a critical role in predicting the effectiveness of oral vitamin E in altering serum lipid parameters.

TABLE 5

MODIFYING VARIABLES FOR THE TOCOPHEROL EFFECT ON CHOLESTEROL REDISTRIBUTION

1. Age less than 35

2. HDL-cholesterol equal to or less than 15% (high risk)

3. Type IV hyperlipoproteinemia
   (elevated VLDL and triglycerides)

4. Body weight no more than 10% above ideal weight
   (if response expected within 30 days)

TABLE 6 provides a comparative analysis of the studies performed to date, specifically focusing on the cholesterol redistribution effect of vitamin E. The data from Hatam and Kayden[6] and the yet to be published New Zealand study[7] have been recompiled to reflect the degree of fulfillment of the modifying variables. Both groups conclude that the effect I originally reported could not be reproduced. However, one can see by these data the minimal fulfillment of the criteria in each case. My latest study, along with numerous off-study, anecdotal instances and the ability to literally "titrate" my own HDL-cholesterol concentration by oral vitamin E, convinces me that the effect is most probably valid. Thus, it is likely beneficial in the prevention of coronary heart disease to the extent that higher HDL-cholesterol levels are correlated with a decreased incidence of coronary heart disease.

The magnitude of the effect is certainly in question. I believe the original data in my first study exaggerated the effect due to the probable low bias of the early electrophoretic methodology for levels below 15%. Now that the methodology is better developed, we rarely see levels below 7%. This low bias of the initial levels (the denominators) exaggerated the percentage change. I now believe that the actual 30-day effect to be expected if all modifying variables are fulfilled is a 50–75% increase in the HDL-cholesterol content. No other explanation is apparent after much deliberation on the subject. I still favor the use of the electrophoretic procedure because in the practice of treating individual patients, the result is graphically represented. It is also directly measured as a relative percent.

In conclusion, it appears, although still based on a very small sampling, that vitamin E beneficially redistributes cholesterol. The true protective effect is the reduction of LDL and VLDL cholesterol as reflected in an increased HDL cholesterol and decreased triglycerides.

TABLE 6

STUDY RESULTS COMPARED WITH RESPECT TO MODIFYING CRITERIA

Study	Subgroup	>35 Years		<35 Years	Number of Additional Criteria Fulfilled					
					3/3		2/3		1/3	
		n	HDL-Cholesterol	n	n	HDL-Cholesterol	n	HDL-Cholesterol	n	HDL-Cholesterol
Hermann 1979[3]	average risk	2	129%	3					3	154%
	high risk	1	238%	4	1	483%	3	375%		
Hatam 1980[6]	average risk	2	95%	4					4	109%
	high risk	2	96%	1					1	93%
	hypercholesterolemia	3	95%	2					2	102%
Hermann 1980[4]	average risk	5	92%	2					2	96%
	high risk	7	127%	0						
New Zealand 1981[7]	average risk	9	85%	0						
	high risk	2	124%	0						
Hermann 1981[5]	average risk	0		5	0		2	138%	3	91%
	high risk	0		2	2	148%				

REFERENCES

1. GORDON, T., W. P. CASTELLI, M. C. HJORTLAND, et al. 1977. High density lipoproteins as a protective factor in coronary heart disease; Framingham Study. Am. J. Med. **62:** 707–714.
2. HULLEY, S. B., R. COHEN & G. WIDDOWSON. 1977. Plasma high-density lipoprotein cholesterol level. Influence of risk factor intervention. J. Am. Med. Assoc. **238:** 2269–2271.
3. HERMANN, W. J., K. WARD & J. A. FAUCETT. 1979. The effect of tocopherol on high-density lipoprotein cholesterol. Am. J. Clin. Pathol. **72:** 848–852.
4. HERMANN, W. J. 1981. Am. J. Clin. Pathol. **76:** 124–126. (Letter in reply to Reference 6.)
5. HERMANN, W. J. Am. J. Clin. Pathol. (In press.) (Letter in reply to Reference 7.)
6. HATAM, L. J. & H. J. KAYDEN. 1981. The failure of alpha-tocopherol supplementation to alter the distribution of lipoprotein cholesterol in normal and hyperlipoproteinemic persons. Am. J. Clin. Pathol. **76:** 122–124.
7. SCHWARTZ, P. L. & I. M. RUTHERFORD. The effect of tocopherol on high-density lipoprotein cholesterol. Am. J. Clin. Pathol. (In press.)

DISCUSSION

H. J. KAYDEN (*New York University School of Medicine, New York, N.Y.*): Dr. Hermann and I have already corresponded in our published data. I was particularly intrigued by the observation that a vitamin whose distribution in lipoproteins is mainly a consequence of the total lipid concentration might have some effect upon the synthesis and distribution of high-density lipoprotein. Therefore, we undertook a study in 10 subjects: 5 normals and 5 subjects, 4 of whom had hypercholesterolemia and 1 of whom had hypertriglyceridemia. Following the protocol exactly as he outlined, we showed no variation at all in the distribution of cholesterol in their lipoproteins. We were able to demonstrate that the vitamin was absorbed and well distributed. I think that what's much more important than the disparity in our respective observations concerns the question of whether there really is a possibility that tocopherol has a role in the synthesis and distribution of a lipoprotein.

There is a lot of confusion about the metabolism of HDL. We know a lot about its apoprotein composition but not a great deal about what controls its levels. I find it extraordinary that any agent could change its levels over such a short period of time. Most of the reports that have been carried out for the value of exercise, such as vigorous jogging, or even alcohol have required a number of weeks. But the one thing I hadn't appreciated before concerns your measurement of the triglyceride concentration in the VLDL. By what method did you make this separation of lipoprotein?

W. J. HERMANN: This is total triglyceride.

H. J. KAYDEN: But not VLDL concentration?

W. J. HERMANN: No. The VLDL is done by staining an electrophoretic strip.

H. J. KAYDEN: Is the VLDL done by the Helena technique?

W. J. HERMANN: No, a Beckman technique that is very similar.

H. J. KAYDEN: Hypertriglyceridemia, which you referred to as type IV, is really an uncommon disorder among the population at large, although it is the most common of the abnormalities of lipoproteins. If you change the diet in those individuals relatively in terms of carbohydrate intake, you can alter the distribution of the triglycerides; and in some subjects, whom we are unable to identify, there is a reciprocal relationship between the concentration of VLDL and HDL.

It does seem to me that the question posed by these studies merits our attention to try to define which part of the population is truly susceptible to the changes. If tocopherol really does have an effect, we should try to learn how that's mediated.

R. E. OLSON (*St. Louis University School of Medicine, St. Louis, Mo.*): Dr. Hermann, I have questions along the same line as those Dr. Kayden has put to you. As I understand your report, what you are saying is that type IV hyperlipidemia in young people responds to vitamin E?

W. J. HERMANN: Yes.

R. E. OLSON: And there is some evidence that because you get no response in people with normal HDL, you get very little response in people who are older. Is that correct?

W. J. HERMANN: It's unpredictable. We've certainly seen people respond, but it's unpredictable.

R. E. OLSON: It seems to me that if this is really true, then you have to do a more refined study, recording actual values for triglycerides. There is a general hypothesis that elevation of HDL-II—which is mobile in athletes, women, and drinkers—changes when there is increased clearance of triglycerides. So the question I have for you is, Did you measure postheparin lipoprotein lipase in any of these subjects, or did you measure, for example, peak triglyceride chylomicron levels after taking a standard fat dose?

W. J. HERMANN: No. These are the types of things that need to be done.

J. J. BARBORIAK (*Medical College of Wisconsin, Milwaukee, Wis.*): I had a group of people with very low levels of high-density lipoprotein cholesterols. They are patients with spinal cord injury. It has been reported repeatedly that they have HDL levels of about 30 mg/dl. We took 19 of these patients and gave them 800 units of vitamin E. Eleven of them had an increase of about 21% over the initial level of 30 mg/dl. There was a subgroup with high initial levels, and they did not respond. We also had a group of joggers with an initial level of about 68 mg/dl, and they did not respond to E. A group of 5 people—3 pharmacists and 2 cardiologists—with an initial average level of 45 mg/dl responded with about a 17% increase. In a group of 14 nurses, the initial level was 66 mg/dl, and they had an increase of 18% over the initial level in the four weeks after the 800 units of vitamin E.

The absolute differences are not great. However, when one looks at the extent of coronary occlusion and the levels of high-density lipoprotein cholesterol, even a few milligrams of HDL make a tremendous difference.

W. J. HERMANN: I would like to make one last comment. I've heard people quote some of these studies wrongly by saying that the total cholesterol is changed. The total cholesterol is extremely stable and is neither reduced nor increased. It's the distribution that's affected.

VITAMIN E SUPPLEMENTATION AND THE RETINOPATHY OF PREMATURITY

Lois Johnson, David Schaffer,* Graham Quinn,*
Donald Goldstein,† Mari Jo Mathis, Chari Otis,
and Thomas R. Boggs, Jr.

Department of Obstetrics and Gynecology
Section on Newborn Pediatrics
Pennsylvania Hospital
Philadelphia, Pennsylvania 19107

This paper will describe a series of studies on the relationship of vitamin E nutrition on the incidence, severity, and long-term outcome of retrolental fibroplasia (RLF) and the further effect of treatment with vitamin E at varying dosage levels and time schedules. The work was done from 1968 to 1980, over which time period the incidence of clinically significant vitamin E deficiency anemia among premature infants (birth weight under 2,000 g) raised on standard formulas and multivitamin drops decreased from something in the range of 20% to less than 1%. The studies involved the premature and intensive-care nurseries of Pennsylvania Hospital under the late Thomas R. Boggs and the outpatient ophthalmology practice of Drs. David Schaffer and Graham Quinn at the Children's Hospital of Philadelphia. Statistical consultation over the 12-year period was provided by Donald Goldstein, Mari Jo Mathis, and Chari Otis. Because it is now generally agreed that RLF, especially in its more common, low-grade form, is more properly referred to as a retinopathy of prematurity, that term and the abbreviation ROP will be used in this paper.

METHODS AND APPROACH

Development of Classification and Scoring Systems for Relating Visual Outcome to Acute Stage Disease, Neonatal Risk Factors, and Therapeutic Interventions

Since 1968, Dr. David Schaffer has been following all premature infants cared for in the Pennsylvania Hospital nurseries with weekly or biweekly eye exams using the indirect ophthalmoscope. Since about 1972, he has supervised a similar surveillance program in the nurseries of the Children's Hospital of Philadelphia and the Hospital of the University of Pennsylvania. At each exam, a description of the retinal findings as well as an assessment of the stage of retinal maturity or grade of ROP was recorded. Examinations were continued until complete regression of active disease or retinal vascular maturity was documented.

If necessary, the surveillance program was continued in the outpatient department. On the basis of this large body of clinical experience, Dr. Schaffer, and later Dr. Quinn, who joined his program in 1977, modified the original classification of Reese, King, and Owens[1,2] to include findings in far peripheral

---

*Department of Ophthalmology, Children's Hospital, Philadelphia, Pa. 19104.
†Population Studies Center, University of Pennsylvania, Philadelphia, Pa. 19104.

0077-8923/82/0393-0473 $01.75/0 © 1982, NYAS

disease and clearly define the characteristics of low-grade ROP for both acute and cicatricial stages. The distinguishing feature of active grade 2 disease in their classification is the demarcation line of Flynn: that of active grade 3, extraretinal neovascularization (ERNV). An initial version of the classification for acute and cicatricial stages of the disease was included in our 1974 report on ROP at Pennsylvania Hospital from 1968 to 1972 and on preliminary results of the 1972 to 1974 clinical trial of the effects of prophylactic vitamin E.[1]

In 1979 the classification system per se was published in an updated version.[2] Two patterns of disease were described. One, by far the most common, is slowly progressive, does not usually exceed a severity of grade 2 (active), and often involves only part of the retina (segmental, as opposed to circumferential, disease). The other is uncommon and characterized by the presence of early dilatation and tortuosity of the posterior pole retinal vessels (i.e., during active grades 1 and 2), a tendency to circumferential involvement of the retina, and rapid progression to severe disease with extensive ERNV and retinal detachment. Disease of this more serious form is termed "plus" ROP, i.e., grade 2-plus active, grade 3-plus active, etc. The most advanced form of grade 2-plus active is defined by gross dilatation and tortuosity of posterior pole vessels and a circumferential (360°) demarcation line. The most advanced form of grade 3-plus active has these features plus extensive four-quadrant ERNV. Regression from grade 3-plus active ROP with extensive ERNV in two or more quadrants is very rare, an outcome of legal blindness or worse occurring in about 70% of victims. Active grades 4 and 5 ROP (partial and complete retinal detachment, respectively, or progressive fibrovascular overgrowth) are reached through the common pathway of 3-plus active disease.

An *incidence severity index* or mean severity ROP score was developed to describe, in one figure, the incidence and severity of acute stage ROP. In its simplest form, it consists of the sum of the highest grade of acute ROP, including 0, in the fellow eyes of each baby. This sum is divided by 1 to give the mean severity score for an individual and by the total number of babies to give the group mean severity. Plus ROP adds 0.5 to the numerical grade, e.g., grade 2 active = 2.0, and grade 2-plus active = 2.5.

The *cicatricial classification* has been addressed with similar care, since the degree of cicatrix is closely correlated with visual outcome. The higher grades of cicatricial (Cic) ROP—grade 3 Cic, in which there is a retinal fold, and grades 4 and 5 Cic, with retinal detachment and fibrous overgrowth—are unequivocal and easily recognized. So also are the more severe examples of grade 2 Cic (dragging of the retina toward a peripheral scar with varying degrees of macular heterotopia). Visual outcome with grade 2 Cic can vary widely depending on the extent and location of scarring. Grade 1-plus Cic, consisting of a far peripheral scar, is a hard finding, but the scar, if small, is easily missed. A wide range of refractive errors, often with anisometropia, is found in association with grade 1-plus Cic. Grade 1 Cic consists of several soft findings, no one of which is diagnostic of previous ROP and not all of which are necessarily present in any one infant. These consist of somewhat tortuous posterior vessels, irregular pigmentation in the region of the previous demarcation line, fine vitreoretinal adhesions, myopia (sometimes severe), and anisometropia. A checklist was worked out to define the constellations of findings that could be called grade 1 Cic ROP. This is important when addressing the matter of sequelae following "regressed" low-grade ROP. In our experience, when regression is complete, as defined by an absence of all cicatricial findings, there is no visual morbidity that can be distinguished from that in the general premature population in whom ROP did not develop in the nursery.[28]

TABLE 1

SCORING SYSTEM FOR LONG-TERM FOLLOW-UP OF ACTIVE ROP

	Right Eye	Left Eye
Grade cicatricial ROP	0 to 5	0 to 5
Refraction or visual acuity*		
Myopia (-0.25 to -6.00)	1 to 3	1 to 3
(correctable to 20/30)		
Visual acuity (corrected)		
20/40 to 20/200	4 to 8	4 to 8
Count fingers to NLP†		
Binocular—strabismus,	0 to 3	
anisometropia, amblyopia		

*Visual acuity deficit is estimated in children under age three years.
†NLP = no light perception.

Finally, an outcome or visual morbidity score was developed. This includes grade of cicatricial disease, refractive error or visual acuity, and presence or absence of anisometropia, amblyopia, and strabismus (TABLE 1). This score is a summation of findings in each eye. Therefore, a child who is blind in one eye but has useful vision in the other can be adequately described (see TABLES 1 and 2). In the more severe grades of active ROP, disparate findings in fellow eyes are not uncommon in both active and cicatricial stages.

The visual morbidity score has been useful in assessing the following:

1. The relationship of pattern and severity of acute stage disease to visual outcome.

TABLE 2

CLINICAL RANKING, MORBIDITY SCORE AND OPHTHALMOLOGIC FINDINGS
AT ONE TO TWO YEAR FOLLOW-UP

Clinical Ranking	Morbidity Score	Representative Clinical Sequelae following Active ROP
A to C	0–8	Cicatricial ROP grade 1 to 1.5. Minimal to no visual handicap. Mild to moderate myopia.
D	9–11	Grade 1.5 to 2 cicatricial ROP; moderate to high myopia. Anisometropia/amblyopia/strabismus.
E	12–14	Grade 2 Cic with high myopia correctable to 20/20 vision. Anisometropia/amblyopia/strabismus.
F	15–17	Cicatricial ROP grade 2 to 3 with high myopia. Visual acuity correctable to only 20/200 in one eye. Anisometropia/amblyopia/strabismus.
G	18–20	Grade 2 to 3 Cic in one eye with corrected visual acuity 20/200. Fellow eye grade 4–5 cicatricial with light perception only.
H	21–22	Grade 4–5 Cic in one eye with light perception at best. Fellow eye grade 3 Cic with count finger vision.
I	23–26	Grade 4–5 Cic in both eyes with or without light perception.

2. The effect of treatment on visual outcome per se and as it relates to changes in pattern and severity of acute stage disease.

3. The relationship of visual outcome to the evolution of premature intensive-care techniques, survival of increased numbers of very immature infants, and the improved ability to recognize and supply the nutritional needs of the critically ill and growing premature.

Survey of Changes in Commercial Formulas Used to Feed Premature Infants—1968 to 1978: Relation to Measured Levels of Vitamin E in Serum in Premature Infants

Since 1968, records have been kept of product labels and manufacturers' brochures with regard to tocopherol, polyunsaturated fatty acid (PUFA), and iron content of commercial formulas used in our nurseries.

Since 1972, we have routinely measured the serum total tocopherol content of premature infants admitted to our nurseries soon after birth and at two- to three-week intervals thereafter. The micro method of Hashim was used.[3] Red blood cell (RBC) hydrogen peroxide fragility and RBC malondialdehyde (MDA) studies have been done in representative infants by the methods of Gordon and Stocks respectively.[4,5]

CLINICAL STUDIES

Since 1968, a surveillance of the incidence and severity of ROP at Pennsylvania Hospital nurseries has been maintained by Drs. Schaffer and Quinn by means of weekly or biweekly eye exams using the indirect ophthalmoscope. Examinations are continued until the retinal vasculature is mature or active retinopathy has regressed or stabilized at some degree of cicatrix. Infants with cicatrix are maintained in continuous long-term follow-up as suggested by Tassman.[6]

January 1, 1968 to February 1, 1972: Background Surveillance

The initial surveillance of incidence and severity of RLF in the Pennsylvania Hospital nurseries covering the period from January 1968 to February 1972 has been described in detail elsewhere.[1] Of the infants who developed active ROP (most of which appeared to regress completely), 40% returned for long-term follow-up between one and two years after a term birth date. It is this follow-up that is of particular importance to this paper.

February 1, 1972 to May 1, 1974: First Clinical Trial of Prophylactic Vitamin E for ROP

Single-blind, alternate infant enrollment, using the Hoffmann-La Roche preparation of parenteral *all-rac-α*-tocopheryl acetate or its placebo on investigational new drug (IND) permit. Weekly or biweekly ophthalmologic examinations with long-term follow-up.

All infants at Pennsylvania Hospital with birth weights under 2,001 g regardless of oxygen need and over 2,001 g with a gestational age under 36 weeks if oxygen therapy were required for over 24 hours were eligible to enter the study. Twins were enrolled as twins even if the larger exceeded the birth weight limit of eligibility. Infants whose parents did not wish to participate in the study or who could not be approached for informed consent until after age 48 hours were admitted to a no-injection control group. Ophthalmologic information was therefore available on all infants. Once informed consent was signed, infants were enrolled within birth weight groups ($\leq$ 1,000 g, 1,001–1,500 g, 1,501–2,000 g, > 2,000 g) and in order of admission to the nursery. Of infants with birth weight 2,000 g or less, 65 to 70% were inborn. Assignment to treatment group was made by nurse research assistants not involved in patient care by entrance of the infant's name on lined enrollment sheets, which they alternately assigned to medication "A" or "B" (vitamin or placebo respectively). If an infant died before the next succeeding line had been filled, that line was assigned to the same treatment (either A or B) as its predecessor. This was done in an effort to assure a more equal distribution of survivors between treatment groups among low birth weight infants whose chances for survival were still poor. (During the two-year period from 1971–72, the mortality rate at Pennsylvania Hospital among inborn and outborn infants was 60 and 70% respectively.) A similar adjustment was made for lines assigned to infants who died before receiving a first eye exam.

Pediatricians, parents, and, in particular, ophthalmologists were completely blinded as to treatment group. Orders were written for medication "A" or "B," which was packaged in identical, single-dose, dark-colored, appropriately labeled vials. Injections were given by the clinical care nursing staff.

Infants enrolled as uninjected controls (group C) were managed in exactly the same way as study infants from the standpoint of nursery routine and serial eye exams. Serum E analyses, however, were done only as indicated on a clinical basis, i.e., once soon after admission to the nursery and at two- to three-week intervals thereafter, when other hematologic tests were being run.

Extensive data were abstracted from the hospital charts for all three groups of babies, including birth weight, gestational age, parity, Apgar score, clinical diagnoses at admission, extent and duration of oxygen and ventilator therapy, arterial blood gas measurements, volume of transfused blood required, complications during the hospital stay, etc.

The dosage of intramuscular medication was 15 mg (0.3 ml) per kg, the initial injection almost always being given within 24 hours of birth. This was repeated at 6- to 12-hour intervals until a serum E level of 1.5 mg/dl was obtained (usually by age 48 hours). A serum E level in the range of 1.5 to 2.0 mg/dl was then maintained by intramuscular (IM) injections given every one, two, or three days as needed. The details of this dosage schedule have been previously published.[1] Placebo-injected infants received comparable volumes at comparable time intervals. When oral feedings were well established, oral medication was used to supplement and then supplant intramuscular medication. However, no oral placebo was available. Treatment was continued until the eyes were mature or active retinopathy had regressed. Treatment was not continued after hospital discharge. Serum E analyses were performed prior to the first injection of study medication, daily until stable, and then twice weekly until hospital discharge. The microcolorimetric method of Hashim,[3] which required between 50 and 100 λ of serum or plasma, was used. Red blood cell H_2O_2 fragility studies were done on the same sample of blood at weekly or biweekly intervals by the method of Gordon.[4]

Ophthalmologists, who were in the nursery only once a week early in the morning, could not distinguish between infants receiving injections and those who did not (i.e., between A and B versus C babies) and had no idea of treatment group assignment with regard to vitamin versus placebo. Nurses giving the injections may have surmised the treatment group assignment, however, since the code was simple. For these reasons the importance of keeping parents and ophthalmologists unaware of treatment group assignment, i.e., "blinded," was repeatedly stressed to the nurses by the research staff. We know of no instance of "unblinding" of the ophthalmologists during either the intake or follow-up phase of the study.

Parents were asked to return for a follow-up exam between their infant's ages one and two years. This procedure was followed whether or not an infant had had ROP in the nursery. However, a consistent effort to maintain the sample was made only among infants who had had signs of retinopathy while in the nursery, since this group was smaller in number and more important.

The incidence and severity of acute stage ROP (severity being defined as sum of ROP grade for fellow eyes) and the visual morbidity at age one to two years were used to compare treatment groups. The mean severity score for a group is defined as the ROP grade sum for each baby, including 0, divided by the number of babies in the group and is therefore a measure of both incidence and severity. The visual morbidity score is defined in TABLE 1.

Intake to this first study, including intake to group C (uninjected controls), was stopped on May 1, 1974, the last four months having been used primarily to enroll infants to this latter group, which was to be used to address the question of vehicle effect. Two reasons dictated this termination. *First,* a new batch of Similac formula containing half again the previous amount of vitamin E had been received in the nursery and old supplies were nearly exhausted. These latter were being used to feed already enrolled babies. New admissions to the nursery were placed on the new formula. *Second,* the number of infants enrolled in the no-injection control group was almost equal to those in the placebo and vitamin groups. The pattern of serum E levels during the nursery stay in these infants was indistinguishable from that of placebo infants, and neither had changed throughout this study period. It was decided therefore to consider subsequent admissions as belonging to a no-injection control group for a future study that would evaluate the effectiveness of a new, more biologically available preparation of parenteral α-tocopherol free alcohol.[7] *Third,* a Bourns respirator had recently been purchased and was beginning to be put to clinical use. This extended our ability to offer intensive care to the sick, very small premature and, as in other nurseries, was to be associated with an increased survival rate among infants at highest risk for ROP.

May 1, 1974 to February 1, 1976: Second Clinical Trial of Prophylactic Vitamin E for ROP

Single (ophthalmology) blind, nonrandomized, no placebo, E treatment periods interspersed with no-injection control period. Parenteral tocopherol free alcohol (or acetate) and oral E alcohol (E-OH) used under Roche IND restrictions to achieve blood E level of 3 mg/dl, ophthalmology protocol and eligibility requirements unchanged.

Our goals for this second study period were:

1. Gain clinical experience with Roche's new E-OH parenteral preparation related to clinical effectiveness and possible deleterious side effects.

2. Verify the findings of the first study.

3. Extend our experience to include larger numbers of small, sick babies in the 1,250-g birth weight range.

4. Gain information on the hypothesis that serum E levels in excess of the usual normal range might be associated with a further decrease in mean severity of ROP.

In collaboration with the Hoffmann-La Roche Department of Medical Research, the following guidelines for this study were established:

1. IM injections of placebo in infants would probably not be justified in infants with birth weights in the range of 1,250 g or less, especially in view of the apparently beneficial effect of vitamin E. Therefore no parenteral placebo should be used.

2. IM injection of a promising, but unproven, therapy such as high-dosage vitamin E was not justified in infants weighing under 1,000 g. In 1974, mortality rates in such infants were in the range of 80% and trauma of any kind was of course a further jeopardy.

3. Since protocol with regard to target serum E level could not be maintained, it would be necessary to exclude infants with birth weights of 1,000 g or less if they required early intensive care and were judged unable to take oral medication for an extended period. This decision would need to be made within 48 hours of hospital admission. (One set of twins met this criterion of exclusion during 1974–75.)

4. Informed consent would be asked only of parents whose infants were born during periods assigned to E treatment; all other infants would fall into an informal control group. Management of E-treated infants would be identical to that of controls except for more frequent monitoring of serum E levels in the former to regulate dosage of the vitamin. The target serum E level in treated infants would be 3.0 mg/dl and was to be achieved through a combination of oral and parenteral treatment by the least number of injections possible.

In addition, it was decided to use the summer months (May through September) for entering control infants and abstracting clinical data from hospital charts on infants enrolled in the just-completed trial using α-tocopheryl acetate. This would maximize the efficiency of our much-curtailed research staff.

Finally, our initial experience with parenteral free E alcohol indicated that, compared to parenteral E acetate, this preparation is moderately irritating as an intramuscular injection. This required us to limit the size and frequency of E alcohol injections to a maximum of 0.4 to 0.5 ml per site and to stipulate that it could be repeated in smaller infants only after three to four days and used only in the thigh muscles. The resulting dosage regimen included use of both parenteral E acetate and E alcohol in small infants requiring parenteral feedings for extended periods. In retrospect, this latter would not really have been necessary since E alcohol is very effective in raising serum E levels and proved to be well tolerated under the new guidelines.

Between ages one and two years, infants cared for in this second treatment period were recalled for ophthalmologic exams and assessment of visual morbidity (see TABLE 1). Effect of treatment was evaluated on the basis of acute stage eye findings and long-term visual sequelae. Admission to this study ended February 1, 1976 and was dictated by loss of research personnel and limitation of funds. Details of admission to this second study are being published elsewhere.

Late 1976 to Mid-1978: Late Treatment of Already Established
Severe ROP (Active Grade 3-Plus)

In late 1976, a respirator-dependent two-month-old infant (birth weight, 960 g) was found to have advanced grade 3-plus active ROP at the first ophthalmologic exam. Her condition had been too critical to allow for an eye exam earlier. The apparent response of this high-risk infant to high-dosage intramuscular and oral vitamin E therapy was striking and prompted us to offer this treatment to other infants. For admission to this study, we required that the patient be referred prior to retinal detachment and have the following retinal findings: a 360° demarcation line, extensive ERNV in two or more quadrants, and prominent posterior pole dilatation and tortuosity. After informed consent was signed, the serum E level was raised as quickly as possible to 5 to 6 mg/dl by a combination of parenteral and oral therapy. It was maintained in that range until the progression of active disease had stopped and retinopathy had clearly begun to regress. This occurred in two to four weeks time in most infants. The dosage was then decreased so as to maintain a level of 3 to 4 mg/dl for another month. A serum E level in the range of 2.0 to 2.5 mg/dl was then maintained until age one year. This level could usually be achieved with an oral dose of 25 to 75 mg/day (0.5 ml one to three times a day).

DISCUSSION AND RESULTS

1968-71 ROP Survey: Sequelae of Low-Grade ROP at Age One to Two Years

The incidence and severity of acute stage retinopathy as distributed between birth weight groups in the Pennsylvania Hospital nurseries from 1968 through 1971 are shown in TABLE 3. In considering the finding presented here, it is important to remember that most very low birth weight (under 1,200-g birth weight) survivors at that time were small-for-gestational-age infants who did not require intensive care by present-day standards. They often needed little or no

TABLE 3

INCIDENCE OF ACTIVE RETINOPATHY OF PREMATURITY:
PENNSYLVANIA HOSPITAL (1968–1971)*

Birth Weight (grams)	Number of Babies	Number with ROP	Active Stages of ROP					Incidence of ROP
			1	2	3	4	5	
759–1000	8	6†	3	0	3	0	0	75.0%
1001–1500	50	16	9	3	3	1	0	32.0%
1501–2000	52	9	5	4	0	0	0	17.3%
2001–2500	37	2	1	1	0	0	0	5.4%
Over 2500	29	0	0	0	0	0	0	0.0%
Totals	176	33	18	8	6	1	0	18.8%

*The study population consisted of all infants with birth weights of 1,500 grams or less regardless of oxygen therapy and all infants with birth weights of greater than 1,500 grams who needed supplemental oxygen. Serum E levels in these infants were in the range of 0.3 mg/dl throughout the hospital stay.
†One of these infants received no O_2; one received 22 hours of 26% O_2.

TABLE 4

SEQUELAE OF LOW-GRADE RESOLVED RETINOPATHY OF PREMATURITY
AT AGE ONE TO TWO YEARS*

Birth Weight (grams)	Grade of Acute ROP od	Grade of Acute ROP os	Morbidity Ranking (score)	Grade of Cic ROP od	Grade of Cic ROP os	Myopia (none to severe) od	Myopia (none to severe) os	Amblyopia	Strabismus	Anisometropia
D 1940	1	1	A (0–2)	0	0	0	0	0	0	0
M 1130	1	1	A (0–2)	1+	0	0	0	0	0	0
G 1250	1	1	C (6–8)	1	0	3	2	0	0	1
H 1500	1	1	C (6–8)	1+	1+	1	1	0	1	0
C 1890	2	2	B (3–5)	1+	1+	1	1	0	0	0
S 1070	2	2	B (3–5)	1+	1+	1	1	0	0	0
MA 1720	2	2	C (6–8)	1+	1+	1	1	1	1	0
MB 1600	2	2	D (9–11)	1+	1+	2	2	1	1	1
R 1247	2	2	D (9–11)	1+	1+	1	2	1	1	1
O 1140	2	2	D (9–11)	2	2	2	2	0	0	1

*Pennsylvania Hospital, infants born 1968–1971. The standard formula for premature infants during the period 1968 through 1971 was Similac with iron, which provided per liter 12 mg iron, 4 IU of *all-rac-α*-tocopherol, and an E:PUFA ratio of 0.3; od is right eye; os is left eye.

oxygen during their stay in the nursery and tolerated cautious, early oral feedings. In contrast, a significant proportion of survivors in the 1,500-g birth weight range had severe respiratory distress and required artificial ventilation. In our nurseries, this was usually accomplished with a negative tank respirator.

As can be seen from TABLE 3, ROP was more common and more severe in the lower birth weight groups. Though present in over one-third of low birth weight infants, it was usually mild in degree and regressed spontaneously. These have been consistent findings by all workers in the field and have not changed over the past 10 to 15 years in spite of advances in neonatal care. What has changed since 1968–72, at least in our nurseries, is the pattern of visual morbidity to be found between 1 and 2 years of age among infants who have had this more common, low-grade form of ROP. Before about 1972, significant visual morbidity, though mild in degree, was the rule among such infants, even though active disease had apparently regressed completely (see TABLE 4). The abnormalities noted at the 1-year follow-up were of the type commonly found among premature infants. Had no scrutiny of the peripheral retina been part of their newborn care, there would have been no reason to attribute the myopia and strabismus found in these infants to ROP save the inconspicuous peripheral findings of low-grade cicatricial disease. These might well have gone unrecognized in another setting. In contrast, FIGURE 1 shows the long-term visual morbidity among infants who had had low-grade ROP in the nursery during the years 1972 to 1976 and compares it with the visual morbidity found among similar infants cared for during the earlier time period. Healing from ROP had been more complete in these later born infants who comprised the study population for our first trial of the effect of prophylactic vitamin E on ROP. This is shown by the highly significant decrease in sequelae of ROP that was found among control and E-treated infants alike. Among E-treated infants, no sequelae whatsoever could be attributed to ROP,

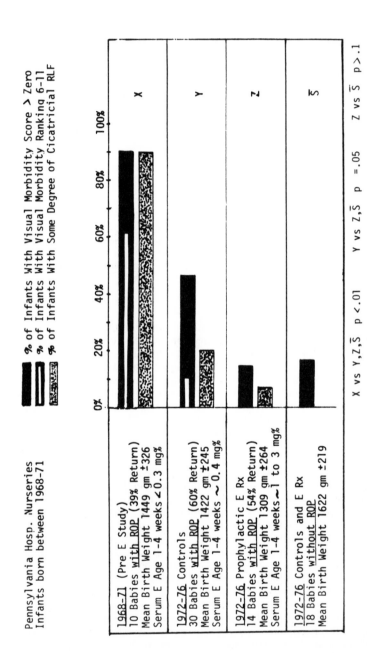

FIGURE 1. Visual morbidity score and incidence of cicatricial ROP at follow-up exam—age one to two years. Findings in infants with mild resolved ROP versus no ROP. Comparison between time periods—effect of high-dosage E treatment.

since they did not differ at age 1 year from infants who had not developed any retinopathy while in the nursery. (The number of returning infants in this no-ROP group is small and embraces treated and untreated infants. It is in all likelihood, however, a representative group.)

We believe the difference in healing between the two time periods in treated and untreated infants alike is primarily due to the growth-modulating and healing properties of vitamin E, which expressed themselves in association with only modest increments in serum E level. Certainly the most important difference in nutrition of premature infants born before 1972 as compared to those born subsequently related to vitamin E. During the mid-1960s, it was common practice to use formulas that were rich in iron, high in polyunsaturated fatty acids, and low in vitamin E throughout the nursery course as well as after discharge. This feeding practice aggravated the subclinical state of E deficiency that is present in the human newborn as well as in the newborn of many mammalian species. This deficiency state is evidenced by meager body stores of the vitamin, low serum E levels, and an increased fragility of RBC membranes on oxidant challenge. The latter is one of the more accurate and readily available biochemical markers of E

TABLE 5

CHANGES IN THE COMPOSITION OF SIMILAC (S-20) FROM 1968 TO 1978

Similac*	E (IU/L)	Percent of Fatty Acids as Linoleic Acid	Fe (mg/L)	E:PUFA Ratio†
1968–72	5 IU	32%	12	0.3
1972–74	9 IU	32%	trace	0.50
1974–75	12 IU	32%	trace	0.66
1975–76	15 IU	32 → 23%	trace	0.7 to 1.1
1977–78	15 IU	23%	trace	1.1

*Similac was the predominant formula used at the Pennsylvania Hospital premature nurseries from 1968 to 1978.

†E:PUFA ratio = mg RRR-α-tocopherol to polyunsaturated fatty acids (linoleic plus linolenic); 1 mg RRR-α-tocopherol = 1.5 IU of vitamin E; 1 mg all-rac-α-tocopheryl acetate = 1.0 IU of vitamin E.

deficiency in humans and is present long before clinical signs of anemia, encephalopathy, or myopathy appear, if indeed they ever do.

Though generally unrecognized until the work of Hassan, Oski, Melhorn, and others,[8-12] clinical E deficiency in the mid-1960s was common among growing premature infants, especially those with birth weights below 1,500 g.[11,12] It reached its peak at about eight weeks after birth and was associated with variable degrees of anemia, especially if iron supplements were started soon after birth.[13] It slowly corrected itself as fat absorption improved and growth rate decreased.

The response of commercial suppliers of infant feedings (and vitamin drops) to this new information was prompt and commendable. The generous E:PUFA ratios of the newer formulas have largely done away with clinical evidence of E deficiency in the premature. (Breast milk from a well-nourished mother also provides a generous supply of E relative to PUFA in most instances.)

The course of formula changes over the 10-year period from 1968 to 1978, using Similac as a representative formula, is presented in TABLE 5. The effect of these changes on serum E levels in healthy prematures born at Pennsylvania Hospital who were able to tolerate early oral feedings is shown in FIGURE 2. Of note are the higher serum E concentrations at birth in babies born in 1978 as compared to 1972. They indicate that there had been an increase in the E content of maternal diets. However, the content of polyunsaturated fat in maternal diets must also have increased, because the RBC membranes of the newborn in 1978 were still abnormally susceptible to oxidative attack as measured by standard hydrogen peroxide assays. Therefore, though presumably endowed with better

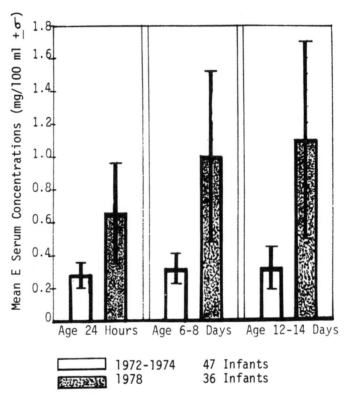

FIGURE 2. Infants with birth weights less than 2,000 g who were not treated with supplemental vitamin E and were able to take early oral feedings.

stores, these more recently born infants would still seem to need the kind of initial boost of vitamin E that is provided by the colostrum of mammalian milk.[29]

The remarkable richness of colostrum and early milk with regard not only to absolute content of α-tocopherol but also of α-tocopherol relative to PUFA is shown in TABLE 6, which is a compilation from work by Quaife, Harris, Herting, Abderhalden, and Jansson.[14-18] Nutritional research continues to demonstrate how well the milk of the mother is adapted to the needs of her newly born.

TABLE 6

CONCENTRATION OF TOTAL TOCOPHEROL RELATIVE TO POLYUNSATURATED FATTY ACID
CONTENT OF COLOSTRUM, TRANSITIONAL, AND MATURE MILK*

	α-Tocopherol (IU/L)	Linoleate (% of fatty acid)	E:PUFA (mg/g)
Human colostrum			
Quaife-Harris[14,15] 1947 & 1950	1.3 to 36	—	—
Jansson et al.[18] 1981 (mean)	10.0 ± 5.5	12.1 ± 1.0	6.23 ± 3.9
Human transitional milk			
Abderhalden[17] 1947	4.0 to 18.5	—	—
Jansson et al.[18] 1981 (mean)	4.8 ± 1.8	12.8 ± 2.8	1.43 ± 0.66
Human mature milk			
Quaife-Harris[14,15] 1947 & 1950	1.0 to 5.0		
Jansson et al.[18] 1981 (mean)	3.2 ± 1.8	12.9 ± 2.2	0.78 ± 0.28
Cow colostrum			
Herting & Drury[16] 1969 (mean)	4.33 to 2.41		2.16 ± 1.43
Cow milk (mature)			
Herting & Drury[16] 1969	0.56 to 0.32		0.21 ± 0.08

*Values are given as range or mean ± standard deviation (SD).

Clinical Trials of Prophylactic Vitamin E for ROP

The results of the two clinical trials of prophylactic vitamin E treatment for ROP are shown in TABLES 7 through 13. TABLE 7 shows incidence and mean severity of ROP for vitamin E, placebo, and no-injection control groups for study 1 infants with birth weights of 2,000 g or less. Vitamin E treatment was associated with a reduction in both incidence and severity of ROP, with the difference in mean severity between groups being significant at p < 0.02 (analysis of variance). From February 1972 to May 1974, no instance of either severe or moderately severe ROP (grade 3 active or worse) was encountered in our nurseries. Therefore the differences seen between E-treated and control infants represent an effect on low-grade retinopathy.

During study 1, the mean serum E level during the nursery stay was 0.36

TABLE 7

EFFECT OF VITAMIN E ON INCIDENCE AND SEVERITY OF ROP: FINDINGS
IN INFANTS WITH COMPLETE ACUTE STAGE EYE DATA*

	Vitamin E	Placebo	No Injection
Number of infants	49	46	41
Number with ROP	11	16	14
Incidence of ROP	22%	35%	34%
Mean severity	0.55	1.02	1.19
Analysis of variance		t (134) = −2.3	
Mean severity		p = 0.012	

*Only infants with birth weights of 2,000 g or less. Pennsylvania Hospital, February 1972 to May 1974.

mg/dl ± 0.143 (standard deviation) for placebo and 0.34 mg/dl ± 0.085 (SD) for no-injection control infants. For E-treated infants, it was 2.0 mg/dl ± 0.478 (SD). Birth weight, gestational age, and requirement for oxygen and transfused blood were similar between groups (TABLE 8). Treatment was associated with a significant decrease in mean severity of ROP (p < 0.02). TABLE 9 shows that this is also true when both study periods are considered together (1972–76).

Considering the second study alone, the same downward trend in incidence and severity of ROP was seen, but as shown in TABLE 10, the differences between groups did not reach the level of statistical significance. Again birth weight, gestational age, and requirement for blood and oxygen were similar between groups. However, in comparison to study 1 infants, infants cared for during the later time period had a somewhat lower mean birth weight (1,582 g vs. 1,662 g) and required much more intensive care. This was reflected in a doubling of the mean number of days of oxygen treatment required and a doubling of the volume of

TABLE 8

EFFECT OF VITAMIN E ON MEAN SEVERITY OF ROP: FINDINGS IN INFANTS
WITH COMPLETE ACUTE STAGE EYE DATA*

	Birth Weight (mean; grams)	Gestation (mean; weeks)	F_{lo_2} >Room Air (mean; days)	Blood Transfused (ml/kg)	ROP Mean Severity (score)
Treated (n = 58)	1681	33.8	2.46	23	0.50
Not treated (n = 103)	1652	33.6	2.91	23	0.94
t-test	0.82	0.14	0.69	0.01	2.10
p (two tailed)	0.604	0.885	0.488	0.991	0.037
p (one tailed)					0.019

*Pennsylvania Hospital, February 1972 to May 1974. Infants with birth weights under 2,000 g, or over 2,000 g if gestational age 36 weeks or less and >24 hours O_2 treatment required. Mean serum E level of treated infants = 2.03 ± 0.478 (SD) from day 4 to discharge.

transfused blood administered per kilogram of body weight. We interpreted this as posing too great an oxidant stress for the vitamin E provided.

Among study 2 E-treated infants, the mean serum E level was 3.1 mg/dl ± 0.958 (SD) as compared to 0.5 mg/dl ± 0.236 (SD) in control infants (p < 0.0001). It is interesting to note that, as shown in TABLE 11, the mean serum E levels in study 2 control infants were significantly higher (p < 0.001) than those of control infants enrolled in study 1.

One infant in study 2 developed blinding ROP, a control infant with a birth weight of 1,640 g who suffered a severe anoxic insult at birth. In addition, one of a pair of 1,000-g twins developed blinding ROP. This set of twins was removed from the study before age two days because it was clear that maintaining treatment protocol would not be possible in the male, who had been assigned to the E group. The male died with bronchopulmonary dysplasia (BPD) at about two months of age. The little girl survived, but with extensive anoxic brain damage. She had originally been assigned to the control group.

TABLE 9

EFFECT OF VITAMIN E ON MEAN SEVERITY OF ROP: FINDINGS IN INFANTS WITH COMPLETE ACUTE STAGE EYE DATA*

	Birth Weight (mean; grams)	Gestation (mean; weeks)	F_{io_2} >Room Air (mean; days)	P_{ao_2} >100 mm Hg (mean; hours)	Blood Transfused (ml/kg)	ROP Mean Severity (score)
Treated (n = 105)	1648	33.5	4.6	8.3	37.5	0.65
Not treated (n = 164)	1619	33.3	4.4	8.8	34.4	1.04
t-test	0.70	0.44	0.13	0.52	0.31	2.17
p (two tailed)	0.485	0.661	0.900	0.601	0.754	0.031
p (one tailed)						0.016

*Pennsylvania Hospital, February 1972 to February 1976. Infants with birth weight under 2,000 g, or over 2,000 g if gestational age 36 weeks or less and >24 hours O_2 treatment required.

TABLE 10

EFFECT OF VITAMIN E ON MEAN SEVERITY OF ROP: FINDINGS IN INFANTS
WITH COMPLETE ACUTE STAGE EYE DATA*

	Birth Weight (mean; grams)	Gestation (mean; weeks)	$F_{i_{O_2}}$ >Room Air (mean; days)	Blood Transfused (ml/kg)	ROP Mean Severity (score)
Treated (n = 47)	1607	33.1	7.16	56	0.83
Not treated (n = 61)	1562	32.6	6.91	54	1.21
t-test	0.72	1.24	0.08	0.07	1.21
p (two tailed)	0.475	0.219	0.934	0.941	0.229†
p (one tailed)		0.11			0.12

*Pennsylvania Hospital, May 1974 to February 1976. Infants with birth weight under 2,000 g, or over 2,000 g if gestational age 36 weeks or less and >24 hours O_2 treatment required. Mean serum E level of treated infants = 3.10 ± 0.958 (SD) from day 4 to discharge.

†If a weighted severity score is used that reflects more accurately the clinical implications of severe versus low-grade ROP, then t = 1.85, p = 0.033 (one tailed).

The experience with this pair of twins convinced us that any definitive study of the effect of vitamin E on the pathogenesis of ROP would require the option of being able to administer parenteral medication by intravenous infusion. The protocol for our three-hospital, double-blind, clinical trial, sponsored by the National Eye Institute, has included this capability. (Intake to this trial ended in May 1981.)

TABLE 12 shows the results of data from the combined trials (studies 1 and 2) using a multiple regression technique. Predictor variables are entered into the equation in order of their contribution to outcome variance. Very weak predictors are not entered at all. The cumulative R^2 value represents the fraction of total outcome variance that can be accounted for by the predictors selected for entrance. Birth weight is by far the most important predictor. Volume of blood received per kilogram of body weight and then treatment group are selected for entrance into the equation. Both have p values in the highly significant range. It is important to note however that the contribution of these two variables to R^2 is

TABLE 11

CHANGING MEAN CONCENTRATIONS OF TOTAL TOCOPHEROL IN SERUM
OF UNTREATED INFANTS AT PENNSYLVANIA HOSPITAL*

	February 1972 to May 1974	May 1974 to February 1976	t-test
Day 0 to 1	0.29 ± 0.118	0.33 ± 0.148	t = 1.806 p = 0.05
Day 5 to discharge	0.35 ± 0.110	0.51 ± 0.236	t = 5.965 p <0.001

*Values represent means ± SD in infants with birth weights of 2,000 g but requiring over 24 hours of oxygen treatment. Serum tocopherol is given in mg/dl ± 1 SD.

TABLE 12

PREDICTION OF INCIDENCE AND SEVERITY (MEAN SEVERITY) OF ROP:
PENNSYLVANIA HOSPITAL, FEBRUARY 1972 TO FEBRUARY 1976

Predictor Variable	R^2	F	p
Birth weight	0.30824	93.587	<0.001
Blood (ml/kg)	0.33438	10.102	<0.001
Type of treatment	0.34545	4.667	<0.001
Days F_{iO_2} over room air	0.34955	2.147	<0.05
Shock	0.35344	1.239	NS
Apnea	0.35625	1.268	NS
Pregnancy complications	0.35389	0.868	NS

*Multiple regression analysis. The dependent variable is mean severity of ROP for all infants. The seven predictors account for only 36% of outcome variance. Includes only infants with complete acute stage eye data ($n = 269$) and birth weights of 2,000 g or less, or over 2,000 g but under 36 weeks gestation and requiring oxygen for over 24 hours.

small in absolute terms and that even with all significant predictors entered, only about 35% of outcome variance is accounted for.

TABLE 13 shows results of the regression analysis for babies with birth weights of 1,500 g or less. Again birth weight is the most powerful predictor followed by treatment group, blood requirement, and shock. When infants are preselected for moderately low birth weight, only 30% of outcome variance is accounted for. Most known risk factors for ROP [e.g., apnea, Apgar, P_{aO_2} sepsis, necrotizing enterocolitis (NEC)] were included in the research data base. Hypercarbia, acidosis, and anoxia were also included but not in the detailed way that recent work suggests they should be.[19-21] However, these problems were not prominent among survivors in the study populations described and their more rigorous inclusion probably would not have added much to the ability to predict mean severity of ROP in an individual infant. The data speak strongly for the existence of individual resistance (or susceptibility) factors and are consistent with the great variability in degree of pathology that results from a given hyperoxic exposure as previously observed in both human and animal studies.[22,23] In recent work with

TABLE 13

PREDICTION OF INCIDENCE AND SEVERITY (MEAN SEVERITY) OF ROP:
PENNSYLVANIA HOSPITAL, FEBRUARY 1972 TO FEBRUARY 1976*

Predictor Variable	R^2	F	p
Birth weight	0.17714	11.180	<0.001
Type of treatment	0.21931	6.482	<0.001
Blood (ml/kg)	0.25995	6.032	<0.001
Shock	0.27963	6.072	<0.001
Pregnancy complications	0.29363	1.748	NS
Days F_{iO_2} over room air	0.29407	0.076	NS
Apnea	0.29446	0.047	NS

*Multiple regression analysis. The dependent variable is severity of ROP in infants $\leq 1,500$ g birth weight. The seven predictor variables account for 29.5% of the total variance. Includes only infants with complete acute stage eye data ($n = 95$) and birth weights of 1,500 g or less. The contribution of birth weight to outcome variance is relatively less when only infants with birth weights of 1,500 g or less are considered.

the kitten model, Phelps and Rosenbaum reported a very high correlation between the litter a kitten belonged to and the appearance of the retina two weeks after hyperoxic exposure.[24] This "queen effect" emphasizes the importance of genetic differences in the pathogenesis of ROP.

Maintenance of serum E levels in the 1.5 to 3.0 mg/dl range was not associated with apparent untoward side effects. The incidence of NEC and culture-proven sepsis during 1972–76 was not different between treatment groups ($\chi^2 = 0.39$, p > 0.3). The incidence of BPD was very low and also did not differ between treatment groups ($\chi^2 = 0.17$, p > 0.5).

Treatment of Already Established Severe ROP

Spontaneous regression from midstage grade 3-plus active ROP (characterized by a 360° demarcation line, obvious dilatation and tortuosity of blood vessels of the posterior retina, and prominent ERNV in two or more quadrants) is rare and incomplete at best. The outlook for vision is poor, with about a 70% chance of legal blindness (best corrected vision 20/200) or worse. More advanced grade 3-plus active ROP invariably goes on to some degree of retinal detachment and has an even worse prognosis.

Against this dismal background, the results of our preliminary work with high-dosage vitamin E treatment of already established midstage grade 3-plus active ROP is very encouraging. During 1976, 1977, and 1978, we treated 10 such infants, first in the Pennsylvania Hospital nurseries and later, on request of the infants' doctors, at Children's Hospital and the Hospital of the University of Pennsylvania. The findings in these 10 infants at the one to two year follow-up are presented in TABLE 14. The visual morbidity score as previously described is used to define outcome. Also presented are the findings at follow-up in 14 untreated infants born during the same time period and cared for in the same nurseries. E treatment had either not been requested or was requested only after major retinal detachment had occurred, which was too late to begin treatment by our protocol. All eye examinations were done by Drs. Schaffer and Quinn, and all infants had been under their ophthalmologic care throughout their hospital course. Infants who exhibited significant tractional phenomena (which is occasionally seen while active disease is still present) or who developed any degree of retinal detachment, whether on E treatment or not, were referred to Dr. William Tassman for consultation and possible surgical intervention. None of the 24 infants in TABLE 14 were treated surgically prior to the one to two year follow-up visit.

A significantly improved visual outcome was associated with high-dosage E treatment (p < 0.02). The incidence of legal blindness (rank G) or worse was decreased from 71% to 40%. A good visual outcome (defined by ranks A through D or scores 0 through 11) was found in 40% of E-treated but in only 14% of non-E-treated infants. One of the E-treated infants had no cicatricial findings whatever and a one-year visual morbidity score of only 2. An intermediate outcome (ranks E and F) was found to be about equally distributed between groups. No adverse side effects other than an occasional sore injection site were associated with E treatment.

Cryotherapy, photocoagulation, and scleral buckling are the only other treatments presently available for severe progressive ROP. Opinions differ as to the optimal timing for these procedures and the value of treatment.[25,26] Certainly the results reported here for high-dosage E treatment compare favorably with results of these other approaches.

It is important to remember that ROP is an anoxic retinopathy. Only the initial injury to the primitive vasoformative tissues of the retina is hyperoxic in nature. The pivotal work of Drs. Kretzer and Hittner reported at this meeting has greatly advanced our understanding of the nature of this hyperoxic insult, especially as it occurs today under conditions of controlled oxygen therapy. It has also provided important insight into the role of vitamin E in modulating the response of vasoformative tissues to changes in oxygen tension.

It is doubtful that vitamin E exerts its beneficial effects in the anoxic stages of ROP in the same way as in the preceding period of hyperoxic insult. The optimal

TABLE 14

VISUAL MORBIDITY SCORE AT AGE ONE TO TWO YEARS IN 24 CHILDREN WHO HAD
ACTIVE GRADE 3-PLUS ROP OR WORSE IN THE NURSERY*

Visual Morbidity	E Treatment 1976–1978 (10 infants)†	No E Treatment 1976–1978 (14 infants)†
Rank A–B Score 0–5	1 (10.0%)	0 —
Rank C–D Score 6–11	3 (30.0%)	2 (14.3%)
Rank E–F Score 12–17	2 (20.0%)	2 (14.3%)
Rank G–H Score 18–22	1 (10.0%)	1 (7.1%)
Rank I Score 23–26	3 (30.0%)	9 (64.3%)
Mean birth weight	1070 g	1176 g

*Infants were cared for in the nurseries of the University of Pennsylvania Neonatal Complex (Hospital of the University of Pennsylvania, Children's Hospital of Philadelphia, and Pennsylvania Hospital). All ophthalmologic examinations were performed by Drs. Schaffer and Quinn.

†Distribution by rank. p < 0.02 (analysis of variance).

serum levels (i.e., dosage regimen) may also be different. That it does function both to decrease the hyperoxic insult and to decrease the extent of neovascularization as a response to anoxia is clear from the kitten work of Phelps and Rosenbaum.[24,27] Extent of neovascularization and tendency to regression and repair versus the tendency to progression and fibrous outgrowth are the main determinants of eventual pathology and are greatly influenced by individual and species differences. Vitamin E appears to be able to favorably influence these phenomena, perhaps through its capacity to modulate growth, decrease scar formation, and promote healing. At the peak of severe acute stage disease, when the eye appears congested and inflamed and there is vascular stasis with leakage of fluid and exudate from abnormal vessels, the functions of vitamin E as antiinflammatory agent and modulator of prostaglandin balance may be important. It should be emphasized, however, that vitamin E, used to raise serum levels well above the physiologic range, is a pharmacologic agent with potential toxic side effects. It should be used on a study protocol and with careful monitoring of serum E levels.

In conclusion, beneficial effects of vitamin E therapy have been demonstrated at several points along the pathogenetic pathway of ROP. These need to be verified and extended to include infants of lower birth weights. The optimal levels of serum vitamin E to be sought at different points of the disease pathway need to be clarified so that preventive and therapeutic regimens can be developed. The improved E nutrition provided by present-day infant formulas appears to have already decreased the incidence of sequelae from low-grade ROP.

SUMMARY

The effect of high-dosage E treatment (Rx) initiated at the stage of 3-plus active disease (target serum E levels, 5–6 mg/dl) was evaluated by a standardized scoring system of visual morbidity at the one to two year eye exam among infants cared for in the University of Pennsylvania Neonatal Complex (1976–1978). The incidence of legal blindness in both eyes or worse was decreased from 71 to 40% in E Rx ($n = 10$) as compared to non-E Rx ($n = 14$) infants, and the number of infants with minimal visual morbidity was increased. Pilot studies (1972–76; target serum E level, 1.5 and 3.0 mg/dl) of the prophylactic effect of E Rx from birth on showed a decrease in mean severity of acute stage disease and a decrease in sequelae at one to two years. A striking difference in visual morbidity following resolved low-grade ROP was seen when prestudy infants (1968–72) who were fed early iron supplements and given formulas with low E:PUFA ratios were compared to non-E Rx as well as to E Rx 1972–76 infants. Vitamin E seems to exert a beneficial effect at all stages of ROP, perhaps because of its broadly based regulatory role.

ACKNOWLEDGMENTS

This study represents the cooperative effort of many people to whom we cannot pay proper recognition, but whose support we gratefully acknowledge. We thank, in particular, the devoted nursing staff of the premature nurseries of the Pennsylvania Hospital, the parents of the infants we were trying to help, and the cheerful, competent members of our past and present research and laboratory staff: Christine Dalin, Rosemary Dworanczyk, Dorothy Grey, Mary Grous, Beverly Harrison, Betty Lamplugh, Tony Mignano, Joan Moshang, and Dorothy Neff. We thank Dorothy Neff and Mary Lou Walsh for secretarial help and Dr. Schaffer's office staff for help with patient follow-up. Finally we thank Soraya Abbassi, M.D., for help of any kind, whenever it was needed.

REFERENCES

1. JOHNSON, L., D. SCHAFFER & T. BOGGS. 1974. The premature infant, vitamin E deficiency and retrolental fibroplasia. Am. J. Clin. Nutr. **27:** 1158.

2. SCHAFFER, D., L. JOHNSON, G. QUINN & T. BOGGS. 1979. A classification of retrolental fibroplasia to evaluate vitamin E therapy. Ophthalmologica **86:** 1749.
3. HASHIM, S. & G. SCHUTTRINGER. 1966. Rapid determination of tocopherol in macro and micro quantities of plasma. Am. J. Clin. Nutr. **19:** 136.
4. GORDON, H., H. NITOWSKY & M. CORNBLATH. 1966. Studies on tocopherol deficiency in infants and children. I. Hemolysis of erythrocytes in hydrogen peroxide. Am. J. Dis. Child. **92:** 164.
5. STOCKS, J., E. OFFERMAN, C. MODELL & T. DORMANDY. 1972. The susceptibility to autooxidation of human red cell lipids in health and disease. Br. J. Hematol. **23:** 713.
6. TASSMAN, W. 1968. Juvenile retinal detachment. J. Pediatr. Ophthalmol. **5:** 160.
7. NEWMARK, H., W. POOL, et al. 1975. Biopharmaceutic factors in parenteral administration of vitamin E. J. Pharm. Sci. **64:** 655.
8. HASSAN, H., S. HASHIM, T. VANITALLIE & W. SEBRELL. 1966. Syndrome in premature infants associated with low plasma vitamin E levels and high polyunsaturated fatty acid diet. Am. J. Clin. Nutr. **19:** 147.
9. OSKI, F. & L. BARNESS. 1967. Vitamin E deficiency: a previously unrecognized cause of hemolytic anemia in the premature infant. J. Pediatr. **70:** 211.
10. MELHORN, D. & S. GROSS. 1971. Vitamin E-dependent anemia in the premature infant. I. Effects of large doses of medicinal iron. J. Pediatr. **79:** 569.
11. MELHORN, D. & S. GROSS. 1971. Vitamin E-dependent anemia in the premature infant. II. Relationships between gestational age and absorption of vitamin E. J. Pediatr. **79:** 581.
12. LO, S., D. FRANK & W. HITZIG. 1973. Vitamin E and hemolytic anaemia in premature infants. Arch. Dis. Child. **48:** 360.
13. WILLIAMS, M., R. SHOTT, P. O'NEAL & F. OSKI. 1975. Role of dietary iron and fat on vitamin E deficiency anemia of infancy. N. Engl. J. Med. **292:** 887.
14. QUAIFE, M. 1947. Tocopherols (vitamin E) in milk: their chemical determination and occurrence in human milk. J. Biol. Chem. **169:** 513.
15. HARRIS, P., M. QUAIFE & P. O'GRADY. 1952. Tocopherol content of human milk and of cow's milk products used for infant feeding. J. Nutr. **46:** 459.
16. HERTING, D. & E. DRURY. 1969. Vitamin E content of milk, milk products, and simulated milks: relevance to infant nutrition. Am. J. Clin. Nutr. **22:** 147.
17. ABDERHALDEN, R. 1947. Vitamin E content of human milk and cow milk. Biochem. Z. **47:** 318.
18. JANSSON, L., B. AKESSON & L. HOLMBERG. 1981. Vitamin E and fatty acid composition of human milk. Am. J. Clin. Nutr. **34:** 8.
19. LUCEY, J., J. HORBAR & M. ONISHI. 1981. Cerebral and retinal hypoperfusion as a possible cause of retrolental fibroplasia—hypothesis to explain non O_2 related RLF. (abst.). Pediatr. Res. **15:** 670.
20. PHELPS, D. & A. ROSENBAUM. 1982. Effect of hypoxemia on recovery from oxygen induced retinopathy in the kitten model. (abst.). Pediatr. Res. **16:** 303A.
21. FLOWER, R., D. BLAKE, et al. 1981. Retrolental fibroplasia: evidence for a role of the prostaglandin cascade in the pathogenesis of oxygen-induced retinopathy in the newborn beagle. Pediatr. Res. **15:** 1293.
22. KINSEY, V. 1956. Retrolental fibroplasia: cooperative study of retrolental fibroplasia and the use of oxygen. Arch. Ophthalmol **56:** 481.
23. ASHTON, N. 1979. Symposium, retrolental fibroplasia. Ophthalmologica **86:** 1695.
24. PHELPS, D. & A. ROSENBAUM. 1977. The role of tocopherol in oxygen-induced retinopathy: kitten model. Pediatrics **59**(suppl.): 998.
25. KALINA, R. 1980. Treatment of retrolental fibroplasia. Surv. Ophthalmol. **24:** 229.
26. BEN-SIRA, I., I. NISSENKORN, E. GRUNWALD & Y. YASSUR. 1980. Treatment of acute retrolental fibroplasia by cryopexy. Br. J. Ophthalmol. **64:** 758.
27. PHELPS, D. & A. ROSENBAUM. 1979. Vitamin E in kitten oxygen-induced retinopathy. II. Blockage of vitreal neovascularization. Arch. Ophthalmol. **97:** 1522.
28. SCHAFFER, D., G. QUINN & L. JOHNSON. 1982. Sequelae of arrested, mild retinopathy of prematurity. Paper presented at the 13th Biannual Meeting of the Gonin Society, Cordoba, Argentina, April.

29. JOHNSON, L., C. DALIN, R. DWORANCYZK & B. HARRISON. 1982. Functional significance of serum vitamin E levels. Pediatr. Res. **16:** 167A.

————————————◆————————————

DISCUSSION

R. J. SOKOL (*Children's Hospital Medical Center, Cincinnati, Ohio*): Could you tell me if there was any change in the way you monitored P_{aO_2} in these patients? Was there any significant difference in the average P_{aO_2} for the groups of patients?

L. JOHNSON: The last patient studied was born in 1976. We did not have a transcutaneous monitor in the nursery at that time. These were all arterial blood gases, and there was no difference in the amount of exposure to P_{aO_2} over 100 mm Hg in each group.

R. J. SOKOL: Were you drawing blood gases as frequently from 1972 to 1976 as you were from 1976 to 1978?

L. JOHNSON: Yes.

D. L. PHELPS (*University of California, Los Angeles, Calif.*): Can I ask a question. When Dr. Tassman says 70% legal blind on your stage 3-plus, does that include his late retinal detachments? In other words, is this a lifetime prognosis?

L. JOHNSON: No. The 70% legally blind figure applies to early visual outcome (age one year or less) and involves almost entirely the infant with grade 3 Cic ROP or worse. Infants with moderate to severe grade 2 Cic ROP, with severe myopia and marked traction on the retina, are the ones at risk for late retinal detachment. As shown in our data, they usually have a visual acuity of 20/20 (best corrected) at age one to two years.

W. A. PRYOR (*Louisiana State University, Baton Rouge, La.*): I know there's quite a literature on RLF, and I was delighted to hear your study. Are there data on the effect of varying amounts of E?

L. JOHNSON: We have been trying to address that problem in our sequential clinical trials. In the larger double-blind trial sponsored by the NEI, for which intake was recently completed, a very high serum E level was maintained to try to definitively learn whether "more E is better" and what side effects may be expected. Our earlier trials, and that of Dr. Hittner, were testing the effect of E in a more physiologic range.

P. M. FARRELL (*University of Wisconsin, Madison, Wis.*): The data you showed on cord blood tocopherol levels in the recent assessment being higher than the earlier values are interesting. I wanted to ask if you would elaborate on this. There seems to be a large standard deviation, so there must have been some infants with very high tocopherol levels.

L. JOHNSON: The large standard deviation probably reflects differences in both maternal diet and placental function. Some infants nowadays do have surprisingly high day-zero serum E levels (up to 0.9 mg/dl). Others, especially those born to mothers with toxemia or placental insufficiency, still have levels of 0.3 mg/dl or less.

H. J. MEVWISSEN (*Albany Medical College, Albany, N.Y.*): How do you explain the fact that one eye is bad and the other eye is not so bad?

L. JOHNSON: I think that local conditions in the eye, probably largely hemodynamic in nature, influence the retinal response both to hyperoxia and to primary and secondary hypoxia. The degree of scarring and fibrous overgrowth seems to be considerably influenced by anoxia secondary not only to degree of endothelial hyperoxic insult but to differences in tissue perfusion as well. Difference in degree of disease between fellow eyes is much more common in severe ROP. The mechanism of action of E at this stage of the disease may be different from its action in the preceding hyperoxic stage, which, in most infants, causes only a mild, reversible, secondary, anoxic retinopathy.

BIOCHEMICAL IMPLICATIONS OF CURRENT
STUDIES ON VITAMIN E*

T. F. Slater

Department of Biochemistry
Brunel University
Uxbridge, Middlesex
UB8 3PH United Kingdom

I have interpreted my brief to try to highlight what I feel are important implications of the presentations given to this meeting, and to indicate my views on some major outstanding problems concerning the biochemistry of vitamin E in relation to cell pathology.

Much, though by no means all, of what we have heard here on the subject of the biochemical actions of vitamin E revolves around its participation in free radical reactions. Such studies reflect the increasing number of examples of toxic agents, or toxic metabolic pathways, that are known to involve free radical intermediates. In many cases, these toxic free radical intermediates are produced by interaction with the reduced nicotinamide-adenine dinucleotide phosphate (NADPH)–cytochrome P_{450} electron-transport chain.[1,2] Such reactive free radical intermediates can damage the integrated metabolism of the cell in many ways,[3] so that it is natural to search for ways to scavenge (or remove) such reactive free radicals; in such reactions vitamin E undoubtedly has an important role to play. A large number of studies over many years have demonstrated the effectiveness of vitamin E as an efficient scavenger of many electrophilic radicals.[4]

In my opinion, one area requiring considerable further study is that relating to the *quantitative* aspects of free radical–scavenger interactions under conditions that are relevant to the biological situation. In other words, to study the kinetics of free radical–scavenger interactions in solution, and to obtain information on the one-electron redox potentials of selected scavenger free radical redox couples. Since reactive free radicals have short half-lives, this means that rapid kinetic procedures must be used for studying such kinetic aspects. One suitable method is pulse radiolysis; a recent review providing useful background information is by Willson.[5]

I will discuss now some data relating to the metabolic activation of CCl_4 to illustrate the results that can be obtained with this technique. This hepatotoxic agent is known to be metabolically activated by the liver NADPH-P_{450} system; the toxic product is believed to be mainly the trichloromethyl radical ($CCl_3^{\cdot}$).[6,7] This free radical has been represented in the literature as being of high chemical reactivity and as being responsible for the increased lipid peroxidation observed during CCl_4 intoxication.[3,6]

However, when $CCl_3^{\cdot}$ was produced by pulse radiolysis under *strictly anaerobic conditions*, it did not react significantly with a variety of compounds tested except molecular oxygen.[8] With oxygen, a diffusion-controlled reaction produced the $CCl_3O_2^{\cdot}$ peroxy radical. The latter species was found to be many times more reactive as an electrophile than was $CCl_3^{\cdot}$ itself.[2,8,9] Thus, the chemical reactivity

*The work of the author referred to here was made possible by generous support from the Cancer Research Campaign and the National Foundation for Cancer Research.

496

of CCl_3^- can be greatly modified by the local concentration of O_2. Similar changes in electrophilicity on reaction with O_2 have been found with corresponding free radicals produced from halothane by pulse radiolysis.[10]

The formation of CCl_3^- in a biomembrane in the presence of O_2 leads to a highly reactive $CCl_3O_2^-$ species that can interact readily with neighboring amino acids, thiols, polyunsaturated fatty acids, etc. Such highly reactive free radicals cannot diffuse very far: their reactivity ensures that they are trapped in their own microenvironment.[11] Similar comments apply, of course, to other highly reactive radicals, like OH^-. Secondary and tertiary products of the interaction of the primary free radical with its surroundings have lower chemical reactivity and can diffuse further. Aldehydic breakdown products resulting from lipid peroxidation in the endoplasmic reticulum may, for example, escape from the cell and cause damaging effects at a distance.

From the above discussion, it is clear that to effectively scavenge such reactive primary free radicals, the scavenger must get to the precise site of radical formation at the time when the free radicals are being produced and in a concentration sufficient to ensure effective competition with neighboring biomolecules. These criteria for effective scavenging have been discussed in a recent review.[12]

Returning to the effect of O_2 on the reactivity of CCl_3^-, these results indicate that certain early features of free radical-mediated damage can be dissociated from each other by the widely differing electrophilicities of the primary vs. the secondary peroxy radical. For example, with CCl_4, the formation of CCl_3^- may be more associated with covalent binding whereas $CCl_3O_2^-$ may be the major initiator of lipid peroxidation. Since scavengers and metabolic inhibitors in general will react at different rates with CCl_3^- than with $CCl_3O_2^-$, differential inhibitions of covalent binding or lipid peroxidation can be observed.[2] Such comments are perhaps relevant to data presented by Dr. Hochstein, who showed that antioxidants like 3,5-di-t-butyl-4-hydroxy toluene can inhibit lipid peroxidation, but not protein iodination, in his H_2O_2/T_4 system.[13]

A number of extremely interesting clinical consequences have been reported at this meeting to follow relatively long-term supplementation with vitamin E. Although I believe it probable that vitamin E is exerting some beneficial effects in such disturbances through its free radical-scavenging properties, other properties and influences of vitamin E must also be borne in mind. For example, the effects of long-term vitamin E supplementation on the pool sizes of other tissue scavengers, any one of which may have more selectivity for the damaging radical species in question than does vitamin E itself. In this regard, I suspect we will have to do more complete balance sheets of tissue antioxidants in cases of vitamin E deficiency and supplementation until we know much more about tissue antioxidant interactions and regenerative pathways.

In addition, high doses of vitamin E, while certainly not diminishing the free radical-scavenging ability of this substance, may well have additional effects quite unrelated to free radical scavenging. The results of Dr. Wolf concerning the effectiveness of phytol on the increased pressure response in a lung-perfusion system are relevant to this theme.[14] Long-term vitamin E administration could well have effects on the polyunsaturated fatty acid content of membranes, on the distribution of polyunsaturated fatty acids in membranes, on membrane pressure and fluidity, as well as on the absorption and transport of other lipid-soluble materials. In my opinion, therefore, it is necessary to be cautious in ascribing long-term high-dose effects of vitamin E more or less solely to an antioxidant or free radical-scavenging property.

To illustrate such speculations with fact, I can refer to recent studies with another free radical scavenger, promethazine. This phenothiazine derivative can interact with $CCl_3O_2^-$ very effectively,[9] and can inhibit CCl_4-stimulated lipid peroxidation in liver microsomes at nM concentration.[15] However, promethazine has several other important effects on CCl_4 toxicity in the whole rat. It can slow the absorption into the blood and the liver uptake of CCl_4 over the first two hours of intoxication;[16] it can also significantly lower body temperature in the presence of CCl_4,[17] and thus decrease the metabolic activation of CCl_4. It can increase the respiratory rate in the presence of CCl_4 and thus increase the rate of exhalation of the toxic agent.[18] Such "secondary" effects are superimposed on its highly efficient action as a scavenger of $CCl_3O_2^-$.

A further complication of the use of some free radical scavengers in biological systems is that the *overall* biological effect may not show a simple dose dependence. Promethazine, for example, is a good scavenger at low concentration (e.g., 1–100 μM in liver microsomal systems), but at higher concentrations, its surface active properties become dominant and may result in substantial membrane damage, to lysosomes for example.[19] Such crossover effects thus have to be borne in mind when rather arbitrarily increasing scavenger concentrations.

An important aspect of free radical-mediated damage to biomembranes is lipid peroxidation, and we have heard a lot during this meeting about malondialdehyde (MDA) values and their assumed relationship to free radical-initiated lipid peroxidation. In fact MDA values do generally correlate reasonably well with the extent of lipid peroxidation as measured by loss of polyunsaturated fatty acid, O_2 uptake, etc.,[20] even though malondialdehyde is a relatively minor product of lipid peroxidation. It is, however, the major aldehyde reacting with thiobarbituric acid in the much used TBA reaction.[21] Malondialdehyde has a number of interesting biological reactivities of its own, including the cross-linking reactions discussed after the paper by Dr. Chiu et al.[22] However, it is only one of many aldehydes produced by lipid peroxidation and, as it is the main one that is positive in the TBA test, the others may be inadvertently overlooked. In a collaborative study with Professor H. Esterbauer (University of Graz, Austria) and Professor M. U. Dianzani (University of Turin, Italy) we have now separated about 40 such aldehydic products of lipid peroxidation,[23] and some, like 4-hydroxy-nonenal, are biologically very reactive in the μM range of concentrations.[24,25] I believe, therefore, that the production and role of such other aldehydic products of lipid peroxidation have also to be considered along with MDA itself.

Another area that I feel deserves much further study concerns the turnover of vitamin E in biomembranes. Dr. Machlin presented extensive data on the buildup and decay of vitamin E in various tissues.[26] But from what I have already said concerning the very restricted diffusibility of reactive free radicals, it is evident that we need some new methodology to study the *local* concentration of vitamin E at sites where free radicals are preferentially formed, around cytochrome P_{450} for example. In addition, we will require information about the turnover of vitamin E in such sites in the sense of its one-electron redox reactions. In the latter respect, the role of other tissue antioxidants/free radical scavengers in assisting and/or preserving the local status of vitamin E has to be considered.

An interaction of vitamin E and C in modifying free radical-mediated disturbances has been suggested on several previous occasions.[27] An effective and direct interaction of vitamin E$^{\cdot}$ with vitamin C can be demonstrated by pulse radiolysis.[28] Clearly, it is of importance to know whether other local membrane antioxidants such as inosine, ubiquinone, or urate can enter such cooperative sequences.

Lastly, in this short personal account, I feel we must explore more thoroughly the basic assumptions that we often make with respect to the nature of the free radical intermediates in biological systems. In my own case, for example, I wrote about the (presumed) high reactivity of CCl_3^- for almost 15 years before the pulse radiolysis data demonstrated the much greater electrophilicity of $CCl_3O_2^-$. In many other schemes currently in the literature we see proposals for OH^-, $O_2^{-\cdot}$, peroxy radicals, perferryl groups, carbenes, singlet oxygen, etc., whereas the hard experimental evidence for the actual production of such species in the systems under study is often lacking. Considerable work has to be invested, in my opinion, to establish unequivocally the reactive radicals involved. In this respect the spin-trapping technique,[29] though not without its own hazards of interpretation, may lead us quickly in the right direction.

I hope my brief remarks are not interpreted as ones of despair at our lack of precise biochemical knowledge with respect to the functions of vitamin E. On the contrary, I believe we are on the verge of very exciting and important advances in cell physiology, biochemistry, and pathology as a result of these studies on vitamin E and free radical scavengers. Not least because of the intrinsic importance of polyunsaturated fatty acids in biomembrane structure and function, and the unique biochemical features resulting from the "switch" of arachidonate peroxidation from the prostaglandin sequence to lipid peroxidation or vice versa.[30] The interaction of vitamin E (and other scavengers) with primary free radicals and with lipid peroxy radicals, and the corresponding interplay with the prostaglandin sequence will, in my view, lead us into new and important areas of study.

REFERENCES

1. MASON, R. P. 1979. Free radical metabolites of foreign compounds and their toxicological significance. *In* Reviews in Biochemical Toxicology. E. Hodgson, J. R. Bend & R. M. Philpot, Eds. **1:** 151–200. Elsevier-North Holland, Inc. New York, N.Y.
2. SLATER, T. F. 1982. Free radicals as reactive intermediates in tissue injury. *In* Biological Reactive Intermediates. Chemical Mechanisms and Biological Effects. R. Snyder, D. V. Parke, J. Kocsis, D. J. Jollow & G. G. Gibson, Eds. **2:** 575–589. Plenum Publishing Corp. New York, N.Y.
3. SLATER, T. F. 1972. Free Radical Mechanisms in Tissue Injury. Pion Ltd. London, England.
4. WITTING, L. A. 1980. Vitamin E and lipid antioxidants in free radical initiated reactions. *In* Free Radicals in Biology. W. A. Pryor, Ed. **4:** 295–319. Academic Press, Inc. New York, N.Y.
5. WILLSON, R. L. 1978. Free radical and tissue damage: mechanistic evidence from radiation studies. *In* Biochemical Mechanisms of Liver Injury. T. F. Slater, Ed.: 123–224. Academic Press. London, England.
6. RECKNAGEL, R. O., E. A. GLENDE & A. M. HRUSZKEWYCZ. 1977. Chemical mechanisms in carbon tetrachloride toxicity. *In* Free Radicals in Biology. W. A. Pryor, Ed. **3:** 97–132. Academic Press, Inc. New York, N.Y.
7. SLATER, T. F. 1981. Interaction sites of CCl_4 with the NADPH–cytochrome P_{450} electron transport chain in rat liver microsomes. *In* Recent Advances in Lipid Peroxidation and Tissue Injury. A. Garner & T. F. Slater, Eds.: 1–28. Brunel University. Uxbridge, England.
8. PACKER, J. E., T. F. SLATER & R. L. WILLSON. 1978. Life Sci. **23:** 2617–2620.
9. PACKER, J. E., R. L. WILLSON, D. BAHNEMANN & K-D. ASMUS. 1980. J. Chem. Soc. Perkin Trans. 2: 296–299.
10. SCHAEFER, M., J. MÖNIG, R. L. WILLSON & T. F. SLATER. Pulse radiolysis studies on halothane free radicals. (Manuscript in preparation.)

11. SLATER, T. F. 1976. Biochemical pathology in microtime. *In* Recent Advances in Biochemical Pathology: Toxic Liver Injury. M. U. Dianzani, G. Ugazio & L. M. Sena, Eds.: 99–108. Minerva Medica. Torino, Italy.

12. SLATER, T. F. 1981. State of the art: free radical scavengers. R. Soc. Med. Int. Congr. Symp. Ser. No. 47: 11–15.

13. HOCHSTEIN, P. 1981. Paper presented at the Conference on Vitamin E: Biochemical, Hematological, and Clinical Aspects, New York, N.Y., Nov. 11–13.

14. WOLF, H. R. D. & H. W. SEEGER. Experimental and clinical results in shock lung treatment with vitamin E. Ann. N.Y. Acad. Sci. (This volume.)

15. SLATER, T. F. & B. C. SAWYER. 1971. Biochem. J. **123**: 823–828.

16. REDDROP, C. J., W. RIESS & T. F. SLATER. 1981. Biochem. Pharmacol. **30**: 1443–1447.

17. REDDROP, C. J. 1980. Concentration, kinetics, metabolism and interactions of CCl_4 and promethazine in the rat. Ph.D. Thesis. Brunel University. Uxbridge, England.

18. REDDROP, C. J., W. RIESS & T. F. SLATER. 1981. Biochem. Pharmacol. **30**: 1449–1455.

19. SLATER, T. F. 1968. Aspects of cellular injury and recovery. *In* The Biological Basis of Medicine. E. E. Bittar & N. Bittar, Eds. **1**: 369–414. Academic Press, Inc. New York, N.Y.

20. BESWICK, P. H., K. CHEESEMAN, G. POLI & T. F. SLATER. 1981. Comparison of methods used for measuring lipid peroxidation in rat liver microsomes and isolated hepatoxytes. *In* Recent Advances in Lipid Peroxidation and Tissue Injury. A. Garner & T. F. Slater, Eds.: 156–176. Brunel University. Uxbridge, England.

21. ESTERBAUER, H. & T. F. SLATER. 1981. IRCS Med. Sci. **9**: 749–750.

22. CHIU, D., E. VICHINSKY, M. YEE, K. KLEMAN & B. LUBIN. Peroxidation, vitamin E, and sickle-cell anemia. Ann. N.Y. Acad. Sci. (This volume.)

23. ESTERBAUER, H. 1982. Aldehydic products of lipid peroxidation. *In* Free Radicals, Lipid Peroxidation and Cancer. D. C. H. McBrien & T. F. Slater, Eds.: 101–122. Academic Press. London, England.

24. BENEDETTI, A., M. COMPORTI & H. ESTERBAUER. 1980. Biochim. Biophys. Acta **620**: 281–296.

25. DIANZANI, M. U. 1982. Biochemical effects of saturated and unsaturated aldehydes. *In* Free Radicals, Lipid Peroxidation and Cancer. D. C. H. McBrien & T. F. Slater, Eds.: 129–151. Academic Press. London, England.

26. MACHLIN, L. J. & E. GABRIEL. Kinetics of tissue α-tocopherol uptake and depletion following administration of high levels of vitamin E. Ann. N.Y. Acad. Sci. (This volume.)

27. TAPPEL, A. L. 1968. Geriatrics **23**: 97–105.

28. PACKER, J. E., T. F. SLATER & R. L. WILLSON. 1979. Nature London **278**: 737–738.

29. JANZEN, E. E. 1980. A critical review of spin trapping in biological systems. *In* Free Radicals in Biology. W. A. Pryor, Ed. **4**: 115–154. Academic Press, Inc. New York, N.Y.

30. SLATER, T. F. & C. BENEDETTO. 1981. Free radical reactions in relation to lipid peroxidation inflammation and prostaglandin metabolism. *In* The Prostaglandin System. F. Berti & G. P. Velo, Eds.: 109–126. Plenum Publishing Corp. New York, N.Y.

CLINICAL IMPLICATIONS OF THE STUDIES PRESENTED AT THE CONFERENCE: AN EVALUATION

Herbert J. Kayden

Department of Medicine
New York University School of Medicine
New York, New York 10016

In reviewing the presentations at this conference, including the poster sessions and the discussions, there are a number of areas that appear to me to be of particular interest, and I should like to emphasize these areas, as well as identify certain observations that merit further study.

I should like to begin with methodology—which reveals some of my own interest and bias. Plasma, platelet, and erythrocyte levels of tocopherol can be accurately measured by spectrophotometry, with or without high-pressure liquid chromatography.[1,2] What is needed now is a consistent form of reporting tocopherol values. Early on, it was necessary to report vitamin E to triglyceride or vitamin E to cholesterol ratios, and a number of investigations have stressed the value of reporting vitamin E levels in plasma related to plasma total lipid concentration.[3,4] However, the sensitivity of newer methods warrants that tocopherol values be reported as accurately as possible. There may be additional merit in recording total plasma lipid levels or total plasma cholesterol levels, if one is interested in surveying groups of individuals for determination of tocopherol distribution curves or to determine if deficiency exists in a population. But to substitute ratios for the original numbers limits the value of the data. It also would be preferable to give the values for the content of tocopherol in erythrocytes as directly analyzed, that is, as $\mu g/10^{10}$ cells or $\mu g/ml$ of cells with known hematocrit, rather than to continue to report data of percent hemolysis upon challenge with hydrogen peroxide.[1] The variations in the technique of carrying out the peroxide hemolysis test are many—ranging from the concentration of peroxide used in the test to the duration of incubation and the method of estimation of degree of hemolysis. Furthermore, hemolysis may be prevented by relatively small additions of tocopherol, far below optimal levels, and I believe it would be preferable to make the direct measurement of the tocopherol content of cellular elements of the blood.

From a number of the presentations of diseases presumably associated with tocopherol deficiency, it is apparent that plasma and red cell measurements yield insufficient data; what is needed is an analysis of the tocopherol level in tissues. For ambulatory humans, we have developed a needle biopsy aspiration method of adipose tissue, which gives a better reflection of tissue stores and which will be helpful in indicating the kinetics of tocopherol uptake and release.[5] The method can also be adapted for the measurement of tocopherol in other tissues obtained from hospitalized humans undergoing surgery or biopsy of other organs, and perhaps also in postmortem material. Such information would be of considerable interest in evaluating the metabolism and storage of tocopherol.

There is renewed interest in studying the absorption from the gastrointestinal tract and the distribution of tocopherol in the serum lipoproteins in man and animals. We need to study the kinetics of transport of tocopherol from lipopro-

501

0077-8923/82/0393–0501 $01.75/0 © 1982, NYAS

teins into the tissues. While absorption of tocopherol in humans appears to be almost exclusively into chylomicrons, the manner and rate of disposition from the chylomicrons to the liver and other tissues are less certain. The kinetics of exchange from very low-density (VLDL) and low-density lipoproteins (LDL) to tissues in humans has not been precisely defined. And what is the role of the high-density lipoproteins? Do they serve to transport tocopherol from the adipose tissue to plasma for redistribution to other tissues if tocopherol intake is reduced?

One additional aspect concerning lipoproteins: it should be noted that some investigators have reported that tocopherol administration (in high doses) alters the distribution of cholesterol between low- and high-density lipoproteins, and may also alter the extent of cholesterol esterification in low-density lipoprotein.[6] Our own observations on a limited sample of normal adults and hyperlipemic subjects showed no effect of tocopherol on plasma lipid distribution.[7] But clearly, further studies are in order, not only to identify the susceptible population, but even more importantly to define the mechanism of tocopherol action upon lipoprotein structure. Does this represent a direct effect of vitamin E upon hepatic synthesis of VLDL and LDL? Does tocopherol have an effect upon the action of the enzyme responsible for cholesterol esterification [lecithin cholesteryl acyl transferase (LCAT)]? And does tocopherol play any role in altering steroid hormone synthesis by the adrenal, ovary, or testis? These are fertile areas for further studies—and the methodology for such studies has been developed in the past decade.

We know that tocopherol is stored in adipose tissue in individuals who consume large amounts of the vitamin, and we know that plasma levels fall if the diet is devoid of tocopherol. But the catabolism of tocopherol has not been delineated either in humans or animals, and there would seem to be merit in studying what *utilization* of tocopherol means.

I am particularly struck by the reports by several groups at this meeting of the defined clinical syndrome associated with cholestasis and low levels of plasma tocopherol; oral treatment with tocopherol does not restore plasma levels to normal in all cases.[8-10] The neurological and muscular abnormalities seem so well defined and shared by all patients and show such a favorable response to tocopherol (given parenterally when required) that it seems appropriate to conclude that tocopherol deficiency that develops in childhood can cause nerve cell damage. We had suspected that deficiency of tocopherol in the genetic disorder abetalipoproteinemia contributed to the neurologic and muscular abnormalities that characterize that disorder, and had begun tocopherol repletion in patients with that disease 17 years ago.[11] The cholestatic state telescopes the time period of development of pathology from years to months, and the astute clinicians caring for those patients have demonstrated the reversibility of the disease process. Similarly, patients with abetalipoproteinemia and neurologic disabilities have shown a beneficial response to the administration of tocopherol.[12] Of even greater importance, children (even infants) recognized to have abetalipoproteinemia are given prophylactic doses of vitamin E, with every indication that large oral doses, given several times a day, prevent the neurologic disorder with its concomitant muscular abnormality and ophthalmoplegia. It would therefore appear that the ataxia and neuromuscular abnormalities seen in the abetalipoproteinemic patient are not a direct consequence of the abnormal genetic information, but represent a secondary result of malabsorption. Having posed this question a decade and a half ago, I am gratified that the original hypothesis was correct.

Another area that merits comment concerns the hematological system, with particular emphasis upon the observations in the newborn and in the premature infant. From the presentations of several groups, it would appear appropriate to recommend that oral tocopherol and vitamin K be given routinely to premature infants. Those premature infants requiring oxygen therapy because of pulmonary disease should be carefully followed for the plasma vitamin E levels, and parenteral tocopherol should be administered when oral administration of the vitamin is ineffective. The low levels of plasma tocopherol in the premature newborn document the limited transfer of the vitamin across the placenta; the low levels of plasma lipids also contribute to the low plasma vitamin E content. The need for tocopherol in managing the anemia that develops is due in part to the change to a higher oxygen tension than existed in utero. It is a tribute to those interested in neonatology that infants at such high risk can be managed and ultimately survive.[13,14]

Another instance of a new clinical area requiring our evaluation of the status of tocopherol in the patient and in the diet concerns the use of total parenteral nutrition for patients who heretofore would long since have succumbed.[15] These include patients with extensive bowel surgery as well as patients with metastatic cancer undergoing chemotherapy. Here, tocopherol deficiency can develop very swiftly due to the peroxidation of the intravenous lipid solutions; this may impose far greater stress than we had previously anticipated. The clinical problems of the very premature infant and of the adult patient requiring total parenteral nutrition represent human conditions in which vitamin E deficiency is a truly potential hazard requiring attention.

As an aside, and acknowledging the success of the second launching of the space shuttle Columbia, it should be noted that the astronauts in that ship do not breathe 100% oxygen. One of the more interesting, and not necessarily widely publicized, observations of the initial space explorations was the red blood cell destruction and relative anemia that occurred in the astronauts who were breathing pure oxygen and who had not been given supplemental tocopherol prior to takeoff for the expected oxygen stress in the pure oxygen atmosphere of the spaceships.

The last decade has witnessed the recognition of the importance of arachidonic acid release from phospholipids and the synthesis of prostaglandins, thromboxanes, and prostacyclins. The role of tocopherol in the cascade from arachidonic acid, following the path of the cycloxygenase to the endoperoxides— or to lipoxygenases to the hydroperoxy fatty acids, must surely be the subject of studies in the coming years.[16] And the studies of the role of vitamin E in platelet metabolism and platelet function are perhaps the most extensive already carried out in human subjects that relate to this area of biochemical investigation.[17,18]

It is clear that I have been highly selective in choosing only a fraction of the areas covered in this conference for comment. This represents my personal interest, and is not meant to be a qualitative judgment. What is more satisfying to me is that in constrast to a conference 10 years ago, the organizers of the present conference were able to select papers that presented solid data, with little anecdotal material and few unsubstantiated clinical studies. Part of this change represents the evolution of scientific activity in all areas; but in the field of vitamin E, it represents the effort of investigators to fully define the role of tocopherol in human metabolism. Their success can be measured by the quality of the papers presented and the vigorous discussion that followed each presentation. I am delighted to have participated in this program and look forward to the next conference on tocopherol.

REFERENCES

1. KAYDEN, H. J., C. K. CHOW & L. BJORNSON. 1973. Spectrophotometric method for determination of tocopherol in red blood cells. J. Lipid Res. **14:** 533–540.
2. HATAM, L. J. & H. J. KAYDEN. 1979. A high-performance liquid chromatographic method for the determination of tocopherol in plasma and cellular elements of the blood. J. Lipid Res. **20:** 639–645.
3. HORWITT, M. K., C. C. HARVEY, C. C. DAHM, JR. & M. T. SEARCH. 1972. Relationship between tocopherol and serum lipid levels for determination of nutritional adequacy. Ann. N.Y. Acad. Sci. **203:** 223–236.
4. FARRELL, P. M., S. L. LEVINE, M. D. MURPHY & A. J. ADAMS. 1978. Plasma tocopherol levels and tocopherol-lipid relationship in a normal population of children as compared to healthy adults. Am. J. Clin. Nutr. **31:** 1720–1726.
5. HATAM, L. & H. J. KAYDEN. Tocopherol levels in needle aspiration biopsies of adipose tissue: normal subjects and abetalipoproteinemic patients. Ann. N.Y. Acad. Sci. (This volume.)
6. HERMANN, W. J., K. WARD & J. FAUCETT. 1979. The effect of tocopherol on high-density lipoprotein cholesterol. A clinical observation. Am. J. Clin. Pathol. **72:** 848–852.
7. HATAM, L. J. & H. J. KAYDEN. 1981. The failure of α-tocopherol supplementation to alter the distribution of lipoprotein cholesterol in normal and hyperlipoproteinemic persons. Am. J. Clin. Pathol. **76:** 122–126.
8. GUGGENHEIM, M. A., S. P. RINGEL, A. SILVERMAN, B. E. GRABERT & H. E. NEVILLE. Progressive neuromuscular disease in children with chronic cholestasis and vitamin E deficiency: clinical and muscle biopsy findings and treatment with α-tocopherol. Ann. N.Y. Acad. Sci. (This volume.)
9. ROSENBLUM, J. L., J. P. KEATING, A. P. PRENSKY & J. S. NELSON. 1981. A progressive, disabling, neurologic syndrome in children with chronic liver disease: a possible result of vitamin E deficiency. N. Engl. J. Med. **304:** 503–508.
10. GRABERT, B. E., M. A. GUGGENHEIM, S. P. RINGEL, H. P. CHASE & H. E. NEVILLE. 1980. Neuromuscular disease related to chronic vitamin E deficiency. Ann. Neurol. **8:** 217.
11. KAYDEN, H. J. & R. SILBER. 1965. The role of vitamin E deficiency in the abnormal hemolysis of acanthocytosis. Trans. Assoc. Am. Phys. **78:** 334–341.
12. MULLER, D. P. R., J. K. LLOYD & A. C. BIRD. 1977. Long-term management of abetalipoproteinemia: possible role for vitamin E. Arch. Dis. Child. **52:** 209–214.
13. EHRENKRANZ, R. A., R. C. ABLOW & J. B. WARSHAW. Effect of vitamin E on the development of oxygen-induced lung injury in neonates. Ann. N.Y. Acad. Sci. (This volume.)
14. CHISWICK, M. L., J. WYNN & N. TONER. Vitamin E and intraventricular hemorrhage in the newborn. Ann. N.Y. Acad. Sci. (This volume.)
15. THURLOW, P. M. & J. P. GRANT. Vitamin E and total parenteral nutrition. Ann. N.Y. Acad. Sci. (This volume.)
16. GOETZL, E. J. 1980. Vitamin E modulates the lipoxygenation of arachidonic acid in leukocytes. Nature **288:** 183–185.
17. KRETZER, F. L., H. M. HITTNER, A. T. JOHNSON, R. S. MEHTA & L. B. GODIO. Vitamin E and retrolental fibroplasia: ultrastructural support of clinical efficacy. Ann. N.Y. Acad. Sci. (This volume.)
18. STEINER, M. & R. MOWER. Mechanism of action of vitamin E on platelet function. Ann. N.Y. Acad. Sci. (This volume.)

Index of Contributors

(Italicized page numbers refer to comments made in discussion.)